30 X

D0758339

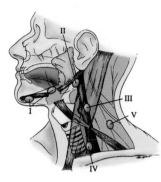

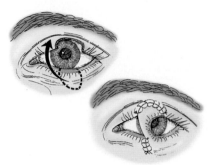

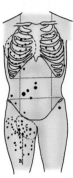

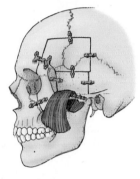

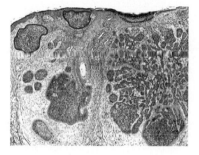

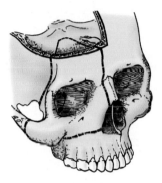

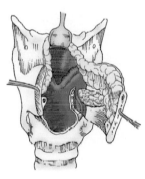

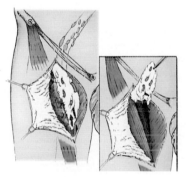

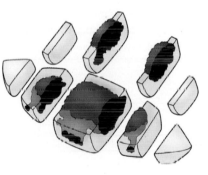

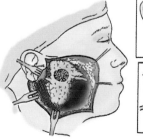

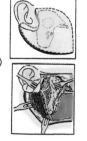

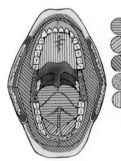

TONGUE

FLOOR OF MOUTH

BUCCAL MUCOSA

RETROMOLAR TRIGONE

HARD PALATE

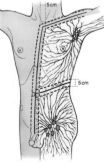

Plastic Surgery

Plastic Surgery
First Edition

Editor:
Joseph G. McCarthy, MD

Editors, Hand Surgery volumes:
James W. May, Jr., MD
J. William Littler, MD

Plastic Surgery

Second Edition

Editor

Stephen J. Mathes, MD
Professor of Surgery
Chief, Division of Plastic Surgery
University of California, San Francisco
School of Medicine
San Francisco, California

Editor, Hand Surgery Volumes

Vincent R. Hentz, MD
Professor of Surgery
Chief, Division of Plastic and Hand Surgery
Stanford University School of Medicine
Stanford, California

With illustrations by Kathy Hirsh and Scott Thorn Barrows, CMI, FAMI

Shireen L. Dunwoody, Editorial Coordinator

VOLUME *V*

TUMORS OF THE HEAD, NECK, AND SKIN

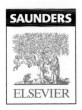

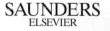

SAUNDERS
ELSEVIER

1600 John F. Kennedy Blvd.
Ste 1800
Philadelphia, PA 19103-2899

PLASTIC SURGERY, 2nd ed.

Volume I 0-7216-8812-8/978-0-7216-8812-1
Volume II 0-7216-8813-6/978-0-7216-8813-8
Volume III 0-7216-8814-4/978-0-7216-8814-5
Volume IV 0-7216-8815-2/978-0-7216-8815-2
Volume V 0-7216-8816-0/978-0-7216-8816-9
Volume VI 0-7216-8817-9/978-0-7216-8817-6
Volume VII 0-7216-8818-7/978-0-7216-8818-3
Volume VIII 0-7216-8819-5/978-0-7216-8819-0
8-Volume Set 0-7216-8811-X/978-0-7216-8811-4

Notice

Knowledge and best practice in this field are constantly changing. As new research and experience broaden our knowledge, changes in practice, treatment and drug therapy may become necessary or appropriate. Readers are advised to check the most current information provided (i) on procedures featured or (ii) by the manufacturer of each product to be administered, to verify the recommended dose or formula, the method and duration of administration, and contraindications. It is the responsibility of the practitioner, relying on his or her own experience and knowledge of the patient, to make diagnoses, to determine dosages and the best treatment for each individual patient, and to take all appropriate safety precautions. To the fullest extent of the law, neither the Publisher nor the Editors assume any liability for any injury and/or damage to persons or property arising out of or related to any use of the material contained in this book.

The Publisher

Previous edition copyrighted 1990.

Library of Congress Cataloging-in-Publication Data
Mathes, Stephen J.
    Plastic surgcry / Stephen J. Mathes ; editor Vincent R. Hentz.—2nd ed.
        p.   cm.
    ISBN 0–7216–8811–X
    1. Surgery, Plastic.   I. Hentz, Vincent R.   II. Title.
RD118.M388 2006
617.9'5— dc21

                                        2003041541

Acquisitions Editors: Sue Hodgson, Allan Ross, Joe Rusko, Judith Fletcher
Senior Developmental Editor: Ann Ruzycka Anderson
Publishing Services Manager: Tina Rebane
Senior Project Manager: Linda Van Pelt
Design Direction: Steven Stave
Cover Designer: Shireen Dunwoody

Printed in China

Last digit is the print number: 9   8   7   6   5   4   3   2   1

This text is dedicated to Mary H. McGrath, who is my inspiration and a source of joy in our daily life together, our adventures at home and away, and our shared enthusiasm and excitement as plastic surgeons.

✦ CONTRIBUTORS

CHARLOTTE E. ARIYAN, MD, PhD
Resident in General Surgery
Yale University–New Haven Hospital
New Haven, Connecticut

STEPHAN ARIYAN, MD, MBA
Clinical Professor of Surgery
   (Plastic Surgery, Otolaryngology)
Yale University School of Medicine
Director, Yale Melanoma Unit
Yale Cancer Center
New Haven, Connecticut

SHAHID R. AZIZ, MD, DMD
Assistant Professor
Department of Oral and Maxillofacial Surgery
University of Medicine and Dentistry of New Jersey
New Jersey Dental School
Newark, New Jersey

RONALD M. BARTON, MD, FACS
Associate Professor of Surgery
Virginia Commonwealth University School of Medicine,
   Medical College of Virginia Campus
Director, Evans-Haynes Burn Unit
Medical College of Virginia Hospital
Richmond, Virginia

GREGORY L. BORAH, MD, DMD, FACS
Professor of Surgery
University of Medicine and Dentistry of New Jersey
Robert Wood Johnson Medical School
Chief, Division of Plastic and Reconstructive Surgery
Robert Wood Johnson Medical Center
New Brunswick, New Jersey

RICHARD CHAFFOO, MD, FACS
Assistant Clinical Professor
Division of Plastic Surgery
Department of Surgery
University of California, San Diego, School of Medicine
San Diego, California
Active Staff, Division of Plastic Surgery
Scripps Memorial Hospital
La Jolla, California

KEITH DENKLER, MD
Associate Clinical Professor of Plastic Surgery
University of California, San Francisco, School of
   Medicine
San Francisco, California
Chief of Medical Staff
Marin General Hospital
Greenbrae, California

STEVEN A. GOLDMAN, MD
Assistant Professor of Plastic Surgery
Case Western Reserve School of Medicine
Staff Physician
University Hospitals of Cleveland
Cleveland, Ohio

JULIANA E. HANSEN, MD, FACS
Associate Professor of Surgery
Oregon Health and Science University School of Medicine
Chief, Division of Plastic and Reconstructive Surgery
Oregon Health and Science University Hospitals and
   Clinics
Portland, Oregon

**IAN T. JACKSON, MD, DSc (Hon), FRCS, FACS
FRACS (Hon)**
Director
Institute for Craniofacial and Reconstructive Surgery
Chief
Department of Plastic Surgery
Director
Training Program
Providence Hospital
Southfield, Michigan

WILLIAM F. KIVETT, MD, FACS
Attending Plastic Surgeon
Sutter Medical Center, Sutter Warrack Hospital,
   HealthSouth Surgery Center, and Beauty & Health
   Medical Center of California
Santa Rosa, California
Palm Drive Hospital
Sebastopol, California

DAVID L. LARSON, MD, FACS
Professor and Chairman
Department of Plastic Surgery
Medical College of Wisconsin
Attending Surgeon
Froedtert and Medical College of Wisconsin Plastic
    Surgery Center
Milwaukee, Wisconsin

PABLO LEÓN, MD
Assistant Professor of Surgery
Division of Plastic and Reconstructive Surgery
Department Surgery
University of California, San Francisco, School of
    Medicine
Chief, Plastic Surgery Section
San Francisco Veterans Affairs Medical Center
San Francisco, California

EDWARD A. LUCE, MD, FACS
Private Practice
The Plastic Surgery Group of Memphis
Memphis, Tennessee

JENNIFER J. MARLER, MD
Assistant Professor of Surgery
Division of Plastic Surgery
University of Cincinnati College of Medicine
Pediatric Surgeon
Cincinnati Children's Hospital Medical Center
Cincinnati, Ohio

JOHN B. MULLIKEN, MD, FACS
Professor of Surgery
Harvard Medical School
Senior Associate in Surgery
Children's Hospital
Boston, Massachusetts

DEEPAK NARAYAN, MS, MD, FRCS (Eng), FRCS (Edin)
Assistant Professor
Department of Surgery
Yale University School of Medicine
New Haven, Connecticut
Chief
Plastic Surgery
Veterans Administration Connecticut Healthcare
    System-West Haven Campus
West Haven, Connecticut

✦ PREFACE

It is a great thing to start life with a small number of really good books which are your very own. *Through the Magic Door* (1908), Sir Arthur Conan Doyle

My meeting for lunch with Joseph McCarthy in Boston in 1998 during the annual meeting of the Society of Plastic Surgery was arranged to discuss the possibility of my becoming the editor of the new edition of *Plastic Surgery.* I was well aware of the responsibility of assuming this giant project. My admiration of the past editors, including Joseph McCarthy for the 1990 edition of *Plastic Surgery* and John Marquis Converse for the 1964 and 1977 editions of *Reconstructive Plastic Surgery,* was great since these texts in my estimation really defined our specialty of plastic surgery and provided the platform for future advances in treating congenital and acquired deformities. My memory of Converse's first edition started with my residency in plastic surgery on my first rotation at the private practice of William Schatten, John Hartley, and John Griffith in Atlanta, Georgia. There, in moments when I was not involved in patient care activities, I would enjoy reading the pages of clinical advice on all subjects related to plastic surgery in the five volumes of *Reconstructive Plastic Surgery.* Subsequently, in 1977, as a faculty member at Washington University, I was privileged to be able to purchase my own copy of the then six-volume edition of *Reconstructive Plastic Surgery,* again edited by Converse. This time, my reading of the exciting pages was less relaxed, since I was using the text as the reference in preparation for my plastic surgery board examinations.

By 1990, I was able to contribute a chapter to *Plastic Surgery,* edited by Joseph McCarthy, and I personally knew most of the contributors, having witnessed the evolution of many of the new advances and unique contributions contained within the then eight volumes. With this background, I was excited and honored to have been recommended as the next editor of this text, which has so well reflected the greatness of the specialty of plastic surgery. My meeting was punctuated by advice regarding the importance of the text and the selection of experts who would provide both guidance and stimulation to future readers on the many subjects important to physicians involved in plastic surgery. The complexity of orchestrating so many contributors in a timely fashion was also emphasized. I left this luncheon inspired to undertake this project, with the anticipation of capturing the best and most innovative surgeons as contributors to achieve an edition in keeping with the unique traditions of excel-

lence of the past editions of *Plastic Surgery* and *Reconstructive Plastic Surgery.*

My first step was to find an academic hand surgeon to edit the two hand volumes. J. William Littler had served as the editor of the hand and upper extremity volume in Converse's two editions of *Reconstructive Plastic Surgery.* Littler was a master hand surgeon and one of the foremost innovators in hand surgery. McCarthy selected a unique combination of academic hand surgeons, James W. May and J. William Littler, to edit the two volumes dedicated to upper extremity and hand surgery in the 1990 edition of *Plastic Surgery.* With the many new techniques related to microvascular surgery, the space devoted to this important aspect of plastic surgery had been expanded into two volumes. Jim May, like Bill Littler, is a master hand surgeon, a gifted teacher, and an innovator in all aspects of plastic surgery and was able to include both his contributions and those of many other hand surgeons, who all took part in advancing this important discipline.

Fortunately, the decision regarding who should be the hand editor for this edition of *Plastic Surgery* was obvious. Vincent R. Hentz is a master hand surgeon and past president of the American Society of Surgery of the Hand. As an accomplished educator and chief of the division of plastic and hand surgery at Stanford, he is the ideal person to follow in the footsteps of Littler and May. In keeping with the many innovations and new techniques in upper extremity and hand surgery, this edition contains two volumes devoted to hand surgery. Of interest, we have shifted the editorial geography from the East Coast (New York City and Boston) to the West Coast (San Francisco and Palo Alto). Unfortunately, despite the improvement in weather characteristics of the western coastline of the United States, the commitment to continue the excellence of this text has kept the editors mostly indoors during the complex editing process necessary to complete these volumes.

The goal of this edition is to cover the scope of plastic surgery. The key was to select the best contributors to define the problems encountered in plastic surgery, to provide both the most current and the most successful solutions, and to deliver the challenge for future innovation in each area of plastic surgery. In this new edition, there are 219 chapters with 293 contributors. Each of the senior authors of the 219 chapters was carefully selected for his or her recognized expertise in the assigned subject of the chapter. Each author has personally contributed to the advancement in knowledge related to his or her area of expertise in our specialty.

The authors selected are inspirational leaders due to their many innovations toward improvement in the management of the plastic surgery patient. After the manuscripts were submitted, each chapter was carefully reviewed by the editors to ensure that all aspects of the authors' assigned topics were adequately covered and well illustrated so that the reader could readily incorporate the chapter content into the practice of plastic surgery.

In the eight volumes included in this edition, all subjects pertinent to the scope of plastic surgery are covered. Many new topics, 67 in all, have been developed or were enlarged from broader subjects and warranted a new individual chapter. Thirteen of these new chapter topics are included in Volume I: General Principles. The enlargement of the volume containing general principles reflects the continuing expansion of our specialty, the emphasis on experimental and clinical research, and the impact of research on the practice of plastic surgery. In the remaining volumes, devoted to specific clinical topics, two new types of chapter formats were added: 25 technique chapters and 7 secondary chapters. The technique chapters are added to complement the overview chapters and are designed to focus on particular techniques currently in use for a clinical problem. Likewise, the secondary chapters are again an extension of the overview chapters on particular subjects but focus on problems that persist despite the application of primary plastic surgery solutions. These secondary chapters are designed to demonstrate areas where operations may fail related to improper patient or technique selection or technique failures. They also discuss procedures to correct unsatisfactory outcomes following primary plastic surgery.

Volumes II through VII are divided into specific topographical areas of plastic surgery. Volume II: The Head and Neck (Part 1) is devoted to cosmetic procedures and contains six new topic chapters, seven new technique chapters, and three new secondary chapters. This volume now contains color illustrations, which will help the reader evaluate problems and results following cosmetic procedures. Many important subjects are expanded and introduced. For instance, there are now five chapters on the face lift, which provide the reader with the ability to compare techniques and focus on specific aspects of the procedure. Volume III: The Head and Neck (Part 2) is dedicated to reconstructive procedures and contains 10 new topics as well as the traditional subjects used in the previous edition. Volume IV: Pediatric Plastic Surgery contains five new topics and provides multispecialty approaches to children presenting with congenital facial anomalies. Volume V: Tumors of the Head, Neck, and Skin has seven new topics. Along with management principles of head and neck cancer, identification and treatment of melanoma and non-melanoma skin cancer have been added in new topic chapters. Volume VI: Trunk and Lower Extremity contains 34 added topics. For example, in the area of postmastectomy reconstruction, 12 new chapters have been added to provide specific diagnostic, management, and technical information on breast reconstruction issues. Similarly, four new chapter topics have been added on body contouring procedures. With emphasis on bariatric surgery and body contouring procedures, these chapters provide a complete array of information on techniques and outcomes. Volume VII: The Hand and Upper Limb (Part 1) contains introductory and general principles related to diagnosis and management of acquired disorders, both traumatic and nontraumatic. Volume VIII: The Hand and Upper Limb (Part 2) contains three parts: congenital anomalies, paralytic disorders, and rehabilitation. The two volumes on hand and upper extremity surgery contain an additional 22 chapters introducing new subjects to this edition of *Plastic Surgery*.

Education involves the process of observation as well as contact with teachers, mentors, colleagues, and students and the literature. Each component is essential to learning a specialty in medicine and maintaining competence in the specialty over the course of one's career. In plastic surgery, the abundance of master surgeons gives everyone the opportunity to observe excellence in technique, during residency and later through educational programs. Contact with teachers and colleagues must be maintained in order to keep abreast of the new innovations in medicine and to measure one's outcomes in the context of standard of care. Our professional society meetings and symposia, both locally and nationally, provide us with this opportunity. Contact with mentors and students is critical for innovation. The physician must seek out these sources of inspiration and stimulation to improve patient care. Collaboration with professionals is a unique opportunity to allow further growth in our specialty and is available in every medical environment. The literature allows the physician to see where we have been, where we are currently, and what the future holds. The physician can hold a piece of literature in the hand and review its message both in critical times, when patient management decisions must be made on a timely basis, and during leisure times, when a subject is studied and carefully measured against personal experience and knowledge acquired through professional contacts. It is hoped that this edition of *Plastic Surgery*, like its predecessors, can serve the purpose of literature in teaching. Its eight volumes contain more than 6800 pages of information carefully formulated by recognized experts in our specialty in plastic surgery. It is designed, as initially stated, to define the current knowledge of plastic surgery and to serve as a platform for future creativity to benefit the patient we see with congenital and acquired deformities.

Stephen J. Mathes, MD, 2005

✦ ACKNOWLEDGMENTS

So many talented and dedicated professionals are necessary to complete a text of this magnitude. It is impossible to really thank everyone adequately, since there are so many people behind the scenes who were silently working toward the completion of this project. However, I shall endeavor to acknowledge the people who provided scientific, technical, and emotional support to make this edition of *Plastic Surgery* possible.

My first contact with the publisher (Saunders, now Elsevier) started with my meeting with Allan Ross and Ann Ruzycka Anderson. Allan Ross, executive editor, was assigned to guide this text to publication. He is a dedicated publishing executive who was most supportive at the inception of this project. Ann Ruzycka Anderson, senior developmental editor, has been working in medical publishing for 20 years. This text was most fortunate to have Allan and Ann assigned as the guiding forces at the onset. Ann states that working on this text is "something exciting, worthwhile, and important" because she is helping to "produce the largest book in medical publishing history."

Because this book took 5 years to complete, there were changes in the personnel involved in the project. Joe Rusko, medical editor, assumed the responsibilities of guiding the development of the text, with Allan Ross taking on the role of consultant. Joe has great enthusiasm and provided great ideas for the format of this book and for associated advertising. During the past year, the project was turned over to the leadership of Sue Hodgson, currently the publishing director and general manager for Elsevier Ltd. With Sue living in London, the project took on a more international outlook, with Sue flying between London, Philadelphia, New York, and San Francisco to keep the project moving ahead to completion. Both Sue Hodgson and Allan Ross have a great deal of success in guiding complex publications to press. Sue has published highly successful books in dermatology, and now, it is hoped, she will be able to make the same claim for the field of plastic surgery. For sure, she can now lay claim to publishing the largest medical book in existence. Recently, Sue Hodgson summed up her role in the publishing industry as follows: "The opportunity to create new products to answer the market's educational needs and handling high-profile and demanding projects are what get me out of bed in the morning." All plastic surgeons who use this text are indebted to the perseverance and commitment of these publishing leaders: Allan Ross, Joe Rusko, and Sue Hodgson.

"The quality of a person's life is in direct proportion to their commitment to excellence, regardless of their chosen field of endeavor."

—Vince Lombardi

After the authors were selected for the 219 chapters, it was obvious that we needed someone special to serve as the editorial coordinator between the editors and the authors. Thanks to the advice of Allan Ross and Ann Ruzycka Anderson, Shireen Dunwoody was recommended for this position. Shireen is an accomplished computer programmer and musician and has served as a senior medical writer, media programmer/editor, and developmental editor since 1991. Among the high-profile medical texts on which she has worked are *Clinical Oncology* (Martin Abeloff et al., editors), *Surgery of the Liver and Biliary Tract* (Leslie Blumgart, editor), and *Fundamentals of Surgery* (John E. Niederhuber, editor). Shireen has worked closely with the editors and our assigned authors during every step of the process—obtaining the manuscripts (including a multitude of meetings and phone calls with authors), helping find artists when needed, confirming references, discovering historical information as related to the many subjects covered in *Plastic Surgery*, and coordinating all these data with the publishing staff in Philadelphia and New York. When asked to describe what this job was like, she described the process as follows: "At times, this project has been a struggle, but most of the time it has been a joy (kind of like raising eight children). On any given day, working on this project has given me a reason to (1) get up in the morning; (2) stay up all night; (3) despise the morning; (4) stay sober; (5) get drunk; (6) laugh; (7) cry; (8) live; (9) lie; (10) rejoice. Who could ask for anything more? It has certainly kept things interesting!" Shireen credits special members of the publishing staff for helping this immense project move ahead at a fairly steady pace. In Philadelphia, Linda Van Pelt, senior project manager, book production, and RoseMarie Klimowicz, freelance copyeditor, have been with this project since its inception. They have both dedicated vast amounts of blood, sweat, tears, and personal time. Ann Ruzycka Anderson has been dedicated to this project since the onset and has also worked closely with Shireen. Judy Fletcher, publishing director, provided the support needed for timely layouts and served as an advocate for this project even when layout or illustrations were changed to maintain the continuity and artistry of the chapters. Finally, Shireen acknowledges her two amazing assistants in Palm Springs, California, Donna Larson and Carla Parnell, who have helped her scan, copy, crop, sort, mail, and stay sane. Without the dedication and brilliance of Shireen Dunwoody in bringing out the best in the editors, publishers, authors, and artists, this text would not have the quality and completeness it now possesses.

My immediate family was always supportive of this project despite the time-consuming work associated with text preparation. I wish to acknowledge and thank my family for their exciting accomplishments, which are a source of pride and enjoyment: Mary, Norma, Paul, Leslie, Isabelle, Peter, David, Brian, Vasso, Zoe, Ned, Erin, Maggie, and Rick.

In any profession, the support and encouragement of one's colleagues are essential for productivity. I wish to thank the faculty in our division of plastic surgery for their specific contributions to the text and their active roles as outstanding teachers for our residents and students at the University of California in San Francisco. The faculty, both full time and clinical, include the following: Bernard Alpert, Jim Anthony, Ramin Behmand, Kyle Bickel, Greg Buncke, K. Ning Chang, Tancredi D'Amore, Keith Denkler, Issa Eschima, Robert Foster, Roger Friedenthal, Gilbert Gradinger, Ronald Gruber, William Hoffman, Clyde Ikeda, Gabriel Kind, Chen Lee, Pablo Leon, Mahesh Mankani, Robert Markeson, Mary McGrath, Sean Moloney, Douglas Ousterhout, John Owsley, Lorne Rosenfield, Vivian Ting, Bryant Toth, Philip Trabulsy, D. Miller Wise, and David Young.

During the time span in which this book was edited, a group of outstanding residents completed their plastic surgery residencies at UCSF. All these residents contributed to both the care of many of the patients included in the chapters written by our faculty and the development of concepts used in the chapters of this edition. Each resident listed has contributed to the advancement of our knowledge in plastic surgery: Delora Mount, Richard Grossman, Jeff Roth, Laura McMillan, Kenneth Bermudez, Marga Massey, Yngvar Hvistendahl, Duc Bui, Te Ning Chang, Hatem Abou-Sayed, Farzad Nahai, Hop Nguyen Le, Clara Lee, Scott Hansen, Jennifer Newman-Keagle, and Wesley Schooler. General surgery residents, research fellows, and students who participated in the project include Lee Alkureishi, Julie Lang, Edward Miranda, and Cristiane Ueno.

Without the dedication of our staff, the preparation of this text would not have been possible. Crystal Munoz served as our office manager during most of the preparation time. My patient coordinators, Marian Liebow and, later, Skye Ingham, are patient advocates and made the arrangements necessary to treat the patients discussed in our chapters. Our nurses, Janet Tanaka and, later, Ann Hutchinson, were essential to the overall care of patients presenting to our clinical practice. Our staff provides the support needed to allow the faculty to have the time necessary to participate in the creative activities expected in academic plastic surgery.

Plastic surgeons depend on visual assessment of problems; thus, illustrations are an essential part of our scientific literature. Numerous artists were involved in the chapters selected by the individual authors. However, two artists were available to all the contributors and provided outstanding art to accompany many of the chapters. Kathy Hirsh, located in Shanghai, China, and Scott Barrows, in Chicago, have worked diligently to provide accurate artistic interpretations of the surgical procedures recommended throughout this text.

"Mental toughness is many things. It is humility because it behooves all of us to remember that simplicity is the sign of greatness and meekness is the sign of true strength. Mental toughness is spartanism with qualities of sacrifice, self-denial, dedication. It is fearlessness, and it is love."

—Vince Lombardi

All the authors who contributed to these volumes exemplify mental toughness. To complete a chapter for a text is often considered an unappreciated task. However, thanks to the great reputation established by the prior editors of this comprehensive work, John M. Converse and Joseph G. McCarthy, and the previous editors of the hand volumes, William Littler and James May, the top plastic surgeons in their respective fields have given their time and efforts to maintain the excellence associated with past editions of this text. Thanks to these contributors, this book provides information at the forefront of innovation and current practice in the specialty of plastic surgery. The contributors and their families are thanked for their perseverance and sacrifice in the completion of these chapters and for their dedication to our specialty, plastic surgery.

SJM

✦ CONTENTS

✦ VOLUME II

The Head and Neck, Part 1

✦ VOLUME III

THE HEAD AND NECK, PART 2

✦ VOLUME IV
Pediatric Plastic Surgery

✦ VOLUME VII

The Hand and Upper Limb, Part 1

INTRODUCTION AND GENERAL PRINCIPLES 1

ACQUIRED DISORDERS— TRAUMATIC 151

Pediatric Tumors

JULIANA E. HANSEN, MD ✦ RICHARD CHAFFOO, MD

Cancer is diagnosed each year in the United States in nearly 12,000 pediatric patients (younger than 19 years) and accounts for 10% of childhood deaths. Although leukemias form the largest group of these pediatric cancers, a significant number represent tumors for which plastic surgical input will be requested.[1] Dealing with childhood maladies is an emotionally charged and challenging situation for all involved. Prompt diagnosis and timely delivery of treatment will optimize these difficult encounters. Familiarity with pediatric-specific tumors is therefore important for plastic surgeons.

Fortunately, the majority of masses seen in children are benign. A mass in the head or neck of an infant or child is most likely to be lymphadenopathy secondary to infection. Within the first year of life, the most common tumors for which plastic surgical consultation is obtained include hemangiomas, cystic hygromas, teratomas, dermoid cysts, and branchial cleft sinuses. Of these, hemangiomas represent the most common benign neoplasm of infancy. They occur in 2.6% of newborns and are present in 12% of children by the age of 1 year.[1]

Malignant neoplasms, rare in the first year of life, present with an incidence of 183 per 1 million live births.[2] Between the ages of 1 and 5 years, the cancers most commonly seen are leukemias, central nervous system tumors, lymphomas, and neuroblastoma. After the age of 5 years, the incidence of leukemia and neuroblastoma decreases, whereas lymphoma, soft tissue sarcomas, thyroid cancer, and salivary gland tumors increase in frequency.

ETIOLOGY

Only a small percentage of pediatric malignant neoplasms have a clear cause. Hereditary factors, infections (viral in particular), parental age, prenatal exposure to certain drugs, and elevated birth weight have all been associated with various types of neoplastic disease. Approximately 3% to 12% of children treated for a malignant disease will develop a second, new cancer within 20 years and overall face a 10-fold increased risk above that of controls.[3] Chemotherapy (alkylating agents in particular) and radiation therapy are thought to be significant risk factors. Exposure to cigarette smoking, electromagnetic fields, parental occupational exposures, and other environmental exposures have also been speculated to play a role in pediatric malignant neoplasms, although few direct causal relationships have been specified. The majority of benign masses have an infectious cause. These manifest either primarily, as in lymphadenitis, abscess, or sialadenitis, or as a result of a secondary infection of a congenital defect, as in an infected branchial cleft cyst.

DIAGNOSTIC STUDIES

Although standard radiographic imaging procedures in children often require general anesthesia, the benefits of imaging of large complex masses greatly outweigh the risks. Computed tomographic scans are essential in the work-up of masses of the head and neck. Magnetic resonance imaging is the procedure of choice for evaluation of soft tissue masses of the extremities. In the pediatric population, core needle biopsies, with or without imaging guidance, have been shown to be effective diagnostic tools.[4,5] Needle localization of small tumors for excisional biopsy has also been shown to be effective in young children.[6]

BENIGN TUMORS

Inflammatory Masses

LYMPHADENOPATHY

Infections of the head and neck in the pediatric population can present as masses that may appear to be neoplasms and may cause airway emergencies. Lymphadenopathy in the superficial neck involving anterior cervical, posterior cervical, and occipital nodes is commonplace after upper respiratory tract infections. *Staphylococcus aureus* and beta-hemolytic streptococcus are the most common bacterial causes. Viral infections also frequently cause lymphadenopathy. Enlargement may persist for months to years. Marked enlargement and obvious acute inflammatory changes warrant additional work-up or treatment. Acute cervical lymphadenitis that presents with erythema, tenderness, and induration over the affected nodes should be treated with antibiotics and incision and drainage if a large quantity of pus is present. When the usual work-up and treatment for infection are not diagnostic, excisional lymph node biopsy should be considered. Granulomatous diseases as well as malignant neoplasms should be sought.

Tuberculosis and other atypical mycobacterial infections are still causes of chronic suppurative lymphadenitis. Scrofula (tuberculous cervical adenitis) is typically seen in children younger than 6 years and presents as painless progressive node enlargement. Open sores, called cold abscesses, may develop over the infected nodes. Skin testing (PPD) may not be helpful with atypical mycobacterial infections because the cross-reactivity is only 15%. Surgical excision of affected nodes rather than incision and drainage should be performed if open wounds are present to prevent the formation of chronic draining fistulas. Once cultures are sent, four-drug therapy including rifampin, isoniazid, ethambutol, and pyrazinamide is instituted urgently for suspected tuberculous infections with positive skin test results. The course of treatment is 6 months, and the antibiotic regimen may be tapered to two drugs once culture and sensitivity results are obtained. Suspected atypical infections are treated with a combination of clarithromycin and ethambutol, rifampin, or ciprofloxacin while results of culture are awaited.[7]

ABSCESSES

Retropharyngeal abscess is seen most often in infants and toddlers and rarely in older children. An infection in this area may cause difficulty in swallowing, respiratory tract obstruction, and neck stiffness. This condition in a young child represents a surgical emergency; drainage and establishment of a stable airway are essential. Peritonsillar abscess may result from untreated tonsillitis. Extension may lead to the development of a lateral pharyngeal abscess, causing a lateral neck mass. Trismus and hoarseness may be seen. Severe disease may be associated with airway obstruction and carotid artery erosion. Ludwig angina develops most commonly as a result of dental caries, and this severe streptococcal or mixed infection can spread rapidly through the floor of the mouth to involve the submaxillary space. Swelling in the submandibular and submental areas, floor of the mouth, and tongue may rapidly cause airway obstruction. Broad-spectrum antibiotics including penicillin should be started immediately. Early infections may not require drainage. In later infections, collections of pus may develop between the deep muscles of the floor of the mouth and tongue.

SIALADENITIS

Swelling, erythema, and tenderness over the parotid or submandibular gland may represent acute, chronic, or recurrent sialadenitis. When acute parotitis develops in the neonate, it is often associated with prematurity and often follows a bout of dehydration. Suppurative parotitis in newborns is usually unilateral but can be bilateral and is caused by *S. aureus, Streptococcus viridans,* or *Streptococcus pyogenes.* Most patients respond to antibiotics and rehydration. Recurrence is rare. Abscess formation after sialadenitis in children, although rare, has been described.[8-11]

Aseptic sialadenitis has also been described in premature infants fed long term by orogastric tubes. Exclusive feeding in this way can reduce reflex salivary gland stimulation, saliva production, and duct clearance, causing functional ductal obstruction and inflammation.[12] Recurrent infections may be seen during childhood, with the age at onset being between 1 and 10 years. Involvement may be unilateral or bilateral, and the average number of episodes is 1.7 per year. A history of excessive histamine-related reactions and reactive airways was a common finding in a series of 30 pediatric patients with recurrent suppurative parotitis.[13] Streptococcus is the most common etiologic agent. The process is usually self-limited, often resolving during teenage years. Parotidectomy has been used to treat those patients with recalcitrant disease.

The submandibular gland is the salivary gland most likely to be affected by chronic sclerosing sialadenitis (also called a Kuttner tumor). The appearance is identical clinically to a glandular neoplasm, and resection of the entire gland may be required for adequate treatment.[14]

PYOGENIC GRANULOMA

Pyogenic granuloma is a rapidly growing, highly vascular lesion. It may develop in children of any age and is also commonly seen in adults. Pyogenic granuloma develops spontaneously or after minor trauma and may arise on either the skin or mucous membranes. The head and neck are the most commonly affected areas, but the upper extremities are also frequently involved (Figs. 105-1 and 105-2). On histologic examination, proliferating capillaries in a fibromyxomatous stroma are seen. The pathognomonic lobular architecture of the lesions has given rise to the less commonly used name of lobular capillary hemangioma.

These highly vascular tumors may grow rapidly to a large size (2 to 3 cm). They may have intermittent bouts of profuse bleeding, even from lesions only millimeters in size. This may result in multiple emergency department visits by anxious parents for what appears to be an otherwise negligible lesion. Treatment can involve cautery alone for smaller lesions, although the recurrence rate has been documented as high as 43.5%.[15] Full-thickness skin excision with primary closure is curative. Shave excision and laser photocoagulation with a vascular laser (argon or KTP) have also produced good results with low recurrence.[16]

Branchial Cleft Anomalies

Failure of fusion of the branchial arches, which develop between the third and sixth weeks of gestation, can cause fistulas, sinus tracks, cysts, cartilaginous rests,

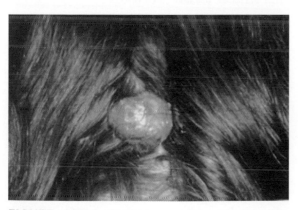

FIGURE 105-1. Pyogenic granuloma of the scalp treated by excision.

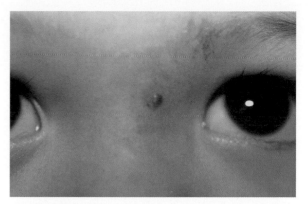

FIGURE 105-2. A 1-year-old with small pyogenic granuloma of the glabellar region causing profuse recurrent bleeding. This was treated by cauterization.

or skin tags. When connections to the pharynx are present, these lesions are susceptible to infection. Presentation of sinuses and fistulas is generally during the first decade of life. Cysts tend to be present in higher, less conspicuous areas of the neck, and a first-time diagnosis of branchial cleft cyst is not uncommonly made in older children, adolescents, and adults.

Anomalies of the second branchial arch are the most common. A complete, nonfused second arch leaves a cleft from the base of the tonsil, paralleling the anterior border of the sternocleidomastoid muscle, to the lower portion of the muscle near its sternal origin. An anomalous track may open anywhere along the upper three quarters of the anterior border of the sternocleidomastoid muscle. This may represent a blind sinus or extend all the way into the tonsillar fossa. Drainage of saliva may be a chronic problem. Cysts may also form along this line but tend to be anterior to the upper portion of the muscle. Treatment requires complete fistulous track excision and is done through one or more short transverse neck incisions.

The first branchial arch is involved far less often than the second (8% of patients). A complete anomalous cleft of the first arch leaves a defect from the external auditory canal, under and along the border of the mandible, to the midline. Fistulous tracks and cysts along this line may extend through the parotid and jeopardize branches of the facial nerve during excision. Two thirds of these lesions present as cysts without tracks. Far fewer are either sinuses with cysts, ending as a cul-de-sac at the mastoid, or complete fistulas. Duplication of the external auditory canal may be present. A preauricular incision extending to the external opening is used for exposure and excision of the complete track.

Third branchial cleft anomalies are rare. The external opening lies along the anterior border of the sternocleidomastoid muscle, as for a cleft of the second arch, but the track runs deep to the carotid artery and toward or through the thyrohyoid membrane.[17-20]

Thyroglossal Duct Remnants

Embryologic thyroid gland development involves the thyroglossal duct, which runs from the foramen cecum, in the posterior midline of the tongue, through the hyoid bone, and down to the central lower neck. Persistence of the thyroglossal duct can be manifested as a cyst anywhere along its course. Thyroid gland remnants may also be present within the cyst or alone. A lingual thyroid may be the only functioning thyroid tissue present. These ductal remnants usually present as a cystic mass below the hyoid in the anterior neck. External openings are generally not seen unless there has been an infection that has spontaneously drained or been surgically drained. Movement with swallowing is characteristic. Surgical excision is recommended for cosmetic reasons or for infection and drainage. Sistrunk[21] in 1920 described the definitive approach, which includes removal of the central portion of the hyoid bone and excision of the track up to the foramen cecum at the base of the tongue. Careful excision of small finger-like accessory ducts coming off the main duct should be done under loupe magnification. Thyroid scans should be performed if there is question about the location of functioning thyroid tissue.[22,23]

Dermoid Cysts

Dermoids are cysts containing both ectoderm and mesoderm. They are epithelium lined and contain varying amounts of hair follicles, sebaceous glands, and connective tissue. Dermoid cysts commonly arise in the head and neck and are present at birth, although they may not become clinically evident until later in life (Fig. 105-3). They probably result from the embryologic inclusion of germ cells between fusing tissue layers. In the head, these cysts frequently extend down to the craniofacial skeleton. Periorbital dermoids may originate from suture lines. The lateral brow is a common place for dermoid cysts originating from the zygomaticofrontal suture. Submandibular dermoids may originate between branchial arch fusion planes. The lateral brow, midline of the nose, and neck are common locations, although all sites may be involved. Dermoid cysts may become large, compressing adjacent structures. They may cause bone erosion, proptosis if they are located in the orbit, airway compression, or swallowing problems when they are located in the neck.

Midline cysts of the nose must be approached with caution because they may extend down through the nasofrontal region to the base of the skull (Fig. 105-4). These masses deserve imaging before surgical excision if they are large or fixed. Axial and coronal

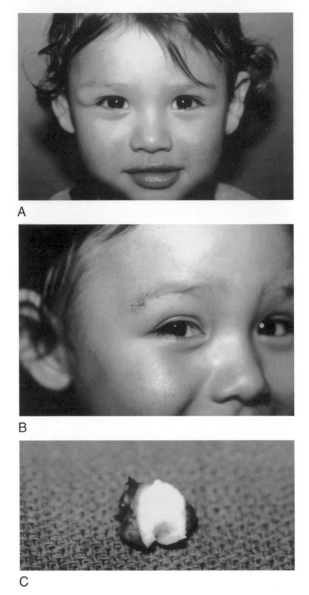

A

B

C

FIGURE 105-3. *A to C,* A 2-year-old with right lateral brow dermoid, present since birth.

computed tomographic scans will help differentiate an extracranial dermoid cyst from one that extends intracranially or from a different type of lesion that emanates from inside the dura. Encephalocele must be ruled out before proceeding with excision of midline masses. Cysts in the orbit should also be imaged to assess involvement of the globe, orbital nerve, or extraocular muscles. Dermoids that are outside of the orbit, mobile, and small may not require any imaging studies before surgical excision. Complete excision is the recommended treatment, and removal of the stalk down to the point of origination is indicated.

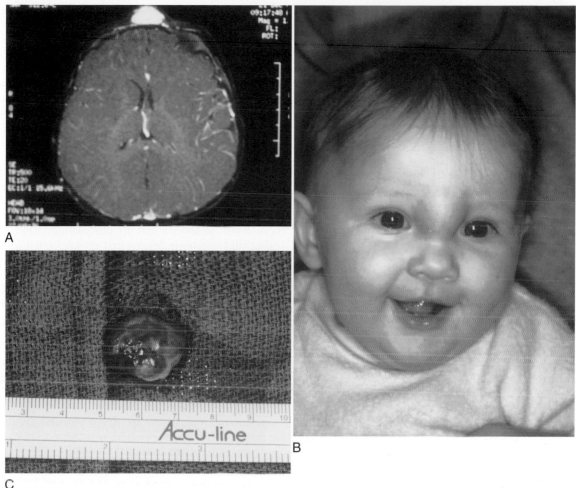

FIGURE 105-4. *A* and *B,* A 5-month-old with 3-cm frontonasal mass. A computed tomographic scan confirmed that there was no intracranial component of this midline lesion. *C,* Excision confirmed the diagnosis of dermoid cyst.

Teratomas

Teratomas are congenital tumors composed of multiple tissue types. They occur in approximately 1 in 4000 births.[24] True teratomas, teratoid tumors, dermoid cysts, and epignathi are all forms of teratomas. True teratomas and teratoid tumors contain tissues from all three germ lines, but only true teratomas have visible differentiation of ectoderm, mesoderm, and endoderm into recognizable structures. Dermoids contain only ectoderm and mesoderm. Epignathi are teratomas that show a high degree of differentiation, resulting in complete organ and limb formation within the tumor.

Approximately 10% of teratomas occur in the head and neck, most commonly in the orbit, glabellar area, sinuses, nasopharynx, and cervical area. Nasopharyngeal teratomas usually arise from the superior or lateral walls of the nasopharynx and are seen at birth or shortly after. They frequently appear as a polypoid

mass (hairy polyp) hanging from a stalk. If large enough, they may present with airway obstruction. Cervical teratomas present as neck masses and are usually seen at birth. They tend to be partially cystic with mixed echogenicity by ultrasound examination. They can enlarge, causing airway obstruction by tracheal compression. Once the diagnosis is made, immediate surgical excision is indicated.

Sacrococcygeal teratoma occurs in 1 in 40,000 live births and accounts for between 37% and 65% of all childhood teratomas.[25] The most common type of sacrococcygeal teratoma is one with a large external component and a minimal presacral component. As the internal (presacral) component predominates, the incidence of malignancy increases. Completely external tumors have an 8% incidence of malignancy. At the time of diagnosis, 17% of sacrococcygeal teratomas are malignant. For completely internal tumors, however, the incidence of malignancy is

38%. Complete surgical excision including the coccyx is the treatment. For malignant tumors, chemotherapy with or without radiation therapy is used adjunctively. Tumors that show a high degree of histologic immaturity should also be treated with adjunctive chemotherapy.

Benign Vascular Tumors

Childhood vascular lesions are classified as either hemangiomas or malformations, as defined by Mulliken. Hemangiomas are the most common benign tumors of infancy with an incidence of 8% to 12%.[26] They may be present at birth (40%) or appear in the neonatal period, most commonly before 8 weeks of life (60%). These lesions are characterized histologically by endothelial cell hyperplasia and proliferation with increased mitotic activity.[27,28]

HEMANGIOMAS

Hemangiomas typically present as a small red or blue mark on the skin that may rapidly increase in size (Fig. 105-5). This change in the clinical appearance of the skin lesion coincides with the proliferative phase of the hemangioma, lasting up to 9 months. During this time, the classic histologic findings of endothelial hyperplasia with abnormal lumen formation are seen. Problems with ulceration may develop in rapidly progressive lesions that are in areas subject to friction.

Involution occurs spontaneously, beginning after 9 months of age. This phase is much slower than the proliferative phase and may take up to 7 to 9 years. Resolution will be complete in more than 50% of children by the age of 5 years and in more than 70% by the age of 7 years.[29] Incomplete regression may occur, or permanent skin changes may result. Residual skin changes such as telangiectasias or scarring are left in 10% to 26% of patients.

Treatment of hemangiomas is reserved for nonhealing ulcerated lesions, compromise of function by large compressive lesions (visual impairment is common), bleeding, high-output cardiac failure, and platelet trapping with coagulopathy. Systemic and intralesional steroid administration is the first line of treatment. Steroids should be started during the proliferative phase to arrest growth and induce early regression; 30% of patients will respond well to steroid use. A response should be evident within 2 to 4 weeks of beginning systemic steroids, and treatment should continue up to 1 month after arrest of the proliferative phase to prevent rebound growth. A slow steroid taper during 2 to 3 months should follow.

Intralesional steroids also have a success rate of approximately 30%. The response rate is faster, and local complications include tissue necrosis, tissue atrophy, and hypopigmentation. Topical steroids have also been used with some success. The response rate is slower than with intralesional injections.

Treatment by pulsed dye laser, yttrium-aluminum-garnet laser, or a combination of the two is used commonly for hemangiomas that are superficial. These appear bright red. This treatment frequently requires several sessions and is done under general anesthesia for young children. Treatment is carried out to lighten the lesion and to arrest the proliferative phase, limiting the size of the hemangioma. Extensive laser treatments can cause scarring.

Surgical excision is seldom considered first-line treatment because of the extensive nature of these lesions, their proximity to vital structures and the facial nerve, and the scarring that results. Surgical excision is reserved for lesions that are obstructing vision or other vital functions, lesions that are associated with platelet trapping, or lesions that are localized and can be completely excised to improve contour and appearance. In patients with large hemangiomas, complete involution may result in areas of significant skin redundancy, requiring later excision and recontouring. Interferon alfa-2 therapy for hemangiomas is currently being studied with interest, but at this time, no clear benefits of this type of treatment have been reported.

VASCULAR MALFORMATIONS

Vascular malformations are developmental abnormalities of the vascular system, usually occurring as sporadic rather than inherited anomalies. They may be composed of capillaries, veins, arteries, lymph channels, or a combination of these. The vascular malformation may be seen at birth or may not be manifested until youth or teenage years (Fig. 105-6).

Capillary malformations (port-wine stains) tend to be present at birth and are seen in 0.3% of newborns. On the face, almost half of capillary malformations will follow one of the trigeminal sensory patterns. These low-flow lesions tend to grow proportionally with the child and may develop a rough nodular texture over time. Laser therapy and surgical excision for limited areas are suitable treatment options.

Venous malformations tend to be soft, nonpulsatile compressible lesions. Expansion with the Valsalva maneuver or tourniquet placement on an extremity is characteristic. Lesions may be located superficially, within the skin or subcutaneous tissues, or isolated to muscle or bone. Growth occurs proportionate to the child or after injury or partial resection.[25] Sclerosants, coagulation, or surgical excision may be indicated for cosmetic or functional reasons.

Arteriovenous malformations are high-flow lesions that are seen less often than capillary or venous malformations. They manifest after birth and cause progressive dilation and tortuosity of the venous vessels. Pulsations or a palpable thrill may be felt and bruits

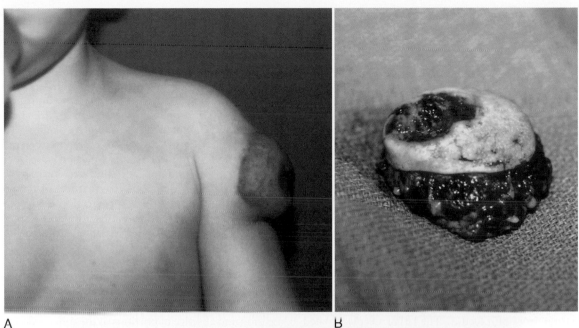

A   B

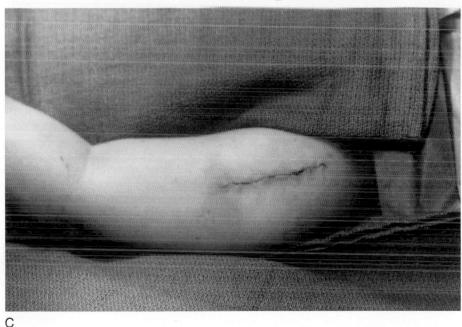

C

FIGURE 105-5. *A,* A 1-year-old girl with hemangioma of the arm with ulceration and bleeding, resulting in multiple emergency department visits. *B* and *C,* The lesion was well circumscribed and easily excised with minimal blood loss.

auscultated over the lesion. Cardiac failure and disseminated intravascular coagulation may complicate large lesions. Angiography is an essential component of the work-up for these malformations. Selective embolization may be used as the sole treatment or in preparation for surgical excision. The use of hypotensive anesthesia and cardiopulmonary bypass must be considered in planning of surgical excision of large

lesions to limit hemorrhage that might otherwise be uncontrollable.

Lymphatic malformations are present at birth in 65% of patients and present by the age of 2 years in 90%.[30] These tumors consisting of anomalous lymphatic channels do not have proliferative capacities but do tend to grow proportionate with the child's development (Fig. 105-7). In addition, they may

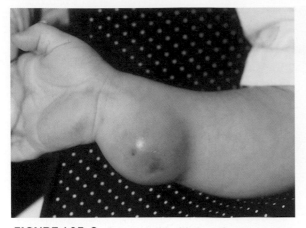

FIGURE 105-6. A 1-year-old with 4-cm forearm mass, enlarging since birth. Exploration revealed a venous malformation.

expand because of increasing fluid accumulation in areas without adequate drainage or enlarge acutely during times of infection. The larger, deeply situated lesions tend to be cystic and involve neurovascular structures, making complete excision difficult. These lesions have a tendency to become infected. Rapid enlargement in the head and neck area can cause a surgical emergency because of airway compromise. Subtotal resection or staged resection is often necessary. Associated soft tissue and skeletal hypertrophy may be seen with lymphatic malformations. Unlike with hemangiomas, spontaneous regression is not seen.

Neurofibromas

Neurogenic tumors, arising from the neural sheath cells, are located along peripheral and cranial nerves.

In children, their presentation may be either solitary or multiple (Fig. 105-8). Multiple neurofibromatosis is most familiar as von Recklinghausen disease. This syndrome of multiple neurofibromas, abnormal skin pigmentation, bone abnormalities, and multiple associated congenital anomalies is inherited in an autosomal dominant pattern with variable penetrance. The incidence is 0.03% of live births. Half of children born with von Recklinghausen disease will be diagnosed at birth by characteristic patterns of pigmentation (café au lait spots), skin tumors, and associated anomalies. Intracranial, abdominal, and thoracic location of tumors may delay diagnosis. The natural history of the syndrome is one of slow progression in the size and number of tumors. Although it is initially benign, there is a significant risk for malignant transformation of 8% to 16%.[31,32]

Plastic surgical involvement may be requested for skin tumors; for tumors involving cranial nerves presenting with facial palsies; and in patients with cranio-orbital neurofibromatosis, in which orbital bone erosion and absence of portions of the sphenoid bone present significant challenges. Children may present with solitary lesions that may be cutaneous or subcutaneous in origin. The patient with elephantiasis neuromatosa will develop severe distortion of the face that may include proptosis. These hanging pedunculated lesions require complete excision for prevention of progressive facial deformity. Because of the extensive nature of these tumors, multiple debulking procedures are more commonly performed.[25] Plexiform lesions arise from major nerve trunks and therefore tend to be deeply located within tissues (Fig. 105-9). In patients with plexiform neurofibroma involving the craniofacial region, computed tomographic scan is essential because these tumors may

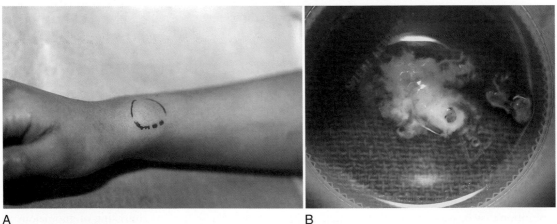

A   B

FIGURE 105-7. *A,* A 5-year-old with 3-cm enlarging forearm mass. Computed tomographic scan was nondiagnostic. *B,* Excisional biopsy was done of this watery, multiloculated cystic lesion, and pathologic examination showed lymphatic malformation.

tumors (Fig. 105-13). Within the pediatric population, it accounts for up to 75% of skin appendage tumors. In a series of 76 pilomatrical neoplasms in a pediatric population, 4 patients with pilomatrical carcinoma were identified (5%).[53] Pilomatrical carcinoma as well as aggressive pilomatrixoma has the tendency to recur after local excision.

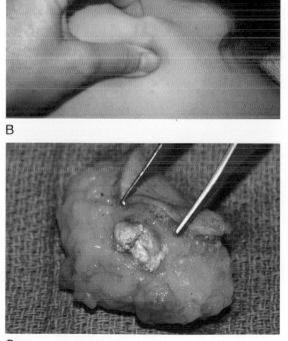

A

B

C

FIGURE 105-13. *A* and *B,* A 12-year-old girl with enlarging pilomatrixoma of the back. *C,* These irregular, firm, chalky subcutaneous lesions require wide excision to prevent recurrence.

Other types of benign cutaneous adnexal tumors include trichoepithelioma, syringoma, cylindromas, syringocystadenoma papilliferum, eccrine acrospiroma, and eccrine and apocrine hidrocystomas. No specific treatment is required for these tumors. If removal is desired, surgical excision is required. Laser resurfacing is not effective.

MALIGNANT NEOPLASMS

Neuroblastoma

Neuroblastoma is the most common malignant tumor seen in infancy. This tumor arises from neural crest cells that form the sympathetic nervous system and adrenal medulla. It presents as a painless, slow-growing mass fixed to underlying structures and may arise anywhere that sympathetic nerve tissue is present. Symptoms may arise from mass effect or from systemic release of catecholamines, causing sweating, pyrexia, diarrhea, and paroxysmal hypertension. Neuroblastoma represents more than 40% of neonatal malignant disease and 10% to 20% of all childhood malignant neoplasms.[54] The adrenal glands and neighboring retroperitoneal sympathetic ganglia are the most common sites of occurrence, representing 65% to 80% of primary tumors; 10% to 15% are seen in the mediastinum, 5% in the cervical region, and 5% in the pelvis. Multiple primary sites may occur in infants. Metastases from hematogenous as well as from lymphogenous spread are not infrequently seen at the time of diagnosis. Children presenting before the age of 1 year tend to have earlier stage disease with the most favorable prognosis. Stage I tumors (confined to the primary site) and stage II tumors (extending outside of the original organ structure but not crossing the midline and with ipsilateral node involvement) have survival rates up to 90%.[55] Treatment involves complete excision. Stage III tumors (primary tumor crosses the midline with bilateral node involvement) and stage IV tumors (distant metastases, bilateral nodes) may require preoperative chemotherapy or radiation therapy to shrink the tumor, offering the best chance for complete resection. Vincristine and cyclophosphamide are the most commonly used chemotherapeutics.[56-61]

Soft Tissue Sarcoma

RHABDOMYOSARCOMA

Rhabdomyosarcoma is a malignant tumor of mesenchymal origin thought to arise from cells committed to a skeletal muscle lineage. About 250 patients are diagnosed with rhabdomyosarcoma yearly in the United States. This is the third most common solid, extracranial tumor of childhood after Wilms tumor and neuroblastoma. Common sites include the head and neck, genitourinary tract, and extremities.[62] Typical presentation is a palpable mass (Fig. 105-14). Treatment should include complete surgical extirpation whenever possible. Survival is increased by the addition of radiation therapy and multiagent chemotherapy.[63] One third of patients will have recurrent metastatic disease, which is often fatal.

FIBROSARCOMA

Fibrosarcoma represents 11% of the soft tissue sarcomas in childhood. This tumor may originate in either soft tissue or bone.[64] Twenty percent of patients have a disease process involving the head and neck, for which survival rates of 80% are reported. Presentation before 5 years of age portends a better prognosis. Distant metastases will develop in 10% of these patients. After 5 years of age, the prognosis is similar to that for adults, with metastatic rates approaching 50%. Wide local excision or en bloc resection without sacrifice of vital structures is the primary therapeutic modality. Preoperative chemotherapy may be helpful in shrinking tumor, facilitating and limiting the extent of the dissection.[65]

SYNOVIAL SARCOMA

Synovial sarcomas typically arise in or near tendons and tendon sheaths as solitary, well-circumscribed lesions. These rare tumors usually present in the lower extremity, upper extremity, and groin. They represent 8% to 10% of all malignant neoplasms of somatic soft tissues and are the most common sarcoma of the hands and feet. Surgical excision including amputation is the treatment of choice. Multimodality adjuvant treatment is used, but the benefits of postoperative chemotherapy and radiation therapy, although promising, are not clearly established yet.[66-68]

ALVEOLAR SOFT PART SARCOMA

Alveolar soft part sarcoma is a rare soft tissue tumor occurring primarily in the skeletal muscles or musculofascial planes of the extremities. It occurs frequently in the trunk, head, and neck. Wide local excision is the mainstay of therapy. Metastases occur to the lungs, bone, and central nervous system. It can recur more than 10 years after primary resection. Survival rates are 82% at 2 years, 59% at 5 years, and 47% at 10 years.[69-71]

HEMANGIOPERICYTOMA

Hemangiopericytomas originate from the vascular pericytes of Zimmerman, histologically related to the glomus tumor. There is a lack of uniformity in appearance, growth, and biologic behavior. The musculoskeletal system and hand are the most common

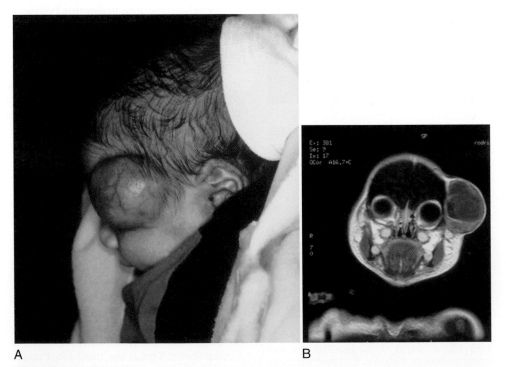

A   B

FIGURE 105-14. *A* and *B,* Newborn with rhabdomyosarcoma. Despite aggressive chemotherapy and surgical resection, he died at the age of 2 years.

primary sites. A painless mass with rapid growth or the appearance of the mass at a site of previous trauma is the typical presentation. Treatment includes wide local excision. Radiation therapy may be effective in providing tumor control. Overall mortality is high (50%), but mortality varies according to the location of presentation.[72-74]

LIPOSARCOMA

Liposarcoma represents 4% of childhood soft tissue tumors. The most common primary sites are the retroperitoneum and peripheral soft tissues. The thigh, inguinal region, shoulder, and buttocks are commonly affected. The tumors start deep between large muscle groups and often reach considerable size before encroachment on subcutaneous tissues. Tumor size and duration do not correlate well with prognosis. Treatment includes wide local excision. The role of chemotherapy and radiation therapy is uncertain.[75-77]

LEIOMYOSARCOMA

Leiomyosarcoma is rarely seen among pediatric patients. The most common location for presentation is in the lower extremity, followed by the head and neck and the trunk. A report of 27 patients with primary gastrointestinal leiomyosarcoma concluded that complete excision was the best treatment. Visceral metastases were rare in this study. Leiomyosarcoma has a favorable long-term prognosis.[78]

MALIGNANT MESENCHYMOMA

Malignant mesenchymoma arises from migratory neural crest cells. It has sporadically been reported to occur in the perineum and extremity bones; however, these tumors are predominantly of the external soft tissues. Size and histologic composition affect prognosis most strongly. Local invasion is often seen. Wide local excision is the treatment of choice.[79]

Malignant Bone Tumors

OSTEOSARCOMA

Osteosarcomas involve the long bones and the jaw bones primarily; they account for 20% of all primary bone malignant neoplasms and 6% of primary maxillary and mandibular malignant tumors. They are rarely seen in childhood. When they do present in the pediatric population, there is a 2:1 female-to-male predilection. Typical presenting signs include painful swelling, paresthesias, alveolar ulceration, trismus, loose teeth, nasal obstruction, and epistaxis, depending on the anatomic site involved. Skin invasion is rare. Treatment includes radical resection of the involved bone and surrounding soft tissue and postoperative radiation therapy. Nodal dissection is added for

clinically positive adenopathy. Distant metastases usually involve the lungs. Five-year survival is 27% for maxillary tumors and 37% for mandibular tumors.[80-84]

EWING SARCOMA

Ewing sarcoma usually involves the long bones or extraskeletal soft tissue. Involvement of the skull and facial bones is infrequent. When the head is affected, the mandible is the most common site of occurrence. Symptoms include severe pain and secondary swelling of the affected bone. Hematogenous spread to the lungs and bone will have occurred in 15% to 30% of patients at the time of presentation. Primary radiation therapy and combined chemotherapy have resulted in 2-year survival rates of up to 56%.[81,82,85]

CHONDROSARCOMA

Chondrosarcoma most commonly arises in the nasal septum, sphenoid sinus, ethmoid complex, maxilla, and nasopharynx. It is seen about half as often as osteosarcoma in the pediatric population. Adequate primary treatment is wide surgical resection. Prognosis is related to the adequacy of the surgical resection and the histologic grade of the tumor. Radiation treatment is reserved for local recurrences and as palliation for distant metastases.[86,87]

Retinoblastoma

Retinoblastoma, a highly malignant tumor arising from the retina, occurs in 1 of 18,000 live births in the United States each year. Bilaterality occurs in 25% to 50% of all patients. The average age at clinical onset is 18 months, and the majority of patients present by the age of 3 years. Two thirds of patients present with leukokoria, or a white pupillary reflex. Globe mobility disturbances are common. Spontaneous hyphema may develop. Invasion into the skull may occur and cause cranial nerve deficits. Enucleation is the procedure of choice in patients with unilateral vitreal involvement. Combination radiation therapy and chemotherapy are used for invasive disease.[88,89]

Salivary Gland Tumors

Salivary gland tumors in childhood typically involve the major salivary glands. The parotid gland is most often involved, followed by the submandibular gland with an incidence of 7:1. Half of all pediatric parotid tumors are either hemangiomas or lymphangiomas. These are present at birth and are seen to increase in size with crying. The skin overlying the hemangioma may be marked by telangiectasias and feel doughy and compressible. By the age of 3 years, 50% of hemangiomas of the parotid will spontaneously involute. Early surgical intervention is reserved for patients with airway obstruction. The most common nonvascular parotid tumor of childhood is the benign mixed tumor. This is best treated by superficial parotidectomy. Mucoepidermoid carcinoma is the most common parotid malignant neoplasm. These tend to be low grade and are treated by total parotidectomy with facial nerve sparing.[90]

Nasopharyngeal Carcinoma

Nasopharyngeal carcinoma represents less than 1% of all childhood malignant neoplasms but appears to be on the rise in African Americans, especially teens. Cervical adenopathy is often the presenting complaint. Nasal obstruction, epistaxis, otalgia, and odynophagia are common accompanying symptoms. Distant metastases at the time of presentation are rare. Cranial nerve involvement signals skull base erosion. Treatment involves surgical resection and irradiation. Adjuvant chemotherapy has not been as clearly demonstrated to be of benefit.

Thyroid Cancer

Thyroid cancer represents the third most common solid tumor in children and adolescents and 3% of all pediatric malignant neoplasms. Patients typically present with an asymptomatic neck mass. Although it is biologically more aggressive and advanced than adult thyroid cancer, paradoxically it has a better prognosis when it is discovered in this age group. Sixty percent to 80% of pediatric patients present with pathologically palpable cervical adenopathy. Fine-needle aspiration is recommended by most authorities to establish a diagnosis and to assist in treatment planning. The dominant histologic type is papillary, follicular variant. Although irradiation is a known risk factor, only a minority of patients have such a history. Surgery remains the standard treatment, although the extent of the thyroid resection remains controversial. Most centers recommend nearly total or total thyroidectomy. Conservative neck dissection is indicated when palpable adenopathy is present. Postoperative radiation therapy and sodium iodide I 131 are indicated in selected patients. The presence of local metastases at initial surgery is most predictive of local recurrence. Local recurrence is also age dependent. In patients who present before 10 years of age, there is a 10% to 35% incidence of recurrence.[91-94]

Breast Cancer

Breast cancer is a rare entity in the pediatric population. History typically includes a painless, enlarging breast mass. Appropriate work-up involves fine-needle aspiration, when feasible, or excisional biopsy.[95] Most breast masses in children represent benign disease.

Fibroadenomas account for a large percentage of palpable breast masses in the pediatric population.[96] In a 25-year period at St. Jude Children's Hospital, 18 pediatric patients were diagnosed with breast cancer; 16 were girls, and 2 were boys. Most patients had metastatic disease (13) secondary to rhabdomyosarcoma, and all died of their disease. Two patients had primary breast cancer, alveolar rhabdomyosarcoma and non-Hodgkin lymphoma, treated by biopsy and chemotherapy. Three patients had secondary breast cancer.[97]

Juvenile papillomatosis of the breast is a benign proliferative condition. It presents as a firm, discrete mass of significant size, between 1 and 8 cm. It may be unilateral or bilateral and develops in women younger than 30 years. In a series of 300 patients with juvenile papillomatosis, 63% were diagnosed in women younger than 20 years; the youngest patients were 15 years old.[98] On histologic examination, multiple cysts, ductal hyperplasia, apocrine metaplasia, and varying degrees of atypia are seen. The association between juvenile papillomatosis and subsequent breast cancer is unclear. Rarely, carcinoma has been diagnosed at the same time. The presence of atypia suggests that this may serve as a precancerous lesion. In the series out of Memorial Sloan-Kettering Cancer Center, 4 patients of 41 (10%) with juvenile papillomatosis developed breast cancer. A significant family history of breast cancer and recurrent bilateral juvenile papillomatosis was seen in all these young women.

Excisional biopsy of discrete breast masses should be done by a circumareolar approach. Particular care must be exercised in diagnosis of a breast mass in the adolescent; a discrete subareolar mass, even if it is unilateral, may represent a physiologic breast bud.

REFERENCES

1. Mulliken J: Cutaneous vascular lesions of children. In Serafin D, Georgiade NG, eds: Pediatric Plastic Surgery. St. Louis, CV Mosby, 1984:137-154.
2. Ross JA, Swensen AR: Prenatal epidemiology of pediatric tumors. Curr Oncol Rep 2000;2:234-241.
3. Albano E, Stork LC, Greffe BS, et al: Neoplastic disease. In Hay W, Groothuis J, Hayward A, Levin M, eds: Current Pediatric Diagnosis and Treatment, 13th ed. Norwalk, Ct, Appleton & Lange, 1997:793-800.
4. Willman JH, White K, Coffin CM: Pediatric core needle biopsy: strengths and limitations in evaluation of masses. Pediatr Dev Pathol 2001;4:46-52.
5. Hussai HK, Kingston JE, Domizio P, et al: Imaging-guided core biopsy for the diagnosis of malignant tumors in pediatric patients. AJR Am J Roentgenol 2001;17:43-47.
6. Hardaway BW, Hoffer FA, Rao BN: Needle localization of small pediatric tumors for surgical biopsy. Pediatr Radiol 2000;30:318-322.
7. Jervis PN, Lee JA, Bull PD: Management of non-tuberculous mycobacterial peri-sialadenitis in children: the Sheffield otolaryngology experience. Clin Otolaryngol 2001;26:243-248.
8. David RB, O'Connel EJ: Suppurative parotitis in children. Am J Dis Child 1970;119:332-335.

9. Pershall KE, Koopmann CF Jr, Coulthard SW: Sialadenitis in children. Int J Pediatr Otorhinolaryngol 1986;11:199-203.

10. Bova R, Walker P: Neonatal submandibular sialadenitis progressing to submandibular gland abscess. Int J Pediatr Otorhinolaryngol 2000;53:73-75.

11. Bafaqeeh SA: Complicated neonatal submandibular suppurative sialadenitis. Int J Pediatr Otorhinolaryngol 1998;44:267-271.

12. Lindgren C, Balihodzic Lucovic V: Aseptic sialadenitis in preterm infants associated with long-term oro-gastric tube feeding. Eur J Pediatr 1998;157:1014-1016.

13. David RB, O'Connel EJ: Suppurative parotitis in children. Am J Dis Child 1970;119:332-335.

14. Williams HK, Connor R, Edmondson H: Chronic sclerosing sialadenitis of the submandibular and parotid glands: a report of a case and review of the literature. Oral Surg Oral Med Oral Pathol Oral Radiol Endod 2000;89:720-723.

15. Patrice SJ, Wiss K, Mulliken JB: Pyogenic granuloma (lobular capillary hemangioma): a clinicopathologic study of 178 cases. Pediatr Dermatol 1991;8:267-276.

16. Kirschner RE, Low DW: Treatment of pyogenic granuloma by shave excision and laser photocoagulation. Plast Reconstr Surg 1999;104:1346-1349.

17. Storoos RJ, Manni JJ: The double auditory meatus—a rare first branchial cleft anomaly: clinical presentation and treatment. Am J Otol 2000;21:837-841.

18. Stulner C, Chambers PA, Telfer MR, Corrigan AM: Management of first branchial cleft anomalies: report of two cases. Br J Oral Maxillofac Surg 2001;39:30-33.

19. Huang RY, Damrose EJ, Alavi S, et al: Third branchial cleft anomaly presenting as a retropharyngeal abscess. Int J Pediatr Otorhinolaryngol 2000;54:167-172.

20. Kenealy JF, Torsiglieri AJ Jr, Tom LW: Branchial cleft anomalies: a five-year retrospective review. Trans Pa Acad Ophthalmol Otolaryngol 1990;42:1022-1025.

21. Sistrunk WE: The surgical treatment of cysts of the thyroglossal tract. Ann Surg 1920;71:121.

22. Sprinzl GM, Koebke J, Wimmers-Klick J, et al: Morphology of the human thyroglossal tract: a histologic and macroscopic study in infants and children. Ann Otol Rhinol Laryngol 2000;109(pt 1):1135-1139.

23. Josephson GD, Spencer WR, Josephson JS: Thyroglossal duct cyst: the New York Eye and Ear Infirmary experience and a literature review. Ear Nose Throat J 1998;77:642-644, 646-647, 651.

24. Sobol S: Surgical management of tumors of the neck. In Thawley SE, Panje WR, Batsakis JG, Lindberg RD, eds: Comprehensive Management of Head and Neck Tumors. Philadelphia, WB Saunders, 1987:1369-1370.

25. Parry SW, Mathes SJ: Reconstruction of posterior trunk defects in the pediatric patient. In Serafin D, Georgiage NG, eds: Pediatric Plastic Surgery. St. Louis, CV Mosby, 1984:887.

26. Lanzkowsky P: Miscellaneous tumors. In Lanzkowsky P, ed: Manual of Pediatric Hematology and Oncology, 2nd ed. New York, Churchill Livingstone, 1995:542.

27. Brown TJ, Friedman J, Levy ML: The diagnosis and treatment of common birthmarks. Clin Plast Surg 1998;25:509-525.

28. Mulliken J, Glowacki J: Hemangiomas and vascular malformations in infants and children: a classification based on endothelial characteristics. Plast Reconstr Surg 1982;69:412-422.

29. Mulliken JB: Diagnosis and natural history of hemangiomas. In Mulliken JB, Young AE, eds: Vascular Birthmarks. Philadelphia, WB Saunders, 1988:59.

30. Mulliken JB: Cutaneous vascular anomalies. In McCarthy JG, ed: Plastic Surgery. Philadelphia, WB Saunders, 1990:3191.

31. Batsakis JG: Tumors of the peripheral nervous system. In Batsakis JG, ed: Tumors of the Head and Neck: Clinical and Pathological Considerations, 2nd ed. Baltimore, Williams & Wilkins, 1979:313-333.

32. Poyhonen M, Niemela S, Herva R: Risk of malignancy and death in neurofibromatosis. Arch Pathol Lab Med 1997;121:139-143.

33. Krastinova-Lolov D, Hamza F: The surgical management of cranio-orbital neurofibromatosis. Ann Plast Surg 1996;36:263-269.

34. Dionne GP, Seemayer TA: Infiltrating lipomas and angiolipomas revisited. Cancer 1974;33:732-738.

35. Slavin SA, Baker DC, McCarthy JG, Mufarrij A: Congenital infiltrating lipomatosis of the face: clinicopathologic evaluation and treatment. Plast Reconstr Surg 1983;72:158-164.

36. Slavin SA, Baker DC, McCarthy JG, Mufarrij A: Congenital infiltrating lipomatosis of the face. Plast Reconstr Surg 1983;72:158-164.

37. Chen CM, Lo LJ, Wong HF: Congenital infiltrating lipomatosis of the face: case report and literature review. Chang Gung Med J 2002;25:194-200.

38. Bouletreau P, Breton P, Freidel M: Congenital infiltrating lipomatosis of the face: case report. J Oral Maxillofac Surg 2000;58:807-810.

39. Gorken C, Alper M, Bilkay V, et al: Congenital infiltrating lipomatosis of the face. J Craniofac Surg 1999;10:365-368.

40. Van Wingerden JJ, Erlank JD, Becker JH: Liposuction for congenital infiltrating lipomatosis of the face. Plast Reconstr Surg 1988;81:989.

41. Dehner LP, Askin FB: Tumors of fibrous origin in childhood. Cancer 1976;38:888-900.

42. Blythe WR, Logan TC, Holmes DK, Drake AF: Fibromatosis colli. Am Fam Physician 1996;54:1965-1967.

43. Sharma S, Mishra K, Khanna G: Fibromatosis colli in infants. Acta Cytol 2003;47:359-362.

44. Ferkel RD, Westin GW, Dawson EG, Oppenheim WL: Muscular torticollis. J Bone Joint Surg Am 1983;65:894-900.

45. Zito J, Fitzpatrick P, Amedee R: Juvenile nasopharyngeal angiofibroma. J La Med Soc 2001;153:395-398.

46. Bales C, Kotapka M, Loerner LA, et al: Craniofacial resection of advanced juvenile nasopharyngeal angiofibroma. Arch Otolaryngol Head Neck Surg 2002;128:1071-1078.

47. Lowlicht RA, Jassin B, Kim M, Sasaki CT: Long-term effects of Le Fort I osteotomy for resection of juvenile nasopharyngeal angiofibromas on maxillary growth and dental sensation. Arch Otolaryngol Head Neck Surg 2001;128:923-927.

48. Allen PW: Recurring digital fibrous tumours of childhood. Pathology 1972;4:215-223.

49. Shapiro L: Infantile digital fibromatosis and aponeurotic fibroma. Case reports of two rare pseudosarcomas and review of the literature. Arch Dermatol 1969;99:37-42.

50. Bloem JJ, Vuzevski ND, Huffstadt AJ: Recurring digital fibroma of infancy. J Bone Joint Surg Br 1974;56:746-751.

51. Riefkohl R, Georgiade N: Facial bone tumors in children. In Serafin D, Georgiade NG, eds: Pediatric Plastic Surgery. St. Louis, CV Mosby, 1984:678.

52. Gross CW, Montgomery WW: Fibrous dysplasia and malignant degeneration. Arch Otolaryngol 1967;85:653-657.

53. Marrogi AJ, Wick MR, Dehner LP: Pilomatrical neoplasms in children and young adults. Am J Dermatopathol 1992;14:87-94.

54. De Lorimier AA, Bragg KU, Linden G: Neuroblastoma in childhood. Am J Dis Child 1969;118:441-450.

55. Breslow N, McCann B: Statistical estimation of prognosis for children with neuroblastoma. Cancer Res 1971;31:2098-2103.

56. Young LW, Rubin P, Hansen RE: The extra-adnexal neuroblastoma: high radiocurability and diagnostic accuracy. Am J Roentgenol Radium Ther Nucl Med 1970;108:75-91.

57. Bodian M: Neuroblastoma. Pediatr Clin North Am 1959;6:449.

58. Fortner J, Nicastri A, Murphy ML: Neuroblastoma: natural history and results of treating 133 cases. Ann Surg 1968;167:132-142.

59. King RL, Storaasli JP, Bolande RP: Neuroblastoma review of 28 cases and presentation of two cases with metastases and long term survival. Am J Roentgenol Radium Ther Nucl Med 1961;85:733-747.
60. Koop CE: The role of surgery in resectable, not resectable, and metastatic neuroblastoma. JAMA 1968;205:157-158.
61. Phillips R: Neuroblastoma. Ann R Coll Surg Engl 1953; 12:27.
62. Dagher R, Halman L: Rhabdomyosarcoma: an overview. Oncologist 1999;4:34-44.
63. Grosfeld JL: Risk-based management: current concepts for treating malignant solid tumors of childhood. J Am Coll Surg 1999;189:407-425.
64. Soule EH, Pritchard DJ: Fibrosarcoma in infants and children. A review of 110 cases. Cancer 1977;40:1711-1721.
65. Trobs R, Meier T, Bennek J, et al: Fibrosarcoma in infants and children: a retrospective analysis—overdiagnosis in earlier years. Pediatr Surg Int 1999;15:123-128.
66. van der Heide HJ, Veth RP, Pruszczynski M, et al: Synovial sarcoma: oncological and functional results. Eur J Surg Oncol 1998;24:114-119.
67. Scully SP, Temple HT, Harrelson JM: Synovial sarcoma of the foot and ankle. Clin Orthop 1999;364:220-226.
68. Ferrari A, Casanova M, Massimino M, et al: Synovial sarcoma: report of a series of 25 consecutive children from a single institution. Med Pediatr Oncol 1999;32:32-37.
69. Park YK, Uhni KK, Kim YW, et al: Primary alveolar soft part sarcoma of bone. Histopathology 1999;35:411-417.
70. Ogose A, Yazawa Y, Ueda T, et al: Alveolar soft part sarcoma in Japan: multi-institutional study of 57 patients from the Japanese Musculoskeletal Oncology Group. Oncology 2003;65:7-13.
71. Pang LM, Roebuck DJ, Griffith JF, et al: Alveolar soft-part sarcoma: a rare soft-tissue malignancy with distinctive clinical and radiological features. Pediatr Radiol 2001;31:196-199.
72. Sabini P, Josephson GD, Yung RT, Dolitsky JN: Hemangiopericytoma presenting as a congenital midline nasal mass. Arch Otolaryngol Head Neck Surg 1998;124:202-204.
73. Carew JF, Singh B, Kravs DH: Hemangiopericytoma of the head and neck. Laryngoscope 1999;109:1409-1411.
74. Backwinkel KD, Diddams JA: Hemangiopericytoma. Cancer 1970;25:896-901.
75. Ribuffo D, Onesti MG, Elia E, et al: Liposarcomas of the thigh. Scand J Plast Reconstr Surg 1998;32:323-330.
76. Ferrari A, Casanova M, Spreafico F, et al: Childhood liposarcoma: a single-institutional twenty-year experience. Pediatr Hematol Oncol 1999;16:415-421.
77. Pollack A, Zagars GK, Goswitz MS, et al: Preoperative vs. postoperative radiotherapy in the treatment of soft tissue sarcomas: a matter of presentation. Int J Radiat Oncol Biol Phys 1998;42:563-572.
78. Kennedy AP Jr, Cameron B, Dorion RP, McGill C: Pediatric intestinal leiomyosarcomas: case report and review of the literature. J Pediatr Surg 1997;32:1234-1236.
79. Freitas AB, Aguiar PH, Miura FK, et al: Malignant ectomesenchymoma. Case report and review of the literature. Pediatr Neurosurg 1999;30:320-330.
80. Rivera-Luna R, De Leon-Bojorge B, Ruano-Aguilar J, et al: Osteosarcoma in children under three years of age. Med Pediatr Oncol 2003;41:99-100.
81. Hoffer FA: Primary skeletal neoplasms: osteosarcoma and Ewing sarcoma. Top Magn Reson Imaging 2002;13:231-239.
82. Pierz KA, Womer RB, Dormans JP: Pediatric bone tumors: osteosarcoma, Ewing's sarcoma, and chondrosarcoma associated with multiple hereditary osteochondromatosis. J Pediatr Orthop 2001;21:412-418.
83. Gadwal SR, Gannon FH, Fanburg-Smith JC, et al: Primary osteosarcoma of the head and neck in pediatric patients: a clinicopathologic study of 22 cases with a review of the literature. Cancer 2001;91:598-605.
84. Meyers PA, Gorlick R: Osteosarcoma. Pediatr Clin North Am 1997;44:973-989.
85. Shamberger RC, Grier HE: Ewing's sarcoma/primitive neuroectodermal tumor of the chest wall. Semin Pediatr Surg 2001;10:153-160.
86. Rozeman LB, Hogendoorn PC, Bovee JV: Diagnosis and prognosis of chondrosarcoma of bone. Expert Rev Mol Diagn 2002;2:461-472.
87. Gadwal SR, Fanburg-Smith JC, Gannon FH, Thompson LD: Primary chondrosarcoma of the head and neck in pediatric patients: a clinicopathologic study of 14 cases with a review of the literature. Cancer 2000;88:2181-2188.
88. De Potter P: Current treatment of retinoblastoma. Curr Opin Ophthalmol 2002;13:331-336.
89. Singh AD, Shields CL, Shields JA: Prognostic factors in retinoblastoma. J Pediatr Ophthalmol Strabismus 2000;37:134-141, quiz 168-169.
90. Rogers DA, Rao BM, Bowman L, et al: Primary malignancy of the salivary gland in children. J Pediatr Surg 1994;29:44-47.
91. Skinner MA: Cancer of the thyroid gland in infants and children. Semin Pediatr Surg 2001;10:119-126.
92. McGregor LM, Rosoff PM: Follicle-derived thyroid cancer in young people: the Duke experience. Pediatr Hematol Oncol 2001;18:89-100.
93. Ben Arush MW, Stein ME, Perez Nahum M, et al: Pediatric thyroid carcinoma: 22 years of experience at the Northern Israel Oncology Center (1973-1995). Pediatr Hematol Oncol 2000;17:85-92.
94. Hung W: Solitary thyroid nodules in 93 children and adolescents: a 35-year experience. Horm Res 1999;52:15-18.
95. Murphy JJ, Morzaria S, Gow KW, Magee JF: Breast cancer in a 6-year old child. J Pediatr Surg 2000;35:765-767.
96. Ciftci AO, Tanyel FC, Buyukpamukcu N, Hicsonmez A: Female breast masses during childhood: a 25-year review. Eur J Pediatr Surg 1998;8:67-70.
97. Rogers DA, Lobe TE, Rao BN, et al: Breast malignancy in children. J Pediatr Surg 1994;29:48-51.
98. Rosen PP, Kimmel M: Juvenile papillomatosis of the breast. Am J Surg Pathol 1990;93:599-603.

CHAPTER 106

Vascular Anomalies

JENNIFER J. MARLER, MD ✦ JOHN B. MULLIKEN, MD

NOMENCLATURE AND NOSOLOGY

The study of vascular anomalies is a rapidly evolving multidisciplinary field that incorporates several surgical and medical specialties. Because these disorders usually involve the skin, the largest organ of the body, the initial consultation is often with a plastic surgeon (or a pediatric dermatologist).

The greatest impediment to development of this field has been a lack of standardized terminology. For centuries, it was believed that vascular birthmarks were imprinted on the unborn child by a mother's emotions or diet. This doctrine of maternal impressions was reflected in words for brightly colored foods applied to vascular anomalies. Adjectives such as "cherry," "strawberry," and "port-wine" have their roots in this folklore.[1] Physicians usually preferred the Latin term *naevus maternus* for vascular birthmarks.

In the middle of the 19th century, the first attempt was made to categorize vascular anomalies histologically by Virchow, the father of cellular pathology. He called them angioma simplex, angioma cavernosum, and angioma racemosum.[2] His student, Wegener, developed a comparable histomorphic subcategorization for "lymphangioma."[3] This nomenclature persisted well into the 20th century. The same word was often applied to entirely different vascular anomalies. Virchow's angioma simplex became synonymous with capillary or strawberry hemangioma. Angioma cavernosum was used indiscriminately for subcutaneous hemangiomas (that regress) and venous malformations (that never regress). Angioma racemosum was modified to racemose (cirsoid) aneurysm or arteriovenous hemangioma, referring to an arteriovenous

malformation, a vascular lesion that expands over time. This confusing nosology has been responsible for improper diagnosis, illogical treatment, and misdirected research.

A biologic classification system, introduced in 1982,[4] dispersed most of the terminologic confusion that obscured the field of vascular anomalies. This scheme evolved from studies that correlated physical findings, natural history, and cellular features.[4] The key to this biologic classification is proper use of the Greek nominative suffix -oma. Once meaning "swelling" or "tumor," -oma in modern times denotes a lesion caused by up-regulated cellular growth. There are two major categories of vascular anomalies, tumors and malformations. Vascular tumors are endothelial neoplasms characterized by increased endothelial turnover. Hemangioma is the most common, a tumor that arises almost exclusively in infants. Other tumors are the hemangioendotheliomas, tufted angioma, hemangiopericytomas, and other rare vascular neoplasms including angiosarcoma. Vascular malformations are the result of abnormal development of vascular elements during embryogenesis and fetal maturation. These may be single-vessel forms (capillary, arterial, lymphatic, or venous) or combined. Unperturbed vascular malformations do not demonstrate increased endothelial turnover. They are designated according to the predominant channel type as capillary malformation, lymphatic malformation, venous malformation, arteriovenous malformation, and complex forms such as capillary-lymphatic-venous malformation. Malformations with an arterial component are rheologically fast flow; the remainder are slow flow in nature.

This biologic classification was accepted at the biennial meeting of the International Society for Vascular

Anomalies in Rome.[5] Differences that distinguish between hemangiomas and vascular malformations have been extended to include radiologic criteria[6-10] and immunohistochemical markers.[11,12] Apparent exceptions to this bipartite system do exist. For example, in rare instances, the shunting of blood by feeding and draining vessels in a large hemangioma can simulate an arteriovenous malformation. Vascular malformations, although fundamentally structural disorders, can exhibit endothelial hyperplasia, possibly triggered by clotting, ischemia, embolization, partial resection, or hormonal influences. Pyogenic granuloma, a tiny acquired vascular tumor, frequently appears in the dermis along with a capillary malformation. Rarely, vascular tumors and vascular malformations can coexist. For example, hemangiomas are common and can occur in a child with a malformation; in the overwhelming number of cases, this association is coincidental. However, these are rare instances of a true pathogenic association of midline hemangioma and structural anomalies.

History and physical examination give a diagnostic accuracy of more than 90% in distinguishing between vascular tumors and vascular malformations.[13] The most likely error in assigning a clinical diagnosis continues to be an inaccurate, imprecise use of terminology. Perhaps the most egregious example is "hemangioma," so often applied generically and indiscriminately to vascular lesions that are entirely different in histology and behavior. "Cavernous hemangioma" is another confusing term; there is no such entity—the lesion is either a deep hemangioma or a venous malformation.

The terms *congenital* and *acquired* should be used with caution in describing vascular anomalies. Hemangioma can be nascent or fully grown in a neonate. Therefore, the word "congenital" should be restricted to vascular lesions that are present and fully expressed at birth. Vascular malformations, although present at birth at a cellular level, may not manifest until childhood or in adult life. "Acquired," a term often used for cutaneous lesions that appear after 1 year of life, is inappropriate for a vascular anomaly that is present but not clinically apparent at birth.

VASCULAR TUMORS

Hemangioma

PATHOGENESIS

Hemangiomas are endothelial tumors with a biologic behavior that is unique in the realm of neoplasia; that is, they grow rapidly, slowly regress, and never recur. They are "angiogenesis dependent," as are all tumors, relying on the recruitment of new blood vessels for their growth.[14] As with other forms of pathologic angiogenesis, control mechanisms governing blood vessel

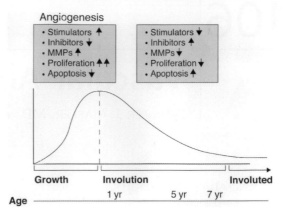

FIGURE 106-1. Life cycle of hemangioma. In the proliferative phase (0 to 1 year), there is increased endothelial turnover, production of angiogenesis stimulators, and levels of remodeling enzymes, such as matrix metalloproteinases (MMPs), necessary for angiogenesis; angiogenesis inhibitors are down-regulated. During the involuting phase (0 to 7 years), there is increased endothelial apoptosis and production of angiogenesis inhibitors; expression of angiogenesis stimulators and remodeling enzymes decreases.

growth are lost. Conceptually, hemangiogenesis could involve either an up-regulation of angiogenic factors or down-regulation of natural inhibitors.

There are three stages in the life cycle of a hemangioma, each characterized by a unique constellation of biologic markers and processes: the proliferating phase (0 to 1 year of age), the involuting phase (1 to 5 years of age), and the involuted phase (after 5 years of age) (Fig. 106-1). These stages are usually clinically apparent and can be documented by light microscopy and immunohistochemistry.[11]

Proliferating Phase

An immature hemangioma is composed of plump, rapidly dividing endothelial cells that form tightly packed sinusoidal channels. Even at this early stage, the endothelial cells express phenotypic markers of mature endothelium, such as CD31, factor VIII-related antigen (von Willebrand factor), *Ulex europaeus* lectin I, and VE-cadherin (an interendothelial adhesion molecule).[11,15,16] Features of activated endothelium, such as up-regulation of the endothelium-specific leukocyte adhesion molecule E-selectin, can be demonstrated.[16] Two known potent angiogenic peptides, vascular endothelial growth factor (VEGF) and basic fibroblast growth factor (bFGF), increase during proliferation.[11,17] Urinary bFGF levels are usually high in infants with proliferating hemangiomas and diminish to normal levels during regression.[18] Other molecules up-regulated during this phase include enzymes involved in extracellular remodeling (type IV collagenase, urokinase, and proteases), monocyte chemoattractant protein, and vitronectin (deposited in the subendothelial space during proliferation).[11,19-22] Other molecules, such as interferon-ß in the epidermis overlying the hemangioma, are down-regulated.[23]

Endothelial cells derived from proliferating-phase hemangioma form vascular channels in tissue culture.[24] Cultured stromal cells extracted from proliferative hemangiomas release a mitogen indistinguishable from VEGF that may function as a paracrine stimulator of endothelium.[25]

Involuting Phase

The hallmarks of regression are decreasing endothelial proliferation, increasing apoptosis, and the beginning of fibrofatty replacement of the hemangioma. By light microscopy, involution is characterized by dilatation of vascular lumens, flattening of endothelial cells, and progressive deposition of perivascular and interlobular or intralobular fibrous tissue to establish a lobular architecture. Smooth muscle actin staining is increased during this phase.[11] Stromal cells (including mast cells, fibroblasts, and macrophages) become more obvious during involution, and there is ultrastructural evidence for paracrine signaling between these cell types.[22,26] It is likely that these cellular events are secondary, initiated as a response to the upsurge of endothelial turnover.

There is evidence for increased expression of native antiangiogenic molecules during regression. Tissue inhibitor of metalloproteinase, a protein that suppresses formation of new blood vessels, is present.[11] Mast cells appear and may secrete modulators that down-regulate endothelial turnover.[11,27] The hyperplastic epidermis overlying the hemangioma begins to produce increasing amounts of interferon-ß,[23] believed to play a role in involution.

The increased proliferation seen in the proliferative phase slows dramatically during the involuting phase. Apoptosis gradually increases, beginning before 1 year of age and peaking at 2 years.[28] The net result is loss of volume of the tumor and increasing softness of the overlying skin.

Involuted Phase

After regression is complete, all that remains are a few tiny capillary-like feeding vessels and draining veins (some of which can be abnormally large) surrounded by islands of fibrofatty tissue admixed with dense collagen and reticular fibers. The endothelium lining these vessels is flat and mature. Multilaminated basement membranes, an ultrastructural hallmark of the proliferating phase, persist around the residual tiny capillary-sized vessels.[26,29]

The biologic switch that initiates the growth of hemangioma and the origin of the endothelial cells in these tumors remain unknown. Our understanding of these has been hampered by the lack of an animal model of the common, spontaneously regressing hemangioma

of infancy. Some authors have proposed a fetal or placental derivation for the tumor. The cellular morphology and protein expression of neonatal hemangioma endothelial cells are more characteristic of embryonic than of neonatal microvascular endothelial cells.[30] Other possible causes of hemangioma are viral and genetic.

Parapox infection in humans causes proliferation of endothelial cells and dilatation of cutaneous blood vessels.[31] The human herpes virus 8, the common agent in Kaposi sarcoma, is not found in hemangiomas.[32] A similar orf virus, avian hemangioma virus, has been identified in spontaneous "hemangioma-like" lesions in hens.[33] Vascular tumors have been induced in laboratory mice and rats with polyoma middle T antigen and polyoma virus.[34,35] Unlike hemangiomas, these vascular tumors exhibit malignant growth, do not regress spontaneously, and cause premature death of the animal. There is a transplantable murine hemangioendothelioma cell line that is associated with thrombocytopenia and anemia.[36] Because this tumor appears to simulate Kasabach-Merritt phenomenon, it has been used to test angiogenic inhibitors,[37] gene gun therapy,[38] and agents that stimulate platelet production.[39]

It is more likely that hemangiogenesis involves a genetic alteration. There is no strong evidence for mendelian inheritance in a study of monozygotic versus dizygotic twins.[40] On occasion, siblings are affected, usually in fair-skinned families with a predisposition to female offspring. There are rare kindreds that suggest familial transmission of hemangiomas in an autosomal dominant pattern with incomplete penetrance and variable expressivity.[41] The lesions in these families are indistinguishable from common "sporadic" hemangioma. In some pedigrees, there appears to be coexistence of hemangioma and vascular malformation in different members of the same family as well as in the same individual. A putative locus has been identified on 5q in three such families.[42]

Another genetic hypothesis imputes a somatic mutation, the local loss or gain of genetic material during fetal development that produces an altered cell line stimulated by autocrine or paracrine signaling. Endothelial cell cultures from proliferative hemangiomas are clonal, and they grow more rapidly than cell cultures of control endothelium.[43] Therefore, it is possible that hemangioma begins as an intrinsic (genetic) alteration in an endothelial cell or progenitor line rather than as an up-regulation by an external stimulus or down-regulation by a local antiangiogenic factor.

CLINICAL FEATURES

Hemangioma is the most common tumor of infancy and childhood, occurring in 4% to 10% of white infants.[44] These lesions are three to five times more common in girls than in boys; an even higher female preponderance is noted in hemangiomas that are problematic or associated with structural abnormalities.[45-48] There is an increased frequency of hemangiomas in premature infants, with a reported incidence of 23% in neonates who weigh less than 1200 g.[49] Hemangiomas are unusual in dark-skinned infants.

Hemangiomas occur most often in the craniofacial region (60%), followed by the trunk (25%) and extremities (15%).[13] Eighty percent of cutaneous hemangiomas are single; 20% are multiple. Multiple cutaneous lesions are often associated with tumors in other organ systems, particularly the liver. Less commonly, extracutaneous hemangiomas arise in the absence of cutaneous tumors.

Hemangiomas generally manifest at approximately 2 weeks after birth. Their appearance is heralded, in 30% to 50% of infants, by a premonitory cutaneous mark that may resemble a pale spot, a telangiectatic or macular red stain, or a bruise-like pseudoecchymotic patch. However, there is wide variability in this timing. Deep or subcutaneous lesions, such as in the parotid or posterior thorax, may not be noted until the infant is several months of age.

The presentation of hemangiomas is variable in size, extent, and morphology (Fig. 106-2). If the superficial dermis is involved, the skin becomes raised, firm, and bosselated with a vivid crimson color. If the hemangioma is confined to the lower dermis, subcutis, or muscle, the overlying skin may be only slightly raised and warm and have a bluish hue. All of these structures may be involved with a superficial raised component overlying a deeper tumor. Hemangioma in an extremity often presents a telangiectatic appearance. The adjectives "cavernous" and "capillary," previously applied to deep and superficial hemangiomas, respectively, are confusing and inaccurate and should be discarded.[1,4]

The three stages of histologic appearance of this tumor correlate with its clinical course (Figs. 106-3 and 106-4).[4]

Proliferating Phase

Hemangiomas grow rapidly during the first 6 to 8 months of life. Frequent observation is needed to document the growth pattern. There are few indicators that predict the eventual volume of a particular hemangioma or that precisely forecast the onset and outcome of involution. Typically, hemangiomas begin to plateau in growth by 10 to 12 months, although some do so earlier and some do so later.

Involuting Phase

After 1 year of age, the growth of the hemangioma slows and for a time is proportionate to that of the child.

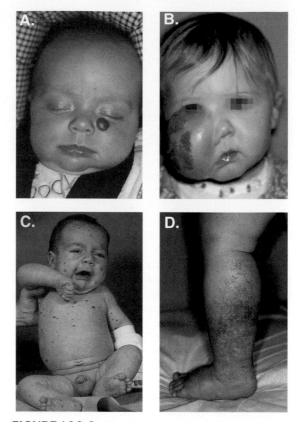

FIGURE 106-2. Morphologic variation of hemangioma. *A,* Localized tumor involving the superficial dermis ("strawberry-like"). *B,* Deep and superficial tumor obstructing the visual axis. *C,* Multiple tiny cutaneous tumors with visceral involvement. *D,* Telangiectatic hemangioma of lateral calf.

The telltale signs of regression appear. The bright crimson color fades to a dull purplish hue. The skin begins to pale, typically beginning at the center of the lesion, and a patchy grayish discoloration arises. The hemangioma is less turgid on palpation.

The involuting phase extends from 1 year until 5 to 7 years of age. The rate of regression is unrelated to the appearance, depth, gender, site, or size of the hemangioma.[13] Typically, the last vestiges of color disappear by 5 to 7 years of age. Involution is complete in 50% of children by 5 years of age and in 70% of children by 7 years, with continued gradual improvement until 10 to 12 years.[50]

Involuted Phase

Nearly normal skin is restored in approximately 50% of children with hemangioma. The involved skin may have telangiectasias and a crepe-like laxity (anetoderma) secondary to destruction of elastic fibers. Yellow discoloration or scarred patches persist if ulceration occurred during the proliferating phase. If

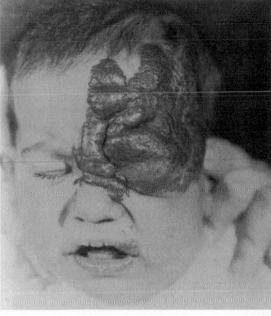

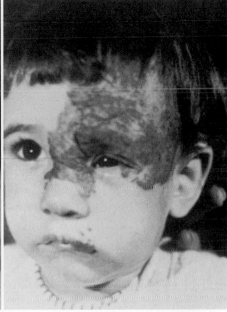

A   B

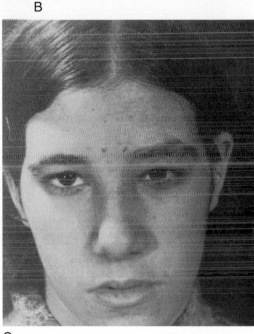

FIGURE 106-3. Involution of a superficial hemangioma. *A,* A newborn with an extensive hemangioma of the face. *B,* At age 4 years, the hemangioma is in its involuting phase. *C,* At age 14 years, involution is complete. There is expansion of the eyebrow; skin texture is excellent. (From Mulliken JB, Young AE: Vascular Birthmarks: Hemangiomas and Malformations. Philadelphia, WB Saunders, 1988.)

C

the tumor was once large and protuberant, there is often a fibrofatty residuum and redundant skin. Hemangioma of the scalp or eyebrow often destroys hair follicles.

Even extensive and bulky subcutaneous hemangiomas can regress totally, whereas a flat, superficial hemangioma can irreversibly alter the cutaneous texture, resulting in an atrophic patch. This variable outcome renders prognostication in infancy difficult.

Hemangiomas rarely cause major skeletal distortion or hypertrophy.[51] A large facial hemangioma can, however, be associated with minor cartilage or bone overgrowth, presumably secondary to increased blood flow. Hemangioma can also produce a mass effect on the local facial skeleton, the nose, an ear, or the jaw. Even extensive hemangiomas of the extremities have not been documented to cause circumferential or longitudinal overgrowth.

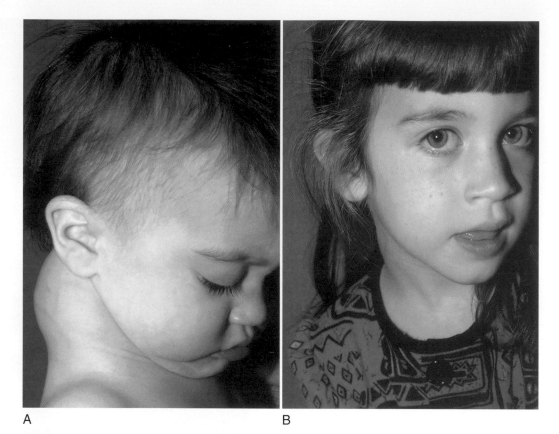

A   B

FIGURE 106-4. Involution of deep hemangioma. *A,* Posterior cervical tumor. *B,* Nearly complete regression at age 4 years.

There are at least two subsets of hemangioma that demonstrate patterns of histologic and biologic behavior unlike that of typical infantile hemangioma (Fig. 106-5). Both are called congenital hemangiomas, meaning that they develop during prenatal life and are fully developed at birth.

One type of congenital hemangioma involutes rapidly during the first few weeks or months of life.[52] These tumors are often raised with a characteristic red-violaceous color and coarse telangiectasias, often with a peripheral pale halo or central pallor. There is often superficial ulceration and, occasionally, signs of rapid arteriovenous shunting that can simulate an arteriovenous malformation, both clinically and radiologically. Their distribution more commonly involves the trunk and extremities. RICH (rapidly involuting congenital hemangioma) is the term that has been proposed for this curious type of neonatal vascular tumor.

A second, less common type of congenital hemangioma persists into late childhood. These lesions are typically ovoid, macular or slightly raised, pale gray with prominent telangiectasias, and warm to palpation. NICH (noninvoluting congenital hemangioma)

is the term that has been proposed for this type of hemangioma.[53]

Hemangiomatosis: Cutaneous and Visceral

Multiple hemangiomas in a single patient have been called disseminated hemangiomatosis, suggesting metastases from a primary tumor (not proved). In these infants, the cutaneous lesions are usually tiny (<5 mm in diameter), firm, and dome-like. Any infant with five or more cutaneous tumors should be suspected of harboring visceral hemangiomas (most commonly in the liver, followed by the brain, gastrointestinal tract, and lung) and screened by ultrasonography or magnetic resonance imaging (MRI), as indicated.

Intrahepatic hemangiomas are more common in female babies. They range from tiny asymptomatic tumors discovered incidentally to large single or multiple lesions with or without cardiac consequences. Two clinical patterns occur. In the first and most common, infants present with congestive heart failure, hepatomegaly, and anemia 1 to 16 weeks after birth.[54] A systolic bruit may be heard over the liver, reflecting the intrahepatic shunting of blood. The diagnosis of intrahepatic arteriovenous malformation must be

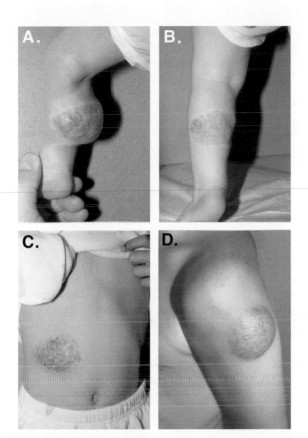

FIGURE 106-5. Two types of congenital hemangioma. *A* and *B,* Rapidly involuting congenital hemangioma of posterior calf demonstrating accelerated regression during a 6-week period. *C* and *D,* Noninvoluting congenital hemangioma on abdomen of a 7-year-old girl and arm of an 8-year-old boy, both unchanged since birth.

excluded in these patients with ultrasonography, MRI, or angiography by an experienced radiologist.

In the second and less common setting, infants present with massive enlargement and jaundice in the absence of significant shunting. These patients develop respiratory failure secondary to upward displacement of the diaphragm and, occasionally, renal failure as a result of impaired vena cava blood return due to increased intra-abdominal pressure (abdominal compartment syndrome).

The mortality rate for hepatic hemangiomas is high—30% to 80%.[55,56] In a series of 43 children with hepatic vascular anomalies treated at our institution during the last 25 years, 90% of these were hemangiomas and 10% were arteriovenous malformations.[54] Malignant neoplasia must be considered in the differential diagnosis of any infant with a hypervascular hepatic lesion, such as hepatoblastoma or metastatic neuroblastoma. An accurate diagnosis is generally possible on the basis of clinical examination and imaging without recourse to biopsy.

Intracranial hemangioma is unusual, unless there are multiple cutaneous and hepatic lesions. These are generally small dural or pial-based hemangiomas, although larger tumors do occur and can cause obstructive hydrocephalus or other neurologic consequences.

DIFFERENTIAL DIAGNOSIS

Two maxims must be remembered in the differential diagnosis of a cutaneous vascular lesion in infancy: not all hemangiomas look like strawberries, and not all strawberries are hemangiomas.[1,57]

Hemangiomas are frequently misdiagnosed (Fig. 106-6). Deep hemangioma, particularly in the cervical or trunk regions, can be mistaken for lymphatic or venous malformation. A macular hemangioma can imitate a capillary malformation (or "port-wine stain"); on the extremity, it can simulate cutis marmorata telangiectasia congenita. Another rare cutaneous variant of hemangioma exhibits persistent fast flow (shunting), leading to confusion with arteriovenous malformation. This variant has a predilection for the extremities and can cause complications, including ulceration, bleeding, thrombosis, and high-output cardiac failure, necessitating embolization and surgical intervention.[57]

Other infantile vascular tumors can be misdiagnosed as hemangioma; these include hemangioendothelioma,[58] tufted angioma,[59] hemangiopericytoma,[60] and fibrosarcoma.[61] If there is any question about the clinical diagnosis, radiologic examination is mandated. Biopsy is indicated if there is any suspicion of malignancy by history, physical examination, or radiologic imaging. Staining for GLUT-1, an erythrocyte-type glucose transporter protein specific for hemangiomas, may be helpful in distinguishing between hemangioma, other tumors, and vascular malformations.[12] Whereas typical infantile hemangiomas demonstrate positive immunohistochemical staining, other infantile vascular tumors do not. Of note, GLUT-1 is negative in the two forms of congenital hemangioma, rapidly involuting and noninvoluting.

ASSOCIATED STRUCTURAL ANOMALIES

Hemangiomas are not usually considered to be part of any recognized syndromes.[62] Moreover, because they are so common, hemangiomas occasionally coexist with but are not necessarily associated with a dysmorphic syndrome. To be designated "associated" with another defect, an abnormality must occur with a frequency of greater than 10%.

However, there are uncommon examples in which hemangiomas do occur in association with malformations, although these abnormalities are not usually of vascular origin (Fig. 106-7). In these instances, the

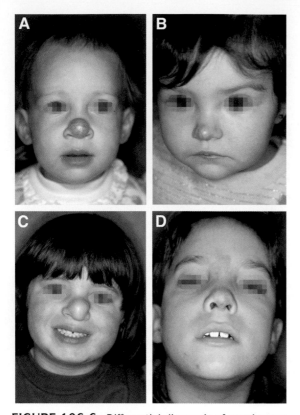

FIGURE 106-6. Differential diagnosis of nasal vascular anomalies. *A,* Hemangioma. *B,* Venous malformation. *C,* Lymphatic malformation. *D,* Arteriovenous malformation. (From Marler JJ, Mulliken JB: Vascular anomalies: classification, diagnosis, and natural history. Facial Plast Surg Clin North Am 2001;9:496.)

female preponderance is even more striking.[46] Associative structural anomalies are most frequently seen with extensive midline hemangioma. Reported ocular associations include microphthalmia, increased retinal vascularity, congenital cataract, and optic nerve hypoplasia.[63] There may be persistent embryonic intracranial and extracranial arteries, hypoplasia or absence of the ipsilateral carotid or vertebral vessels,[64] aneurysmal dilatation of the carotid artery,[65] coarctation and right-sided aortic arch,[66-68] or dilatation of the carotid siphon. Cerebrovascular occlusive disease can develop in these infants.[65] Dandy-Walker malformation or other cystic malformations of the posterior fossa can occur.[63,69] Sternal clefting or a supraumbilical raphe may be seen in association with extensive facial and cervicothoracic hemangiomas.[46]

Lumbosacral hemangioma is one of several ectodermal lesions known to signal underlying occult spinal dysraphism, which includes lipomeningocele, tethered spinal cord, and diastematomyelia.[70,71] A curious "fawn tail" (acrochordon) can be found in the center of a lumbar hemangioma. Ultrasonography is used to screen infants younger than 4 months for occult spinal dysraphism. MRI is generally necessary to identify spinal cord abnormalities. We have encountered hemangioma in the dural (thecal) lining of the spinal cord.

There are rare instances in which pelvic or perineal hemangiomas may be associated with urogenital and anorectal anomalies, such as anterior or vestibular anus, hemiclitoris, atrophic or absent labia minora, and hypospadias.[70,72]

RADIOLOGIC FEATURES

Ultrasonography

The hallmarks of a proliferating hemangioma are localized, dense parenchyma and fast flow. Hemangiomas show decreased arterial resistance, increased venous velocity, and a discrete soft tissue mass.[73,74] Ultrasonography is useful in differentiating a deep hemangioma from a lymphatic or venous malformation, but even an experienced ultrasonographer may have

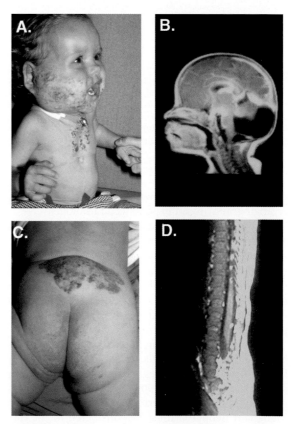

FIGURE 106-7. Structural anomalies associated with hemangioma. *A,* Sternal cleft with cervicofacial hemangioma necessitating tracheostomy. *B,* Sagittal MRI of posterior fossa cyst (Dandy-Walker anomaly). *C* and *D,* Lumbosacral hemangioma overlying tethered cord, depicted by MRI.

difficulty distinguishing a proliferating hemangioma from an arteriovenous malformation because both are fast flow. Sonography is useful for documenting the response of hemangiomas to pharmacologic therapy, particularly following the change in intrahepatic hemangiomas.

MRI

On MRI, hemangiomas appear to be a parenchymatous (solid) tissue of intermediate density on T1-weighted spin echo images and moderate hyperintensity on T2-weighted spin echo images (Fig. 106-8). Flow voids, prominent within and around the tumor, are indicative of rapid flow (shunting) between feeding arteries and dilated draining veins.[7,75] Gradient-recalled echo sequences confirm the presence of fast-flow vessels.

Intracranial hemangiomas are more commonly detected with more frequent use of MRI. These are usually located on the dura, but choroidal and intraparenchymal tumors can also occur. Hemangioma in the involuting phase exhibits progressively less flow with decreasing size and number of feeding and draining vessels. Lobularity becomes more obvious, and fatty tissue can be a prominent feature. Involuted cutaneous hemangioma may appear as an avascular fatty mass.

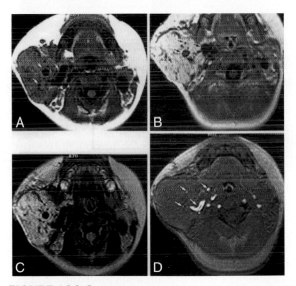

FIGURE 106-8. MRI imaging of hemangioma. *A,* Axial T1-weighted image demonstrates flow voids *(arrows),* indicating dilated feeding and draining vessels. *B,* T1-weighted image after intravenous administration of gadolinium shows uniform contrast enhancement. *C,* T2-weighted sequence, also with uniform signal enhancement. *D,* Gradient-recalled echo sequence confirms the presence of enlarged feeding and draining vessels. (From Burrows PE, Laor T, Paltiel H, Robertson RL: Diagnostic imaging in the evaluation of vascular birthmarks in pediatric dermatology. Dermatol Clin 1998;16:460.)

Nuclear Scanning

Radionuclide scanning, with technetium Tc 99m-tagged red blood cells, can be used to document deep multiple hemangiomas in the gastrointestinal tract or central nervous system.

MANAGEMENT

Observation

Most hemangiomas are small and harmless tumors, and they should be allowed to undergo proliferation and involution under careful monitoring by a pediatrician. Such lesions will leave normal or slightly blemished skin. Parents should be reassured and educated about the natural course of these banal tumors.

An infant with hemangioma is usually referred to a vascular anomalies specialist by a pediatrician or pediatric dermatologist because of the hemangioma's large size, rapid growth, dangerous location, or potential for other complications. The consultant must recognize and address the parents' concerns about the enlarging tumor on their infant. Parental reactions of disbelief, fear, and mourning are common and similar in intensity to parental reactions to permanent malformations.[76] Even if the proper decision is not to intervene, this does not mean that nothing should be done. The parents must be given a thorough explanation of the natural history of the particular hemangioma. It is helpful to show photographs to illustrate the expected progression and result of regression. It is also important for photographs to be taken at initial consultation and during the evolution of the hemangioma. Parents often choose to do their own serial photography, and these pictures frequently compose a personal album that documents the child's improvement. Parents may ask to meet other families who have children with similar conditions.

Facial hemangiomas, regardless of size, typically cause the most distress to caretakers. Parents relate their experiences of how strangers (and occasionally even well-intentioned relatives) have made rude, unsolicited comments. Parental responses are variable. These episodes can lead to social isolation of the infant in an attempt to protect the child from unpleasant comments or stares.

Unfortunately, there are few prognostic indicators, and the consultant must rely on experience.[77] Frequent visits and re-evaluation of the hemangioma are usually necessary, particularly if the tumor is potentially problematic. It is important to establish a supportive relationship with the infant's parents, to be available for their questions as they arise, and to gain their confidence. This helps sustain their hope that their baby will, indeed, get better. Desperate parents often consult the Internet for medical assistance, deriving information that is anecdotal, neither edited nor peer reviewed, and of variable accuracy.

When to Intervene

The hemangiomatous spectrum ranges from small tumors that regress fully without sequelae and require no treatment to endangering tumors that require therapy because of serious complications. In the middle of the spectrum are the nonproblematic hemangiomas that often stimulate debate about whether to treat or not. Specialists differ on the indications for intervention for such hemangiomas.

Local Treatment for Ulceration or Bleeding

Spontaneous epithelial breakdown, crusting, ulceration, and necrosis occur in 5% of cutaneous hemangiomas.[78] Ulceration can arise at any anatomic site but is most common in lesions involving the lips, perineum, anogenital area, and extremities (Fig. 106-9). Pain causes the infant to be irritable, to feed inadequately, and to sleep poorly. Ulcerated sites may become secondarily infected, leading to cellulitis, septicemia, and in some instances death.[79]

Cleaning along with a daily application of hydrated petrolatum or a topical antibiotic is useful for small or superficial ulcerations. Topical viscous lidocaine may be applied intermittently to relieve pain. If there is an eschar on the surface of the hemangioma, sharp débridement to healthy underlying tissue is indicated. This should be followed by wet-to-dry dressings to stimulate granulation tissue or, alternatively, hydrocolloid dressings. Dressings are often difficult to secure in locations where ulceration is common.

Superficial ulceration usually heals within days to weeks, whereas deep ulceration can take weeks to heal. Pharmacologic treatment with corticosteroid can accelerate healing and minimize recurrence. Flashlamp pulsed dye laser (two applications, 4 to 6 weeks apart) is also reported to alleviate pain and to aid healing.[80,81] If possible, total resection of an ulcerated hemangioma is the most expeditious treatment. Excision should be considered if primary closure is possible and if the resulting scar would be predictably the same after surgical removal of the regressed hemangioma later in childhood. Resection in infancy is most often indicated for ulcerated tumors of the scalp, chest, or extremity and rarely for facial lesions. After involution of hemangioma, scarring is predictably worse in areas of ulceration compared with previously nonulcerated areas (see Fig. 106-9).

Punctate bleeding from a bosselated hemangioma is a rare complication that can be frightening to parents. They should be instructed to compress the bleeding area with a clean pad, holding pressure for 10 minutes by the clock. In rare instances, a suture is needed to control a local bleeding site.

Pharmacologic Therapy for Complications

The precise frequency of endangering and life-threatening complications caused by hemangiomas is

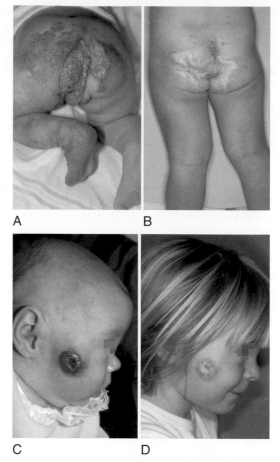

FIGURE 106-9. Ulcerated hemangioma. *A,* Tumor of extremity and buttocks that healed with dressings. *B,* Scarring in involuting phase, patient at age 5 years. *C,* Ulcerated cheek lesion. *D,* Scarring at site 4 years later.

unknown; it has been estimated to be 10%.[47] Complications include destruction, distortion, and obstruction; these occur principally in the cervicofacial region. The complication rate is unrelated to the size of the hemangioma; even small hemangiomas can obstruct a vital structure, such as the eye or subglottis.

Ulceration can destroy part of an eyelid, ear, nose, or lip. Periorbital hemangioma can block the visual axis, causing deprivation amblyopia, or extend into the retrobulbar space, leading to ocular proptosis. More commonly, a small hemangioma involving the upper eyelid or supraorbital area can distort the growing cornea, producing astigmatic amblyopia. Any infant with a periorbital hemangioma should be examined promptly by a pediatric ophthalmologist.

Subglottic hemangioma is a common life-threatening lesion. The symptoms are typically hoarseness and, later, biphasic stridor, generally manifesting between birth and 12 weeks of age. Approximately 50% of these infants have a cutaneous cervical hemangioma, often in the "beard distribution."[82] Evaluation of an infant with a cervicofacial hemangioma should include assessment of the airway. If pharmacologic therapy fails, tracheostomy may be necessary to maintain the airway.[83]

Hemangiomas can also produce cardiovascular complications. High-output congestive heart failure is potentially life-threatening and usually caused by a hepatic hemangioma, although a large cutaneous hemangioma can also divert blood flow. Gastrointestinal tumors can be single, multifocal, or diffuse, carpeting the bowel and mesentery. Bleeding from single and multiple mucosal lesions is generally responsive to pharmacologic treatment or locally invasive measures, either endoscopic or surgical. However, diffuse infiltrative hemangioma of the bowel can cause life-threatening hemorrhage. Surgical resection is not possible in most instances. Management generally relies on repeated transfusion, parenteral nutrition, and antiangiogenic drug therapy to hasten involution. Caution in diagnosis is necessary. Vascular malformations of the gastrointestinal tract are more common than hemangiomas and do not respond to pharmacologic treatment.

INTRALESIONAL CORTICOSTEROID INJECTION. Intralesional injection of corticosteroid should be considered for a small, well-localized cutaneous hemangioma, typically for lesions on the nasal tip, cheek, lip, or eyelid. The rationale is to minimize cutaneous expansion and size of the tumor. Triamcinolone (25 mg/mL) is injected slowly at a low pressure with a 3-mL syringe and 25-gauge needle. The dosage is 3 to 5 mg/kg per injection. When possible, the periphery of the lesion should be compressed (by the ring of an instrument) to minimize the chances for embolization of the colloidal particles.

Overdosage can cause subcutaneous atrophy, but this is temporary. Three to five injections administered at 6- to 8-week intervals are usually needed. The response rate is similar to that for systemic corticosteroid.[84,85] Intralesional injection of corticosteroid can effectively stabilize a small ulcerated hemangioma with subsequent healing. Systemic corticosteroid should be given for a large ulcerated tumor.

Intralesional injection for periorbital hemangioma should be done cautiously. There are two reported cases of blindness, presumed to be due to embolic occlusion of the retinal artery,[86] in addition to a report of eyelid necrosis.[87] Potent topical corticosteroid resulted in improvement in one small series of patients with periocular lesions.[88]

SYSTEMIC CORTICOSTEROID THERAPY. Orally administered corticosteroid is the first-line treatment for problematic, endangering, or life-threatening hemangiomas. Prednisone or prednisolone is administered at 2 to 3 mg/kg per day, in the morning, for 2 weeks. An equivalent dose of intravenously administered corticosteroid can effect a rapid change in a sensitive tumor in an acute situation, such as a narrowed upper airway, occluded visual field, intestinal bleeding, or high-output cardiac failure. If there is a response, the dosage is tapered slowly, usually every 2 to 4 weeks, and the drug is terminated when the child is 10 to 11 months of age. There is sometimes minor rebound growth after corticosteroid is discontinued; this may warrant another 4 to 6 weeks of therapy. Rebound growth can happen if the dose is lowered too quickly or administered on alternate days. Live vaccines (such as polio, measles, mumps, rubella, and varicella) should be withheld during steroid treatment.

In the authors' practice, the sensitivity of hemangioma to steroids is as high as 90%, manifesting as stabilization of growth or accelerated regression (Fig. 106-10). Some investigators claim that results are improved by increasing the dosage to 5 mg/kg per day.[89-91] However, there are no prospective, controlled studies to support this protocol, and steroid complications are more likely at this dosage.[48]

Side effects can occur with corticosteroid. Cushingoid facies is expected and happens in virtually all

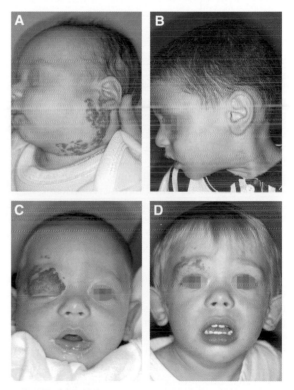

FIGURE 106-10. Corticosteroid treatment. *A,* Cheek lesion with superficial and deep components at age 1 month, before 7-month course of oral prednisolone. *C,* Hemangioma producing obstructive amblyopia at age 2 months, treated with an 18-month course of oral prednisolone. *B and D,* Patient at age 2 years.

infants. This subsides as the dose is tapered toward the end of therapy. Parents should be cautioned that some infants receiving corticosteroid therapy become irritable. Others develop gastrointestinal reflux and discomfort; this responds to orally administered histamine receptor blockers, such as omeprazole.

In a retrospective study of corticosteroid treatment of hemangiomas, 35% of infants exhibited a slowing in the rate of height gain and 25% had diminished weight gain. Approximately 15% of children had accelerated weight gain while receiving the therapy. However, all children returned to their pretreatment curves for height and weight by 14 to 24 months of age. There was no increased incidence of infection, hypertension, or bone resorption at a dose of 2 to 3 mg/kg per day. The only major complications encountered, steroid myopathy and infection, occurred in a few infants who were given a prolonged high dose (in the range of 5 mg/kg per day).[48]

INTERFERON ALFA. Recombinant interferon alfa, 2a or 2b, is considered the second-line drug for endangering hemangiomas.[18,92-98] Some investigators use this as a first-line therapy. However, in our experience, the side effects of interferon alfa are more serious than those of corticosteroids, and it should be reserved for hemangiomas that are recalcitrant to corticosteroid therapy.

Indications for interferon therapy include failure of response to corticosteroid, contraindications to prolonged systemic corticosteroid, complications of corticosteroid, and the rare instance of parental refusal to use corticosteroid. Interferon should be initiated and the corticosteroid rapidly tapered and stopped within a few weeks. There is no evidence that interferon and corticosteroid are synergistic, and therefore they are not coadministered.[99]

The rationale for interferon therapy is that it is antiangiogenic, among its numerous effects. Interferon decreases bFGF mRNA and total protein.[100,101] Increased levels of urinary bFGF are present in children with hemangiomas and other vascular tumors[18]; this decreases in response to interferon (or corticosteroid) therapy.[102]

The empiric dose for interferon is 2 to 3 million units/m^2, injected subcutaneously every day. The response is generally slower in comparison to the more dramatic effect frequently observed with corticosteroid. The absolute dose of interferon should be titrated upward as the infant gains weight, especially if there is rebound growth. However, the interferon dose often does not have to be adjusted as natural regression begins. Usually 6 to 12 months of interferon treatment is necessary. Interferon therapy is successful for more than 80% of hemangiomas, even for tumors that fail to respond to corticosteroid (Fig. 106-11).

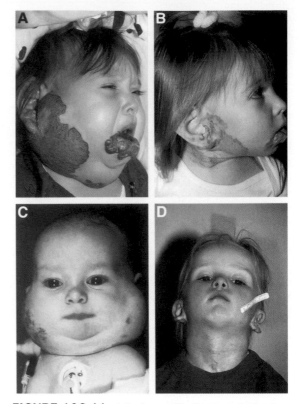

FIGURE 106-11. Interferon alfa therapy. *A,* Cervicofacial hemangioma refractory to corticosteroid treatment. *B,* After 10 months of interferon alfa. *C,* Cervicofacial and subglottic hemangioma unresponsive to corticosteroid in infant given a 10-month course of interferon alfa. *D,* Appearance at age 4 years.

Interferon typically causes a low-grade fever for the first 1 to 2 weeks. Pretreatment with acetaminophen or ibuprofen, 1 to 2 hours before injection, usually ameliorates this febrile reaction. Interferon causes several reversible toxicities, including an up to fivefold elevation of hepatic transaminases, transient neutropenia, and anemia.[98,103] Interferon does not need to be discontinued because of minor neutropenia or elevation of hepatic enzymes. Neutropenia at these doses is ascribed to margination of leukocytes, not to true bone marrow suppression, and it usually resolves. Infants receiving interferon grow and gain weight normally.

Spastic diplegia is the most serious possible toxicity of interferon therapy.[103,104] It has an estimated incidence of 5%, but in our experience, it is significantly higher, on the order of 20%. Infants who are younger than 6 months when interferon therapy is initiated are particularly vulnerable. All children who are treated with interferon should be observed by a neurologist, with an evaluation at the onset of therapy and periodic re-examination during the course of therapy. If long tract signs appear, interferon should be discontinued, or the dose should be lowered if the life-threatening condition caused by the hemangioma persists. In general, spastic diplegia improves after the termination of interferon therapy. The mechanism for this serious complication is unknown.

Other Therapies

Chemotherapy, specifically vincristine and cyclophosphamide, has been effective for life-threatening vascular tumors, including hemangioma. There is no role for irradiation in the management of cutaneous hemangiomas, and its value in managing intrahepatic hemangiomas is debatable.[105]

EMBOLIC THERAPY. Embolization is used for hemangiomas that cause severe congestive heart failure and do not respond promptly enough to drug therapy. Hepatic hemangiomas are the most common lesions that require embolization. Because of the variable angioarchitecture of these tumors, appropriate techniques and occlusive materials vary. The effectiveness of embolization in controlling congestive heart failure depends on the ability of the operator to occlude a large percentage of the shunts. Improvement in cardiac function is often transient. It is best to continue antiangiogenic therapy, even after an apparently successful embolization. Rarely, embolization of the feeding arteries is indicated in infants with complicated cutaneous or musculocutaneous vascular tumors, but the benefit is likely to be transient unless adjunctive pharmacotherapy or repeated embolization is used.

LASER THERAPY. Photocoagulation of hemangiomas has a popular appeal. Its role is a frequent subject of explanation to patients and discussion among physicians. Some investigators advocate prompt lasering of nascent hemangioma in the belief that this will prevent the growth of the tumor and its complications.[106] However, flashlamp pulsed dye laser (577 to 585 nm) penetrates only 0.75 to 1.2 mm into the dermis. Therefore, only the superficial portion of the hemangioma is affected, resulting in some lightening. However, superficial hemangiomas are the very tumors that do not cause problems and would be expected to regress in time, leaving nearly normal skin.[107] Most hemangiomas begin, ab initio, in or deep to the middle dermis. Furthermore, these tumors often arise in a field rather than in a tiny focus with centrifugal spread. As a result, most cutaneous hemangiomas are beyond the reach of the laser beam, even at their earliest manifestation. There is no evidence that even repeated laser application will diminish the bulk or accelerate involution of the deep portion of a hemangioma.[108,109] Furthermore, overzealous lasering can cause ulceration, partial-thickness skin loss, and consequent scarring. Hypopigmentation can also occur. There is no controversy about the usefulness of pulsed dye laser for telangiec-

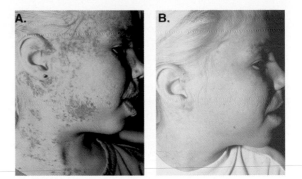

FIGURE 106-12. Laser therapy. *A,* Superficial hemangioma with telangiectasia. *B,* Appearance after five laser sessions.

tasias that often persist during and after involution (Fig. 106-12).

Continuous wave carbon dioxide laser is used for excision of subglottic hemangioma.[110] Another strategy is intralesional laser photocoagulation with a bare fiber (Nd:YAG) inserted through multiple needle passages into the tumor.[111,112] In experienced hands, intralesional laser photocoagulation can be effective, particularly if rapid shrinkage is needed, as for an obstructing tumor of the upper eyelid.[111,113] However, this technique carries a risk of thermal damage and ulceration.[114]

Operative Management

If every hemangioma began as a localized nest of cells, the ideal treatment would logically be prompt excision before the tumor extends into the surrounding dermis. However, there are two flaws with this logic and an additional practical problem. First, the hemangioma that is small when it is first seen is usually destined to remain diminutive. In this instance, excision may leave a more obvious scar than the skin changes that follow natural involution. Second, a particular hemangioma's size and distribution seem to be predetermined as a "field transformation" that may include skin, subcutaneous tissue, and muscle. Therefore, an extensive nascent lesion is out of the bounds of surgical excision at the outset. Finally, most infants do not come to medical attention until the hemangioma has reached a size at which resection would be disfiguring.

Most hemangiomas should be left alone, allowing proliferation and involution to run their course. Drug therapy is indicated for large, problematic, or endangering hemangiomas. Nevertheless, excision can be considered in each of the three stages of the hemangioma life cycle. The windows for surgical therapy are conveniently divided into the three phases that correlate with infancy, early childhood, and late childhood to early adolescence.

INFANCY (PROLIFERATIVE PHASE). There are relative indications for excision of hemangioma during the proliferative phase. These include obstruction, usually visual or subglottic; deformation, such as periorbital distortion with secondary astigmatic amblyopia; bleeding or ulceration unresponsive to topical or systemic therapy; and anticipated scar from ulceration that would be more pronounced than that after surgical resection.

An obstructive hemangioma of the upper eyelid or brow that does not respond to pharmacologic therapy can be either excised or debulked.[115,116] Other candidates for resection include well-localized or pedunculated lesions, particularly those that bleed or are ulcerated. Healing of a deep ulceration is often slow with use of topical therapy; the infant is in constant pain. An ulcerated hemangioma of the scalp usually results in alopecia. The scalp and thoracic skin are lax in an infant, facilitating excision and primary closure of an ulcerated tumor in these locations (Fig. 106-13).

EARLY CHILDHOOD (INVOLUTING PHASE). More commonly, staged or total excision of a large or protuberant involuting-phase hemangioma is undertaken during the preschool period (Fig. 106-14). Children at this age begin to become aware of their body (facial) differences. A child with an obvious hemangioma, albeit involuting, may develop low self-esteem. The surgical scar must be weighed against the child's (not the parents') emotional distress. Excision of a hemangioma in early childhood is indicated if it is obvious that resection is inevitable (e.g., a consequence of postulceration scarring, expanded and inelastic skin, and fibrofatty residuum), if the scar would be the same were excision postponed until the involuted phase, if the scar is easily hidden, or if staged excision or reconstruction is necessary.[117]

Every child's hemangioma presents a unique problem and deserves individual consideration. Conventional resection techniques do not always apply. Lenticular excision with linear closure is the traditional method for removal of a spheroidal lesion. Indeed, this is useful in several locations, such as transverse excision of a lesion in the labial mucosa or upper eyelid. Staged resection is often necessary, and ultimately, a lenticular excision must extend beyond the lesional border into normal skin to avoid formation of "dog-ears." Furthermore, lenticular excision with linear closure causes a central flattening that is particularly noticeable in a convex facial area, such as the cheek or forehead. To minimize the scar, circular excision and intradermal pursestring closure should be the first consideration. Circular excision can be done in stages, and lenticular excision is often chosen as the last procedure. The final scar will be markedly shorter than after single or staged lenticular excision.[118]

Hemangiomas in certain anatomic areas need special attention. These are discussed by region.

Forehead. Because the goal is the shortest possible transverse scar, circular excision with pursestring closure is often the best initial procedure. This will minimize distortion of the eyebrow. It is difficult to correct for expanded (or missing) hair follicles caused by the hemangioma.

Eyelid. A tarsal crease incision is generally best. Because there is often distortion in three dimensions, staged resection is often necessary to correct palpebral length, height, and ciliary margin and to adjust the levator aponeurosis.

Cheek. Circular excision with pursestring closure is usually preferred, often with a final lenticular excision of the scar in the axis of the relaxed cutaneous tension lines.

Lips. Inelastic skin, the result of hemangiomatous dermal proliferation, makes it difficult to correct labial form in both repose and animation. Hemangiomatous involvement often results in a bulky, fibrofatty vermilion-mucosa. Staged excisions and reconstruction generally give optimal results. Fusiform excision inside the vermilion-mucosal line or at the vermilion-cutaneous junction causes least obvious scarring. When needed, vertical scars on the upper lip are best placed on the philtral ridge or melolabial fold. Vertical scars on the lower lip should be avoided because extra skin and vermilion are needed for a full smile. Mucosal advancement may be needed if the lower labial vermilion is destroyed by scar.

Ear. Localized retroauricular hemangioma can cause a protruding ear, and this may be an indication for early excision to avoid a permanent auricular deformity. More diffuse auricular hemangiomas cause macrotia, usually best corrected by excision in the involuted phase. Auricular staged reconstruction is done if the auricle has been destroyed during the proliferating phase.

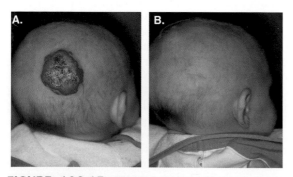

FIGURE 106-13. Surgical treatment. *A*, Ulcerated hemangioma of scalp that bled frequently. *B*, Six weeks after surgical excision.

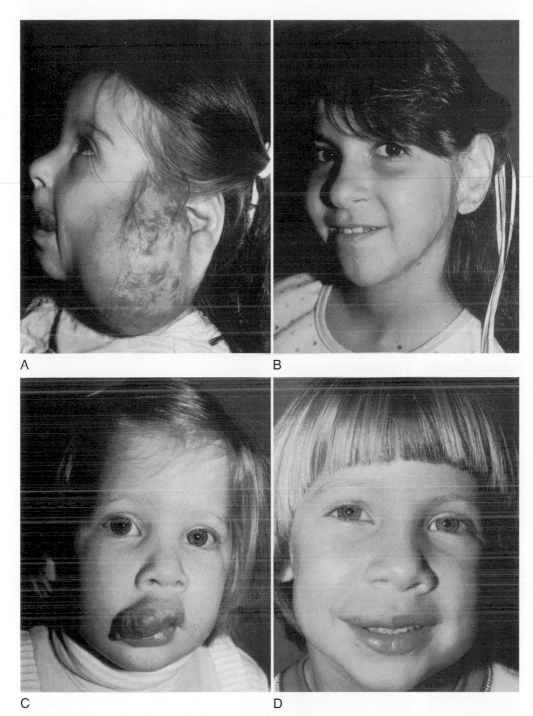

A

B

C

D

FIGURE 106-14. Operative therapy for hemangioma in early childhood. *A,* A large facial hemangioma in a 2$\frac{1}{2}$-year-old girl. *B,* Redundant skin and tumor were excised at age 4 years; dissection was performed superficial to the seventh cranial nerve. Appearance at age 10 years. Note the auricular enlargement, a rare example of skeletal hypertrophy secondary to a hemangioma. *C,* A 5-year-old girl with involuting-phase hemangioma of the lip. Even with complete regression, excess mucosa and submucosa remain. *D,* One year after contour excision. (From Mulliken JB, Young AE: Vascular Birthmarks: Hemangiomas and Malformations. Philadelphia, WB Saunders, 1988.)

Neck. Hemangioma grows in three dimensions, and thus cervical hemangioma, like labial hemangioma, is a sculptural problem in both the third and fourth dimensions. There must be sufficient tissue to allow full extension and to accommodate movement and growth. Excision is best done in the transverse axis (cervical relaxed cutaneous tension lines). Excision in the vertical axis is sometimes necessary, either at the preauricular join with the neck or in the midline with Z-plastic closure.

Nose. The nose is a psychologically sensitive focus. Nasal tip hemangiomas are notoriously slow to evidence regression, and they often leave behind a bulbous mass of fibrofatty tissue. Resection can often be done through unilateral or bilateral rim incisions. If the lobule and columella are overexpanded and skin must be removed, an open rhinoplasty approach is used. Approximation of the splayed alar cartilages should be done in conjunction with removal of a nasal hemangioma (Fig. 106-15). Care should be taken

not to overresect domal tissue or nasal tip skin. With continued evolution and shrinkage, a blunted nasal tip can result. Conservative staged resection is recommended.

LATE CHILDHOOD (INVOLUTED PHASE). It may be best to postpone the removal of the hemangiomatous residuum until the involuted phase (Fig. 106-16). Eventually, the involuted skin can look remarkably normal, particularly if the hemangioma involved only the reticular dermis. However, the skin is often atrophic and contains tiny telangiectatic vessels. If ulceration occurred during the proliferative phase, this area becomes a hypopigmented or yellow-tan scar. A once protrusive hemangioma generally leaves behind irrevocably expanded skin or fibrofatty tissue.

Thus, indications for resection during late childhood include damaged skin, abnormal contour, and distortion. Resection may be possible in a single stage, but more often the procedures are staged to minimize distortion and scarring. Staged excision is particularly useful for involuted hemangiomas of the lips, cheek, glabella, and scalp (see Fig. 106-16). Blepharoplasty and rhytidoplasty types of excisions are helpful to tighten the loose, crepe-like skin that may remain after involution of a large facial hemangioma. Ptosis correction and eyelid revision are often necessary after regression of an upper eyelid lesion. Uncommonly, there is both extensive scarring and loss of tissue so that more complicated reconstructive techniques are needed.

Other Vascular Tumors: Evaluation and Treatment

PYOGENIC GRANULOMA

Pyogenic granuloma is a common acquired vascular tumor in the pediatric age group. These lesions can occur anywhere but typically arise in the central face (Fig. 106-17). They are rare before the age of 6 months,[119] generally occurring in older children (mean age, 6.7 years) and adults. There is often no history of trauma or a preexisting dermatologic condition; however, they can appear in a capillary stain.

Pyogenic granuloma grows quickly, starting as a sessile papule and evolving into a pedunculated structure connected to the underlying dermis by a narrow stalk. These lesions generally remain small (average diameter, 6.5 mm). The surface epithelium often crusts over, followed by slough of the superficial tissue. Exfoliation without recurrence is rare.

Anxious parents often bring their child to a physician's office or emergency department after a bleeding episode. Pyogenic granuloma has been confused with hemangioma. Pathologists have muddied the terminologic waters even more by referring to these lesions as lobular capillary hemangioma. The treatment of

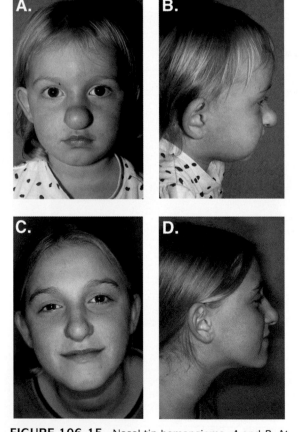

FIGURE 106-15. Nasal tip hemangioma. *A* and *B,* At 3 years of age, there has been some improvement in the bulbous tip. *C* and *D,* At age 14 years, 1 year after open tip exposure, excision, apposition of alar cartilages, and skin sculpting.

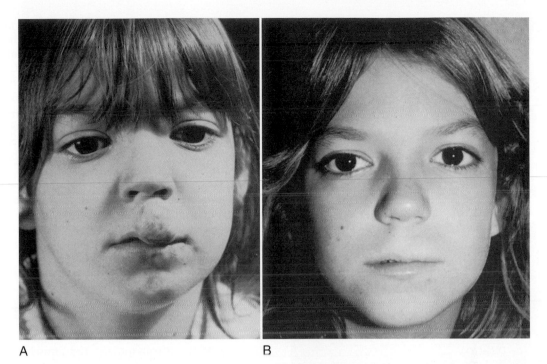

A   B

FIGURE 106-16. Excision of an individual hemangioma during late childhood. *A,* A 7-year-old girl with residual hemangioma of the upper lip (despite 275 rad given during the early proliferative phase). *B,* At age 11 years after two-stage excision in the transverse and vertical axes. (From Mulliken JB, Young AE: Vascular Birthmarks: Hemangiomas and Malformations. Philadelphia, WB Saunders, 1988.)

pyogenic granulomas is curettage, shave excision and laser phototherapy,[120] or full-thickness excision.[119]

KAPOSIFORM HEMANGIOENDOTHELIOMA: KASABACH-MERRITT PHENOMENON

Since the report in 1940, the double eponym Kasabach-Merritt syndrome has been used to describe profound thrombocytopenia, petechiae, and bleeding in the presence of a "giant hemangioma." Only recently has it been recognized that persistent, profound thrombocytope-nia is never associated with the common hemangioma of infancy. Rather, it occurs with a more invasive type of infantile vascular tumor called kaposiform hemangioendothelioma (KHE).[121-123] Furthermore, this coagulopathy is best designated Kasabach-Merritt phenomenon, rather than a syndrome, because the mechanism for platelet trapping is not yet understood and the condition is likely to be pathogenically heterogeneous.

The tumor is usually present at birth, although it can also appear postnatally. The sexes are equally

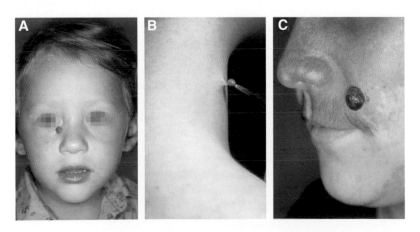

FIGURE 106-17. Pyogenic granuloma. *A,* Bleeding, friable lesion present for 2 months, 1 cm inferior to the medial canthus. *B,* Cervical lesion with slender stalk of tissue. *C,* Pyogenic granuloma frequently arises in a capillary malformation, such as in this 16-year-old boy with Sturge-Weber syndrome.

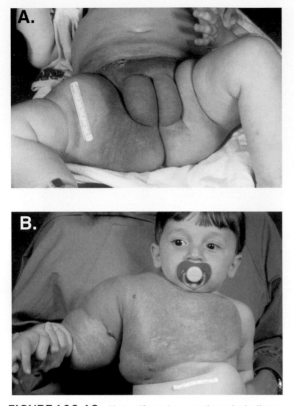

FIGURE 106-18. Kaposiform hemangioendothelioma. *A,* Note brawny, indurated character of the perineal tumor in this 13-month-old girl. *B,* Kaposiform hemangioendothelioma in right upper extremity of a 15-month-old boy who subsequently died of complications from the disease.

affected, unlike with common hemangioma. The tumors are unifocal and commonly involve the trunk, shoulder girdle, thigh, perineum, or retroperitoneum and, less commonly, the head and neck region. The overlying skin is a brawny deep red-purple, tense, edematous, and warm (Fig. 106-18). There is ecchymosis over and around the tumor. Histopathologic examination shows aggressive infiltration of normal tissue by sheets or nodules of slender, spindle-shaped endothelial cells, dilated lymphatic spaces, and coexistent slit-like vascular spaces filled with hemosiderin and fragmented red blood cells.

An infant with Kasabach-Merritt phenomenon is at risk for hemorrhage—intracranial, pleuropulmonic, intraperitoneal, or gastrointestinal. Thrombocytopenia is profound ($<10,000/mm^3$), and generalized petechiae are present. Fibrinogen is markedly low, and fibrin split products (D-dimer) are increased. The prothrombin and activated partial thromboplastin times are variably but minimally elevated. In rare instances, KHE can present without thrombocytopenia or coagulopathy.

MRI clearly differentiates KHE from common hemangioma.[123] As with all vascular tumors, there is enhancement, increased signal on T2-weighted images, and dilated feeding and draining vessels. Unlike hemangioma, KHE has a poorly defined margin with extension through tissues, including muscle, and relatively small vessels relative to the size of the tumor. There is a stranding pattern of T2 hyperintensity in the subcutaneous tissues that resembles lymphedema or lymphatic malformation; this is thought to be due to obstruction or lymphatic invasion. Signal voids (without flow-related enhancement) are believed to represent hemosiderin or other blood products. The postgadolinium T1-weighted sequence demonstrates enhancement, as in the T2 pattern, consistent with tumor extension in lymphatics or subcutaneous septa. Frequently, osteolysis is noted adjacent to the bone, although the tumor is rarely present within the bone.[123]

Treatment

Biopsy is rarely indicated for a coagulopathic vascular tumor. KHE is usually too large and diffusely infiltrative to resect. There are two caveats in managing thrombocytopenia associated with these tumors: platelet transfusion should be avoided unless there is active bleeding or an invasive procedure is indicated; and heparin should not be given because it can stimulate growth of the tumor, aggravate the platelet trapping, and worsen the bleeding. Administration of platelets can produce sudden swelling of the tumor, and in a cervical KHE, this can cause airway obstruction.

Although several pharmacologic therapies have been successful in controlling KHE, no single drug is consistently effective. First-line therapy is systemic corticosteroid, as discussed before for hemangioma; second-line treatment is interferon. Both of these therapies are less effective in treating KHE than hemangioma. Interferon is successful in approximately 50% of infants with KHE and Kasabach-Merritt phenomenon. Vincristine has also been effective in some patients. The mortality rate remains high, 20% to 30%, particularly for the retroperitoneal tumor. KHE often continues to proliferate into early childhood with some regression in mid-childhood. Even if drug therapy is successful in correcting the coagulopathy and shrinking the tumor, long-term follow-up evaluation often reveals persistent although usually asymptomatic tumor.[124]

TUFTED ANGIOMA

Tufted angioma, also known as angioblastoma of Nakagawa, is a tumor that has overlapping clinical and histologic features with KHE, suggesting that tufted angioma and KHE are on a spectrum.[5,59,123] Like KHE, it affects both sexes equally and has a similar anatomic distribution. It can be congenital or acquired (appearing in childhood). The congenital type presents as an ecchymotic plaque or mass and can be associated with Kasabach-Merritt phenomenon. The late-appearing tufted angioma is usually an erythematous macule or plaque, with reddish papules.[5] The microscopic findings are distinctive, consisting of small "cannon-ball" tufts of capillaries in the middle to deep dermis. Imaging and treatment are identical to those for KHE. Well-localized tufted angioma can sometimes be resected.

VASCULAR MALFORMATIONS

Vascular malformations result from errors of embryonic and fetal development. The classification of these anomalies is based on the clinical, radiologic, and histologic appearance of the abnormal channels, which may be either hematic or lymphatic in nature. Thus, a vascular malformation can be slow flow (i.e., capillary, lymphatic, or venous) or fast flow (i.e., arterial). If there are combinations of these elements, the malformation is named accordingly: arteriovenous, lymphatic-venous, or capillary-lymphatic-venous.

Capillary Malformations

PATHOGENESIS

The pathogenesis of capillary malformations (CMs) is not understood. The 19th century "neurovegetative theory" asserted that the primary embryonic defect responsible for such a vascular birthmark occurs in the developing autonomic nervous system.[125] There are several clinical findings that support this hypothesis. The geographic patterns of CMs are often segmental or dermatomal (particularly with branches of the trigeminal nerve), suggesting a relationship to the developing peripheral nervous system. The occasional finding of hyperhidrosis in an area of CM supports such an association. Neuroectoderm is known to contribute to the pericytic and smooth muscle layers of vascular walls.[126,127] The neurogenic hypothesis is supported by the finding of decreased perivascular neural density in CMs[128] and abnormal patterns of innervation of leptomeningeal vessels in Sturge-Weber syndrome.[129] The cutaneous flush of a CM may, in part, be due to an inability of these vessels to constrict secondary to diminished sympathetic innervation.

CLINICAL PRESENTATION

CMs occur anywhere on the body and can be localized or extensive. Rarely, they are multiple, such as in Sturge-Weber syndrome. Historically, CMs have been called port-wine stain or claret stain, terms that are now outdated. They should not be confused with nevus flammeus neonatorum, the most common vascular birthmark, seen in 50% of white neonates. Such irregular macular stains are popularly referred to as angel kiss on the forehead, eyelids, nose, and upper lip or stork bite in the nuchal area. These predictably fade, representing a minor transient dilatation of dermal vessels. If they persist, such a birthmark must be relabeled CM.

CMs have an equal gender distribution; the birth prevalence is 0.3%.[130] The cutaneous discoloration is usually but not always evident at birth; the stain may be hidden by the erythema of neonatal skin. Facial CMs often occur in a dermatomal distribution. Forty-five percent of facial port-wine stains are restricted to one of the three trigeminal dermatomes (Fig. 106-19).[131]

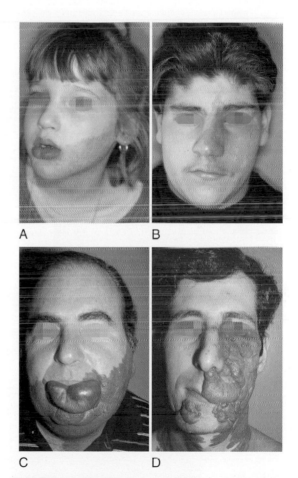

FIGURE 106-19. Facial capillary malformation. *A,* Young girl with a left V3 CM. *B,* Adolescent boy with left V2 capillary staining. *C,* Middle-aged man with V3 CM; note color, labial hypertrophy, and nodularity, changes frequently seen with aging. *D,* Man with left V2, V3, and cervical involvement; note maxillary overgrowth, bilabial hypertrophy, buphthalmos, and cutaneous fibrovascular thickening.

Conversely, 55% of facial CMs are noted to overlap sensory dermatomes, to cross the midline, or to occur bilaterally. The mucous membranes are often contiguously involved. Facial CMs typically become a deeper hue and are prone to nodular expansion as the affected individual ages. In the lower face and midface, there can be maxillary or mandibular overgrowth with labial hypertrophy and gingival hyperplasia. In all patients with an upper facial CM, a diagnosis of Sturge-Weber syndrome should be considered on initial presentation.

Cutaneous CM in the trunk and limbs is also associated with hypertrophy of the soft tissue and underlying skeleton. An extensive CM in an extremity can occur with increased circumference and limb length discrepancy (Fig. 106-20). CMs in these distributions rarely demonstrate the evolution of textural and color changes seen in facial CMs.

CMs often accompany developmental defects of the central neural axis. An occipital CM, often with an associated hair tuft, can overlie an encephalocele or ectopic meninges. A capillary stain on the posterior thorax can signify an underlying arteriovenous malformation of the spinal cord (Cobb syndrome).[132-134] A CM over the cervical or lumbosacral spine is a red flag for occult spinal dysraphism, lipomeningocele, tethered spinal cord, and diastematomyelia.[77] There may be subtle signs of neurogenic bladder dysfunction or lower extremity weakness, and therefore careful neurologic examination, spinal radiographic imaging, and bladder function studies are indicated.[135]

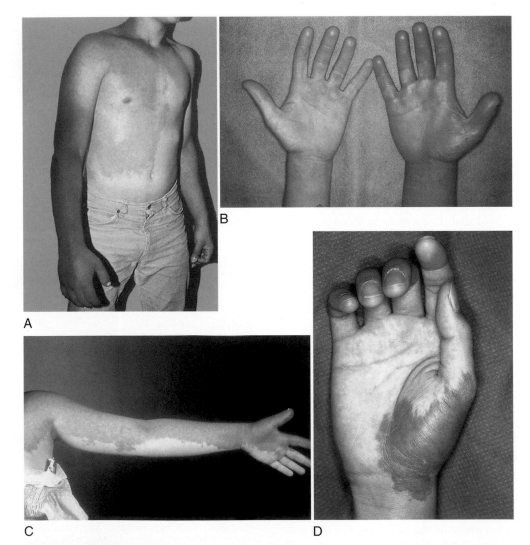

FIGURE 106-20. Extremity capillary malformation. *A* and *B,* Diffuse extremity CM with overgrowth in an adult man. Affected hand compared with unaffected counterpart. *C,* Dermatomal CM pattern in upper extremity. *D,* Limited patchy CM of right hand.

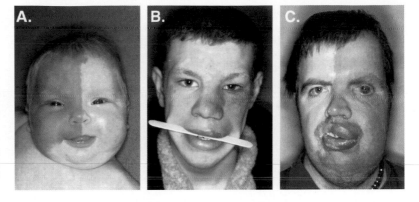

FIGURE 106-21. Sturge-Weber syndrome. *A,* Unilateral V1 and V2 CM in an infant. *B,* Unilateral V1 CM with maxillary overgrowth and occlusal cant in adolescent boy. *C,* Unilateral V1, V2, and V3 involvement with ipsilateral diffuse soft tissue and skeletal overgrowth and glaucoma of the left eye. All patients have leptomeningeal involvement.

Sturge-Weber Syndrome

Sturge-Weber syndrome is composed of a facial CM with ipsilateral ocular and leptomeningeal vascular anomalies. The capillary stain can be in the ophthalmic (V1), extend into the maxillary (V2), or involve all three trigeminal dermatomes (Fig. 106-21).[131] Patients with maxillary or mandibular involvement alone are at low risk for having ophthalmic and intracranial anomalies and should not be described as having Sturge-Weber syndrome.

The leptomeningeal anomalies can be capillary, venous, or arteriovenous malformations. Small foci can be silent, but extensive pial vascular lesions can cause refractory seizures, contralateral hemiplegia, and variably delayed motor and cognitive development. Resection of involved brain may be necessary if seizures cannot be controlled by medication. The anomalous choroidal vascularity can lead to retinal detachment, glaucoma, and blindness. Therefore, periodic ophthalmoscopic examination and tonometry are essential in observing children with Sturge-Weber syndrome. Glaucoma must be detected before irreversible ocular damage ensues. Ophthalmic examination should be performed every 6 months until the age of 2 years and then yearly in children at risk.

RADIOLOGIC FEATURES

The radiologic features of cutaneous CM are nonspecific. Areas of soft tissue and skeletal hypertrophy can be seen by MRI and computed tomography (CT). MRI best demonstrates pial vascular enhancement in a child thought to have Sturge-Weber syndrome. CT is less sensitive, although cerebral atrophy and prominent cortical sulci are seen with both modalities. Pial vascular anomalies are believed to contribute to the later development of gyriform calcifications in the outer layer of the cerebral cortex, most commonly in the temporal and occipital lobes. Angiographic findings include parenchymal blush (likely to be secondary to stasis of contrast material) and cortical venous occlusion and collaterals.

MANAGEMENT

Scarring the skin to diminish the color of a CM has been tried in various forms: multiple parallel incisions,[136] electric current delivered by acupuncture needles (galvanopuncture),[137] electrocoagulation,[138] ultraviolet lamp,[139,140] radiation therapy,[141] rubbing with sandpaper,[142] and freezing.[143,144] The concept of camouflaging a CM by tattooing is credited to Pauli (1835), a full century before tattooing was rediscovered.[145-147] None of these methods yielded satisfying results.[148,149]

Current management of CM is cosmetic camouflage and laser photocoagulation, but there is still a place for excision and grafting.

Cosmetics

There remains a place for external camouflage with cosmetic creams in the treatment of CM (Fig. 106-22). Two well-known products are Covermark (Lydia O'Leary) and Dermablend (Flori Roberts). It requires about 20 minutes to apply the foundation, additional creams, and setting powder. Daily use of makeup

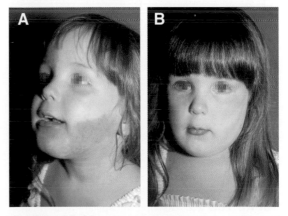

FIGURE 106-22. Makeup camouflage of capillary malformation. Effective disguise of unilateral V3 CM is achieved by makeup in this young child.

demands a patient's full commitment and may be rejected by children. When there is nodularity and hypertrophy of the stained skin in older patients, the appearance is less satisfactory. Only 28% to 39% of patients with CM report consistently using external cosmetic cover.[150,151]

Laser

The modern way to deliver thermal energy to fade a CM is tunable flashlamp pulsed dye laser. The wavelength is set at 585 nm; the chromophore is oxyhemoglobin. Depth of penetration is limited to 1.2 mm. Timing of therapy is controversial. Some authors report improved results when laser therapy is initiated in infancy[152]; others find that age makes no difference.[153]

In general, significant lightening occurs in approximately 80% of patients (Fig. 106-23).[154,155] The outcome is better on the face (lateral more so than medial) than on the trunk. Multiple sessions may be required. The lesion darkens again in up to 50% of patients between 3 and 4 years after treatment.[154] The addition of cryogen spray cooling is reported to yield improved results in patients with CMs as this permits the use of higher laser fluences.[17]

Improvement with laser is less in Asian patients with facial CMs; only 13.6% show 50% or more lightening on objective scoring.[156] A higher rate of complications, including pigmentary changes and hypertrophic scarring, is reported in individuals with darker skin.[156,157]

Operative Management

Small fibrovascular nodules are easily excised. Patients with more extensive fibronodular hypertrophy can benefit from resection and resurfacing with split- or full-thickness skin grafts patterned to fit the aesthetic facial units (Fig. 106-24).[158,159] The grafts should be har-

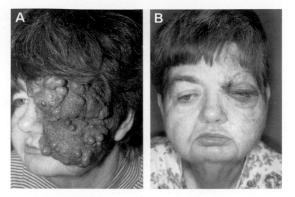

FIGURE 106-24. Excision of facial capillary malformation, followed by resurfacing with skin grafts. *A,* Profound thickening and nodularity of this unilateral V1 and V2 CM obscure this patient's vision. *B,* After staged excision of the forehead, eyelids, and cheeks and resurfacing with skin grafts.

vested from color-matched areas, such as the retroauricular region, supraclavicular areas, or scalp. Clodius and Smahel[160] recommend harvesting scalp skin from the mastoid region 10 to 14 days after epilation.

Unfortunately, excision and resurfacing of a facial CM give a border effect with normal skin that calls attention to the reconstruction. Other potential sequelae include hypertrophic scarring at the edge of the graft, unpredictable pigmentation, and abnormal texture. Cutaneous expansion may be used before the excision of a moderate-sized CM to permit linear closure along the border of a facial unit.[161]

Contour resection is effective to correct macrocheilia and labial ptosis.[162] Orthognathic procedures are indicated for occlusal canting, as the result of hemimaxillary vertical overgrowth, or for mandibular prognathism.

CUTIS MARMORATA TELANGIECTASIA CONGENITA

Cutis marmorata telangiectasia congenita (CMTC) is a distinct pathologic entity, first described by vanLohuizen.[163] This rare vascular anomaly manifests as congenital livid cutaneous marbling, even at normal temperatures, that becomes more pronounced with lower temperatures or with crying. The involved skin is depressed in a serpiginous reticulated pattern and has a distinctive deep purple color (Fig. 106-25). Ulceration may be present. CMTC occurs in a localized, segmental, or generalized distribution, more frequently involving the trunk and extremities than the face or scalp. In one reported series, CMTC was unilateral in 65% of patients and involved a lower extremity in 69% of patients.[164] The affected extremity is

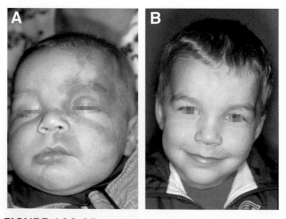

FIGURE 106-23. Lasering of capillary malformation. There is obvious lightening of the patchy unilateral V1 and V2 CM after multiple sessions with the Nd:YAG laser.

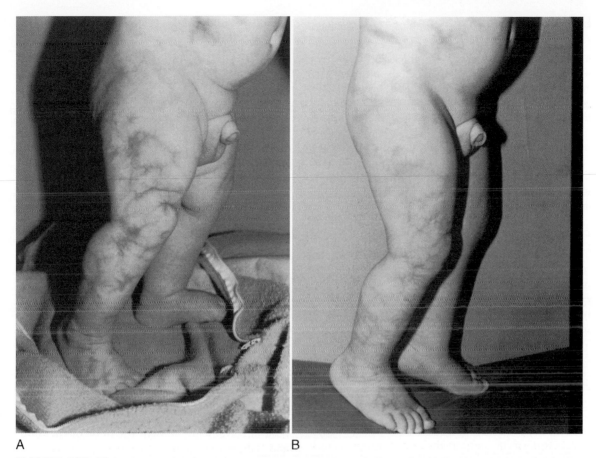

A   B

FIGURE 106-25. Cutis marmorata telangiectasia congenita. *A,* CMTC in a 5-month-old boy. Note the serpiginous and discolored craters of the leg and trunk. *B,* Improvement apparent at 1 year of age. The venous ectasia, skin atrophy, and pigmentation usually persist into adulthood. (From Mulliken JB, Young AE: Vascular Birthmarks: Hemangiomas and Malformations. Philadelphia, WB Saunders, 1988.)

often hypoplastic compared with the nonaffected counterpart.[165,166]

Differential diagnosis includes cutis marmorata (or livedo reticularis) and a telangiectatic variant of hemangioma. Cutis marmorata is merely an accentuated pattern of normal cutaneous vascularity. It is seen as a transient mottling pattern when the child is placed in a low-temperature environment but disappears on warming. Telangiectatic hemangioma, most often seen on an extremity, has a fine, variegated pattern. It is not associated with depression of the involved skin and it regresses, as do the other forms of hemangioma.[57]

Almost all affected infants with CMTC show improvement during the first year of life continuing into adolescence.[1,167] However, atrophy and pigmentation often persist into adulthood in association with ectasia of the superficial veins in the involved limb.

CMTC occurs sporadically in an equal gender distribution.[164,168,169] There are reports suggesting that it may be an autosomal dominant disorder of low

penetrance.[170,171] An alternative theory proposes that CMTC is secondary to the mosaic distribution of an autosomal lethal gene.[172]

There are reported instances of CMTC in association with hypoplasia of the iliac and femoral veins[173] and with congenital glaucoma.[169,174-176] A clinically discrete condition has been described comprising CMTC and macrocephaly. Findings in the macrocephaly-CMTC syndrome include segmental overgrowth, macrosomia, and capillary staining of the philtrum in addition to macrocephaly and CMTC.[177] These children have a high risk for neurologic abnormalities, including developmental delay, mental retardation, megalencephaly, and hydrocephalus.[178] CMTC has also been identified as a component of Adams-Oliver syndrome (i.e., aplasia cutis congenita of the scalp and transverse terminal limb defects).[179,180] Adams-Oliver syndrome with CMTC is thought to be genetic; reported pedigrees support an autosomal recessive pattern of inheritance.[181]

Lymphatic Malformations

Lymphatic malformations (LMs) manifest in various forms, from a localized sponge-like lesion to diffuse involvement of an anatomic region or multiple organ systems. Radiologically and histologically, they are characterized as microcystic, macrocystic, or combined. In the 19th century, these were called lymphangioma for microcystic forms and cystic hygroma for macrocystic forms. These terms are outdated and should no longer be used. The word "lymphangioma" incorrectly implies a "proliferating tumor" and has contributed to the terminologic chaos in the field of vascular anomalies.

PATHOGENESIS

The pathogenesis of LM is easily imagined, but the etiology is unknown. The lymphatic system develops during the sixth week of embryonic life, while the crown-rump length measures 6 to 8 mm. Paired jugular lymph sacs appear first, followed by mesenteric, cisterna chyli, and posterior lymph sacs. These enlarge and become connected by the developing thoracic duct. A second stage of maturation involves the transformation of the sacs into primary lymph nodes and the centrifugal spread of peripheral lymphatics.[182,183] The beginning of the century was marked by controversy in regard to the origin of the lymphatic sacs, believed by some to be venous[184] and by others to be mesenchymal. Investigations support the centrifugal or venous origin for these anomalous lymphatic structures.[185,186]

One etiologic theory for LMs is that either anlagen of the sacs or their sprouting lymphatic channels become "pinched off" from the main lymphatic system, leading to aberrant collections of lymphatic fluid-filled spaces, expansion, and fibrosis. Another theory attributes LMs to abnormal budding of the lymphatic system with a loss of connection to the central lymph channels or to development of lymphatic tissue in aberrant locations.

Understanding of the molecular basis for LMs is in its infancy. The VEGF receptor 3 (VEGFR3, also called Flt4) is restricted to the lymphatic endothelium during development.[185] VEGF3 knockout mice die at embryonic day 9 with major venous anomalies, just before lymphatics sprout.[187] Abnormally distended lymphatic but not hematic channels are found in mice that overexpress the VEGFR3 ligand VEGF-C.[188] No genetic basis has been determined for LMs. However, lymphedema, a generalized type of lymphatic anomaly in the limbs, can be hereditary (Milroy syndrome), and two chromosomal loci have been mapped, one on 5q and the other on 16q.[189-192]

CLINICAL PRESENTATION

An LM is usually noted at birth or within 2 years of life. On occasion, LMs first become evident in later childhood, adolescence, or even adulthood.[193] Prenatal ultrasonography can detect relatively large lesions as early as the second trimester, although LMs are frequently misdiagnosed as other pathologic entities, such as teratoma.[194] True LMs seen antenatally must be differentiated from "posterior nuchal translucency" or "cystic hygroma," obstetric terms reserved for nuchal fluid accumulations in the first trimester. Fetuses with posterior nuchal translucency and fetal hydrops have a poor prognosis. Most are aneuploid; they frequently die in utero or may have Turner or Noonan syndrome.[195,196]

LMs most commonly occur in the cervicofacial region, axilla-chest, mediastinum, retroperitoneum, buttock, and perineum (Fig. 106-26). The overlying skin is usually normal and has a bluish hue. Dermal involvement can manifest as puckering (deep cutaneous dimpling) or tiny pathognomonic vesicles. These vesicles resemble minute blisters that become dark red as a result of intravesicular bleeding.

Facial LMs are localized or diffuse, and they are often associated with skeletal overgrowth (Fig. 106-27). Orbital LMs are reported to cause proptosis in 85%, ptosis in 73%, and restrictive eye movements in 46% of patients.[197] LM in the lower face is the most common cause of macrocheilia, macrotia, and macromelia.[1] Cervicofacial LM may be unilateral or bilateral, often with varying degrees of mandibular bone involvement.[51] LM in the floor of the mouth and tongue manifests as macroglossia, vesicles, and intermittent swelling. An open-bite deformity typically results, often with extensive caries because of limited access for dental hygiene. In the neck, LM occurs most frequently in the anterior cervical triangle.[198] Speech and swallowing may be impaired, and the possibility of oropharyngeal obstruction is always of concern. Tracheostomy may be necessary in early infancy. Similarly, involvement of the supraglottic upper airway by cervical LMs may necessitate neonatal tracheostomy. The mediastinum is often involved in cervical LM.

Multifocal LM

Multifocal lymphatic disease is a term for involvement of multiple organ systems by LM (the old term is lymphangiomatosis). The most typical pattern includes recurrent chylous pleural effusion, scattered osteolytic bone lesions, and splenic involvement. Other terms for the skeletal presentation include Gorham-Stout syndrome, disappearing bone disease, and phantom bone disease.[199]

RADIOLOGIC FEATURES

On CT scan, LMs are depicted as low-density cystic lesions, most often multilocular with septa of variable thickness. MRI is used to outline the extent

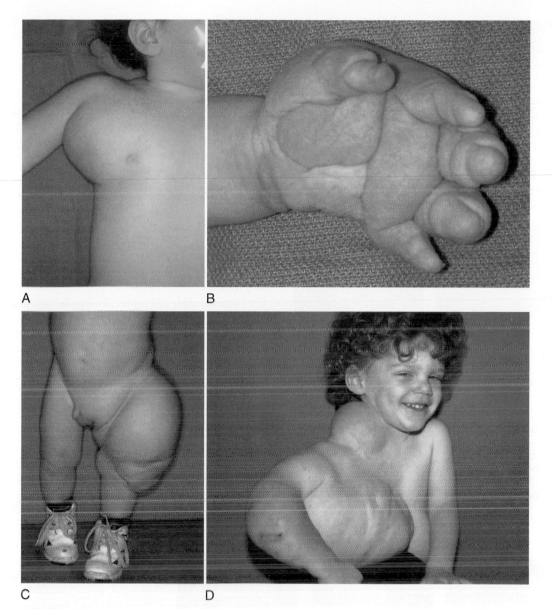

A   B

C   D

FIGURE 106-26. Extremity lymphatic malformation. *A,* Axillary LM. *B,* Hand LM. *C,* Lower extremity and groin LM. *D,* Axillary and right upper extremity LM causing subluxation of shoulder.

of the anomaly and to distinguish lymphatic from venous malformation (Fig. 106-28). On T2-weighted images, the mean signal intensity of an LM is greater than that of muscle, cerebrospinal fluid, and fat.[9] Gadolinium enhancement of T1-weighted images demonstrates intralesional contrast material in a venous malformation, but not in LM. Enhancement of the rim of the cysts is pathognomonic. Ultrasonography can be helpful in diagnosing macrocystic LM, distinguishing it from other subcutaneous masses, and detecting recent hemorrhage.[74]

MANAGEMENT

Management of LM is directed at treatment of sequelae such as bleeding and recurrent infection, correction of contour, and improvement in function.

Antibiotic Therapy

LM can enlarge abruptly secondary to intralesional hemorrhage; this happens in 8% to 12.6% of lesions.[198] There is sudden swelling and ecchymosis. In an orbital LM, rupture and hemorrhage into the lymphatic spaces produce the typical subconjunctival "chocolate cysts"

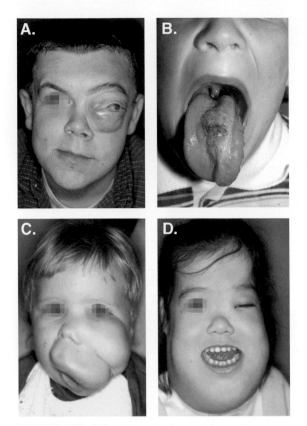

FIGURE 106-27. Morphologic variations of lymphatic malformation. *A,* LM involving orbit, with proptosis, enophthalmos, and chemosis. *B,* Lingual LM with macroglossia. Note vesicles on the dorsal tongue surface. *C,* Predominantly left-sided cervicofacial LM. *D,* Diffuse infiltrating LM involving bilateral mandible, tongue, floor of mouth, and right orbit.

or ocular proptosis. Intralesional bleeding is a predisposing factor for infection. Prophylactic antibiotics should be considered.

Cellulitis is common in LMs, particularly those in the head, neck, and perineum. Sepsis can also occur in mesenteric and retroperitoneal LM.[200,201] This typically manifests as rapid expansion of the lesion with erythema, fever, tenderness, and tenseness (Fig. 106-29). Prompt initiation of antibiotic therapy, aimed at the presumptive offending microbial flora (either oral or gut organisms), is necessary. Oral administration may be effective; often, systemic antibiotics are needed. Infection can be life-threatening in children with parapharyngeal or paratracheal LMs, requiring intubation if there is no tracheostomy. The clinical course is often protracted, and infection frequently recurs. After the inflammatory period, the involved area usually remains firm and edematous for months.

Prophylactic antibiotics are generally not indicated for patients with LMs. Parents can be given a prescription for a broad-spectrum antimicrobial with instructions to administer the drug and to seek medical consultation at the first signs of infection. Dental hygiene is an important prophylactic measure in children with facial LMs because carious primary teeth are a likely source of bacterial contamination. If the palatine tonsils are thought to be the origin of repeated sepsis, tonsillectomy should be considered.

Sclerotherapy

Historically, a variety of agents have been instilled into the cystic spaces of LMs in the hope of causing obliteration and shrinkage. Solutions tested have included boiling water,[202] sodium morrhuate,[203] hypertonic salt

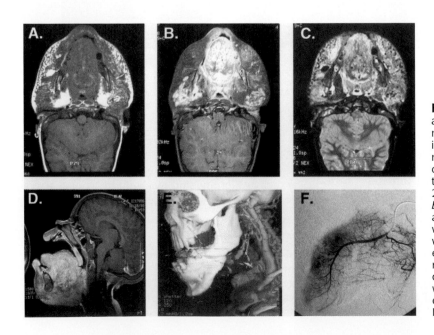

FIGURE 106-28. MRI, CT, and angiographic images of lymphatic malformation. Lymphatic anomaly involving the mandible, floor of mouth, and tongue in a 3-year-old child (morphologically similar to the patient depicted in Figure 106-27D). *A,* T1-weighted MRI sequence. *B,* T1-weighted MRI sequence after administration of gadolinium. *C,* T2-weighted image. *D,* Sagittal T1-weighted sequence with gadolinium enhancement. *E,* Three-dimensional reconstructed CT scan demonstrates diffuse mandibular enlargement with open-bite deformity. *F,* Tongue enlargement with increased vascularity seen in angiographic view.

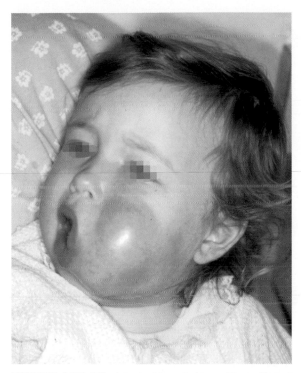

FIGURE 106-29. Infected lymphatic malformation of the cheek. Note swelling and erythema.

or sugar solutions,[204] and iodized oil.[205] None has been successful.

During the last 3 decades, intralesional injection of bleomycin was tried.[206] A success rate of greater than 80% was reported for patients with LMs of the head and neck.[207-209] OK-432 is another intralesional agent used to treat LMs. OK-432 is a lyophilized mixture of attenuated group A *Streptococcus pyogenes* of human origin. Its mode of action is not fully understood. It has been shown to increase a variety of cytokines,[210,211] the production of matrix metalloproteinases,[212] and the proliferation and cytokine production of lymphokine-activated killer cells.[213]

The most dramatic responses follow intralesional injection of OK-432 for macrocystic LM,[214] facial LM,[215] orbital LM,[216] and LMs of the infratemporal or cervical area.[217] The only side effects reported are fevers lasting 2 to 4 days and a local inflammatory reaction of 3 to 7 days' duration. OK-432 has also been injected into recurrent LM after surgical resection.[218,219] It is less effective in diffuse or microcystic cervicofacial LMs.[217] It has been used in neonates,[216,220] and there is a single report documenting successful sclerotherapy of a fetal cervical LM during the second trimester.[221]

Laser

Argon, neodymium:yttrium-aluminum-garnet (Nd:YAG), or carbon dioxide laser can be used to coagu-late troublesome lymphatic vesicles on the surface of the tongue or oral mucosa.[222,223] Unfortunately, the vesicles usually recur.

Operative Management

Procedures are indicated for respiratory obstruction, nutrition, and distortion caused by LM. A newborn with a cervicofacial LM often presents with respiratory obstruction secondary to involvement of the tongue and floor of mouth. This situation can warrant immediate tracheostomy. Aspiration or incision and drainage of a cystic sublingual lesion is an emergency manuever[224]; however, this is rarely more than a temporizing measure.[225] Prenatal diagnosis of cervicofacial LM affords an opportunity for controlled cesarean delivery of an affected infant. The airway can be assessed while the neonate is supported by the placental circulation. Observation, elective intubation, or tracheostomy is selected on the basis of the findings.[226-228] A large cervicofacial LM can also compromise function of the tongue and upper alimentary tract, necessitating placement of a feeding tube. Central line access may be required for total parenteral nutrition in patients with multifocal lymphatic anomalies and chylothorax or chylous ascites.[229]

Resection is the mainstay of treatment for LM (Fig. 106-30). Resection of an LM can usually be deferred until the infant is several months old or in early childhood. The older infant is better able to tolerate prolonged anesthesia. The tedious dissection of delicate neurovascular structures is easier in an older child.

The operative goal is complete resection. Unfortunately, this is rarely possible because the LM involves tissues that are apparently normal and structures that must be preserved. For a diffuse malformation, staged excision is recommended, limiting each procedure to a defined anatomic area (Fig. 106-31). Reoperation on a previously resected area is arduous; LM can develop venous flow after surgical intervention, making repeated resection more difficult. Other guidelines for resection of LM are restricting the extent of dissection to one anatomic region and, if possible, limiting blood loss to the patient's circulating blood volume. Postoperative wound complications are common, such as prolonged drainage and swelling, in addition to the likelihood of fluid recollection and infection weeks later. An elastic compression garment should be fabricated before resection to be available immediately after the procedure. A more custom "refitting" can be done after resolution of postoperative edema. The patient and family should be counseled on use of such a garment.

Additional surgical considerations are particular to the affected region. A coronal incision is used for a frontal-temporal-orbital LM. Preservation of vision may be one indication for resection early. LM in the upper eyelid is removed through an incision in the

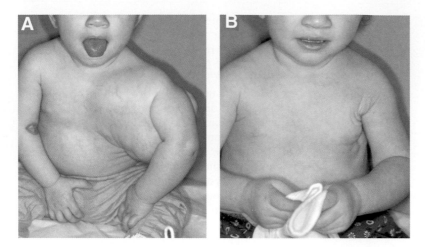

FIGURE 106-30. Single-stage surgical treatment of a lymphatic malformation. *A*, LM of chest wall and axilla. *B*, After resection.

upper tarsal fold. Conjunctival lesions can be locally excised; reformation of cysts is common. Removal of a hemifacial LM is usually done through a preauricular incision and cervical extension, if necessary, with meticulous dissection of the facial nerve in continuity with the superficial portion of the parotid gland.

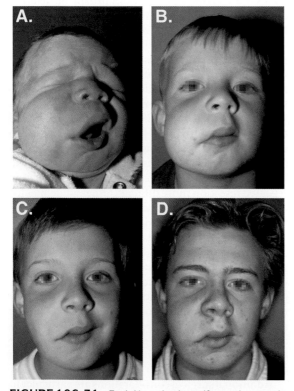

FIGURE 106-31. Facial lymphatic malformation requiring staged resections. Patient at 1 month of age *(A)*, 5 years of age *(B)*, 10 years of age *(C)*, and 18 years of age *(D)*. Multiple resections were necessary to debulk the cheek and to correct the position of the oral commissure.

Other approaches to facial LM include direct excision of affected tissue through a melolabial incision[230] and transoral resection for LM in the medial cheek. Labial LM is resected through a transverse mucosal incision.

Cervical LM requires a radical neck type of dissection with identification and preservation of the spinal accessory, hypoglossal, lingual, and vagus nerves in addition to the marginal mandibular branch of the facial nerve and cervical sympathetic chain. The specimen can be divided during dissection to facilitate exposure and dissection of these structures. The internal jugular vein is usually taken, but the sternocleidomastoid muscle can be preserved if it is not riddled with lymphatic cysts. Although cervical LM can involve the axilla, excision of this area should be undertaken as a separate procedure.

Surgical reduction of macroglossia may be necessary to restore the tongue in the oral cavity or indicated because of an open-bite deformity.[231] However, there is no direct evidence that resection of affected tissue from the tongue will diminish mandibular overgrowth. Osseous hypertrophy and distortion can interfere with dental occlusion and cause facial asymmetry. Skeletal contour reduction, osteotomies of the facial skeleton, and orthognathic procedures are used to correct these bone and occlusal abnormalities. Although the procedures are usually reserved until adolescence, earlier intervention should be considered.[232]

All components of the brachial plexus must be identified and preserved during excision of an axillary LM. An axillary LM extending into the upper extremity usually necessitates staged excision.[233,234] Thoracic wall LMs may be extensive, although they can usually be excised widely, permitting linear closure by advancing skin flaps.

Lymphangioma circumscriptum is the Latin term for superficial cutaneous-subcutaneous lymphatic anomaly. This typically presents anywhere in the posterior cervical area, shoulder, axilla, or lower extremity as multiple vesicular excrescences that irritate the patient, bleed repeatedly, and often drain clear fluid. These abnormal superficial dermal vesicles communicate with blind-ended lymphatic cisterns deep in the subcutaneous plane.[235] Definitive treatment necessitates excision of both skin and subcutaneous tissue down to fascia. Frozen sections may aid in determining margins.[236] The defect may require primary closure with a skin graft or flap. Failure to adequately excise the anomalous lymphatic tissue will result in recurrence as vesicles reappear in the scar or at the juncture of skin and graft or flap.

The outcome of surgical excision depends on the location and extent of the LM. Recurrence has been reported more frequently for craniofacial LM than for other sites.[237] Recurrence is most likely caused by leaving abnormal tissue behind, with subsequent regeneration of anomalous channels. In head and neck lesions, a recurrent or residual lesion is seen more frequently with suprahyoid than with infrahyoid lesions.[238]

Venous Malformations

PATHOGENESIS

Venous malformation (VM) is composed of thin-walled, dilated, sponge-like channels of variable size and mural thickness. There is a normal-appearing endothelial lining; it is the smooth muscle architecture that is abnormal. Smooth muscle alpha-actin staining demonstrates decreased smooth muscle cells that are arranged in clumps rather than concentrically. This mural abnormality probably accounts for the tendency of these malformations to gradually expand over time. In addition, intralesional clotting often occurs, ranging from simple fibrin deposition to the later-appearing pathognomonic calcified "phleboliths." Varying degrees of fibrovascular ingrowth may be noted in these mural thrombi.

There is evidence for a genetic basis for certain types of VMs, such as in Turner syndrome, in which patients can have VMs of the intestine and feet.[239,240] Well-documented pedigrees of familial VMs have been reported; in general, these involve multifocal lesions. Familial multiple glomangioma is an autosomal dominant disorder with high penetrance that manifests in multiple, often tender, blue nodular dermal lesions.[241] Glomangiomas are histologically distinguishable from typical VMs by the presence of numerous glomus cells lining the ectactic vascular channels. The gene for this vascular disorder is glomulin (GLMN) on chromosome 1p21-22.[242,243] The lesions, either scattered or in large clusters of protuberant nodules, typically involve the extremities. They have a deep purple, matted cobblestone appearance that helps distinguish them clinically from banal VM. They tend to be more painful on palpation.

Familial cutaneous-mucosal VM is another autosomal dominant condition characterized by dome-shaped lesions ranging from several millimeters to several centimeters in size.[244] Cerebral cavernous VMs are also familial, and in a small subgroup, hyperkeratotic capillary-venous lesions of the skin are present.[245] The gene for this disorder is KRIT1.[246] Patients with this disorder continue to develop new intracranial lesions during their adult life and remain at significant risk for intracranial hemorrhage.[247]

Blue rubber bleb nevus syndrome (a catchy but cumbersome term coined by Bean[248]) is a rare, sporadic disorder consisting of cutaneous and gastrointestinal VMs. This is the most common vascular anomaly responsible for chronic gastrointestinal hemorrhage. Most cases are sporadic, but autosomal dominant inheritance has been reported. The genetic locus is yet to be identified.[249] The cutaneous lesions are soft and dome shaped or nodular; they have a predilection to occur on the trunk, palms, and soles (Fig. 106-32).[249] The lesions increase in size and number with age. Orthopedic problems can result.[250] The gastrointestinal lesions are widely distributed, most commonly in the small bowel, ranging in number from a few to several hundred per patient. In addition to bleeding, these lesions can cause intussusception and other types of obstruction.[251] Lesions are also frequently present in the liver, gallbladder, mesentery, and retroperitoneum.

CLINICAL PRESENTATION

Venous anomalies are the most common type of vascular malformation. By definition slow-flow anomalies, they present in myriad forms. Although VMs are congenital, they may not become obvious until later in childhood. In general, they are bluish, soft, and compressible. They principally occur in skin and subcutaneous tissues but can also primarily involve muscle, abdominal viscera, joint structures, and the central nervous system. They range in size from tiny lesions to large abnormalities that can distort structures in the face, extremities, or trunk and may involve several contiguous anatomic regions (Fig. 106-33). Most VMs are solitary, although multiple cutaneous and visceral lesions also occur. These multifocal forms can be inherited.

VMs grow commensurately with the child and expand slowly but may enlarge rapidly with thrombosis. They are easily compressed, expanding when the affected area is dependent or after a Valsalva maneuver if the VM is in the head and neck region. Phlebothrombosis is common, leading to distention, firmness, and frequently pain in affected soft tissues. Pain and stiffness, particularly in head and neck lesions, are often most pronounced on awakening in the morning, presumably because of stasis and swelling. Phleboliths, diagnosed as radiopaque nodules on

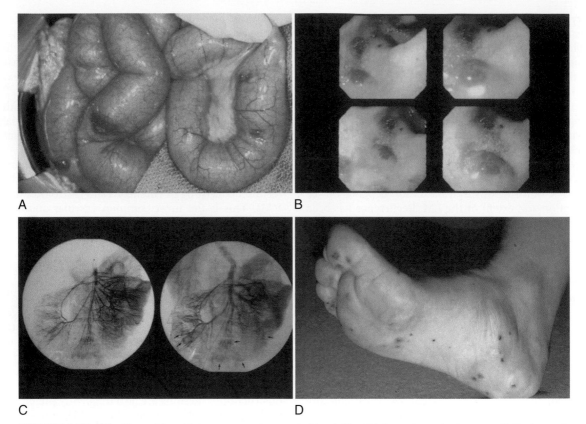

FIGURE 106-32. Blue rubber bleb nevus syndrome. *A,* Blood-filled blebs on intestinal serosa. *B,* Endoscopic view of blebs. *C,* Angiographic view of intestinal blebs demonstrating lesions in venous phase. *D,* Plantar surface lesions typical of this disorder.

plain radiography, can be seen in children as young as 2 years.

Head and Neck

Cervicofacial VMs are often unilateral. They can produce a mass effect resulting in facial asymmetry and progressive distortion of features. Intraorbital VMs expand the orbital cavity and may communicate with VMs of the infratemporal fossa and cheek through the sphenomaxillary fissure. As a result, the patient can have exophthalmia when the head is dependent and enophthalmia when standing upright.[77] Oral VMs tend to cause dental malalignment due to a mass effect. A buccal VM can involve the tongue, palate, and oropharynx but rarely impedes speech or swallowing. Pharyngeal, tracheolaryngeal, and deep cervical-oropharyngeal VMs may compress and deviate the upper airway to cause insidious obstructive sleep apnea.

Extremities

VM in an extremity may be limited to the skin and subcutis or extend into underlying muscles, joints and bone, or both. Limb length discrepancy can occur, or there can be hypoplasia of the affected side due, in part, to chronic disuse secondary to pain. Intraosseous VM causes structural weakening of the bony diaphysis, predisposing to pathologic fracture. VM in the synovial lining of the knee, often incorrectly referred to as synovial hemangioma, causes repeated bloody effusions and episodic joint pain.[252-254] Hemarthrosis is particularly troublesome in children with VM-associated coagulopathy. Hemosiderin arthropathy leads to severe degenerative arthritis.

Bowel

VMs of the gastrointestinal tract can be located anywhere from mouth to anus, with a unifocal, multifocal, or diffuse distribution.[255] Structurally, they may be polypoid, sessile, or nodular, involving any or all layers of the bowel wall. Unifocal lesions range from pinpoint mucosal anomalies to massive VMs that replace entire sections of gut. The most common distribution is surrounding the left colon, rectum, and nearby pelvic and retroperitoneal structures. Foregut lesions can be associated with central mesenteric and portal venous anomalies. The most common presentation is chronic bleeding and anemia.

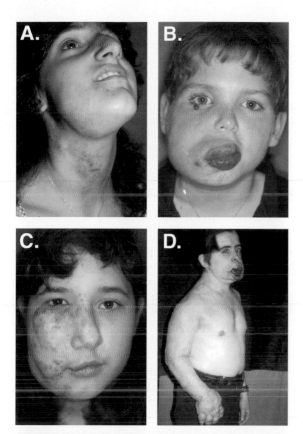

FIGURE 106-33. Morphologic variations of venous malformation. *A,* Superficial VM of neck. *B,* Deep VM causing cheek enlargement, bilabial hypertrophy, and nodule on lower eyelid. *C,* VM of glomovenous type; note cobblestone appearance. *D,* VM involving entire upper extremity and face bilaterally.

guished from lymphatic malformations by the presence of intravascular contrast material on T1 images. Phleboliths or thrombi are seen as signal voids on all MRI sequences but are emphasized on gradient or "susceptibility" sequences. Flow-sensitive sequences show no evidence of increased arterial flow. Magnetic resonance venography is useful for detailing deep venous anatomy, particularly for extremity VM. Doppler ultrasonography also aids in diagnosis of a soft tissue VM. These lesions appear as hypoechoic, heterogeneous, compressible masses with monophasic low-velocity flow. Phleboliths are reported in 8% of patients on ultrasonography.[260] Venography may be required for a complete assessment in patients with extensive VM. Bowel lesions are best visualized directly by endoscopy when possible. Other techniques for radiologic evaluation include MRI, ^{99m}Tc-red blood cell radionuclide scanning, and angiography.

MANAGEMENT

Indications for treatment of VM include appearance, functional problems, and pain. The principal therapeutic modalities are elastic compression, sclerotherapy, and surgical resection or a combined approach.

Conservative Therapy

Elastic compression aids in reducing swelling and pain in an involved extremity. A custom garment can be worn while the patient is upright and removed during

Coagulation

Coagulation studies should be obtained in any patient with an extensive VM, particularly if there is a history of easy bruising or intraoperative bleeding. Stagnation within a VM causes a localized intravascular coagulopathy with resulting prolongation of prothrombin time, decreased fibrinogen (150 to 200 mg/dL), and elevated fibrin split products.[256-259] The activated partial thromboplastin time is generally normal. The platelet count may be slightly decreased, in the 100,000 to 150,000/mm³ range. This coagulopathy is distinct from Kasabach-Merritt phenomenon occurring in association with kaposiform hemangioendothelioma and presenting with platelet counts of less than 10,000 to 20,000/mm³.

RADIOLOGIC FEATURES

MRI is the most informative imaging technique for documenting the nature and extent of a VM (Fig. 106-34). Lesions are hyperintense on T2 images, distin-

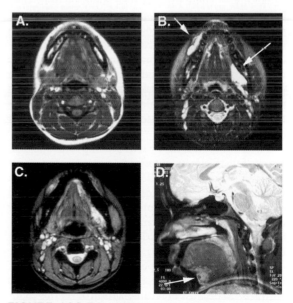

FIGURE 106-34. MRI of oral venous malformation. *A,* VM difficult to distinguish on transverse T1-weighted sequence. *B,* Involvement of tissue superficial and deep to mandible seen on contrast sequence *(arrows).* *C* and *D,* T2-weighted transverse and lateral sequences. Dark circular phlebolith outlined *(arrow).*

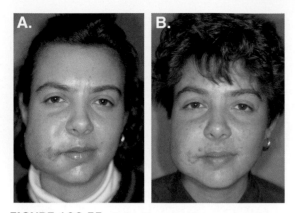

FIGURE 106-35. Sclerotherapy of venous malformation. *A,* Before treatment. *B,* After several sessions of sclerotherapy with ethanol.

recumbency. A baby aspirin taken daily provides some prophylaxis against painful thromboses.

Sclerotherapy

Sclerotherapy, the mainstay of treatment, is the injection of an agent to induce inflammation and obliteration of affected veins (Fig. 106-35). For small cutaneous or mucosal lesions, 1% sodium tetradecyl sulfate (Sotradecol) is effective.[261-263]

For large VMs, sclerotherapy should be done under general anesthesia with real-time fluoroscopic monitoring. Ultrasonography is also helpful in guiding sclerotherapy.[264] These procedures should be done only by an experienced interventional radiologist. In the United States, absolute ethanol is the most common sclerosant. Ethibloc has been used by interventionalists outside of the United States; this agent is a mixture of alcohol, contrast medium, and zein (a corn protein).[265,266] Lipiodol, a contrast agent, can be added to absolute ethanol.[267] An alcohol-containing ethyl cellulose gel has also been used for injection treatment of VMs.[268]

Local complications of sclerotherapy include blistering, full-thickness cutaneous necrosis, and nerve injury.[269] Systemic complications include hemolysis with subsequent hemoglobinuria, anaphylaxis, and cardiac arrest. A number of maneuvers can minimize the passage of the sclerosant into the systemic circulation, including compression and the use of tourniquets for extremity VMs.

Multiple sclerotherapeutic sessions, generally done at bimonthly intervals, are often necessary to shrink a VM because of recanalization of venous channels after initial obliteration. The success rate is reasonably high; in one series, 76% of patients had marked improvement or cure.[269] Other authors report similarly encouraging results for varying subsets of patients.[270,271]

Laser

Successful intralesional photocoagulation with bare-fiber Nd:YAG laser has been reported for patients with tongue and lip VMs.[272] In a retrospective study of facial VMs treated with argon, yellow dye, or YAG:KTP laser, satisfaction of patients was high, but recurrences were common, requiring additional treatment.[273] Intense pulsed light source technology has been reported to be effective for VMs, with small lesions requiring only two or three treatments.[274] A combination of surface laser photocoagulation and sclerotherapy can be used to treat VM of the airway.[275]

Operative Management

In general, it is preferable to shrink a VM by sclerotherapy before scheduling surgical resection.[269] Excision of a small, well-localized VM is usually successful in these cases (Fig. 106-36). In some locations, such as the hand and forearm, staged subtotal resection can be accomplished without preoperative sclerotherapy.

Gastrointestinal VMs present with chronic bleeding, attendant anemia, and transfusion requirements.

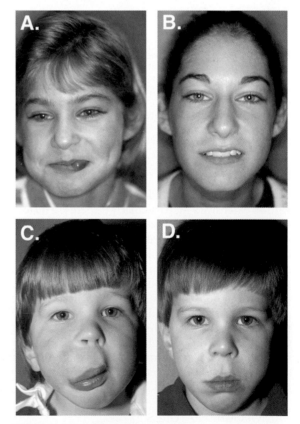

FIGURE 106-36. Sclerotherapy of venous malformation followed by resection. *A* and *C,* Before any intervention. *B* and *D,* Combined approach; lesion initially sclerosed and later surgically excised.

Whenever possible, complete resection is necessary. Excision of multifocal lesions in the gut, such as those seen in blue rubber bleb nevus syndrome, requires a commitment to identifying and removing every VM, of which there may be hundreds. Intraoperative endoscopy is used for direct visualization and transillumination of lesions, and multiple enterotomies are preferred to bowel resection to preserve bowel length.[255] Diffuse colorectal and pelvic VMs are monitored if bleeding or pain is minimal; sclerotherapy may be necessary.[276] Surgical procedures include colostomy to divert the fecal stream or colectomy with endorectal mucosectomy and an anal pull-through procedure.[277]

Arteriovenous Malformations

PATHOGENESIS

The pathogenesis of arteriovenous malformations (AVMs) is not understood. They are believed to result from errors of vascular development between the fourth and sixth weeks of embryonic gestation. Halsted[278] believed that they result from failure of arteriovenous channels in the primitive retiform plexus to regress.

Tissue in the epicenter of an AVM, termed the nidus, reveals close juxtaposition of medium-sized arteries, veins, and vessels. It is difficult, by light microscopy, to determine whether any particular abnormal vascular channel is part of the original (primary) malformation or secondarily altered by increased flow and pressure. In time, the veins become "arterialized" and exhibit intimal thickening, increased smooth muscle within the media, and dilatation of the vasa vasorum.[279] There is also progressive dilatation of the proximal arteries, with fibrosis, thinning of the media, and diminished elastic tissue.[279]

Several mechanisms have been proposed to account for the tendency of AVMs to expand to involve previously quiescent adjacent tissue. Reid[279] believed that the thin-walled arteries and veins rupture into one another, secondary to increased pressure and flow, forming new fistulous connections, an explanation for the rapid enlargement of arteriovenous anomalies that occurs after trauma or during pregnancy. Other authors have proposed that local ischemia plays a role, a result of the "steal phenomenon." It is well known that an AVM can enlarge rapidly after proximal ligation.[280-282] Hurwitz[283] proposed that the failure of enlargement of residual malformation after microvascular tissue transfer may be a result of enhanced vascularity of the reconstructed field. An intrinsic cellular abnormality has been implicated. Endothelial cells cultured from surgical AVM specimens demonstrated a higher proliferation rate, were less responsive to cytokines, and expressed a *c-ets-1* proto-oncogene, suggesting defective regulation of proliferation possibly resulting in reduced apoptosis.[284]

AVMs can cause cardiac enlargement and result in high-output cardiac failure by the direct communication between the high-resistance, high-pressure arterial system and the low-pressure, low-resistance venous system. Arteriovenous fistulas enlarge slowly and the distal vascular bed dilates as more blood is sequestered into the circuits, causing distention of the fistulas and communicating veins. The rheologic changes also stimulate the development of collateral circulation in the region of the AVM. The arteries primarily involved gradually dilate further and become tortuous (presumably because their walls are structurally faulty). The veins also dilate; there is progressive fibrosis within the intima, media, and adventitia. If the fistulas between the arterial and venous circuits are quickly occluded, the heart slows—the reflex bradycardic phenomenon first observed by Nicoladoni.[285]

CLINICAL PRESENTATION

Intracranial AVM is the most common, followed by extracranial head and neck, extremity, truncal, and visceral sites.[286] AVMs are usually noted at birth but are frequently misdiagnosed because of their innocent appearance. Usually, they are mistaken for a port-wine stain or hemangioma. Fast flow typically becomes evident during childhood. The cutaneous stain becomes more erythematous and develops local warmth, a palpable thrill, and a bruit (Fig. 106-37). A mass may expand beneath the capillary stain, occasionally with rapid enlargement after trauma or during puberty.

Later consequences of arteriovenous shunting include ischemic signs and symptoms and indolent ulceration. Intractable pain and intermittent bleeding may ensue. In the lower extremity, dry brown-violaceous plaques, known histologically as pseudo-Kaposi sarcoma, may appear. An extensive AVM can cause increased cardiac output and, ultimately, congestive heart failure. A clinical staging system, introduced by Schobinger in 1990,[287] is useful for documenting the presentation and evolution of an AVM (Table 106-1).

RADIOLOGIC FEATURES

Clinical diagnosis is confirmed by ultrasonography and color Doppler examination. On CT scan and MRI, which best document the extent of the vascular malformation, AVM is characterized by the presence of feeding and draining vessels (Fig. 106-38).[7,288] Enlarged vessels appear as areas of contrast enhancement on CT scan, as signal flow voids (black tubular structures) on spin echo MRI, and as areas of signal enhancement (white tubular structures) on gradient sequences, including magnetic resonance angiography. The intervening nidus may or may not be visible, depending on the size of the channels. AVM does not have "parenchy-

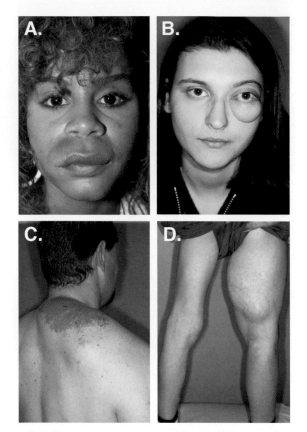

FIGURE 106-37. Morphologic variations of arteriovenous malformation. *A*, Upper lip AVM with cutaneous blush and labial enlargement. *B*, Globe involvement with proptosis. *C*, Shoulder AVM with overlying cutaneous stain. *D*, Posterior upper thigh AVM that is warm and pulsatile.

mal mass," as is seen with hemangioma, but some signal abnormalities may be evident on MRI, possibly related to a fibrofatty matrix or edema. CT and MRI frequently demonstrate increased fat, increased size and sometimes signal abnormality of affected muscle, and bone changes (including sclerosis, lytic defects, and signal changes).

Angiography shows variable degrees of arterial dilatation and tortuosity, arteriovenous shunting, and dilated draining veins. Feeding arteries may have aneurysms in older patients. Discrete fistulas can sometimes be visualized within diffuse AVM. In young children with diffuse AVM, a discrete nidus may not be identifiable.

MANAGEMENT

Except for fast-flow lesions, which may present with cardiac overload in infancy, soft tissue AVM rarely requires treatment during infancy and early childhood. Once the diagnostic evaluation is complete, the child should be observed annually. For patients with a lower extremity AVM, evaluation should include periodic assessment for limb length discrepancy. When a limb length disparity exists, a shoe-lift may be indicated to prevent limping and scoliosis. Distal femoral epiphysiodesis is necessary in older children with a major length difference.

There is discussion about the timing of resection for stage I AVMs. In rare instances, surgical excision of a well-localized stage I AVM may be warranted (Fig. 106-39). More often, intervention is done in a later stage in the natural history of an AVM, when distortion or symptoms, such as pain and ulceration, develop.

The mainstays of management are embolization, sclerotherapy, surgical resection, and reconstruction. Ligation or proximal embolization of feeding vessels should never be done. Such maneuvers deny access for embolization and result in the rapid recruitment of new vessels from adjacent arteries to supply the nidus. Angiography precedes interventional therapy or surgical extirpation for precise delineation of feeding and draining vessels. Embolization can be with coils or glue, accessing the malformation from proximal arterial or retrograde venous approaches. Sclerotherapy is another approach that may be used if tortuous arteries or feeding vessels have been ligated. This involves direct puncture of the nidus during local arterial and venous occlusion.

Complete resection is often not possible or would result in severe disfigurement, particularly in a young patient. In these instances, embolization or sclerotherapy may be used to control symptoms, such as pain, bleeding, and congestive heart failure. Typically, embolization provides only transient improvement because of recruitment of new vessels by the nidus. However, apparent "cures" have been reported with

TABLE 106-1 ✦ CLINICAL STAGING SYSTEM FOR DOCUMENTING THE PRESENTATION AND EVOLUTION OF AN AVM[290]

Stage I (quiescence)	Pink-blue stain, warmth, and arteriovenous shunting by Doppler study
Stage II (expansion)	Same as stage I plus enlargement, pulsations, thrill, bruit, and tense and tortuous veins
Stage III (destruction)	Same as stage II plus dystrophic skin changes, ulceration, tissue necrosis, bleeding, or persistent pain
Stage IV (decompensation)	Same as stage III plus cardiac failure

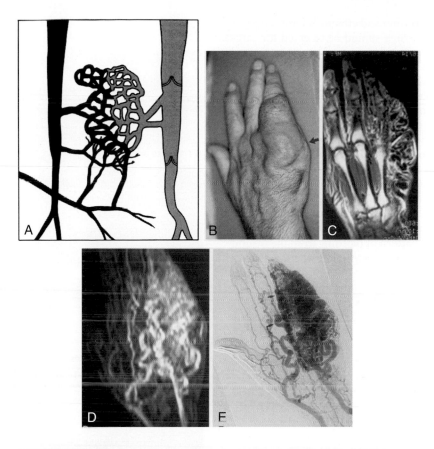

FIGURE 106-38. Imaging of arteriovenous malformation. *A*, Typical AVM demonstrating feeding arteries (black lines), draining veins (gray lines), and the typical intervening nidus composed of a plexiform vascular network. *B*, AVM of the hand in a 50-year-old man who previously underwent amputation of the small finger. *C*, T1-weighted MRI sequence demonstrating soft tissue thickening with tortuous black flow voids indicating vessels within, feeding, and draining the AVM. *D*, Magnetic resonance angiogram of the hand demonstrating AVM and dilated feeding arteries. *E*, Brachial arteriogram with digital subtraction angiography delineates AVM and aneurysmal dysplastic changes in the digital arteries. (From Burrows PE, Laor T, Paltiel H, Robertson RI : Diagnostic imaging in the evaluation of vascular birthmarks in pediatric dermatology. Dermatol Clin 1998;16:466.)

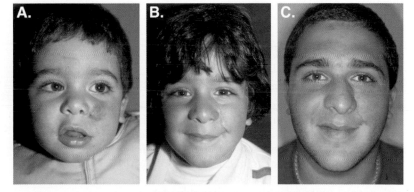

FIGURE 106-39. Early excision of arteriovenous malformation. *A*, AVM of face in infant. *B*, Five-year follow-up after surgical excision of the AVM. *C*, Follow-up during adolescence.

combined embolization and ethanol sclerotherapy.[289] This combined therapy should be reserved for carefully selected patients and performed by an experienced interventional radiologist because of the risks of severe neurologic and soft tissue damage.

When possible, embolization is done 24 to 72 hours before resection. This gives temporary occlusion of the nidus and facilitates the surgical procedure. While bleeding is minimized, the limits of resection are not diminished. The surgical goal is complete resection, unlike staged resection applicable to slow-flow vascular malformations, to minimize the chances of recurrence. The nidus, and usually involved skin, must be widely excised. Study of early magnetic resonance images and angiograms is helpful in planning the excision. The pattern of bleeding from the wound edges is the best way to determine whether the resection is adequate. Intraoperative frozen sections from the resection margins may be helpful. Linear wound closure is sometimes possible (Fig. 106-40). Primary closure often requires skin grafting (Fig. 106-41) or tissue transfer. If there is any concern about the adequacy of resection, temporary coverage with a split-thickness skin graft can be an interim measure.

Combined embolization and surgical resection is most successful for stage I or stage II well-localized AVMs.[290] Follow-up evaluation is necessary for years with clinical examination supplemented by ultrasonography or MRI. The chances of recurrence are high, and experienced surgeons recognize that a "cure" can be judged only after many years. Interestingly, recurrence has been observed to involve free flap tissue used to reconstruct a defect after incomplete excision of AVM.

Unfortunately, many AVMs are not localized. They permeate deep craniofacial structures, infiltrate the pelvic tissues, or penetrate all tissue planes of an extremity.[234] In these cases, surgical resection is rarely indicated, and embolization for palliation is the only course. These patients await the possibility of pharmacologic therapy.

Complex-Combined Malformations

EPONYMOUS VASCULAR DISORDERS

Bannayan-Riley-Ruvalcaba Syndrome

Three entities, Riley-Smith, Bannayan-Zonana, and Ruvalcaba-Myhre-Smith, once considered distinct, have been integrated as Bannayan-Riley-Ruvalcaba syndrome to reflect their overlapping clinical features.[291] The characteristic clinical features of Bannayan-Riley-Ruvalcaba syndrome are macrocephaly with normal ventricular size, multiple subcutaneous or visceral lipomas (encapsulated or diffusely

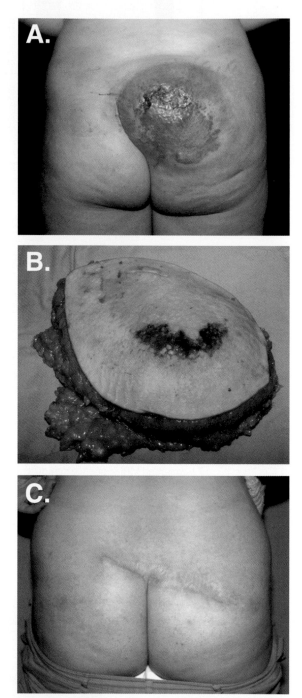

FIGURE 106-40. Delayed excision of AVM. *A,* Buttock AVM with ischemic changes typical of stage III AVM. *B,* Malformation was widely excised after embolization. *C,* Result after delayed closure with skin grafting. The AVM recurred 15 years later during the patient's third pregnancy.

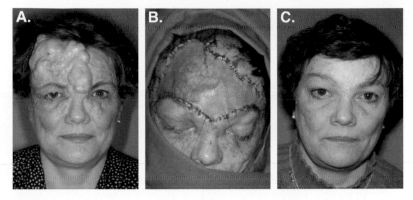

FIGURE 106-41. Cirsoid aneurysm of the scalp. *A,* Preoperative view. Note tortuous and dilated vessels. *B,* Full-thickness skin graft applied to forehead after resection. *C,* Postoperative appearance of patient 1 year later.

infiltrated), vascular anomalies, and skeletal abnormalities. At least half of the patients have central nervous system abnormalities, such as hypotonia, minor to moderate mental retardation, and seizures.[292] Additional features include hamartomatous polyps of the distal ileum and colon,[293] Hashimoto thyroiditis, and retinal abnormalities.[294] The cutaneous vascular lesions, reported to be capillary, venous, and possibly arteriovenous, are usually a minor component of the syndrome. Other cutaneous lesions include, in decreasing frequency, lentigines of the penis, facial verrucae, acanthosis nigricans, and multiple acrochordons.

This autosomal dominant disorder is caused by germline mutations in *PTEN*, a tumor suppressor gene that maps to 10q23.[295] Mutations in *PTEN* are also found in Cowden syndrome, an autosomal dominant disorder characterized by multiple hamartomas and neoplasias of ectodermal, mesodermal, and endodermal origin.[296,297] Phenotypic and genetic overlap between these two disorders has led to a proposal that Cowden and Bannayan-Riley-Ruvalcaba syndromes belong to a single genetic entity, termed *PTEN*-hamartoma tumor syndrome.[298]

Proteus Syndrome

Proteus syndrome refers to a sporadic, progressive vascular, skeletal, and soft tissue condition that lies at the interface of vascular anomalies and overgrowth syndromes. Its name is not eponymous but reflects an elusive understanding of this disorder; Proteus, the Greek god, was able to assume any shape or form to elude capture.

In response to the protean manifestations of this disorder, a consensus workshop was held at the National Institutes of Health in 1998 to recommend diagnostic criteria, differential diagnosis, and guidelines for the evaluation of patients.[299] The diagnostic criteria include three mandatory general criteria: a mosaic or asymmetric distribution of lesions, a progressive course, and sporadic occurrence.[299] In addi-

tion, some number of "category signs" must be present. These include verrucous (linear) nevus, lipomas and lipomatosis, macrocephaly (calvarial hyperostoses), asymmetric limbs with partial gigantism of the hands or feet, and curious cerebriform plantar thickening ("moccasin" feet) (Fig. 106-42). As a rule, Proteus syndrome is not present at birth. Its features suggest that this syndrome may be the result of a dominant lethal gene that survives by somatic mosaicism.[299] Interestingly, germline and germline mosaic *PTEN* mutations were found in a patient with a "Proteus-like" condition manifesting diffuse pelvic and bilateral lower extremity AVMs.[298]

Maffucci Syndrome

Maffucci syndrome denotes the coexistence of exophytic cutaneous venous malformations with bone exostoses and enchondromas.[300] This extremely rare condition typically presents in early to middle childhood. The osseous lesions appear first, most often in the hands, feet, long bones of the extremity, ribs, pelvis, and cranium.[301] There is often a history of recurrent fractures secondary to enchondromatous weakening of bone diaphyses; this occurs before the development of cutaneous vascular lesions. Typically, the patient is initially diagnosed with Ollier syndrome.

The venous malformations involve the subcutaneous tissues and bones and are generally distributed in the extremities. They can be unilateral or bilateral (Fig. 106-43). Their distribution does not necessarily correlate with that of the enchondromas. They are most commonly located on distal extremities, the hands and feet, reported to be 57.1% and 41%, respectively.[302] However, they may occur anywhere and have been reported in the leptomeninges, eyes, and lungs and throughout the gastrointestinal tract from mouth to anus.[248,303-308]

These patients often develop spindle cell hemangioendotheliomas within the venous malformations. These are thought to be a reactive vascular proliferation rather than a true tumor.[309] Malignant transfor-

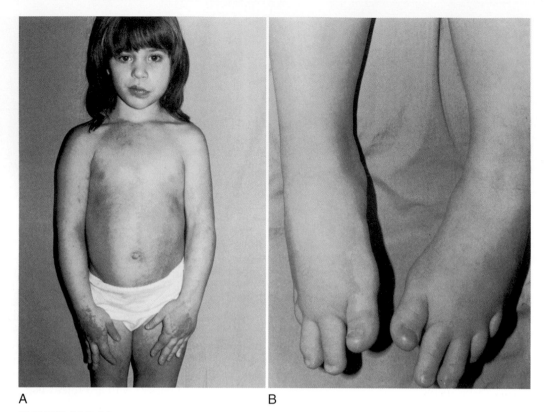

A   B

FIGURE 106-42. Proteus syndrome. *A* and *B,* A 5-year-old girl with left hemicraniofacial hypertrophy (including premature dental eruption), widespread cutaneous capillary staining, and asymmetric gigantism of the fingers and toes. (From Mulliken JB: Cutaneous vascular malformations. In McCarthy JG, ed: Plastic Surgery. Philadelphia, WB Saunders, 1990:3191.)

mation, usually chondrosarcoma, occurs in 20% to 30% of patients.[302,310] Chondrosarcomas arise from sites of enchondromas and have been reported at a variety of anatomic sites, including the cranium.[311] The average age at development of chondrosarcomas is 40 years but ranges from 13 to 69 years.[301,302,310] A majority of the chondrosarcomas are histologically low grade and often cured by surgical resection.[312,313]

The tumors in Maffucci syndrome were once thought to be exclusively mesodermal, but 30% of the tumors are of nonmesodermal origin, including ovarian tumors, hepatic adenocarcinomas, acute myelocytic and lymphoid leukemias, and pituitary and adrenal cortical adenomas.[314] Whereas the genetic basis for this disorder is not understood, this neoplastic evidence suggests that the mutation for Maffucci syndrome may involve a tumor suppressor gene.

SLOW-FLOW CAPILLARY-LYMPHATIC-VENOUS MALFORMATION (KLIPPEL-TRÉNAUNAY SYNDROME)

Klippel-Trénaunay syndrome is an old eponym for capillary-lymphatic-venous malformation (CLVM).

Unfortunately, it is often incorrectly called Klippel-Trénaunay-Weber, invoking Parkes Weber syndrome, a fast-flow vascular malformation. This disorder, diagnosed prenatally or at birth, presents with soft tissue and skeletal hypertrophy of an extremity (either in isolation or bilaterally) and may also involve the trunk. There is tremendous variability in the presentation of this disorder, from a slightly enlarged extremity with a capillary stain to a grotesquely enlarged limb with malformed digits (Fig. 106-44).

The capillary malformation component is distributed in a geographic pattern over the lateral side of the extremity, buttock, or thorax. It can be contiguous or patchy in nature. Whereas the capillary malformation is typically macular in a neonate, later it becomes studded with hemolymphatic vesicles. The venous component of CLVM manifests as abnormal drainage of the affected area. In the lower extremity, the lateral veins enlarge as a child grows, the result of incompetent valves and deep venous anomalies. There is frequently a large lateral vein, termed the vein of Servelle. The deep venous system, although occasionally normal, is often anomalous or may be entirely absent. The lymphatic abnormalities

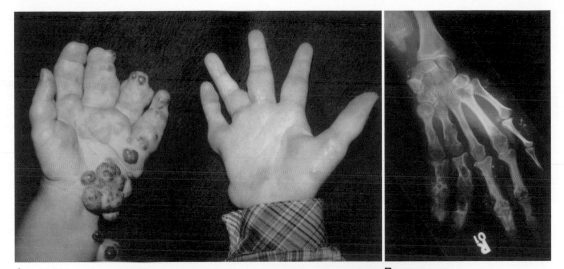

A   B

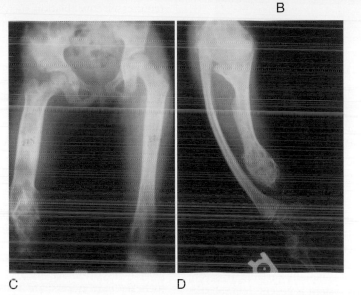

C   D

FIGURE 106-43. Maffucci syndrome. *A,* Bilateral venous malformations in hands, more pronounced on left. Radiographs demonstrate enchondromas in hand *(B),* femur *(C),* and tibia *(D).*

include hypoplasia, macrocysts, lymphoceles, and lymphedema.

Hypertrophy of an affected extremity involves bone and soft tissue structures. In general, there is progressive axial overgrowth in childhood. Sometimes the contralateral foot or hand is enlarged, often with a macrodactylous component and frequently in the absence of a capillary stain. In about 10% of patients with classic CLVM, the involved limb is short or hypotrophic.

Pelvic involvement is common with CLVM of the lower extremity. It is usually asymptomatic, although hematuria, bladder outlet obstruction, chronic cystitis secondary to intestinal flora, constipation, and hematochezia can occur. Upper extremity or truncal

CLVM can involve the posterior mediastinum and retropleural space, although this is rarely symptomatic. Thrombophlebitis occurs in 20% to 45% of patients and pulmonary embolism in 4% to 25%.[315-318]

Imaging

Plain radiographic scanograms are used to assess the length of the extremities. MRI documents the specific types and distribution of the abnormal lymphatic and venous components and soft tissue overgrowth (Fig. 106-45). Magnetic resonance venography is used to document the abnormal superficial and deep venous drainage.[319] The MRI findings are variable, reflecting the heterogeneous severity of this disorder. The lymphatic component of CLVM tends to be macrocystic

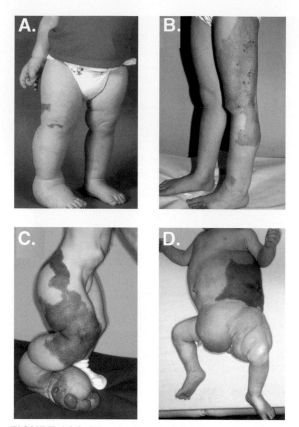

FIGURE 106-44. Morphologic forms of CLVM. Spectrum of lower extremity lesions.

anomalies, and weeping from vesicles in the capillary-lymphatic component.

OVERGROWTH. Overgrowth manifests as increased girth, axial elongation, or distortion of the limb. Limb circumference and axial length should be followed clinically in all patients, generally on an annual basis. A slightly increased limb girth is rarely a clinical problem, but axial overgrowth of the lower extremity requires careful monitoring. By 2 years of age, radiologic surveillance of leg length by plain radiography or CT scanography should be instituted. If the leg length discrepancy is more than 1.5 cm, a shoe-lift for the shorter limb can prevent limping and scoliosis. Epiphysiodesis of the distal femoral growth plate is typically done around 11 years of age. Axial overgrowth of the upper limb does not warrant intervention.

Grotesque congenital enlargement of the foot requires selective ablation, such as ray, midfoot, or Syme amputation, to permit an infant to wear proper shoes. Custom-fitted orthopedic shoes may be needed for these children. Massive circumferential enlargement of the calf, thigh, or buttock can be improved by staged contour resection. Hand involvement may necessitate procedures to improve function, such as digital or palmar debulking or ray resection of a massively enlarged digit.

Thoracic wall and abdominal CLVM is usually resected in stages. Because it is generally not an emergent problem in a neonate, staged contour resections can be initiated in early childhood. When the thoracic wall is involved, a breast bud is often affected and must be addressed in the surgical planning. Intrathoracic extension rarely requires resection unless there is restriction of mediastinal or pulmonary structures. Intestinal involvement, likewise, seldom requires surgical intervention. In rare instances, profound hematochezia may necessitate resection with a colonic pull-through procedure.

The nature of the overgrown tissue is variable, from purely fatty masses to admixed fibrous stroma and lymphatic macrocysts. Neurovascular structures should be preserved. Patients and parents should be counseled that postoperative healing may be problematic. Prolonged drainage should be expected, often necessitating a lengthy postoperative course.

SEQUELAE OF VENOUS ANOMALIES. Management of sequelae of venous involvement is conservative.[316,317] An elastic compressive stocking is recommended for patients with symptomatic venous insufficiency. Superficial varicose or incompetent veins can cause leg fatigue, heaviness, or an inability to wear shoes because of enlarged dorsal veins on the foot. Treatment options for these problems include sclerotherapy, excision, and selected venous ligation. Sclerotherapy is helpful in obliterating troublesome superficial veins or shrinking focal venous

in the pelvis and thighs and microcystic in the abdominal wall, buttock, and distal limb. It can be predominantly subcutaneous or diffusely infiltrative in muscle. The venous component is equally variable. In severe cases, the deep venous system is absent, hypoplastic, or interrupted with venous drainage occurring through dilated, valveless, superficial veins. The pathognomonic marginal vein (of Servelle) is identified in the subcutaneous fat of the lateral calf and thigh, communicating with the deep venous system at multiple levels.

Contrast venography is used in selected patients to delineate the venous drainage of an extremity before resection or sclerotherapy is considered. It is technically challenging in these patients, however, and may require multiple injections with various compressive maneuvers. Angiography may reveal small, discrete arteriovenous fistulas in the proximal extremity, but this finding is not clinically significant. Lymphoscintigraphy is also unlikely to help in the management of these patients.

Management

Treatment is aimed at the sequelae of this complex malformation, such as overgrowth, consequences of venous

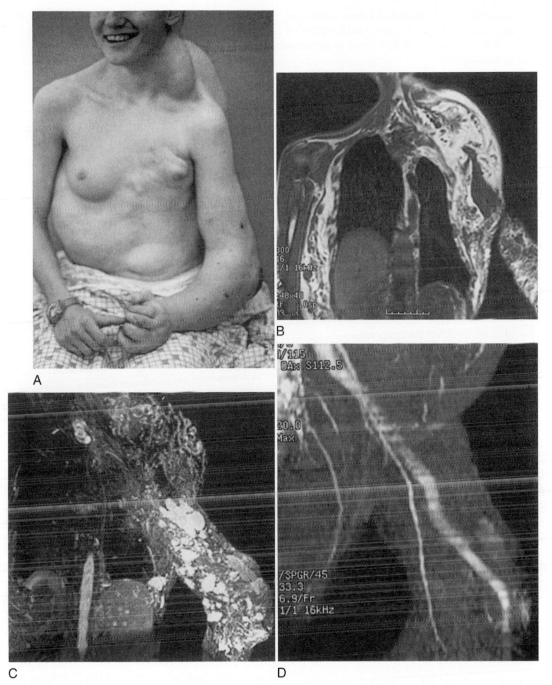

FIGURE 106-45. Imaging of CLVM. *A,* Upper extremity CLVM in a 17-year-old girl. *B,* T1-weighted coronal MRI with high signal tissue in the neck, left arm, and chest wall bilaterally representative of abnormal fat. *C,* T2-weighted coronal MRI demonstrates cystic lymphatic components within the malformation. *D,* Magnetic resonance venogram reveals large anomalous venous channel in left arm. (From Burrows PE, Laor T, Paltiel H, Robertson RL: Diagnostic imaging in the evaluation of vascular birthmarks in pediatric dermatology. Dermatol Clin 1998;16:478.)

malformations or lymphatic cysts in these combined malformations. Direct surgical excision of affected veins as well as subfascial endoscopic ligation of perforators may also be considered.

Before any surgical intervention for CLVM, the anatomy of the deep venous system must be thoroughly evaluated. Unless a deep system is present and functioning, sclerotherapy, excision, or ligation may predispose to venous congestion in an affected extremity. In patients who lack a functional deep system but have recalcitrant symptoms, reconstruction of a deep system, if possible, should precede any other intervention.[316]

BLEEDING FROM LYMPHATIC VESICLES. Intermittent oozing from lymphatic vesicles in areas of capillary malformation is an annoying problem for many patients. Compression with custom-fitted elastic garments helps flatten the vesicles. If this fails, the direct injection of vesicles with 1% sodium tetradecyl sulfate can be effective, but it often has to be repeated. Laser photocoagulation has not been effective. If bleeding persists, other alternatives include excision of underlying veins or subfascial ligation of the perforators feeding the area of the vesicles, embolization of microfistulas by interventional radiology techniques, and excision of the area of vesicular capillary malformation and replacement with a split-thickness skin graft.

FAST-FLOW CAPILLARY-ARTERIOVENOUS MALFORMATION (PARKES WEBER SYNDROME)

Parkes Weber syndrome, first described in 1907, is a timeworn eponym for complex high-flow AVM that permeates throughout a limb. This malformation is evident at birth with symmetric enlargement and pink staining of the involved limb. The lower limb is more frequently involved than the upper. The cutaneous stain tends to be confluent rather than patchy and is typically warmer than a banal capillary malformation (Fig. 106-46). The diagnosis is confirmed by the detection of a bruit or thrill. In extreme cases, a neonate may be in cardiac failure.

Imaging

Overgrowth in an affected extremity is subcutaneous, muscular, and bony with diffuse microfistulas. The enlarged limb muscles and bones exhibit an abnormal signal and enhancement. Magnetic resonance angiography and venography show generalized arterial and venous dilatation. Angiography can demonstrate discrete arteriovenous shunts, particularly around joint structures. Anomalous superficial veins resembling those seen in CLVM may be present.

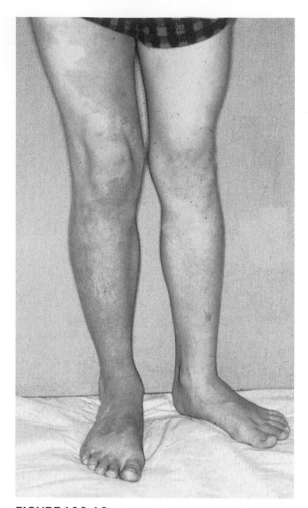

FIGURE 106-46. Parkes Weber syndrome. Dense capillary staining of lower extremity with overgrowth of length and girth. Limb is warm because of diffuse microarteriovenous shunting in skin and muscle.

Management

In rare instances, an infant with capillary-arteriovenous malformation presents in the neonatal period with high-output congestive heart failure and anasarca secondary to shunting through arteriovenous fistulas in the involved extremity. This situation mandates emergent embolization with permanent occlusive agents, often followed by repeated procedures.

Typically, these children are observed annually with careful monitoring for axial overgrowth and development of cutaneous problems. Baseline ultrasonography and color Doppler evaluation of the arterial flow are indicated when the child is 3 or 4 years of age. Treatment is predicated on symptoms. Embolization may be useful for pain or cutaneous ischemic changes.

CONCLUSION

Patients with vascular anomalies have all too often been medical "nomads." During infancy and childhood, their parents took them from one physician to another, and no one seemed to understand the condition. In the past, the problem was often that these vascular anomalies lay in the interface between several medical and surgical specialties. No single specialist had sufficient knowledge to treat the wide variety of vascular disorders.

During the past decade, terminologic confusion has been replaced with an evolving standardization in the field of vascular anomalies. Interested specialists can now communicate effectively with one another. Vascular anomaly teams, composed of various disciplines on the basis of local interest, enthusiasm, and capabilities, are evolving in many major referral centers. These teams are in a unique position because the collective knowledge of such a group provides a forum for problems that otherwise appear "too complicated" or "insoluble." In addition, they serve as a focus for clinical and basic research in this field. The development of databases to record specific information about diagnoses, natural histories, treatments, and responses to treatments will allow outcome studies of larger groups and help guide implementation of specific therapies.

The Internet has had an impact on the referral pattern and care of these patients, allowing individuals with uncommon disorders to unite, share information, and seek knowledge. Family support groups have arisen to fill a need, and many of these have provided admirable service to both families and physicians.

REFERENCES

1. Mulliken JB, Young A: Vascular Birthmarks: Hemangiomas and Malformations. Philadelphia, WB Saunders, 1988.
2. Virchow R: Angioma in die Krankhaften Geschwulste, vol 3. Berlin, Hirschwald, 1863:306-425.
3. Wegener G: Über Lymphangiome. Arch Klin Chir 1877;20:641-707.
4. Mulliken JB, Glowacki J: Hemangiomas and vascular malformations in infants and children: a classification based on endothelial characteristics. Plast Reconstr Surg 1982;69:412-422.
5. Enjolras O, Mulliken JB: Vascular tumors and vascular malformations (new issues). Adv Dermatol 1998;13:375-423.
6. Burrows PE, Mulliken JB, Fellows KE, Strand RD: Childhood hemangiomas and vascular malformations: angiographic differentiation. AJR Am J Roentgenol 1983;141:483-488.
7. Meyer JS, Hoffer FA, Barnes PD, Mulliken JB: Biological classification of soft-tissue vascular anomalies: MR correlation. AJR Am J Roentgenol 1991;157:559-564.
8. Huston JD, Forbes GS, Ruefenacht DA, et al: Magnetic resonance imaging of facial vascular anomalies. Mayo Clin Proc 1992;67:739-747.
9. Burrows PE, Laor T, Paltiel H, Robertson RL: Diagnostic imaging in the evaluation of vascular birthmarks. Dermatol Clin 1998;16:455-488.
10. Dubois J, Garel L, Grignon A, et al: Imaging of hemangiomas and vascular malformations in children. Acad Radiol 1998;5:390-400.
11. Takahashi K, Mulliken JB, Kozakewich HP, et al: Cellular markers that distinguish the phases of hemangioma during infancy and childhood. J Clin Invest 1994;93:2357-2364.
12. North PE, Waner M, Mizeracki A, Mihm MC Jr: GLUT1: a newly discovered immunohistochemical marker for juvenile hemangiomas. Hum Pathol 2000;31:11-22.
13. Finn MC, Glowacki J, Mulliken JB: Congenital vascular lesions: clinical application of a new classification. J Pediatr Surg 1983;18:894-900.
14. Folkman JB, Mulliken J, Ezekowitz RAB: Angiogenesis and hemangiomas. In Oldham K, Colombani P, Foglio R, eds: Surgery of Infants and Children: Scientific Principles and Practice. Philadelphia, Lippincott-Raven, 1997:569-579.
15. Gonzalez-Crussi F, Reyes-Mugica M: Cellular hemangiomas (hemangioendotheliomas) in infants. Light microscopic, immunohistochemical, and ultrastructural observations. Am J Surg Pathol 1991;15:769-778.
16. Kräling BM, Razon MJ, Boon LM, et al: E-selectin is present in proliferating endothelial cells in human hemangiomas. Am J Pathol 1996;148:1181-1191.
17. Chang J, Most D, Bresnick S, et al: Proliferative hemangiomas: analysis of cytokine gene expression and angiogenesis. Plast Reconstr Surg 1999;103:1-9.
18. Chang E, Boyd A, Nelson CC, et al: Successful treatment of infantile hemangiomas with interferon-alpha-2b. J Pediatr Hematol Oncol 1997;19:237-244.
19. Isik FF, Rand RP, Gruss JS, et al: Monocyte chemoattractant protein-1 mRNA expression in hemangiomas and vascular malformations. J Surg Res 1996;61:71-76.
20. Jang YC, Arumugam S, Ferguson M, et al: Changes in matrix composition during the growth and regression of human hemangiomas. J Surg Res 1998;80:9-15.
21. Hasan Q, Ruger BM, Tan ST, et al: Clusterin/apJ expression during the development of hemangioma. Hum Pathol 2000;31:691-697.
22. Tan ST, Velickovic M, Ruger BM, Davis PF: Cellular and extracellular markers of hemangioma. Plast Reconstr Surg 2000;106:529-538.
23. Bielenberg DR, Bucana CD, Sanchez R, et al: Progressive growth of infantile cutaneous hemangiomas is directly correlated with hyperplasia and angiogenesis of adjacent epidermis and inversely correlated with expression of the endogenous angiogenesis inhibitor, IFN-beta. Int J Oncol 1999;14:401-408.
24. Mulliken JB, Zetter BR, Folkman J: In vitro characteristics of endothelium from hemangiomas and vascular malformations. Surgery 1982;92:348-353.
25. Berard M, Sordello S, Ortega N, et al: Vascular endothelial growth factor confers a growth advantage in vitro and in vivo to stromal cells cultured from neonatal hemangiomas. Am J Pathol 1997;150:1315-1326.
26. Dethlefsen SM, Mulliken JB, Glowacki J: An ultrastructural study of mast cell interactions in hemangiomas. Ultrastruct Pathol 1986;10:175-183.
27. Glowacki J, Mulliken JB: Mast cells in hemangiomas and vascular malformations. Pediatrics 1982;70:48-51.
28. Razon MJ, Kräling BM, Mulliken JB, Bischoff J: Increased apoptosis coincides with onset of involution in infantile hemangioma. Microcirculation 1998;5:189-195.
29. Höpfel-Kreiner I: Histogenesis of hemangiomas: an ultrastructural study on capillary and cavernous hemangiomas of the skin. Pathol Res Pract 1980;170:70-90.
30. Dosanjh A, Chang J, Bresnick S, et al: In vitro characteristics of neonatal hemangioma endothelial cells: similarities and differences between normal neonatal and fetal endothelial cells. J Cutan Pathol 2000;27:441-450.

31. Lyttle DJ, Fraser KM, Fleming SB, et al: Homologs of vascular endothelial growth factor are encoded by the poxvirus orf virus. J Virol 1994;68:84-92.

32. Dupin N, Enjolras O, Wassef M, et al: Absence of HHV-8 virus detected in immature hemangiomas in infants. Ann Dermatol Venereol 1998;125:98-99.

33. Soffer D, Resnick-Roguel N, Eldor A, Kotler M: Multifocal vascular tumors in fowl induced by a newly isolated retrovirus. Cancer Res 1990;50:4787-4793.

34. Williams RL, Risau W, Zerwes HG, et al: Endothelioma cells expressing the polyoma middle T oncogene induce hemangiomas by host cell recruitment. Cell 1989;57:1053-1063.

35. Liekens S, Verbeken E, Vandeputte M, et al: A novel animal model for hemangiomas: inhibition of hemangioma development by the angiogenesis inhibitor TNP-470. Cancer Res 1999;59:2376-2383.

36. Hoak JC, Warner ED, Cheng HF, et al: Hemangioma with thrombocytopenia and microangiopathic anemia (Kasabach-Merritt syndrome): an animal model. J Lab Clin Med 1971;77:941-950.

37. Lannutti BJ, Gately ST, Quevedo ME, et al: Human angiostatin inhibits murine hemangioendothelioma tumor growth in vivo. Cancer Res 1997;57:5277-5280.

38. Wang C, Quevedo ME, Lannutti BJ, et al: In vivo gene therapy with interleukin-12 inhibits primary vascular tumor growth and induces apoptosis in a mouse model. J Invest Dermatol 1999;112:775-781.

39. Verheul HM, Panigrahy D, Flynn E, et al: Treatment of the Kasabach-Merritt syndrome with pegylated recombinant human megakaryocyte growth and development factor in mice: elevated platelet counts, prolonged survival, and tumor growth inhibition. Pediatr Res 1999;46:562-565.

40. Cheung DS, Warman ML, Mulliken JB: Hemangioma in twins. Ann Plast Surg 1997;38:269-274.

41. Blei F, Walter J, Orlow SJ, Marchuk DA: Familial segregation of hemangiomas and vascular malformations as an autosomal dominant trait [published erratum appears in Arch Dermatol 1998;134:1425]. Arch Dermatol 1998;134:718-722.

42. Walter JW, Blei F, Anderson JL, et al: Genetic mapping of a novel familial form of infantile hemangioma. Am J Med Genet 1999;82:77-83.

43. Boye E, Yu Y, Paranya G, et al: Clonality and altered behavior of endothelial cells from hemangiomas. J Clin Invest 2001;107:745-752.

44. Holmdahl K: Cutaneous hemangiomas in premature and mature infants. Acta Paediatr 1955;44:70-79.

45. Enjolras O, Riché MC, Merland JJ, Escande JP: Management of alarming hemangiomas in infancy: a review of 25 cases. Pediatrics 1990;85:491-498.

46. Gorlin RJ, Kantaputra P, Aughton DJ, Mulliken JB: Marked female predilection in some syndromes associated with facial hemangiomas. Am J Med Genet 1994;52:130-135.

47. Enjolras O, Gelbert F: Superficial hemangiomas: associations and management. Pediatr Dermatol 1997;14:173-179.

48. Boon LM, MacDonald DM, Mulliken JB: Complications of systemic corticosteroid therapy for problematic hemangioma. Plast Reconstr Surg 1999;104:1616-1623.

49. Amir J, Metzker A, Krikler R, Reisner SH: Strawberry hemangioma in preterm infants. Pediatr Dermatol 1986;3:331-332.

50. Bowers R, Graham E, Tomlinson K: The natural history of the strawberry nevus. Arch Dermatol 1960;82:667-680.

51. Boyd JB, Mulliken JB, Kaban LB, et al: Skeletal changes associated with vascular malformations. Plast Reconstr Surg 1984;74:789-797.

52. Boon LM, Enjolras O, Mulliken JB: Congenital hemangioma: evidence of accelerated involution. J Pediatr 1996;128:329-335.

53. Enjolras O, Mulliken JB, Boon LM, et al: Non-involuting hemangioma: a rare cutaneous vascular anomaly. Plast Reconstr Surg 2001;107:1647-1654.

54. Boon LM, Burrows PE, Paltiel HJ, et al: Hepatic vascular anomalies in infancy: a twenty-seven-year experience. J Pediatr 1996;129:346-354.

55. Berman B, Lim H: Concurrent cutaneous and hepatic hemangiomata in infancy: report of a case and a review of the literature. J Dermatol Surg Oncol 1978;4:869-873.

56. Selby DM, Stocker JT, Waclawiw MA, et al: Infantile hemangioendothelioma of the liver. Hepatology 1994;20:39-45.

57. Martinez-Perez D, Fein NA, Boon LM, Mulliken JB: Not all hemangiomas look like strawberries: uncommon presentations of the most common tumor of infancy. Pediatr Dermatol 1995;12:1-6.

58. Vin-Christian K, McCalmont TH, Frieden IJ: Kaposiform hemangioendothelioma. An aggressive, locally invasive vascular tumor that can mimic hemangioma of infancy. Arch Dermatol 1997;133:1573-1578.

59. Jones EW, Orkin M: Tufted angioma (angioblastoma). A benign progressive angioma, not to be confused with Kaposi's sarcoma or low-grade angiosarcoma. J Am Acad Dermatol 1989;20:214-225.

60. Chung KC, Weiss SW, Kuzon WM Jr: Multifocal congenital hemangiopericytomas associated with Kasabach-Merritt syndrome. Br J Plast Surg 1995;48:240-242.

61. Boon LM, Fishman SJ, Lund DP, Mulliken JB: Congenital fibrosarcoma masquerading as congenital hemangioma: report of two cases. J Pediatr Surg 1995;30:1378-1381.

62. Burns A, Kaplan L, Mulliken J: Is there an association between hemangiomas and syndromes with dysmorphic features? Pediatrics 1991;88:1257-1267.

63. Frieden IJ, Reese V, Cohen D: PHACE syndrome. The association of posterior fossa brain malformations, hemangiomas, arterial anomalies, coarctation of the aorta and cardiac defects, and eye abnormalities. Arch Dermatol 1996;132:307-311.

64. Pascual-Castroviejo I, Viano J, Moreno F, et al: Hemangiomas of the head, neck, and chest with associated vascular and brain anomalies: a complex neurocutaneous syndrome. AJNR Am J Neuroradiol 1996;17:461-471.

65. Burrows PE, Robertson RL, Mulliken JB, et al: Cerebral vasculopathy and neurologic sequelae in infants with cervicofacial hemangioma: report of eight patients. Radiology 1998;207:601-607.

66. Schneeweiss A, Blieden LC, Shem-Tov A, et al: Coarctation of the aorta with congenital hemangioma of the face and neck and aneurysm or dilatation of a subclavian or innominate artery. A new syndrome? Chest 1982;82:186-187.

67. Vaillant L, Lorette G, Chantepie A, et al: Multiple cutaneous hemangiomas and coarctation of the aorta with right aortic arch. Pediatrics 1988;81:707-710.

68. Kishnani P, Iafolla AK, McConkie-Rosell A, et al: Hemangioma, supraumbilical midline raphe, and coarctation of the aorta with a right aortic arch: single causal entity? Am J Med Genet 1995;59:44-48.

69. Reese V, Frieden IJ, Paller AS, et al: Association of facial hemangiomas with Dandy-Walker and other posterior fossa malformations. J Pediatr 1993;122:379-384.

70. Goldberg NS, Hebert AA, Esterly NB: Sacral hemangiomas and multiple congenital abnormalities. Arch Dermatol 1986;122:684-687.

71. Albright AL, Gartner JC, Wiener ES: Lumbar cutaneous hemangiomas as indicators of tethered spinal cords. Pediatrics 1989;83:977-980.

72. Bouchard S, Yazbeck S, Lallier M: Perineal hemangioma, anorectal malformation, and genital anomaly: a new association? J Pediatr Surg 1999;34:1133-1135.

73. Dubois J, Patriquin HB, Garel L, et al: Soft-tissue hemangiomas in infants and children: diagnosis using Doppler sonography. AJR Am J Roentgenol 1998;171:247-252.

74. Paltiel HJ, Burrows PE, Kozakewich HP, et al: Soft-tissue vascular anomalies: utility of US for diagnosis. Radiology 2000;214:747-754.

75. Barton DJ, Miller JH, Allwright SJ, Sloan GM: Distinguishing soft-tissue hemangiomas from vascular malformations using technetium-labeled red blood cell scintigraphy. Plast Reconstr Surg 1992;89:46-52.

76. Tanner JL, Dechert MP, Frieden IJ: Growing up with a facial hemangioma: parent and child coping and adaptation. Pediatrics 1998;101:446-452.

77. Enjolras O, Mulliken JB: The current management of vascular birthmarks. Pediatr Dermatol 1993;10:311-313.

78. Margileth AM, Museles M: Cutaneous hemangiomas in children. Diagnosis and conservative management. JAMA 1965;194:523-526.

79. Drolet BA, Esterly NB, Frieden IJ: Hemangiomas in children. N Engl J Med 1999;341:173-181.

80. Achauer BM, VanderKam VM: Ulcerated anogenital hemangioma of infancy. Plast Reconstr Surg 1991;87:861-866.

81. Morelli JG, Tan OT, Yohn JJ, Weston WL: Treatment of ulcerated hemangiomas infancy. Arch Pediatr Adolesc Med 1994;148:1104-1105.

82. Orlow SJ, Isakoff MS, Blei F: Increased risk of symptomatic hemangiomas of the airway in association with cutaneous hemangiomas in a "beard" distribution. J Pediatr 1997;131:643-646.

83. Sherrington CA, Sim DK, Freezer NJ, Robertson CF: Subglottic haemangioma. Arch Dis Child 1997;76:458-459.

84. Reyes BA, Vazquez-Botet M, Capo H: Intralesional steroids in cutaneous hemangioma. J Dermatol Surg Oncol 1989;15:828-832.

85. Sloan GM, Reinisch JF, Nichter LS, et al: Intralesional corticosteroid therapy for infantile hemangiomas. Plast Reconstr Surg 1989;83:459-467.

86. Ruttum MS, Abrams GW, Harris GJ, Ellis MK: Bilateral retinal embolization associated with intralesional corticosteroid injection for capillary hemangioma of infancy. J Pediatr Ophthalmol Strabismus 1993;30:4-7.

87. Sutula FC, Glover AT: Eyelid necrosis following intralesional corticosteroid injection for capillary hemangioma. Ophthalmic Surg 1987;18:103-105.

88. Elsas FJ, Lewis AR: Topical treatment of periocular capillary hemangioma. J Pediatr Ophthalmol Strabismus 1994;31:153-156.

89. Ozsoylu S: Megadose methylprednisolone for diffuse infantile haemangiomatosis [letter]. Eur J Pediatr 1992;151:389.

90. Ozsoylu S: Oral megadose methylprednisolone for the treatment of giant hemangiomas [letter]. J Pediatr Hematol Oncol 1995;17:85.

91. Sadan N, Wolach B: Treatment of hemangiomas of infants with high doses of prednisone [see comments]. J Pediatr 1996;128:141-146.

92. White CW, Wolf SJ, Korones DL, et al: Treatment of childhood angiomatous diseases with recombinant interferon alfa-2a. J Pediatr 1991;118:59-66.

93. Ezekowitz RA, Mulliken JB, Folkman J: Interferon alfa 2a therapy for life-threatening hemangiomas of infancy [published erratum appear in N Engl J Med 1994;330:300 and 1995;333:595-596]. N Engl J Med 1992;326:1456-1463.

94. Ricketts RR, Hatley RM, Corden BJ, et al: Interferon alpha-2a for the treatment of complex hemangiomas of childhood and infancy. Ann Surg 1994;219:605-612.

95. Soumekh B, Adams GL, Shapiro RS: Treatment of head and neck hemangiomas with recombinant interferon alpha-2B. Ann Otol Rhinol Laryngol 1994;105:201-206.

96. Deb G, Donfrancesco A, DeSio L, Standoli L: Treatment of hemangiomas of infants and babies with interferon alfa 2a: preliminary results. Int J Pediatr Hematol Oncol 1996;3:109-113.

97. Tamayo L, Ortiz DM, Orozco-Covarrubias L, et al: Therapeutic efficacy of interferon alfa-2b in infants with life-threatening giant hemangiomas. Arch Dermatol 1997;133:1567-1571.

98. Greinwald JH, Burke DK, Bonthius DJ, et al: An update on the treatment of hemangiomas in children with interferon alfa-2a. Arch Otolaryngol Head Neck Surg 1999;125:21-27.

99. Mulliken JB, Boon LM, Takahashi K, et al: Pharmacologic therapy for endangering hemangiomas. Curr Opin Dermatol 1995;2:109-113.

100. Singh RK, Gutman M, Bucana CD, et al: Interferons alpha and beta down-regulate the expression of basic fibroblast growth factor in human carcinomas. Proc Natl Acad Sci USA 1995;92:4562-4566.

101. Dinney CP, Bielenberg DR, Perrotte P, et al: Inhibition of basic fibroblast growth factor expression, angiogenesis, and growth of human bladder carcinoma in mice by systemic interferon-alpha administration. Cancer Res 1998;58:808-814.

102. Kaban LB, Mulliken JB, Ezekowitz RA, et al: Antiangiogenic therapy of a recurrent giant cell tumor of the mandible with interferon alfa-2a. Pediatrics 1999;103:1145-1149.

103. Dubois J, Hershon L, Carmant L, et al: Toxicity profile of interferon alfa-2b in children: a prospective evaluation. J Pediatr 1999;135:782-785.

104. Barlow CF, Priebe CJ, Mulliken JB, et al: Spastic diplegia as a complication of interferon alfa-2a treatment of hemangiomas of infancy. J Pediatr 1998;132:527-530.

105. Iyer CP, Stanley P, Mahour GH: Hepatic hemangiomas in infants and children: a review of 30 cases. Am Surg 1996;62:356-360.

106. Garden JM, Bakus AD, Paller AS: Treatment of cutaneous hemangiomas by the flashlamp-pumped pulsed dye laser: prospective analysis. J Pediatr 1992;120:555-560.

107. Mulliken JB: A plea for a biologic approach to hemangiomas of infancy [editorial]. Arch Dermatol 1991;127:243-244.

108. Ashinoff R, Geronemus RG: Failure of the flashlamp-pumped pulsed dye laser to prevent progression to deep hemangioma. Pediatr Dermatol 1993;10:77-80.

109. Scheepers JH, Quaba AA: Does the pulsed tunable dye laser have a role in the management of infantile hemangiomas? Observations based on 3 years' experience. Plast Reconstr Surg 1995;95:305-312.

110. Sie KC, McGill T, Healy GB: Subglottic hemangioma: ten years' experience with the carbon dioxide laser. Ann Otol Rhinol Laryngol 1994;103:167-172.

111. Berlien HP, Muller G, Waldschmidt J: Lasers in pediatric surgery. Prog Pediatr Surg 1990;25:5-22.

112. Achauer BM, Celikoz B, VanderKam VM: Intralesional bare fiber laser treatment of hemangioma of infancy. Plast Reconstr Surg 1998;101:1212-1217.

113. Achauer BM, Chang CJ, VanderKam VM, Baybo A: Intralesional photocoagulation of periorbital hemangiomas. Plast Reconstr Surg 1999;103:11-16.

114. Mulliken JB: Intralesional photocoagulation of periorbital hemangiomas [discussion]. Plast Reconstr Surg 1999;103:17-19.

115. Thomson HG, Ward CM, Crawford JS, Stigmar G: Hemangioma of the eyelid: visual complications and prophylactic concepts. Plast Reconstr Surg 1979;63:641-647.

116. Deans RM, Harris GJ, Kivlin JD: Surgical dissection of capillary hemangiomas. An alternative to intralesional corticosteroids. Arch Ophthalmol 1992;110:1743-1747.

117. Mulliken JB: Special symposium: management of hemangiomas. Frieden IJ, ed. Pediatr Dermatol 1997;14:760-762.

118. Mulliken JB, Rogers GF, Marler JJ: Circular excision of hemangioma and purse-string closure: the smallest possible scar. Plast Reconstr Surg 2002;109:1544-1554.
119. Patrice SJ, Wiss K, Mulliken JB: Pyogenic granuloma (lobular capillary hemangioma): a clinicopathologic study of 178 cases. Pediatr Dermatol 1991;8:267-276.
120. Kirschner RE, Low DW: Treatment of pyogenic granuloma by shave excision and laser photocoagulation. Plast Reconstr Surg 1999;104:1346-1349.
121. Zukerberg LR, Nickoloff BJ, Weiss SW: Kaposiform hemangioendothelioma of infancy and childhood. An aggressive neoplasm associated with Kasabach-Merritt syndrome and lymphangiomatosis. Am J Surg Pathol 1993;17:321-328.
122. Enjolras O, Wassef M, Mazoyer E, et al: Infants with Kasabach-Merritt syndrome do not have true hemangiomas. J Pediatr 1997;130:631-640.
123. Sarkar M, Mulliken JB, Kozakewich HP, et al: Thrombocytopenic coagulopathy (Kasabach-Merritt phenomenon) is associated with kaposiform hemangioendothelioma and not with common infantile hemangioma. Plast Reconstr Surg 1997;100:1377-1386.
124. Enjolras O, Mulliken JB, Wassef M, et al: Residual lesions after Kasabach-Merritt phenomenon in 41 patients. J Am Acad Dermatol 2000;42:225-235.
125. Trelat U, Monod A: De l'hypertrophie unilaterale partielle ou totale du corps. Arch Gen Med 1869;13:636.
126. Johnston M: Radioautographic study of the migration and fate of cranial neural crests in the chick embryo. Anat Rec 1966;156:143-155.
127. Nozue T, Tsuzaki M: Further studies on distribution of neural crest cells in prenatal or postnatal development in mice. Okajimas Folia Anat Jpn 1974;51:131-160.
128. Smoller BR, Rosen S: Port-wine stains. A disease of altered neural modulation of blood vessels? Arch Dermatol 1986;122:177-179.
129. Cunha e Sa M, Barroso CP, Caldas MC, et al: Innervation pattern of malformative cortical vessels in Sturge-Weber disease: an histochemical, immunohistochemical, and ultrastructural study. Neurosurgery 1997;41:872-876.
130. Jacobs AH, Walton RG: The incidence of birthmarks in the neonate. Pediatrics 1976;58:218-222.
131. Enjolras O, Riché MC, Merland JJ: Facial port-wine stains and Sturge-Weber syndrome. Pediatrics 1985;76:48-51.
132. Cobb S: Haemangioma of the spinal cord associated with skin nevi of the same metamere. Ann Surg 1915;62:641.
133. Doppman JL, Wirth FP Jr, Di Chiro G, Ommaya AK: Value of cutaneous angiomas in the arteriographic localization of spinal-cord arteriovenous malformations. N Engl J Med 1969;281:1440-1444.
134. Jessen RT, Thompson S, Smith EB: Cobb syndrome. Arch Dermatol 1977;113:1587-1590.
135. Bauer S: Pediatric neurology. In Krane R, Siroky M, eds: Clinical Neurourology. Boston, Little, Brown, 1988.
136. Squire B: An improvement in the treatment of port-wine mark by linear scarification. Br Med J 1879;2:732.
137. Beard G: Cases of naevi treated by electrolysis. N Y Med J 1877;26:616.
138. Morton E: The treatment of naevi and other cutaneous lesions by electrolysis, cautery and refrigeration. Lancet 1909;2:1658.
139. Kromayer EL: Die Behandlung der roten Muttermale mit Licht und Radium nach Erfahrungen und 40 Fallen. Dtsch Med Wochenschr 1910;36:299.
140. MacCollum D: Treatment of hemangiomas. Am J Surg 1935;29:32.
141. Bowers R: Treatment of haemangiomatous naevi with thorium X. Br Med J 1951;1:121.
142. Jonsson G: New method of treating capillary haemangiomas. Acta Chir Scand 1947;95:275.
143. Morel-Fatio D: Essai de traitement des angiomes plans par poncage coloré de la peau congelée. Ann Chir Plast 1964;19:326-329.
144. Goldwyn RM, Rosoff CB: Cryosurgery for large hemangiomas in adults. Plast Reconstr Surg 1969;43:605-611.
145. Brown J, Cannon B, McDowell A: Permanent pigment injection of capillary hemangiomata. Plast Reconstr Surg 1946;1:106.
146. Conway H: Evolution of treatment of capillary hemangiomas of the face with further observation on the value of camouflage by permanent pigment injection (tattooing). Surgery 1948;23:389.
147. Conway H, McKinney P, Climo M: Permanent camouflage of vascular nevi of the face by intradermal injection of insoluble pigments (tattooing): experience through twenty years with 1022 cases. Plast Reconstr Surg 1967;40:457-462.
148. Thomson HG, Wright AM: Surgical tattooing of the port-wine stain. Operative technique, results, and critique. Plast Reconstr Surg 1971;48:113-120.
149. Grabb WC, MacCollum M, Tan NG: Results from tattooing port-wine hemangiomas. A long-term follow-up. Plast Reconstr Surg 1977;59:667-669.
150. Cosman B: Clinical experience in the laser therapy of port wine stains. Lasers Surg Med 1980;1:133-152.
151. Mills CM, Lanigan SW, Hughes J, Anstey AV: Demographic study of port wine stain patients attending a laser clinic: family history, prevalence of naevus anaemicus and results of prior treatment. Clin Exp Dermatol 1997;22:166-168.
152. Tan OT, Sherwood K, Gilchrest BA: Treatment of children with port-wine stains using the flashlamp-pulsed tunable dye laser. N Engl J Med 1989;320:416-421.
153. van der Horst CM, Koster PH, de Borgie CA, et al: Effect of the timing of treatment of port-wine stains with the flashlamp-pumped pulsed-dye laser. N Engl J Med 1998;338:1028-1033.
154. Orten SS, Waner M, Flock S, et al: Port-wine stains. An assessment of 5 years of treatment. Arch Otolaryngol Head Neck Surg 1996;122:1174-1179.
155. Dummer R, Graf P, Greif C, Burg G: Treatment of vascular lesions using the VersaPulse variable pulse width frequency doubled neodymium:YAG laser. Dermatology 1998;197:158-161.
156. Chan HH, Chan E, Kono T, et al: The use of variable pulse width frequency doubled Nd:YAG 532 nm laser in the treatment of port-wine stain in Chinese patients. Dermatol Surg 2000;26:657-661.
157. Sommer S, Sheehan-Dare RA: Pulsed dye laser treatment of port-wine stains in pigmented skin. J Am Acad Dermatol 2000;42:667-671.
158. Clodius L: Excision and grafting of extensive facial haemangiomas. Br J Plast Surg 1977;30:185-196.
159. Clodius L: Surgery for the facial port-wine stain: technique and results. Ann Plast Surg 1986;16:457-471.
160. Clodius L, Smahel J: Resurfacing denuded areas of the beard with full thickness scalp grafts. Br J Plast Surg 1979;32:295-299.
161. Argenta LC, Watanabe MJ, Grabb WC: The use of tissue expansion in head and neck reconstruction. Ann Plast Surg 1983;11:31-37.
162. Zide BM, Glat PM, Stile FL, Longaker MT: Vascular lip enlargement: Part II. Port-wine macrocheilia—tenets of therapy based on normative values. Plast Reconstr Surg 1997;100:1674-1681.
163. vanLohuizen C: Über eine seltene angeborene Hautanomalie (cutis marmorata telangiectatica congenita). Acta Derm Venereol 1922;3:202.
164. Amitai DB, Fichman S, Merlob P, et al: Cutis marmorata telangiectatica congenita: clinical findings in 85 patients. Pediatr Dermatol 2000;17:100-104.

165. Fitzsimmons JS, Starks M: Cutis marmorata telangiectatica congenita or congenital generalized phlebectasia. Arch Dis Child 1970;45:724-726.

166. Dutkowsky JP, Kasser JR, Kaplan LC: Leg length discrepancy associated with vivid cutis marmorata. J Pediatr Orthop 1993;13:456-458.

167. Devillers AC, de Waard-van der Spek FB, Oranje AP: Cutis marmorata telangiectatica congenita: clinical features in 35 cases. Arch Dermatol 1999;135:34-38.

168. Way BH, Herrmann J, Gilbert EF, et al: Cutis marmorata telangiectatica congenita. J Cutan Pathol 1974;1:10-25.

169. South DA, Jacobs AH: Cutis marmorata telangiectatica congenita (congenital generalized phlebectasia). J Pediatr 1978;93:944-949.

170. Andreev VC, Pramatarov K: Cutis marmorata telangiectatica congenita in two sisters. Br J Dermatol 1979;101:345-350.

171. Kurczynski TW: Hereditary cutis marmorata telangiectatica congenita. Pediatrics 1982;70:52-53.

172. Hamm H: Cutaneous mosaicism of lethal mutations. Am J Med Genet 1999;85:342-345.

173. Morgan JM, Naisby GP, Carmichael AJ: Cutis marmorata telangiectatica congenita with hypoplasia of the right iliac and femoral veins. Br J Dermatol 1997;137:119-122.

174. Petrozzi JW, Rahn EK, Mofenson H, Greensher J: Cutis marmorata telangiectatica congenita. Arch Dermatol 1970;101:74-77.

175. Kremer I, Metzker A, Yassur Y: Intraoperative suprachoroidal hemorrhage in congenital glaucoma associated with cutis marmorata telangiectatica congenita. Arch Ophthalmol 1991;109:1199-1200.

176. Weilepp AE, Eichenfield LF: Association of glaucoma with cutis marmorata telangiectatica congenita: a localized anatomic malformation. J Am Acad Dermatol 1996;35:276-278.

177. Robertson SP, Gattas M, Rogers M, Ades LC: Macrocephaly-cutis marmorata telangiectatica congenita: report of five patients and a review of the literature. Clin Dysmorphol 2000;9:1-9.

178. Moore CA, Toriello HV, Abuelo DN, et al: Macrocephaly-cutis marmorata telangiectatica congenita: a distinct disorder with developmental delay and connective tissue abnormalities. Am J Med Genet 1997;70:67-73.

179. Toriello HV, Graff RG, Florentine MF, et al: Scalp and limb defects with cutis marmorata telangiectatica congenita: Adams-Oliver syndrome? Am J Med Genet 1988;29:269-276.

180. Bork K, Pfeifle J: Multifocal aplasia cutis congenita, distal limb hemimelia, and cutis marmorata telangiectatica in a patient with Adams-Oliver syndrome. Br J Dermatol 1992;127:160-163.

181. Dyall-Smith D, Ramsden A, Laurie S: Adams-Oliver syndrome: aplasia cutis congenita, terminal transverse limb defects and cutis marmorata telangiectatica congenita. Australas J Dermatol 1994;35:19-22.

182. Sabin F: On the development of the superficial lymphatics in the skin of the pig. Am J Anat 1904;3:183.

183. Sabin F: The lymphatic system in human embryos, with a consideration of the morphology of the system as a whole. Am J Anat 1909;9:43.

184. Sabin F: On the origin of the lymphatic system from the veins and the development of the lymph hearts and thoracic duct in the pig. Am J Anat 1905;1:367.

185. Kaipainen A, Korhonen J, Mustonen T, et al: Expression of the fms-like tyrosine kinase 4 gene becomes restricted to lymphatic endothelium during development. Proc Natl Acad Sci USA 1995;92:3566-3570.

186. Wigle JT, Oliver G: Prox1 function is required for the development of the murine lymphatic system. Cell 1999;98:769-778.

187. Dumont DJ, Fong GH, Puri MC, et al: Vascularization of the mouse embryo: a study of flk-1, tek, tie, and vascular endothelial growth factor expression during development. Dev Dyn 1995;203:80-92.

188. Jeltsch M, Kaipainen A, Joukov V, et al: Hyperplasia of lymphatic vessels in VEGF-C transgenic mice [published erratum appears in Science 1997;277:463]. Science 1997;276:1423-1425.

189. Ferrell RE, Levinson KL, Esman JH, et al: Hereditary lymphedema: evidence for linkage and genetic heterogeneity. Hum Mol Genet 1998;7:2073-2078.

190. Evans AL, Brice G, Sotirova V, et al: Mapping of primary congenital lymphedema to the 5q35.3 region. Am J Hum Genet 1999;64:547-555.

191. Kimak M, Karkkainen M, Alitalo K, et al: Mutations in the vascular endothelial growth factor receptor (VEGF-3;Flt4) cause hereditary lymphedema [abstract]. Am J Hum Genet 1999;65:253.

192. Mangion J, Rahman N, Mansour S, et al: A gene for lymphedema-distichiasis maps to 16q24.3. Am J Hum Genet 1999;65:427-432.

193. Nussbaum M, Buchwald RP: Adult cystic hygroma. Am J Otolaryngol 1981;2:159-162.

194. Marler JJ, Fishman SJ, Upton J, et al: Prenatal diagnosis of vascular anomalies. J Pediatr Surg 2002;37:318-326.

195. Fukada Y, Yasumizu T, Takizawa M, et al: The prognosis of fetuses with transient nuchal translucency in the first and early second trimester. Acta Obstet Gynecol Scand 1997;76:913-916.

196. Shulman LP, Phillips OP, Emerson DS, et al: Fetal "space-suit" hydrops in the first trimester: differentiating risk for chromosome abnormalities by delineating characteristics of nuchal translucency. Prenat Diagn 2000;20:30-32.

197. Tunc M, Sadri E, Char DH: Orbital lymphangioma: an analysis of 26 patients. Br J Ophthalmol 1999;83:76-80.

198. Ninh T, Ninh T: Cystic hygroma in children: report of 126 cases. J Pediatr Surg 1974;9:191-195.

199. Gorham L, Stout A: Massive osteolysis (acute spontaneous absorption of bone, phantom bone, disappearing bone): its relation to hemangiomatosis. J Bone Joint Surg Am 1955;37:986-1004.

200. Ricca RJ: Infected mesenteric lymphangioma. N Y State J Med 1991;91:359-361.

201. Nuzzo G, Lemmo G, Marrocco-Trischitta MM, et al: Retroperitoneal cystic lymphangioma. J Surg Oncol 1996;61:234-237.

202. Reder F: Hemangioma and lymphangioma, their response to the injection of boiling water. Med Rec N Y 1920;98:519.

203. Harrower G: Treatment of cystic hygroma of the neck by sodium morrhuate. Br Med J 1933;2:148.

204. Gross R, Goeringer C: Cystic hygroma of the neck. Report of twenty-seven cases. Surg Gynecol Obstet 1939;59:48.

205. Vaughan A: Cystic hygroma of the neck. Am J Dis Child 1934;48:149.

206. Ikeda K, Suita S, Hayashida Y, Yakabe S: Massive infiltrating cystic hygroma of the neck in infancy with special reference to bleomycin therapy. Z Kinderchir 1977;20:227.

207. Okada A, Kubota A, Fukuzawa M, et al: Injection of bleomycin as a primary therapy of cystic lymphangioma. J Pediatr Surg 1992;27:440-443.

208. Orford J, Barker A, Thonell S, et al: Bleomycin therapy for cystic hygroma. J Pediatr Surg 1995;30:1282-1287.

209. Zhong PQ, Zhi FX, Li R, et al: Long-term results of intratumorous bleomycin-A5 injection for head and neck lymphangioma. Oral Surg Oral Med Oral Pathol Oral Radiol Endod 1998;86:139-144.

210. Kataoka M, Morishita R, Hiramatsu J, et al: OK-432 induces production of neutrophil chemotactic factors in malignant pleural effusion. Intern Med 1995;34:352-356.

211. Fujimoto T, Duda RB, Szilvasi A, et al: Streptococcal preparation OK-432 is a potent inducer of IL-12 and a T helper cell 1 dominant state. J Immunol 1997;158:5619-5626.

212. Ueno T, Sujaku K, Tamaki S, et al: OK-432 treatment increases matrix metalloproteinase-9 production and improves dimethylnitrosamine-induced liver cirrhosis in rats. Int J Mol Med 1999;3:497-503.

213. Yamamoto K, Tanaka R, Yoshida S, et al: Effects of OK-432 on the proliferation and cytotoxicity of lymphokine-activated killer (LAK) cells. J Immunother 1999;22:33-40.

214. Luzzatto C, Midrio P, Tchaprassian Z, Guglielmi M: Sclerosing treatment of lymphangiomas with OK-432. Arch Dis Child 2000;82:316-318.

215. Brewis C, Pracy JP, Albert DM: Treatment of lymphangiomas of the head and neck in children by intralesional injection of OK-432 (Picibanil). Clin Otolaryngol 2000;25:130-134.

216. Suzuki Y, Obana A, Gohto Y, et al: Management of orbital lymphangioma using intralesional injection of OK-432. Br J Ophthalmol 2000;84:614-617.

217. Greinwald JH, Burke DK, Sato Y, et al: Treatment of lymphangiomas in children: an update of Picibanil (OK-432) sclerotherapy. Otolaryngol Head Neck Surg 1999;121:381-387.

218. Ogita S, Tsuto T, Nakamura K, et al: OK-432 therapy in 64 patients with lymphangioma. J Pediatr Surg 1994;29:784-785.

219. Ogita S, Tsuto T, Tokiwa K, Takahashi T: Intracystic injection of OK-432: a new sclerosing therapy for cystic hygroma in children. Br J Surg 1987;74:690-691.

220. Samuel M, McCarthy L, Boddy SA: Efficacy and safety of OK-432 sclerotherapy for giant cystic hygroma in a newborn. Fetal Diagn Ther 2000;15:93-96.

221. Watari H, Yamada H, Fujino T, et al: A case of intrauterine medical treatment for cystic hygroma. Eur J Obstet Gynecol Reprod Biol 1996;70:201-203.

222. Apfelberg DB, Greene RA, Maser MR, et al: Results of argon laser exposure of capillary hemangiomas of infancy—preliminary report. Plast Reconstr Surg 1981;67:188-193.

223. White JM, Chaudhry SI, Kudler JJ, et al: Nd:YAG and CO_2 laser therapy of oral mucosal lesions. J Clin Laser Med Surg 1998;16:299-304.

224. Fonkalsrud EW: Surgical management of congenital malformations of the lymphatic system. Am J Surg 1974;128:152-159.

225. Chait D, Yonkers AJ, Beddoe GM, Yarington CT Jr: Management of cystic hygromas. Surg Gynecol Obstet 1974;139:55-58.

226. Hubbard AM, Crombleholme TM, Adzick NS: Prenatal MRI evaluation of giant neck masses in preparation for the fetal exit procedure. Am J Perinatol 1998;15:253-257.

227. Suzuki N, Tsuchida Y, Takahashi A, et al: Prenatally diagnosed cystic lymphangioma in infants. J Pediatr Surg 1998;33:1599-1604.

228. Liechty KW, Crombleholme TM, Weiner S, et al: The ex utero intrapartum treatment procedure for a large fetal neck mass in a twin gestation. Obstet Gynecol 1999;93:824-825.

229. Cochran WJ, Klish WJ, Brown MR, et al: Chylous ascites in infants and children: a case report and literature review. J Pediatr Gastroenterol Nutr 1985;4:668-673.

230. Witt PD, Martin DS, Marsh JL: Aesthetic considerations in extirpation of melolabial lymphatic malformations in children. Plast Reconstr Surg 1995;96:48-57.

231. Dingman R, Grabb W: Lymphangioma of the tongue. Plast Reconstr Surg 1961;27:214-223.

232. Padwa BL, Hayward PG, Ferraro NF, Mulliken JB: Cervicofacial lymphatic malformation: clinical course, surgical intervention, and pathogenesis of skeletal hypertrophy. Plast Reconstr Surg 1995;95:951-960.

233. Upton J, Mulliken JB, Murray JE: Classification and rationale for management of vascular anomalies in the upper extremity. J Hand Surg Am 1985;10:970-975.

234. Upton J, Coombs CJ, Mulliken JB, et al: Vascular malformations of the upper limb: a review of 270 patients. J Hand Surg Am 1999;24:1019-1035.

235. Whimster IW: The pathology of lymphangioma circumscriptum. Br J Dermatol 1976;94:473-486.

236. Bauer BS, Kernahan DA, Hugo NE: Lymphangioma circumscriptum—a clinicopathological review. Ann Plast Surg 1981;7:318-326.

237. Alqahtani A, Nguyen LT, Flageole H, et al: 25 years' experience with lymphangiomas in children. J Pediatr Surg 1999;34:1164-1168.

238. Charabi B, Bretlau P, Bille M, Holmelund M: Cystic hygroma of the head and neck—a long-term follow-up of 44 cases. Acta Otolaryngol Suppl 2000;543:248-250.

239. Burge DM, Middleton AW, Kamath R, Fasher BJ: Intestinal haemorrhage in Turner's syndrome. Arch Dis Child 1981;56:557-558.

240. Weiss SW: Pedal hemangioma (venous malformation) occurring in Turner's syndrome: an additional manifestation of the syndrome. Hum Pathol 1988;19:1015-1018.

241. Rudolph R: Familial multiple glomangiomas. Ann Plast Surg 1993;30:183-185.

242. Boon LM, Brouillard P, Irrthum A, et al: A gene for inherited cutaneous venous anomalies localizes to chromosome 1p21-22. Am J Hum Genet 1999;65:125-133.

243. Brouillard P, Boon LM, Mulliken JB, et al: Mutations in a novel factor, glomulin, are responsible for glomuvenous malformations ("glomangiomas"). Am J Hum Genet 2002;70:866-874.

244. Boon LM, Mulliken JB, Vikkula M, et al: Assignment of a locus for dominantly inherited venous malformations to chromosome 9p. Hum Mol Genet 1994;3:1583-1587.

245. Labauge P, Enjolras O, Bonerandi JJ, et al: An association between autosomal dominant cerebral cavernomas and a distinctive hyperkeratotic cutaneous vascular malformation in 4 families. Ann Neurol 1999;45:250-254.

246. Laberge-le Couteulx S, Jung HH, et al: Truncated mutations in CCM1, encoding KRIT1, cause cavernous angiomas. Nat Genet 1999;23:189-193.

247. Labauge P, Brunereau L, Levy C, et al: The natural history of familial cerebral cavernomas: a retrospective MRI study of 40 patients. Neuroradiology 2000;42:327-332.

248. Bean W: Dyschondroplasia and hemangiomata. Arch Intern Med 1955;95:767.

249. Oranje AP: Blue rubber bleb nevus syndrome. Pediatr Dermatol 1986;3:304-310.

250. McCarthy JC, Goldberg MJ, Zimbler S: Orthopaedic dysfunction in the blue rubber-bleb nevus syndrome. J Bone Joint Surg Am 1982;64:280-283.

251. Tyrrel RT, Baumgartner BR, Montemayor KA: Blue rubber bleb nevus syndrome: CT diagnosis of intussusception. AJR Am J Roentgenol 1990;154:105-106.

252. Greenspan A, Azouz EM, Matthews J 2nd, Decarie JC: Synovial hemangioma: imaging features in eight histologically proven cases, review of the literature, and differential diagnosis. Skeletal Radiol 1995;24:583-590.

253. Pinar H, Bozkurt M, Baktiroglu L, Karaoglan O: Intraarticular hemangioma of the knee with meniscal and bony attachment. Arthroscopy 1997;13:507-510.

254. Price NJ, Cundy PJ: Synovial hemangioma of the knee. J Pediatr Orthop 1997;17:74-77.

255. Fishman SJ, Burrows PE, Leichtner AM, Mulliken JB: Gastrointestinal manifestations of vascular anomalies in childhood: varied etiologies require multiple therapeutic modalities. J Pediatr Surg 1998;33:1163-1167.

256. Bick RL: Vascular disorders associated with thrombohemorrhagic phenomena. Semin Thromb Hemost 1979;5:167-183.

257. Hofhuis WJ, Oranje AP, Bouquet J, Sinaasappel M: Blue rubber-bleb naevus syndrome: report of a case with consumption coagulopathy complicated by manifest thrombosis. Eur J Pediatr 1990;149:526-528.

258. Enjolras O, Ciabrini D, Mazoyer E, et al: Extensive pure venous malformations in the upper or lower limb: a review of 27 cases. J Am Acad Dermatol 1997;36:219-225.

259. Platokouki H, Aronis S, Mitsika A, et al: Diffuse splenic and visceral hemangiomas complicated by chronic consumption coagulopathy. Acta Paediatr Jpn 1998;40:381-384.

260. Trop I, Dubois J, Guibaud L, et al: Soft-tissue venous malformations in pediatric and young adult patients: diagnosis with Doppler US. Radiology 1999;212:841-845.

261. O'Donovan JC, Donaldson JS, Morello FP, et al: Symptomatic hemangiomas and venous malformations in infants, children, and young adults: treatment with percutaneous injection of sodium tetradecyl sulfate. AJR Am J Roentgenol 1997;169:723-729.

262. Siniluoto TM, Svendsen PA, Wikholm GM, et al: Percutaneous sclerotherapy of venous malformations of the head and neck using sodium tetradecyl sulphate (sotradecol). Scand J Plast Reconstr Surg Hand Surg 1997;31:145-150.

263. Gelbert F, Enjolras O, Deffrenne D, et al: Percutaneous sclerotherapy for venous malformation of the lips: a retrospective study of 23 patients [in process citation]. Neuroradiology 2000;42:692-696.

264. Yamaki T, Nozaki M, Sasaki K: Color duplex-guided sclerotherapy for the treatment of venous malformations. Dermatol Surg 2000;26:323-328.

265. Dubois JM, Sebag GH, De Prost Y, et al: Soft-tissue venous malformations in children: percutaneous sclerotherapy with Ethibloc. Radiology 1991;180:195-198.

266. Esteban MJ, Gutierrez C, Gomez J, et al: Treatment with Ethibloc of lymphangiomas and venous angiomas. Cir Pediatr 1996;9:158-162.

267. Suh JS, Shin KH, Na JB, et al: Venous malformations: sclerotherapy with a mixture of ethanol and lipiodol. Cardiovasc Intervent Radiol 1997;20:268-273.

268. Dompmartin A, Labbe D, Theron J, et al: The use of an alcohol gel of ethyl cellulose in the treatment of venous malformations [in French]. Rev Stomatol Chir Maxillofac 2000;101:30-32.

269. Berenguer B, Burrows PE, Zurakowski D, Mulliken JB: Sclerotherapy of craniofacial venous malformations: complications and results. Plast Reconstr Surg 1999;104:1-11.

270. de Lorimier AA: Sclerotherapy for venous malformations. J Pediatr Surg 1995;30:188-193.

271. Pappas DC Jr, Persky MS, Berenstein A: Evaluation and treatment of head and neck venous vascular malformations. Ear Nose Throat J 1998;77:914-916, 918-922.

272. Chang CJ, Fisher DM, Chen YR: Intralesional photocoagulation of vascular anomalies of the tongue. Br J Plast Surg 1999;52:178-181.

273. Derby LD, Low DW: Laser treatment of facial venous vascular malformations. Ann Plast Surg 1997;38:371-378.

274. Raulin C, Werner S: Treatment of venous malformations with an intense pulsed light source (IPLS) technology: a retrospective study. Lasers Surg Med 1999;25:170-177.

275. Ohlms LA, Forsen J, Burrows PE: Venous malformation of the pediatric airway. Int J Pediatr Otorhinolaryngol 1996;37:99-114.

276. Keljo DJ, Yakes WF, Andersen JM, Timmons CF: Recognition and treatment of venous malformations of the rectum. J Pediatr Gastroenterol Nutr 1996;23:442-446.

277. Fishman SJ, Shamberger RC, Fox VL, Burrows PE: Endorectal pull-through abates gastrointestinal hemorrhage from colorectal venous malformations [in process citation]. J Pediatr Surg 2000;35:982-984.

278. Halsted W: Congenital arteriovenous and lymphaticovenous fistulae: unique clinical and experimental observations. Trans Am Surg Assoc 1919;37:262.

279. Reid M: Abnormal arteriovenous communications, acquired and congenital. II. The origin and nature of arteriovenous aneurysms, cirsoid aneurysms and simple angiomas. Arch Surg 1925;10:601.

280. Reinhoff WJ: Congenital arteriovenous fistula: an embryological study with report of a case. Bull Johns Hopkins Hosp 1924;35:271.

281. Coleman CJ: Diagnosis and treatment of congenital arteriovenous fistulas of the head and neck. Am J Surg 1973;47:354.

282. Braverman I, Keh A, Jacobson B: Ultrastructure and three-dimensional organization of the telangiectases of hereditary hemorrhagic telangiectasia. J Invest Dermatol 1990;95:422-427.

283. Hurwitz D, Kerber C: Hemodynamic considerations in the treatment of arteriovenous malformations of the face and scalp. Plast Reconstr Surg 1981;67:421-434.

284. Wautier MP, Boval B, Chappey O, et al: Cultured endothelial cells from human arteriovenous malformations have defective growth regulation. Blood 1999;94:2020-2028.

285. Nicoladoni C: Phlebarteriectasie der rechten oberen Extremitat. Arch Klin Chir 1875;18:252.

286. Gomes M, Bernatz P: Arteriovenous fistulae: a review and ten-year experience at the Mayo Clinic. Mayo Clin Proc 1970;45:81-102.

287. Mulliken JB: Vascular anomalies. In Aston SJ, Beasley RW, Thorne CHM, eds: Grabb and Smith's Plastic Surgery. Philadelphia, Lippincott-Raven, 1997:191-204.

288. Cohen J, Weinreb J, Redman H: Arteriovenous malformations of the extremities: MR imaging. Radiology 1996;158:475-479.

289. Yakes WF, Rossi P, Odink H: How I do it. Arteriovenous malformation management. Cardiovasc Intervent Radiol 1996;19:65-71.

290. Kohout MP, Hansen M, Pribaz JJ, Mulliken JB: Arteriovenous malformations of the head and neck: natural history and management. Plast Reconstr Surg 1998;102:643-654.

291. Cohen MM Jr: Bannayan Riley-Ruvalcaba syndrome: renaming three formerly recognized syndromes as one etiologic entity [letter]. Am J Med Genet 1990;35:291-292.

292. Fargnoli MC, Orlow SJ, Semel-Concepcion J, Bolognia JL: Clinicopathologic findings in the Bannayan-Riley-Ruvalcaba syndrome. Arch Dermatol 1996;132:1214-1218.

293. Gorlin RJ, Cohen MM Jr, Condon LM, Burke BA: Bannayan-Riley-Ruvalcaba syndrome. Am J Med Genet 1992;44:307-314.

294. DiLiberti J, D'Agostino A, Ruvalcaba R, Schimschock J: A new lipid storage myopathy observed in individuals with Ruvalcaba-Myhre-Smith syndrome. Am J Med Genet 1984;18:163-167.

295. Marsh DJ, Dahia PL, Zheng Z, et al: Germline mutations in PTEN are present in Bannayan-Zonana syndrome [letter]. Nat Genet 1997;16:333-334.

296. Starink TM, van der Veen JP, Arwert F, et al: The Cowden syndrome: a clinical and genetic study in 21 patients. Clin Genet 1986;29:222-233.

297. Liaw D, Marsh DJ, Li J, et al: Germline mutations of the PTEN gene in Cowden disease, an inherited breast and thyroid cancer syndrome. Nat Genet 1997;16:64-67.

298. Zhou XP, Marsh DJ, Hampel H, et al: Germline and germline mosaic PTEN mutations associated with a Proteus-like syndrome of hemihypertrophy, lower limb asymmetry, arteriovenous malformations and lipomatosis. Hum Mol Genet 2000;9:765-768.

299. Biesecker LG, Happle R, Mulliken JB, et al: Proteus syndrome: diagnostic criteria, differential diagnosis, and patient evaluation. Am J Med Genet 1999;84:389-395.

300. Maffucci A: Di un caso di encondroma ed angioma multiplo contribuzione al a genesi embrionale dei tumor. Movimento Med Chir (Naples) 1881;3:399.

301. Lewis R, Ketcham A: Maffucci's syndrome: functional and neoplastic significance. J Bone Joint Surg Am 1973;55:1465-1479.

302. Kaplan RP, Wang JT, Amron DM, Kaplan L: Maffucci's syndrome: two case reports with a literature review. J Am Acad Dermatol 1993;29:894-899.

303. Cameron A, McMillan D: Lipomatosis of skeletal muscle in Maffucci's syndrome. J Bone Joint Surg Br 1956;38:693-698.

304. Kennedy J: Dyschondroplasia and hemangiomata (Maffucci's syndrome): report of a case with oral and intracranial lesions. Br J Dent 1973;135:18-21.

305. Loewinger R, Lichenstein J, Dodson W, et al: Maffucci's syndrome: a mesenchymal dysplasia with multiple tumor syndrome. Br J Dermatol 1977;96:317.

306. Lowell S, Mathey R: Head and neck manifestations of Maffucci's syndrome. Arch Otolaryngol 1979;105:427.

307. Moorthy A: Oral manifestations in Maffucci's syndrome. Br Dent J 1983;155:160.

308. Johnson TE, Nasr AM, Nalbandian RM, Cappelen-Smith J: Enchondromatosis and hemangioma (Maffucci's syndrome) with orbital involvement. Am J Ophthalmol 1990;110:153-159.

309. Perkins P, Weiss SW: Spindle cell hemangioendothelioma. An analysis of 78 cases with reassessment of its pathogenesis and biologic behavior. Am J Surg Pathol 1996;20:1196-1204.

310. Sun TC, Swee RG, Shives TC, Unni KK: Chondrosarcoma in Maffucci's syndrome. J Bone Joint Surg Am 1985;67:1214-1219.

311. Dahlin D, Henderson E: Chondrosarcoma, a surgical and pathological problem. Review of 212 cases. J Bone Joint Surg Am 1956;38:1025.

312. Coley B, Higinbotham N: Secondary chondrosarcoma. Ann Surg 1954;139:547-549.

313. Cook P, Evans P: Chondrosarcoma of the skull in Maffucci's syndrome. Br J Radiol 1977;50:833-836.

314. Albregts A, Rapini R: Malignancy in Maffucci's syndrome. Dermatol Clin 1995;13:73-78.

315. Baskerville PA, Ackroyd JS, Lea Thomas M, Browse NL: The Klippel-Trénaunay syndrome: clinical, radiological and haemodynamic features and management. Br J Surg 1985;72:232-236.

316. Gloviczki P, Stanson AW, Stickler GB, et al: Klippel-Trénaunay syndrome: the risks and benefits of vascular interventions. Surgery 1991;110:469-479.

317. Samuel M, Spitz L: Klippel-Trénaunay syndrome: clinical features, complications and management in children. Br J Surg 1995;82:757-761.

318. Jacob AG, Driscoll DJ, Shaughnessy WJ, et al: Klippel-Trénaunay syndrome: spectrum and management. Mayo Clin Proc 1998;73:28-36.

319. Laor T, Burrows PE, Hoffer FA: Magnetic resonance venography of congenital vascular malformations of the extremities. Pediatr Radiol 1996;26:371-380.

Salivary Gland Tumors

STEPHAN ARIYAN, MD, MBA ✦ DEEPAK NARAYAN, MD
✦ CHARLOTTE E. ARIYAN, MD, PhD

ANATOMY

Salivary glands are arranged as lobules of mucinous cells (producing mucus), serous cells (producing thin salivary fluid), or combinations of serous and mucinous cells. The serous cells are small and have basophilic cytoplasm; mucinous cells are larger and oval and have a larger eosinophilic cytoplasm.

Parotid Gland

The parotid gland is the largest of the salivary glands and is located on the face between the zygomatic arch and the angle of the mandible. On histologic evaluation, the parotid is virtually totally serous glands (Fig. 107-1). Although the gland has a dense sheath overlying its surface, which is derived from the submuscular aponeurotic system, it is not an encapsulated gland. It has multiple small segments, growths, and islands of tissue that are found within the subcutaneous tissue of the face. Furthermore, the parotid gland is not segmented into "lobes." Rather, it is a single-lobed, C-shaped gland wrapping itself from its location over the mandible around the ascending ramus to a location deep to the ramus, called the deeper segment (Fig. 107-2). The gland overlying the mandible is separated by the plane made by the branches of the facial nerve coursing within the gland, hence the "superficial segment" overlying the facial nerve.

The facial nerve exits the skull at the stylomastoid foramen, posterior to the styloid process, and gives off its first branch, the posterior auricular nerve. This nerve innervates the auricularis muscle (allowing some patients to wiggle their ears) and gives a branch to the posterior belly of the digastric muscle (the anterior belly is innervated by a branch of the trigeminal nerve) and another branch to the stylohyoid muscle. The remainder of the main trunk of the facial nerve penetrates the mass of the parotid gland to arborize into its five remaining branches (Fig. 107-3):

1. temporal branch to the frontalis muscle;
2. zygomatic branch to the orbicularis oculi muscle;
3. buccal branch to the muscles of the cheek and upper lip;
4. mandibular branch to the muscles of the lower lip and chin; and
5. cervical branch to the platysma muscle.

The main secretory duct of the gland, the Stensen duct, courses through the structures of the cheek to empty into the oral cavity through its orifice in the buccal mucosa at the level of the crown of the upper first and second molar teeth. The course of this duct through the cheek is along an imaginary line drawn from the tragus to the curve of the lateral nares.

Several lymph nodes are associated with the external surface of the parotid gland, and some may be imbedded within this surface tissue. A lymph node can occasionally be found in the segment deep to the facial nerve.

Submandibular Gland

The submandibular glands (also called the submaxillary glands) lie bilaterally deep to the horizontal body

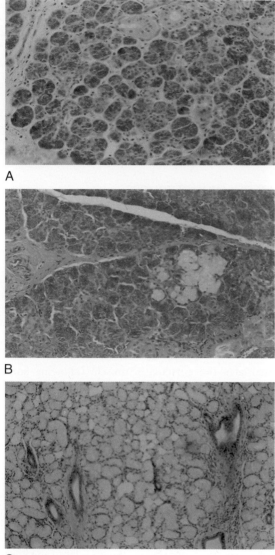

FIGURE 107-1. The parotid gland is composed of essentially only serous glands *(A)*, the submandibular gland is a mixture of serous and mucous glands *(B)*, and the sublingual gland is virtually all mucous glands *(C)*.

overlying the submandibular gland as it crosses the facial vessels. There is also usually a lymph node associated with the external surface of the submandibular gland.

Sublingual Gland

This gland is the smallest of the salivary glands and is frequently half the size of the submandibular gland. It is under the mucosal surface of the lateral floor of the mouth, along the lingual surface of the mandible, anterior to the submandibular gland. The gland has several secretory ducts that empty to the oral cavity through the oral mucosa, although on occasion they can become confluent and empty as a single duct into the Wharton duct. On histologic evaluation, the sublingual glands are composed predominantly of mucous glands (see Fig. 107-1*C*).

Minor Salivary Glands

The oral cavity is also interspersed with a number of small aggregates of salivary tissue in the palate, the lip, the buccal mucosa, or the oral mucosa.

EPIDEMIOLOGY

The incidence of salivary gland tumor in the United States is in the range of 1 to 3 per 100,000 population.[1] This represents less than 3% of all tumors of the body, and the largest bulk of these salivary gland tumors are found in the parotid gland. In fact, the proportion of tumors of the parotid gland compared with the submandibular gland and sublingual gland is $100:10:1$.[2]

Although most salivary gland tumors are found in the parotid gland, 80% are benign.[3] On the other hand, 40% of tumors of the submandibular gland and 60% of tumors of the sublingual gland are found to be malignant (Table 107-1).[4] Whereas tumors of the minor salivary glands are uncommon, 60% to 80% are

of the mandible and are about one fourth to one third the size of the parotid gland. They secrete saliva through the left and right Wharton ducts, which course under the lateral floor of the mouth; each duct exits into the oral cavity just short of the midline along the root of the undersurface of the tongue. On histologic evaluation, the submandibular gland is composed of a mixture of serous and mucous glands (see Fig. 107-1*B*).

The mandibular branch of the facial nerve is found under the platysma muscle, coursing 1 to 2 cm below and parallel to the body of the mandible and

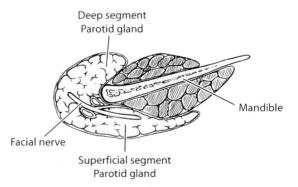

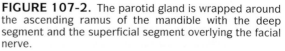

FIGURE 107-2. The parotid gland is wrapped around the ascending ramus of the mandible with the deep segment and the superficial segment overlying the facial nerve.

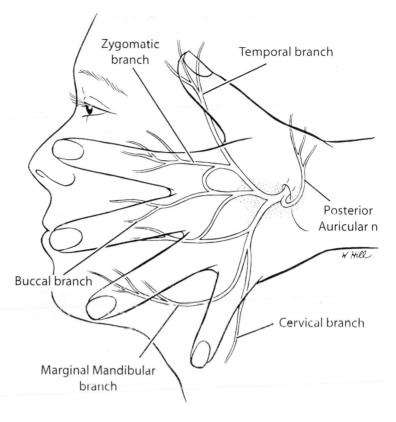

FIGURE 107-3. The facial nerve exits the skull giving off one branch, the posterior auricular nerve to the auricularis muscle, and then proceeds to penetrate the parotid gland to give its next five branches. An easy way to remember these branches and their location is depicted by the five fingers of the hand superimposed on the face.

malignant.[5-7] No etiologic factors have been found for the development of tumors of the salivary glands. However, it has been shown that there is a high incidence of malignant tumors of the salivary glands among patients who had been exposed to radiation.[8]

An association between radiation exposure and salivary gland tumors was first identified in survivors of the atomic bomb in Hiroshima, Japan. One investigation selected 66 patients for a study to evaluate whether there was an increased incidence of malignant salivary gland tumors among individuals with exposure to radiation. Among the atomic bomb survivors, 52.8% (19 of 36) had malignant salivary gland tumors, whereas only 16.7% (5 of 30) of the nonexposed population developed malignant tumors.[9] A further analysis of the data determined that the risk was highest for, but not limited to, mucoepidermoid tumors.[10] These reports have been followed by a study of survivors evaluating

dose of radiation exposure from the atomic bomb. In this study, there was an increase only in mucoepidermoid and Warthin tumors among individuals with an increased radiation dose (estimated radiation dose according to the densitometry system, 1986; high-exposure relative risk of 9.3 for mucoepidermoid carcinoma [11 cases] and 4.1 for Warthin tumor [12 cases]).[11]

On the other hand, low-dose radiation has also been shown to be associated with subsequent malignant transformation of salivary glands. A retrospective analysis of Israeli children who were treated with low-dose radiation for tinea capitis at the time of their immigration between 1949 and 1960 revealed an increase in parotid tumors (4 per 1000 in the irradiated group versus 0 per 1000 in the population control group).[12] In another study, a population of patients receiving x-ray therapy for acne in Los Angeles had an increased incidence of malignant parotid tumors. Those patients who had received more than 15 such treatments had a relative risk of 8.0, and it is estimated that 28% of malignant tumors that occurred in Los Angeles from 1976 to 1984 were attributable to radiation.[13] All these reports suggest that there is a lag phase between the radiation exposure and the malignant transformation of the salivary and endocrine glands. To explore this further, a study of patients who had received head and neck irradiation to the tonsillar area and the

TABLE 107-1 ✦ TUMORS OF SALIVARY GLAND

	Benign	Malignant
Parotid	80%	20%
Submaxillary	60%	40%
Sublingual	40%	60%
Minor salivary glands	20%	80%

nasopharynx demonstrated the interval between radiation exposure and tumor diagnosis to be 7 to 32 years.[14] For these reasons, it is essential that patients who have received radiation be continually observed for the potential development of subsequent salivary gland tumors.

The interpretation of an enlarged salivary gland may prove to be a difficult clinical diagnosis. One of the reasons for this is that many benign enlargements are reactive inflammations, or salivary cysts. Nevertheless, each should be evaluated carefully and methodically with selected examination and tests.

DIAGNOSTIC STUDIES
Fine-Needle Aspiration

Fine-needle aspiration (FNA) biopsy of salivary gland tumors is an area of controversy because the presence of the tumor itself, in the view of many surgeons, is indication enough to operate. Proponents of the technique argue that FNA is valuable in preoperative counseling of the patient about possible facial nerve sacrifice, prognosis, and the necessity for adjunctive procedures such as neck dissection if the tumor proves to be malignant (e.g., for high-grade mucoepidermoid carcinoma). In addition, FNA may save the patient an unnecessary operation by differentiating an inflammatory from a neoplastic lesion or by making a diagnosis of a Warthin tumor in a patient who poses a poor surgical risk, enabling observation alone.

Germane to this discussion is the accuracy of FNA in the context of salivary gland tumors. The sensitivity and specificity of FNA for salivary gland tumors reported in the literature range from a high of 99% sensitivity and 100% specificity as reported by Bhatia[15] to a low of 90% sensitivity and 75% specificity as reported by Cohen et al.[16] In general, however, recent series document a trend toward a higher degree of sensitivity and specificity.[17,18] A higher degree of accuracy has been reported for benign tumors.[19-21]

The common diagnostic pitfalls involve distinction between benign oncocytic tumors and acinic cell carcinomas, pleomorphic adenomas and adenoid cystic carcinomas, high-grade mucoepidermoid carcinoma and metastatic squamous cell carcinoma, and low-grade mucoepidermoid carcinoma and Warthin tumor (Fig. 107-4). Mucoepidermoid carcinomas appear to be the most difficult to diagnose by FNA.[22] In an effort to improve diagnostic accuracy of aspirates, special immunohistochemical stains such as glial fibrillary acidic protein for pleomorphic adenomas[23] and silver staining of nucleolar organizer regions have been used.[24]

A diagnosis of lymphoma by FNA necessitates an open biopsy or a superficial parotidectomy to evaluate nodal architecture and to obtain adequate tissue

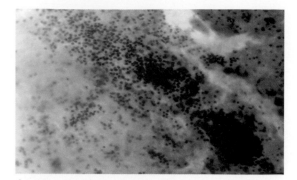

A

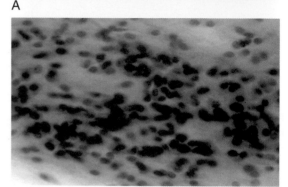

B

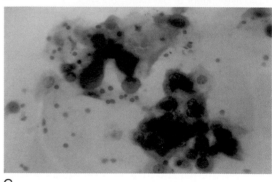

C

FIGURE 107-4. Cytology of fine-needle aspiration specimens showing collections of serous cells mixed with mesenchymal stroma *(A)* representing pleomorphic adenoma, malignant squamous cells *(B)* representing mucoepidermoid carcinoma, and lymphocytic collections *(C)* and salivary gland with cluster of lymphoid tissue representing Warthin tumor.

for immunohistochemical characterization to classify the lymphoma properly.

FNA is essentially free of complications. Hemorrhage and necrosis of the tumor after aspiration of a lymphoma[21] and a Warthin tumor[25] have been reported, but such occurrences are exceedingly rare. The concerns about needle track seeding have been specifically addressed by several authors,[21,26,27] who have found no cause for alarm because of its exceedingly low occurrence.

The technique of FNA reported in 1981 is still recommended.[28] A 21-gauge needle is affixed to a 10-mL controlled syringe; no air is retained in the syringe barrel, and negative pressure is applied by withdrawing the plunger. A minimum of two passes are made into the tumor. The needle is withdrawn and removed from the syringe, air is drawn into the cylinder, the needle is reapplied to the syringe, and a tiny droplet of specimen is applied to the glass slide to prepare a slide smear. The slides are placed immediately into a jar of absolute or 95% alcohol. Next, alcohol is withdrawn through the needle into the syringe and flushed a few times into another jar of absolute alcohol to prepare a cell block.

Imaging Modalities

The introduction of high-resolution imaging in the form of computed tomographic (CT) scans and magnetic resonance imaging (MRI) has revolutionized our ability to define the extent of various pathologic processes throughout the body, and the salivary glands are no exception. Paradoxically, despite the level of technical advancement achieved, these modalities are not routinely used in the management of salivary gland tumors, partly because a histologic diagnosis based on these images is still not possible given the current degree of sophistication. Additional imaging techniques that have been used in defining salivary gland disease include ultrasonography, sialography, and technetium scans.

COMPUTED TOMOGRAPHY

The ready availability and the cost of this imaging modality account for the popularity of CT scans if additional imaging studies are required by the clinician. The ultimate choice of a CT scan or MRI may be dictated by nonclinical factors, but the consensus is that CT scans are better in a patient with a history of inflammatory disorder, whereas MRI is the modality of choice for palpable masses.[29,30] Specific clinical scenarios, as discussed, may mandate the use of CT scans.

CT scans are particularly sensitive in the detection of calcium deposits in the salivary glands, a property that is useful in the diagnosis of elusive ductal calculi. This represents a marked advantage over MRI. Along the same lines, although extraglandular tumor spread is equally well visualized by both modalities, demonstration of subtle bone erosion or sclerosis requires the use of CT scans. Involvement of tumor into soft tissue is better visualized by MRI. Cystic salivary lesions are another area in which CT scans hold an advantage over MRI. The high water content in a majority of salivary gland tumors is presumed to be the cause of the inability of routine MRIs to distinguish between a cyst and a solid mass.

Artifacts from dental implants can have a negative impact on the quality of CT images. This can be mitigated by special views, however. The facial nerve is not routinely imaged in CT scans, which can represent a disadvantage in dealing with tumors with a predilection for perineural spread.

MAGNETIC RESONANCE IMAGING

The distinction between benign and malignant tumors on MRI is predicated on the difference in water content between the two types of tumors. The distinction is not absolute, however. Som and Curtin[30] pointed out that high-grade malignant tumors tend to have low to intermediate signal intensities on all imaging sequences. Well-differentiated tumors, on the other hand, which include benign tumors and low-grade malignant tumors, tend to have a low T1 and high T2 signal intensity (Table 107-2). This is explained by the fact that low-grade malignant tumors are generally differentiated well enough to produce secretory products, which therefore yields a higher net water content, reflected by a high T2 signal.

Contrast agents were developed to improve image resolution on MRI; among these, gadolinium-containing compounds are the most widely used. Gadolinium chelates were developed because of the high relaxivity of the gadolinium ion coupled with the relatively low toxicity of the complex with chelation of the metal ion.[31] Gadolinium therefore enhances lesion identification and characterization. Some authors have suggested that the routine use of gadolinium in magnetic resonance studies of the salivary glands improves the quality of data obtained. The consensus, however, is that this adjunct is not necessary for the majority of the cases.[30]

Kramer and Mafee[32] noted that the intensity of the signal of the parotid gland is slightly less than that of subcutaneous fat and greater relative to muscle on T1-weighted, proton density–weighted, and T2-weighted images. In addition, the submandibular gland has a

TABLE 107-2 ♦ DISTINCTION BETWEEN BENIGN AND MALIGNANT TUMORS BY MRI

	T1	T2
Lymphoma	Low	High
Malignancy (high grade)	Low	Low
Lipoma	Fat signal	Fat signal
Warthin tumor	Intermediate	High
Pleomorphic adenomas	Low to intermediate	High
Hemangioma*	Intermediate	High

*Signal voids representing large-vessel phleboliths are characteristic. Venous malformations are best diagnosed by MRI; true arteriovenous fistulas require an arteriogram for diagnosis.

slightly lower signal intensity than the sublingual gland on proton density–weighted and T2-weighted sequences. This enables the distinction of the deep segment of the submandibular gland from the sublingual gland. These authors recommend conventional transverse T1-weighted and fast spin echo or short T1 inversion recovery T2-weighted techniques without gadolinium for tumors. Intravenous injection of paramagnetic contrast material, however, is extremely useful in evaluating perineural spread and cervical node involvement. MRI is particularly advantageous in delineating the margins of a lesion, thereby enabling clinicians to distinguish between multiple masses and lobulated solitary lesions. These differences in signal intensity as seen by MRI help differentiate between the various neoplasms involving the salivary gland (see Table 107-2).

ULTRASONOGRAPHY

Ultrasonography is most helpful in distinguishing solid from cystic lesions. Cystic lesions that are identified with ultrasonography include simple lymphoepithelial cysts, cystic hygromas involving the salivary glands, ranulas, sialoceles, and multiple lymphoepithelial cysts associated with human immunodeficiency virus (HIV) infection. However, the diagnostic capabilities of this modality are inferior to those of CT and MRI in solid masses. Color Doppler studies attempting to correlate pathologic processes with flow patterns have likewise proven disappointing.

TECHNETIUM SCAN

The ability of salivary glands to concentrate technetium Tc 99m pertechnetate forms the basis for the use of this nuclear medicine technique in imaging of salivary glands. The increased metabolic activity of the cells composing Warthin tumor produces the characteristic image of increased uptake. Oncocytomas are other lesions that may take up this tracer in excess of surrounding gland. Rarely, oncocytic rests in pleomorphic adenomas and oncocytic tumor metastases might also mimic this picture. Aside from Warthin tumor, ^{99m}Tc scans are not useful in salivary gland imaging.

SIALOGRAPHY

Sialography is an invasive procedure that involves identification of the ductal opening of the gland to be studied, cannulation, injection of contrast material, and obtaining views in different planes. Sialograms and contrast delineation of the ductal structure of a salivary gland have little application today in the face of nearly perfect images produced by MRIs and CT scans.[33] Sialograms are useful in demonstrating ductal calculi and ductal disruptions secondary to trauma. Sialography is said to be more sensitive than MRI in the diagnosis of Sjögren syndrome in the early stages of the disease.[30] The sialographic appearance of Sjögren syndrome is characterized by a uniformly distributed, punctate accumulation of contrast material throughout the gland, graphically described as a "leafless fruit-laden tree."[30]

CLASSIFICATION OF TUMORS

The simplest way to classify salivary gland tumors is by their histologic cell types (epithelial or nonepithelial) and by their behavior patterns (benign or malignant) (Table 107-3).

Non-neoplastic Lesions

SIALADENOSIS. The salivary gland can enlarge for nutritional reasons not related to neoplastic cellular changes. These enlargements have been found in association with cirrhosis and malnutrition.

SIALADENITIS. The gland can become enlarged from inflammatory conditions. These can be due to trauma to the maxillofacial area, viruses (most commonly mumps or HIV),[34] or bacteria (most commonly *Staphylococcus aureus*), which can lead to abscess formation (Fig. 107-5). Unusual causes of enlargement have been found to be related to sarcoidosis,[35,36] in which case multiple salivary glands may be found to be enlarged.

TABLE 107-3 ✦ SALIVARY GLAND TUMORS

Primary Tumors	
Benign	
Epithelial	Pleomorphic adenoma (benign mixed tumor)
	Monomorphic adenoma
	Papillary cystadenoma lymphomatosum (Warthin tumor)
	Oncocytoma
Nonepithelial	Hemangioma
Malignant	
Epithelial	Mucoepidermoid carcinoma
	Adenoid cystic carcinoma (cylindroma)
	Acinic cell carcinoma
	Malignant mixed tumor
	Squamous cell carcinoma
	Adenocarcinoma
	Oncocytic carcinoma
Nonepithelial	Lymphoma
Metastatic Tumors to Salivary Glands	
	Kidney
	Breast
	Lung
	Colon

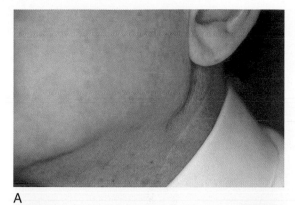
A

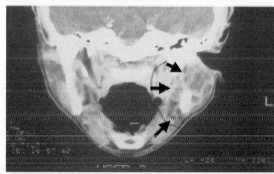
B

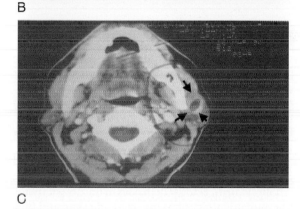
C

FIGURE 107-5. An abscess of the parotid gland is seen as a smooth mass at the angle of the jaw *(A)*. The CT scans *(B* and *C)* show a multiloculated collection.

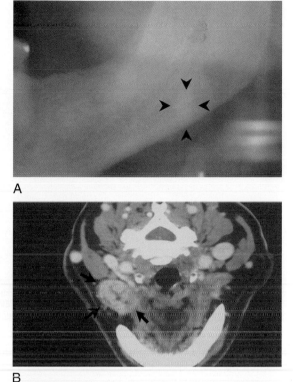
A

B

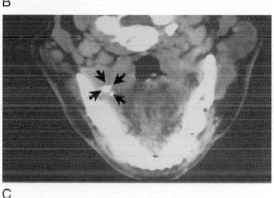
C

FIGURE 107-6. A radiograph of the mandible *(A)* shows a calcified stone. The CT scans show the enlarged submandibular gland *(B)* and the calcified stone *(C)*.

SIALOLITHIASIS. Stones in the ducts of the salivary glands (Fig. 107-6) are a common condition leading to a mass within the gland or enlargement of the gland secondary to obstruction of salivary flow. Most of these are found in the submandibular gland (Fig. 107-7), and a lesser number are found in the parotid gland. A sialogram may sometimes show no stones but rather a stenosis from previous trauma that leads to obstructed or restricted flow (Fig. 107-8).

MUCOCELE. These retention cysts of mucus production are most commonly found in the minor salivary glands. These are frequently located in the lower

lip, and they sometimes develop after trauma to the lip, laceration and suture repair, or secondary healing.

NECROTIZING SIALOMETAPLASIA. This is an unusual and clinically disturbing lesion that has an uncertain cause. It may or may not be related to trauma to the oral mucosa but is manifest as an enlarging and often painless ulceration.[37,38] It is more commonly found in the palatal mucosa (Fig. 107-9) but can also be seen in the buccal mucosa or the lips. It is a self-limited process and heals on its own, or it may be diagnosed by histologic examination after it is removed for not healing.

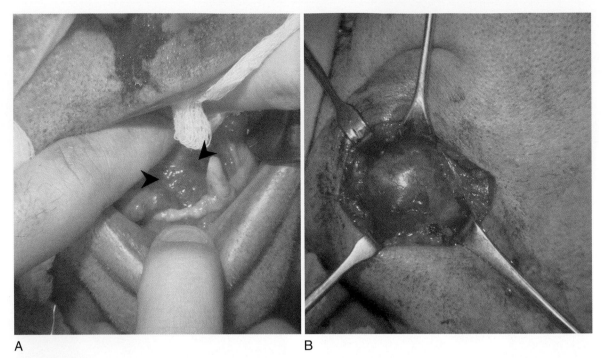

A   B

FIGURE 107-7. An obstructed edematous Wharton duct in the floor of the mouth *(A)* has led to an enlarged salivary cyst *(B)* within the submandibular gland.

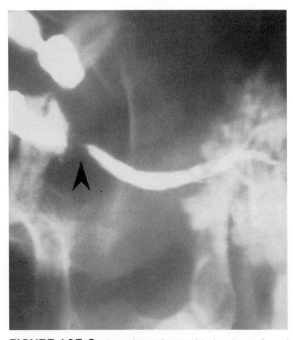

FIGURE 107-8. An enlarged parotid gland was found to be due to stenosis of the Stensen duct when radiopaque dye is injected in a sialogram.

Benign Neoplastic Lesions

Pleomorphic Adenoma. Also known as the benign mixed tumor, pleomorphic adenoma is the most common tumor of salivary glands. The tumor was originally believed to be "mixed" neoplastic cells derived from both duct epithelial cells and myoepithelial cells. However, it is now known to be a neoplasm of purely ectodermal cells.

These tumors most commonly occur in the parotid gland (80% to 90% of cases) and appear as painless, "rubbery" firm, 1- to 2-cm masses in the deeper tissue. They are not attached to the overlying skin, and they do not cause any muscle dysfunction by pressure on the motor branches of the facial nerve. They can rarely be found bilaterally.[39]

On histologic examination, there is a distribution of mostly epithelial and stromal (mesenchymal) cells. These mesenchymal areas of the tumor may consist of chondroid or hyalinized stroma that has the appearance of hyaline cartilage on histologic examination.

A preoperative diagnosis may be made by cytologic examination of a biopsy sample from FNA. The diagnosis is usually made after the tumor mass is removed with surrounding normal gland by means of resection of the entire segment of the parotid gland superficial to the plane of the facial nerve (Fig. 107-10). This procedure will usually result in a low incidence of recurrence (1%).[40] On occasion, the tumor is in the deep

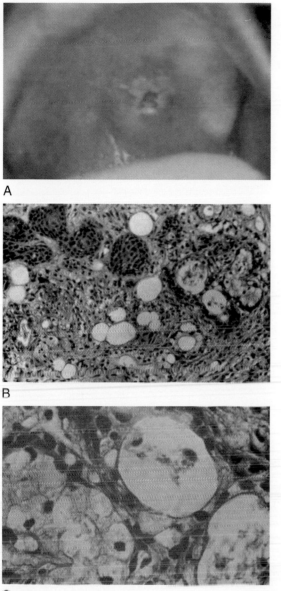

FIGURE 107-9. Necrotizing sialometaplasia presenting as an ulcer with sharp margins in the palate *(A)* of a 56-year-old man. Histologic examination of this lesion under low power *(B)* shows liquefaction and necrosis of mucinous glands and marked inflammatory response. High-power view *(C)* shows destruction of gland, release of mucin, and acute inflammation. (From Gahhos F, Enriquez RE, Ariyan S, et al: Necrotizing sialometaplasia: report of five cases. Plast Reconstr Surg 1983;71:650.)

segment of the parotid gland (Fig. 107-11), requiring dissection of the facial nerve to protect the nerve and subsequently to remove the deep tumor.

Recurrent pleomorphic adenomas are uncommon but require careful management. They are best controlled by aggressive surgical removal and total

parotidectomy when necessary to achieve long-term control rates of better than 90%.[41] Postoperative radiation therapy has been shown to be effective in improving control rates in those patients at high risk for recurrence. Recurrence may also occasionally (less than 1%) be manifested as a transformation to malignant mixed tumor.[42,43]

MONOMORPHIC ADENOMA. Although related to pleomorphic adenoma (benign mixed tumor), these tumors are usually manifested as single-cell variants of the benign mixed tumor. These tumors have been classified differently by a variety of authors, but the most widely used classification is that of Batsakis,[44] which describes the tumor to be derived from the duct cells. As such, they are either purely epithelial (basal cell adenoma) (Fig. 107-12) or purely mesenchymal (myoepithelioma) tumors. On histologic examination, these tumors are found to grow by expansion against the salivary gland tissue and not by infiltration. Batsakis believes that if left alone, these tumors would eventually develop into the pleomorphic variant of the adenoma.

The behavior of this tumor is benign. If the tumor is removed surgically, recurrence is as acceptably low as that of the pleomorphic variant. Malignant transformations are believed to be rare.

WARTHIN TUMOR (PAPILLARY CYSTADENOMA LYMPHOMATOSUM). This benign tumor is the second most common tumor of parotid glands. It is found almost exclusively in the parotid gland and is most commonly found in men between 50 and 60 years old.[45] It is clinically detected as a smooth mass, 3 to 4 cm in diameter, in the superficial segment of the gland (Fig. 107-13); it may be found bilaterally in about 10% of the patients.[46,47]

These tumors are derived from the proliferation of lymphoid tissues of periparotid or intraparotid lymph nodes. As such, they are believed to be proliferative tumors rather than neoplastic tumors. The diagnosis can be aided preoperatively by technetium scans because the tumor consistently concentrates this isotope and gives the appearance of a "hot gland."[48] A preoperative FNA biopsy may show the lymphoid tissue and confirm the diagnosis. The tumor can be surgically removed with a narrow margin of glandular tissue. Recurrences after resection are rare[49] and may represent multicentric foci of lymphoid proliferation.[22] Alternatively, the tumor may be left alone if the diagnosis is confirmed preoperatively and if the patient is willing to accept the facial appearance of fullness.

ONCOCYTOMA. This is a benign neoplasm of the oncocytes and represents less than 1% of all salivary gland tumors.[50] It is usually found in the parotid gland as an encapsulated lobular mass, often in elderly

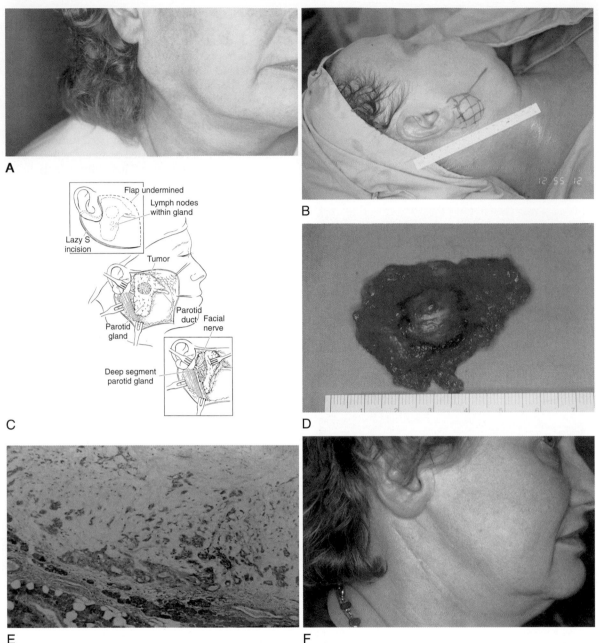

FIGURE 107-10. A large pleomorphic adenoma *(A* and *B)* at the angle of the jaw was removed with the superficial segment of the parotid gland *(C).* The horizontal plane of dissection is along the branches of the facial nerve *(C).* The tumor is removed with the superficial segment of the gland *(D).* Histologic examination *(E)* shows chondroid material (upper half). A shallowness is seen postoperatively at the site of the resected segment of the gland *(F).*

patients. It is believed by some to be a result of aging tissue in salivary glands rather than a true neoplastic development.

Resection of the involved segment of the parotid gland is usually curative. Recurrences or malignant transformations are rare,[51] in which case resection with a good margin of normal tissue is required.

HEMANGIOMA. These tumors are found mostly in the parotid glands, and 50% of these tumors are diagnosed in children.[52] In fact, they are the predominant tumor of parotid glands in children (Fig. 107-14). The tumors are present at birth and are usually identified within the first few months of life. The lesions are capillary, cavernous, or mixed vascular malformations.

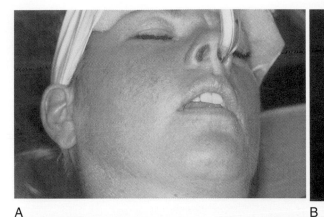

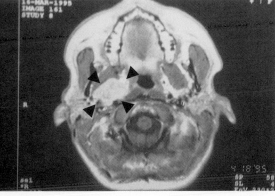

A

B

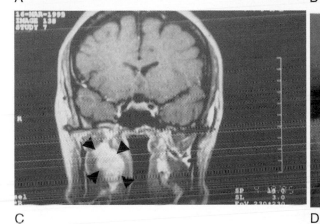

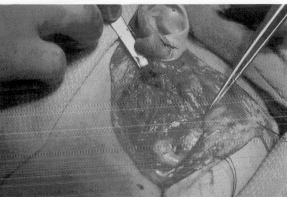

C

D

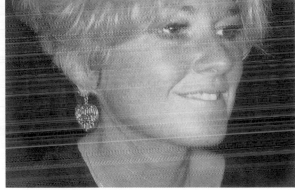

E

FIGURE 107-11. A small mass at the region of the angle of the jaw (A) is seen to be a large tumor of the deep segment of the parotid gland on MRI (B and C). This required a dissection and retraction of the facial nerve to remove the tumor with the deep segment of the gland (D). There is no hollow in the cheek postoperatively (E) because most of the superficial segment was retained.

The capillary hemangiomas are the most common and often grow rapidly for the first 6 months before undergoing spontaneous resolution during the next 5 to 6 years.

The cavernous or mixed vascular malformations may continue to grow. There is no indication for treatment with ionizing radiation, laser treatments, or freezing. When the tumor is expanding, a course of oral prednisone has been shown to be effective.[53] If regression is noted after 2 weeks, another week of treatment is indicated, followed by tapering of the dose. If the growth continues despite treatment, early surgical removal is indicated to prevent physical occlusion of the external auditory canal (Fig. 107-15).

Malignant Neoplastic Lesions

MUCOEPIDERMOID CARCINOMA. This tumor arises from the excretory ducts of the glands and represents the most common malignant tumor of salivary glands (Tables 107-4 and 107-5). Mucoepidermoid carcinoma is the most common malignant tumor to occur in the

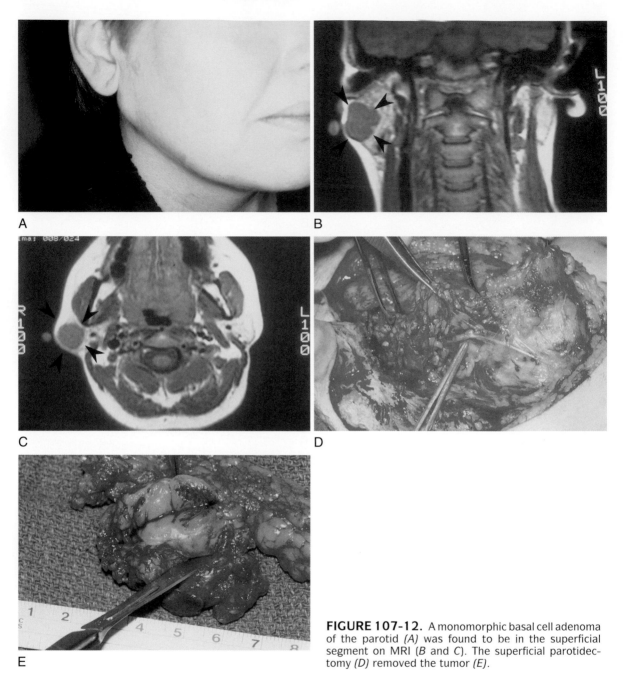

FIGURE 107-12. A monomorphic basal cell adenoma of the parotid *(A)* was found to be in the superficial segment on MRI *(B* and *C)*. The superficial parotidectomy *(D)* removed the tumor *(E)*.

TABLE 107-4 ✦ MALIGNANT TUMORS OF PAROTID GLAND

Type	Percentage
Mucoepidermoid	24
Adenoid cystic	16
Acinic cell	15
Adenocarcinoma	13
Squamous cell	5
Undifferentiated	27

TABLE 107-5 ✦ MALIGNANT TUMORS OF SUBMAXILLARY GLAND AND SUBLINGUAL GLANDS

Type	Submandibular	Sublingual
Adenoid cystic	50%	45%
Mucoepidermoid	25%	40%
Adenocarcinoma	20%	
Malignant mixed	5%	

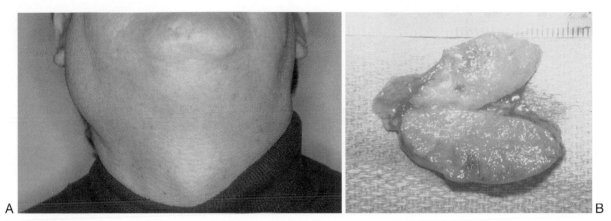

FIGURE 107-13. A unilateral Warthin tumor in a middle-aged man *(A)* was removed and shows the cystic lymphoid tissue on cut section of the tumor *(B)*.

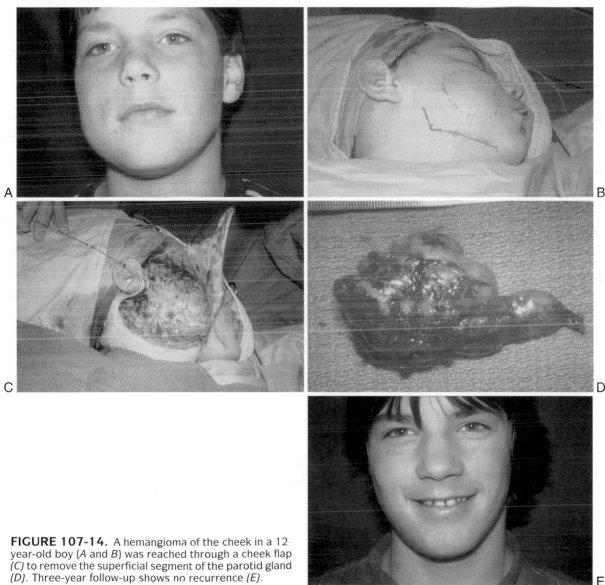

FIGURE 107-14. A hemangioma of the cheek in a 12-year-old boy *(A* and *B)* was reached through a cheek flap *(C)* to remove the superficial segment of the parotid gland *(D)*. Three-year follow-up shows no recurrence *(E)*.

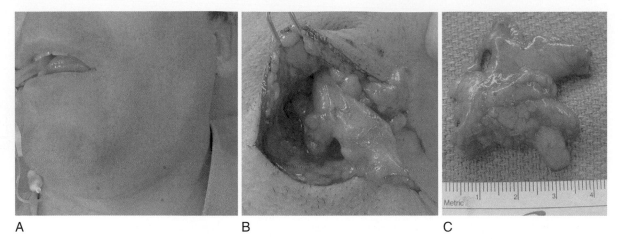

A   B   C

FIGURE 107-15. Soft mass on the cheek overlying the parotid gland *(A)* was diagnosed as a lipoma. The tumor can be dissected out from the gland surface along its tissue planes *(B)*. This tumor was multilobulated *(C),* requiring slow and meticulous dissection of all its extensions from the surrounding tissue.

parotid gland. The tumor appears grossly as a slow-growing, firm to hard mass within the salivary gland. If the tumor is neglected by the patient and grows larger, there may be associated pain (from sensory nerve involvement) or ipsilateral weakness of certain facial muscles (due to tumor infiltration into branches of the facial nerve).

The tumors are characterized histologically by the presence of mucin-producing cells, squamous cells of the ducts or acini, and other cells with little differentiation and scant cytoplasm. They are classified as low-grade, intermediate-grade, or high-grade malignant lesions on the basis of the histologic evaluation of the cell types predominating in the tumor.[54,55]

Low-grade lesions have predominantly mucous cells and well-formed glandular cysts. Intermediate-grade lesions have a combination of the cell types (but cystic or glandular changes are infrequent), are locally invasive, and may metastasize. High-grade lesions have predominantly solid areas of squamous cells, with little or no glandular cysts or mucous cells. These tumors have a greater tendency to invade adjacent tissue, grow rapidly, and metastasize.

The treatment of these tumors should be guided by the grade of differentiation. The behavior of low-grade tumors can be similar to that of pleomorphic adenoma, and the incidence of occult microscopic metastases to regional nodes is less than 10%. Therefore, this variant of the tumor can be treated with superficial parotidectomy alone (Fig. 107-16) if the frozen section of the tumor reveals no tumor at the margins. If the permanent sections after the operation show evidence of tumor at the margins, postoperative radiation therapy is indicated to decrease the chance of recurrence. These patients then need to be observed for evidence of future recurrence or cervical node involvement.

The intermediate-grade tumors have a more aggressive behavior with regard to local or regional involvement. In general, these tumors should be resected with preservation of the facial nerve if it is not involved with tumor. If a sample of the submandibular or jugulodigastric nodes shows any evidence of tumor, a cervical lymph node dissection is indicated. Because the recurrence rate is reported to be 15% to 20%, postoperative radiation therapy to the tumor site and neck should be considered. The 5-year cure rate of intermediate-grade mucoepidermoid carcinoma is reported to be as high as 90%.

High-grade tumors are even more aggressive in their behavior. They have a greater tendency to metastasize to regional neck nodes (60%) and can infiltrate facial nerves (25%), leading to facial weakness. The treatment of these tumors requires a more aggressive approach with a total parotidectomy and resection of any facial nerve branches that are involved with the tumor (Fig. 107-17). Facial nerve grafting with a segment of the great auricular nerve may be indicated. Because of the high incidence of cervical node metastases (Table 107-6), neck dissection is indicated for control. These patients should then be treated with a

TABLE 107-6 ✦ INCIDENCE OF NECK NODE METASTASES BY TUMOR TYPE

Type	Percentage
Squamous cell	70
Mucoepidermoid (high grade)	60
Malignant mixed	30-50
Acinic cell	30
Adenocarcinoma	25
Adenoid cystic	10-15

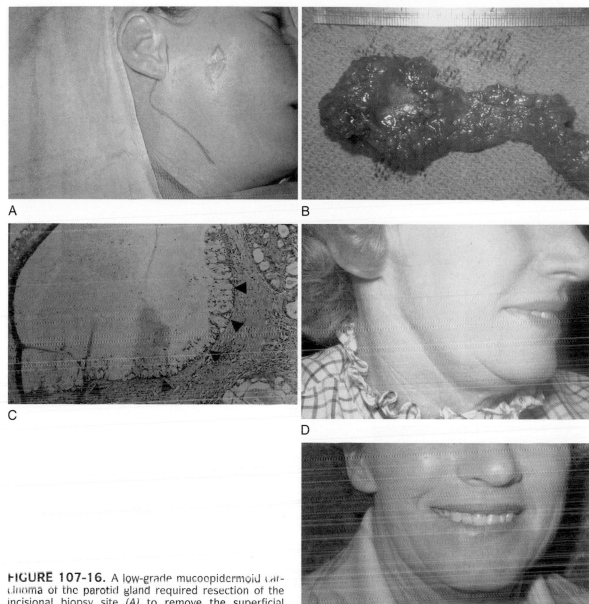

FIGURE 107-16. A low-grade mucoepidermoid carcinoma of the parotid gland required resection of the incisional biopsy site *(A)* to remove the superficial segment of the parotid gland and tumor *(B)*. Histologic examination *(C)* shows well-differentiated cells *(arrows)* lining a mucin-producing gland. Six years after surgery *(D* and *E)*, there is no evidence of recurrence.

full course of postoperative radiation therapy to the site of the primary tumor and to the neck (Fig. 107-18).[56]

ADENOID CYSTIC CARCINOMA (CYLINDROMA). This is the second most common malignant tumor found in the parotid gland and the most common in the submandibular and sublingual glands (see Tables 107-4 and 107-5). This tumor gets its name from its characteristic histologic pattern of cystic or cribriform arrangement that gives a "Swiss cheese" appearance. The tumor appears clinically as a firm 1- to 3-cm lesion that is fixed. It has a marked affinity for perineural inva-

sion (Fig. 107-19), leading to facial weakness and paralysis in 25% to 30% of the patients.[57,58] Lymph node metastases are usually uncommon (10% to 15%); lymph node involvement is usually limited to the first echelon of nodes adjacent to the tumor.[58,59]

The surgical treatment of this insidious tumor requires aggressive resection of the gland to remove the tumor. Because of the affinity of the tumor for neural invasion both locally and at significant distances from the primary tumor, any nerves in the path of the tumor should be resected.[60] This may require resection of the main trunk of the facial nerve, even into

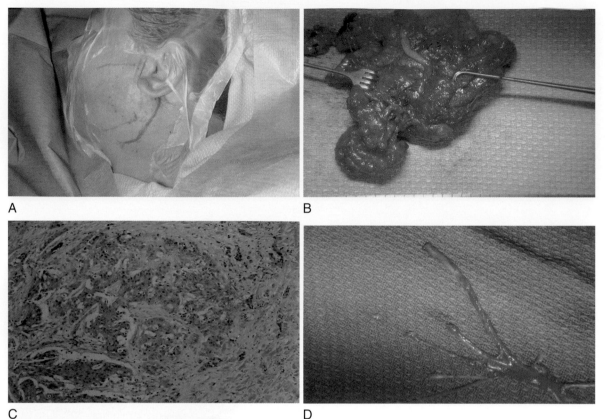

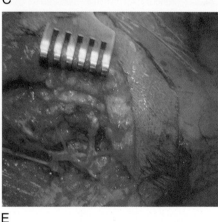

FIGURE 107-17. A high-grade mucoepidermoid carcinoma of the parotid gland *(A)* necessitated total parotidectomy with resection of the facial nerve *(B)*. Histologic examination *(C)* shows poorly differentiated epidermal cells and no mucous glands. The greater auricular nerve *(D)* was used to graft the facial nerve branches *(E)*.

the temporal bone if it is involved. Otherwise, in these extensive cases, the recurrences would involve the skull base and cranial nerves as the tumor spreads into the central nervous system.

Adenoid cystic carcinomas are considered radioresistant in that the recurrences cannot be "cured" with radiation therapy. However, radiation therapy as an adjuvant to surgery can suppress or slow the growth rate.[61] Therefore, this treatment modality has also been helpful in cases of unresectable recurrences.

Adenoid cystic carcinomas behave in an unpredictable fashion. Some tumors grow rapidly and lead to the patient's early demise; others may exhibit very slow growth of pulmonary metastases lasting 20 years. Studies have reported 5-year survival rates of 75% to 80%, but the 10-year survival rates are 10% to 30%, and the 15-year survival rates are 1% to 10%.

ACINIC CELL CARCINOMA. These are malignant tumors of the acinic cells of salivary glands and are found overwhelmingly in the parotid gland. They are solid tumors 1 to 3 cm in diameter but may also appear as cystic masses. The tumor can be multifocal, and 3% of these lesions are found bilaterally.[62]

Acinic cell carcinomas have an aggressive biologic behavior with finger-like extensions of growth into

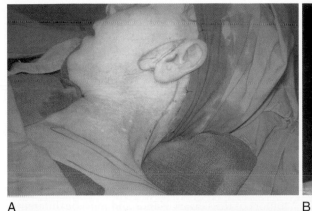

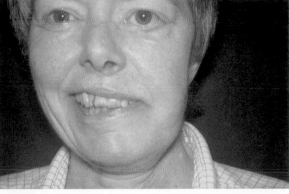

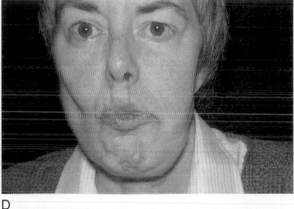

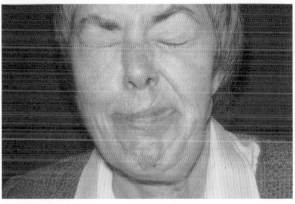

FIGURE 107-18. A recurrent mucoepidermoid carcinoma of the parotid gland *(A)* was treated with total parotidectomy, resection of facial nerve with nerve graft, cervical node dissection, and postoperative radiation therapy. The postoperative left facial palsy *(B* and *C)* improved during the next 12 months *(D* and *E)*.

the adjacent tissues. Lymph node involvement is found in 30% of the patients, and the tumor metastasizes commonly to lung, liver, and bones. Therefore, the treatment of this tumor requires aggressive resection with total parotidectomy, resection of the facial nerve and repair with nerve grafts, and complete neck dissection if nodes are palpable. In patients with clinically negative nodes, elective lymphadenectomy may be considered in selected patients. Radiation therapy does not seem to be effective in controlling recurrences.

ADENOCARCINOMA. These tumors are classified by the very nature of being excluded from the preceding categories of glandular malignant tumors. Their true incidence is not known, but they probably represent about 3% to 5% of all salivary gland tumors (Fig. 107-20).

These tumors appear as hard infiltrating masses that grow slowly. At the time of diagnosis, they are often associated with facial nerve involvement, cervical node metastases, or systemic organ metastases.

When these tumors are in the parotid gland, the treatment is wide resection with sacrifice of the facial

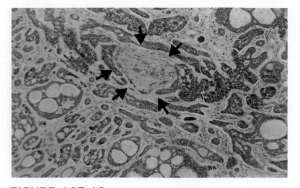

FIGURE 107-19. Adenoid cystic carcinoma showing cystic and cribriform pattern typically described as Swiss cheese. The center of this section shows the tumor cells invading nerve *(arrows)*.

nerve, nerve grafting, and cervical node dissection. Post-operative radiation therapy should be considered because of the frequent and rapid onset of recurrences. The prognosis is poor, with 5-year survivals reported at 25% to 50%.[63]

MALIGNANT MIXED TUMORS. These tumors are most commonly malignant transformation from a benign pleomorphic adenoma. Although it is believed that malignant cells may develop primarily with the basic pattern of a mixed tumor, the consensus remains that malignant mixed tumors and carcinomas arising in a pleomorphic adenoma are one and the same.

However, there is a difference between the recurrent benign mixed tumor, which is composed of well-circumscribed nodules growing in scar tissue and shows benign cytologic patterns, and the malignant mixed tumor, which is not circumscribed but shows invasion into adjacent tissue and nerves.[64]

The treatment of this lesion is aggressive total parotidectomy and resection of the facial nerve with nerve grafting. However, diagnosis of this tumor may be difficult with frozen section, for it may initially be interpreted as a pleomorphic adenoma, with the subsequent permanent sections showing the features of malignant cells and aggressive invasion. The prognosis of this tumor is poor, with 5-year survival rates reported to be about 40%.[65]

SQUAMOUS CELL CARCINOMA. These are rare tumors of the salivary glands and must be differentiated from squamous cell carcinomas metastatic to salivary glands or underdiagnosed mucoepidermoid carcinoma. The true squamous cell carcinomas represent cancers arising from the salivary ducts themselves. These tumors have a high propensity for regional nodal spread.[66]

ONCOCYTIC CARCINOMA. This is a malignant variant of the oncocytoma (itself representing only 1% of all salivary gland tumors), making this a rare tumor. It should be treated with aggressive local resection and cervical nodal dissection if lymph nodes are found to be involved.

LYMPHOMA. This tumor represents the local manifestation of a systemic disease. When it involves salivary glands, it almost always involves the parotid gland, as this is the only salivary gland that contains lymph nodes or lymphoid tissue. These tumors are removed by excisional biopsy of the lymph node (Fig. 107-21) and are evaluated histologically for diagnosis and classification of the type of lymphoma.

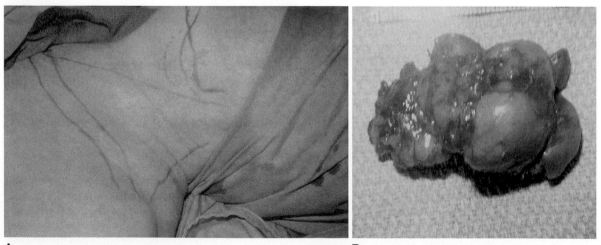

A   B

FIGURE 107-20. Submandibular gland *(A)* was removed and found to be an adenocarcinoma *(B)*.

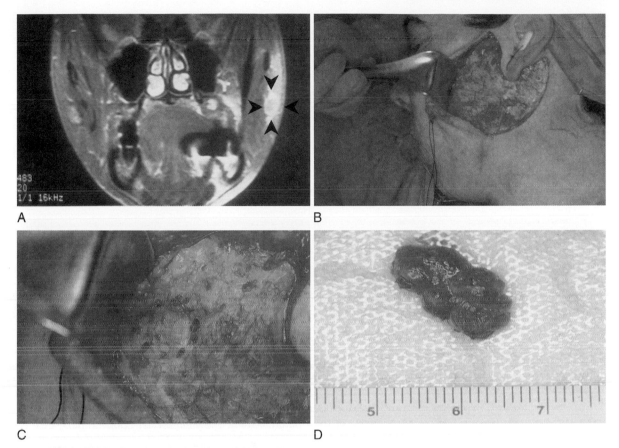

FIGURE 107-21. An MRI of the cheek identified a lymph node in the parotid gland *(A)*. A preoperative needle biopsy showed atypical lymphocytes. The mass was found in the superficial segment of the parotid *(B* and *C)*; it was removed and found to be a lymph node *(D)* harboring a lymphoma.

There is now an increasing incidence of acquired immunodeficiency syndrome (AIDS) diagnosed by the lymph node manifestation of this viral disease.[34] Parotid gland swelling is often found in patients with HIV infection, and this manifestation can also be the initial presentation of the disease. Most commonly, the swelling is bilateral and painless, and it is a benign cystic lesion. The etiology has been postulated to be compression due to intraparotid lymphadenopathy and swelling as a result of the autoimmune phenomena.[67,68] Of note, this benign lesion has been found to be a reservoir of HIV-1.[69] Treatment of this disease is nonsurgical (other than the excision of the nodal tissue for diagnosis) and is dictated by the histologic diagnosis of the node. In addition, patients with AIDS have been found to harbor Kaposi sarcoma of the parotid gland.[70]

Metastatic Tumors

Metastases to salivary glands account for 5% to 10% of salivary gland tumors. The parotid is the salivary gland most commonly involved with these metastases because of its rich lymphoid tissue. For that reason, it is easy to understand that lymphatic metastases to the parotid gland most commonly arise from other malignant neoplasms in the head and neck area. A comprehensive series on metastasis to the parotid gland was performed by Conley and Arena in 1963.[71] Of the 81 cases of metastasis to the parotid, 46% were melanoma, 37% were squamous cell carcinoma, and 14% were other malignant tumors. Sarcomas were the most common in this small last group, but it also included cylindroma of the ear canal and basal cell carcinoma.

Hematogenous spread to salivary glands can also be seen, and the parotid gland is again the most commonly involved. Whereas any cancer can spread to the parotid gland, the most common have been reported to be adenocarcinomas of the thyroid.

Frey Syndrome

Postgustatory sweating (Frey syndrome) is caused by the interconnection of the cut parasympathetic nerve

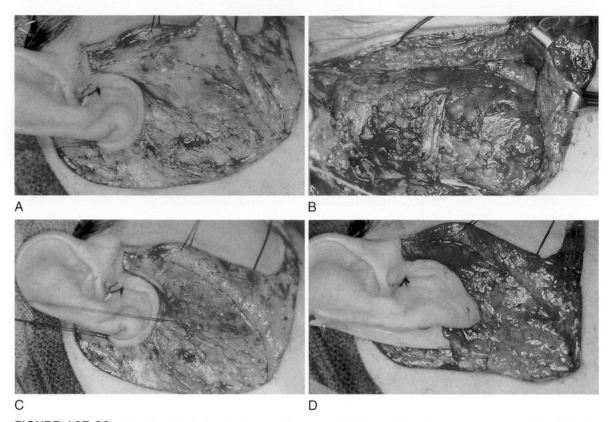

FIGURE 107-22. After the cheek flap is elevated for a parotidectomy, the submuscular aponeurotic system is elevated *(A)* and preserved. After completion of the parotidectomy *(B)*, the submuscular aponeurotic system is placed back over the exposed parotid resection *(C)* before the cheek flap is closed. If the peripheral edge of the submuscular aponeurotic system is preserved and rolled under, it can serve as soft tissue to fill the hollow of the resected gland *(D)*.

fibers of the surgically open and raw parotid gland to the cut sympathetic nerve fibers to the sweat glands of the overlying skin flap of the cheek. Because the sympathetic nerve fibers to the sweat glands are cholinergic fibers, when the patient eats food, the parasympathetic fibers of the gland stimulate the cholinergic fibers of the sweat gland to secrete. The patient then complains of sweating from the cheek on the operative side when eating.

This entity is often minimal and the incidence is reported in the literature to range from 7% to 50%,[72-74] depending on the degree of symptoms necessary for diagnosis. On occasion, there may be profuse sweating requiring intervention. In such cases, re-elevation of the cheek flap will cut these fibers and scarring from the procedure may relieve the symptoms. It is best at these operations to place a sheet of fascia (fascia lata or temporalis fascia) in the intervening space.

Since 1978, our incidence of this syndrome has been reduced by elevating the submuscular aponeurotic system that overlies the parotid gland (Fig. 107-22A) before performing the parotidectomy. The submuscular aponeurotic system is then placed over the exposed remaining deeper segments of the parotid gland (Fig. 107-22B to D) to separate the parasympathetic nerves of the gland from the sympathetic nerves of the skin. Folding over the edges of the submuscular aponeurotic system can also help fill the hollow of the resected superficial segment of the gland.

REFERENCES

1. Eneroth EM: Salivary gland tumors in the parotid gland, submandibular gland and the palate region. Cancer 1971;27:1415.
2. Thackray AC: Salivary gland tumors. Proc R Soc Med 1968;61:1089.
3. Saunders JR, Hirata RM, Jaques DA: Salivary glands. Surg Clin North Am 1986;66:59.
4. Spiro RH, Hajdu SI, Strong EW: Tumors of the submaxillary gland. Am J Surg 1991;162:330.
5. Spiro RH, Thaler HT, Hicks WF, et al: The importance of clinical staging of minor salivary gland carcinoma. Am J Surg 1991;162:330.

6. Beckhardt RN, Weber RS, Zane R, et al: Minor salivary gland tumors of the palate: clinical and pathologic correlates of outcomes. Laryngoscope 1995;105:1155.

7. Neely MM, Rohrer MD, Young SK: Tumors of minor salivary glands and the analysis of 106 cases. J Okla Dent Assoc 1996;86:50.

8. Saka T, Hayaski Y, Takahara O, et al: Salivary gland tumors among atomic bomb survivors. Cancer 1971;27:1415.

9. Takeichi N, Hirose F, Yamamoto H: Salivary gland tumors in atomic bomb survivors, Hiroshima, Japan. Cancer 1976;38:2462.

10. Pogoda J, Preston-Martin S: Comment on "Incidence of salivary gland tumors among atomic bomb survivors, 1950-1987. Evaluation of radiation-related risk" by Land et al (Radiat Res 146:28-36, 1996). Radiat Res 1996;146:356.

11. Land C, Saku T, Hayashi Y, et al: Incidence of salivary gland tumors among atomic bomb survivors, 1950-1987. Evaluation of radiation-related risk. Radiat Res 1996;146:28.

12. Modan B, Baidatz D, Mart H, et al: Radiation-induced head and neck tumours. Lancet 1974;1:277.

13. Preston-Martin S: Prior x-ray therapy for acne related to tumors of the parotid gland. Arch Dermatol 1989;125:921.

14. Scheider A, Favus M, Stachura M, et al: Salivary gland neoplasms as a late consequence of head and neck irradiation. Ann Intern Med 1977;87:160.

15. Bhatia A: Fine-needle aspiration cytology in the diagnosis of mass lesions of the salivary gland. Indian J Cancer 1993;30:26.

16. Cohen MB, Resnicek MJ, Miller TR: Fine-needle aspiration of salivary glands. Pathol Annu 1992;27:213.

17. Stewart CJ, MacKenzie K, McGarry GW, Mowat A: Fine-needle aspiration cytology of salivary gland: a review of 341 cases. Diagn Cytopathol 2000;22:139.

18. Orell SR: Diagnostic difficulties in the interpretation of fine-needle aspirates of salivary gland lesions: the problem revisited. Cytopathology 1995;6:285.

19. Cohen MB, Ljung BM, Boles R: Salivary gland tumors. Fine-needle aspiration vs frozen-section diagnosis. Arch Otolaryngol Head Neck Surg 1986;112:867.

20. Frable MS, Frable WJ: Fine-needle aspiration biopsy of salivary glands. Laryngoscope 1991;101:245.

21. Rodriguez HP, Silver CE, Moisa JJ, Chacho MS: Fine-needle aspiration of parotid tumors. Am J Surg 1989;158:342.

22. Chan MKM, McGuire LJ, King W, et al: Cytodiagnosis of 112 salivary gland lesions. Acta Cytol 1991;36:353.

23. Ostrezega N, Cheng N, Layfield L: Glial fibrillary acid protein immunoreactivity in fine-needle aspiration of salivary gland lesions, a useful adjunct for the diagnosis of salivary gland neoplasms. Diagn Cytopathol 1989;5:145.

24. Cardillo MR: Ag-NOR technique in fine-needle aspiration cytology of salivary gland masses. Acta Cytol 1991;36:147.

25. Kern SB: Necrosis of Warthin's tumor following fine-needle aspiration. Acta Cytol 1988;32:207.

26. O'Dwyer P, Farrar WB, James AG, et al: Needle aspiration biopsy of major salivary gland tumors. Cancer 1986;57:554.

27. Qizilbash AH, Sianos J, Young JEM, Archibald SG: Fine-needle aspiration biopsy cytology of major salivary glands. Acta Cytol 1985;29:503.

28. Shaha AR, Webber C, Dimaio T, Jaffee BM: Needle aspiration biopsy in salivary gland lesions. Am J Surg 1990;160:373.

29. Casselman JW, Mancuso AA: Major salivary gland masses. Comparison of MR imaging and CT. Radiology 1987;165:183.

30. Som PM, Curtin HD: Head and Neck Imaging, vol 2, 3rd ed. Salivary Glands. St. Louis, Mosby, 1996:833-846.

31. Runge VM, Nelson KL: Contrast agents. In Stark DD, Bradley WG, eds: Magnetic Resonance Imaging, 3rd ed. St. Louis, Mosby, 1999:264.

32. Kramer LA, Mafee M: Magnetic resonance imaging of the salivary gland. In Stark DD, Bradley WG, eds: Magnetic Resonance Imaging, 3rd ed. St. Louis, Mosby, 1999:1771-1783.

33. Silvers AR, Som PM: Salivary glands. Radiol Clin North Am 1998;36:941.

34. Shaha AR, DiMaio T, Webber C, et al: Benign lymphoepithelial lesions of the parotid. Am J Surg 1993;166:403.

35. Harvey J, Catoggio L, Gallagher PJ, et al: Salivary gland biopsy in sarcoidosis. Sarcoidosis 1989;6:47.

36. James DG, Sharma OP: Parotid gland sarcoidosis. Sarcoidosis Vasc Diffuse Lung Dis 2000;17:27.

37. Gahhos F, Enriquez RE, Ariyan S, et al: Necrotizing sialometaplasia: report of five cases. Plast Reconstr Surg 1983;71:650.

38. Fowler CB, Brannon RB: Subacute necrotizing sialadenitis: report of seven cases and a review of the literature. Oral Surg Oral Med Oral Pathol Oral Radiol Endod 2000;89:600.

39. Norlin R: Bilateral mixed tumors of the parotid initially regarded as pharyngeal neoplasm. Pract Otorhinolaryngol 1965;27:298.

40. Laccourreye H, Laccourreye O, Cauchois R, et al: Total conservative parotidectomy for primary benign pleomorphic adenoma of the parotid gland: a 25-year experience with 229 patients. Laryngoscope 1994;104:1487.

41. Carew JF, Spiro RH, Singh B, et al: Treatment of recurrent pleomorphic adenomas of the parotid gland. Otolaryngol Head Neck Surg 1999;121:539.

42. McGrath MH: Malignant transformation in concurrent benign mixed tumors of parotid and submaxillary glands. Plast Reconstr Surg 1980;65:676.

43. Foote FW, Frazell EL: Tumors of the major salivary glands. Cancer 1953;6:1065.

44. Batsakis JG: Tumors of the Head and Neck, 2nd ed. Baltimore, Williams & Wilkins, 1979:50-54.

45. Yoo GH, Eisele DW, Askin FB, et al: Warthin's tumor: a 40-year experience at the Johns Hopkins Hospital. Laryngoscope 1994;104:799.

46. Ebbs SR, Webb AJ: Adenolymphoma of the parotid: aetiology, diagnosis, and treatment. Br J Surg 1986;73:627.

47. Lam KH, Ho HC, Ho CM: Multifocal nature of adenolymphoma of the parotid. Br J Surg 1994;81:161.

48. Higashi T, Murahashi H, Ikuta H, et al: Identification of Warthin's tumor with technetium-99m pertechnetate. Clin Nucl Med 1987;12:796.

49. Leverstein H, van der Wal JE, Tiwari RM, et al: Results of the surgical management and histopathological evaluation of 88 parotid gland Warthin's tumours. Clin Otolaryngol 1997;22:500.

50. Paulino AF, Havos AG: Oncocytic and oncocytoid tumors of the salivary glands. Semin Diagn Pathol 1999;16:98.

51. Johns ME, Batsakis JG, Short CD: Oncocytic and oncocytoid tumors of the salivary glands. Laryngoscope 1973;83:1940.

52. William HB: Hemangiomas of the parotid gland in children. Plast Reconstr Surg 1975;56:29.

53. Fost NC, Esterly NB: Successful treatment of juvenile hemangiomas with prednisone. J Pediatr 1968;72:351.

54. Hicks MJ, el-Naggar AK, Flaitz CM, et al: Histocytologic grading of mucoepidermoid carcinoma of major salivary glands in prognosis and survival: a clinicopathologic and flow cystometric investigation. Head Neck 1995;17:89.

55. Goode RK, Auclair PL, Ellis GL: Mucoepidermoid carcinoma of the major salivary glands: clinical and histopathologic analysis of 234 cases with evaluation of grading criteria. Cancer 1998;82:1217.

56. Garden AS, el-Naggar AK, Morrison WH, et al: Postoperative radiotherapy for malignant tumors of the parotid gland. Int J Radiat Oncol Biol Phys 1997;37:97.

57. Sur RK, Donde B, Levin V, et al: Adenoid cystic carcinoma of the salivary glands: a review of 10 years. Laryngoscope 1997;107:1276.

58. Jones AS, Hamilton JW, Rowley H, et al: Adenoid cystic carcinoma of the head and neck. Clin Otolaryngol 1997;22:434.

59. Allen MS, Marsh WL: Lymph node involvement by direct extension in adenoid cystic carcinoma: absence of classic embolic lymph node metastasis. Cancer 1976;38:2017.

60. Casler JD, Conley JJ: Surgical management of adenoid cystic carcinoma in the parotid gland. Otolaryngol Head Neck Surg 1992;106:332.
61. Avery CM, Moody AB, McKinna FE, et al: Combined treatment of adenoid cystic carcinoma of the salivary glands. Int J Oral Maxillofac Surg 2000;29:277.
62. Levin JM, Robinson DW, Lin F: Acinic cell carcinoma: collective review including bilateral cases. Arch Surg 1975;110:64.
63. Blanck C, Eneroth CM, Jakobsson PA: Mucus-producing adenopapillary (non-epidermoid) carcinoma of the parotid gland. Cancer 1971;28:676.
64. LiVolsi VA, Perzin KH: Malignant mixed tumors arising in salivary glands. I. Carcinomas arising in benign mixed tumors: a clinicopathologic study. Cancer 1977;39:2209.
65. Spiro RH, Huvos AG, Strong EW: Malignant mixed tumor of salivary origin: a clinicopathologic study of 146 cases. Cancer 1977;39:388.
66. Spiro RH, Huvos AG, Strong EW: Cancer of the parotid gland: a clinicopathologic study of 288 primary cases. Am J Surg 1975;130:452.
67. Ulrisch R, Jaffe E: Sjögren's syndrome–like illness associated with the acquired immunodeficiency syndrome–related complex. Hum Pathol 1987;18:1063.
68. Ioachim H: Salivary gland lymphadenopathies associated with AIDS. Hum Pathol 1988;19:616.
69. Uccini S, Riva E, Antonelli G, et al: The benign cystic lymphoepithelial lesion of the parotid gland is a viral reservoir in HIV type 1–infected patients. AIDS Res Hum Retrovir 1999;15:1339.
70. Mukherjee A, Silver C, Rosario P, Gerst P: Kaposi's sarcoma of the parotid gland in acquired immunodeficiency syndrome. Am Surg 1998;64:259.
71. Conley J, Arena S: Parotid gland as a focus of metastasis. Arch Surg 1963;87:757.
72. Leverstein H, van der Wal JE, Tiwari RM, et al: Surgical management of 246 previously untreated pleomorphic adenomas of the parotid gland. Br J Surg 1997;84:399.
73. Dulguerov P, Quinodoz D, Cosendai G, et al: Prevention of Frey syndrome during parotidectomy. Arch Otolaryngol Head Neck Surg 1999;125:833.
74. Laskawi R, Ellies M, Rodel R, et al: Gustatory sweating: clinical implications and etiologic aspects. J Oral Maxillofac Surg 1999;57:642.

Tumors of the Craniofacial Skeleton

Ian T. Jackson, MD, DSc (Hon), FRCS, FACS, FRACS (Hon)

Under the heading of craniofacial skeletal tumors are multiple benign and malignant lesions. The rare and not so rare conditions are considered, and the surgical approach for resection is described. The techniques learned in correction of craniofacial anomalies have allowed better tumor exposure, more effective resection, and much improved reconstruction. It also seems that in long-term follow-up, the prognosis for these conditions has improved.

CYSTS AND TUMORS OF THE MANDIBLE AND MAXILLA

If tumors of the paranasal sinuses are excluded, most tumors can be classified as odontogenic or nonodontogenic. Odontogenic lesions are composed of cells normally involved in dental development and are either cysts or tumors. Several classifications have been developed. In the classification of Reichart and Ries,[1] the histogenetic, organogenetic, and embryologic aspects of tooth development are used in four hypotheses that describe the formative process of benign odontogenic tumors (Table 108-1). The ectomesenchyme, which gives rise to odontoblasts and cementoblasts, is distinguished from mesenchymal tissue. Four histogenetic cell groups are used in this classification to describe the various types of odontogenic tumors: ameloblastic, ectomesenchymal, mesenchymal, and neuroectodermal. Combining the four histogenetic cell groups into pairs further facilitates both understanding and the systematic grouping of these neoplasms (Table 108-2). Nonodontogenic refers to all other jaw tumors.

Cysts of the Jaws

Jaw cysts are of two types: those arising from odontogenic epithelium (odontogenic cysts); and those arising from oral epithelium (fissural cysts), which occur at sites of embryonic fusion. Nonepithelial cysts, a third category, include traumatic and aneurysmal bone cysts.[2] Why these occur is unknown; it may be related to inflammation, age,[3] mechanical trauma, systemic disease, and increased local vascularity.[4] Keratocysts

TABLE 108-1 ✦ FOUR HYPOTHESES TO DESCRIBE THE GENESIS OF BENIGN ODONTOGENIC TUMORS

Hypothesis 1

Each neoplasm is characterized histogenetically and organogenetically by its mother tissue.

Hypothesis 2

In the tooth, a histogenetic distinction is made between ectomesenchymal cells (odontoblasts and cementoblasts) and mesenchymal cells that reveal mesodermal properties (supporting tissue, vessels, musculature).

Hypothesis 3

In each neoplastic cell, the same differentiation potentials (morphologic, metabolic, and inductive) are present in the mother cell.

Hypothesis 4

All odontogenic tumors are neoplasms in the sense of either autonomous or regulated proliferation of tumor cells.

From Reichart PA, Ries P: Consideration on the classification of odontogenic tumours. Int J Oral Surg 1983;12:323. Reproduced by permission of the International Association of Oral and Maxillofacial Surgeons.

can be aggressive and destroy significant areas of the jaws, cause dentition problems, and destroy neighboring structures. Tooth root resorption is not usually caused by cysts; when this is seen, it suggests a neoplastic process.

The lining of cysts may undergo malignant or ameloblastic change. Thus, it should always be sent for histologic examination.[5]

Cysts are not painful unless they become infected. They may cause no problems, but if they become large, a painless swelling is noted. There can be dental disruption, destruction of bone, facial deformity, or pathologic fractures.

ODONTOGENIC CYSTS

These are divided into developmental and inflammatory.

Developmental Odontogenic Cysts

GINGIVAL CYST. These cysts occur in the infant palate and alveolar ridges.[6] Those in the palate are fissural; alveolar lesions are derived from dental lamina.[7] They may be solitary or multiple and are usually small (<5 mm in diameter). These cysts contain keratin and usually resolve without treatment.[8]

In adults, gingival cysts are rare.[5] Again, they arise from dental lamina,[9] are painless, grow slowly, and are only 1 to 1.5 mm in diameter.[10] They are soft and

TABLE 108-2 ✦ HISTOGENESIS OF BENIGN ODONTOGENIC TUMORS

	Ameloblastic	Ectomesenchymal	Mesenchymal	Neuroectodermal (in strict sense)
Ameloblastic	Ameloblastoma Adenomatoid odontogenic tumor Calcifying epithelial odontogenic tumor			
Ectomesenchymal	Ameloblastic fibroma Ameloblastic fibro-odontoma Complex odontoma Cementoblastoma	Compound odontoma Dentinoma Odontogenic fibroma Odontogenic myxoma		
Mesenchymal	"Adamantine" hemangioma	Periapical cementoma dysplasia Gigantiform cementoma Cementifying fibroma	Fibroma Lipoma Hemangioma	
Neuroectodermal (in strict sense)	Ameloblastoma with neurinoma	"Central pacinian neurofibroma"	Neurofibroma	Neuroblastoma Melanotic neuroectodermal tumor of infancy
		in strict sense		in extended sense
		odontogenic tumors		

From Reichart PA, Ries P: Consideration on the classification of odontogenic tumours. Int J Oral Surg 1983;12:323. Reproduced by permission of the International Association of Oral and Maxillofacial Surgeons.

fluctuant. On radiologic examination, there is bone erosion. They rarely recur after excision.

LATERAL PERIODONTAL CYST. These cysts also arise from the dental lamina[9] and account for approximately 2% of odontogenic cysts.[5] They are asymptomatic and radiologically oval, translucent, and adjacent to a tooth root. They are usually less than 1 cm in diameter. The mandibular canine or premolar is most commonly involved.[11]

On histologic evaluation, these cysts are lined by thin, nonkeratinizing squamous epithelium.[9] The tooth is healthy, and treatment is enucleation of the cyst.

DENTIGEROUS CYST. An alternative name is follicular cyst; it makes up 18% of jaw cysts. Dentigerous cysts are asymptomatic and radiologically translucent. They encircle the crowns of unerupted teeth.[12] These cysts can become infected and cause a painful swelling. Their size varies from 2 to 10 cm. Large lesions can displace teeth and resorb roots. They mostly occur in the mandible in the region of the third molar.[13] In the maxilla, they tend to occur in the canine area.

They are lined by nonkeratinizing stratified squamous epithelium and rarely become malignant.[5]

ODONTOGENIC KERATINOCYST. The alternative term is primordial cyst; this seems to develop from dental lamina rests and basal cell hamartomas of the overlying oral mucosa.[2] It makes up 9% of odontogenic cysts.

On histologic evaluation, the cyst is composed of keratinizing stratified squamous epithelium that may show dysplastic change.[14] The size varies from 1 to 9 cm, and it can cause jaw expansion. It may perforate the cortex and is seen in association with the nevoid basal cell carcinoma of Gorlin and Goltz.[15] The recurrence rate after excision is 20% to 60%.[16]

Odontogenic keratinocysts can occur at any age, commonly between 20 and 50 years; men are affected twice as often as women are.[14] The mandible is more often involved than the maxilla. In the maxilla, they usually occur posteriorly and can grow enough to cross the midline.

The presentation is that of swelling and drainage and sometimes pain, paresthesia, and trismus. On radiologic examination, the cyst is radiolucent, is unilocular or multilocular, and has sclerotic margins. In 7% of patients, there are multiple cysts, especially in Gorlin syndrome. This syndrome is inherited as an autosomal dominant trait with marked penetrance and variable expressivity. Basal cells occur at an early age and are multiple; they are associated with jaw cysts, skeletal anomalies, calcification of the falx cerebri, nasal deformity, and palmar or plantar pits.[15]

Treatment consists of enucleation with aggressive curettage of the resulting cavity and close follow-up.

Ellis and Fonseca[17] have suggested that if the lesion recurs, it should be resected with 1-cm margins. The overlying oral mucosa must be excised at the enucleation, and inaccessible areas are cauterized with Carnoy solution.[18]

There is a variety of keratocyst that bursts out of the ascending ramus into the infratemporal fossa. This can erode the base of the skull and invade the middle cranial fossa. There is trismus and pain and a typical appearance on radiography and computed tomographic (CT) scan (Fig. 108-1).

Treatment is total parotidectomy with preservation of the facial nerve and, if possible, en bloc excision of the involved mandible, infratemporal fossa, and base of skull and any extension into the middle cranial fossa. Failure to do this invites recurrence, which is inoperable. Death is usually due to involvement of the cavernous sinus and resulting hemorrhage.

CALCIFYING ODONTOGENIC CYST (GORLIN CYST). This cystic lesion makes up 2% of jaw cysts.[19] It can be cystic or solid. It is similar histologically to the cutaneous lesion, the calcifying epithelioma of Malherbe.[20] The epithelial lining has ghost cells together with keratinization and calcification. On radiologic examination, it is a cyst containing calcified material.[2] In some, there is extensive ameloblastic proliferation of the epithelium.[20]

The majority occur in bone at any age but most commonly between the ages of 20 and 40 years. They affect the maxilla and mandible equally.[21] Most of these occur anterior to the first molar. They are painless, grow slowly, and are usually 1 to 8 cm in diameter. They should be resected, followed by aggressive curettage; with this, recurrence is rare.[2]

Inflammatory Odontogenic Cysts

RADICULAR CYST. These are the most common jaw cysts, ranging from 55% to 74%.[2,22] They begin as a periapical granuloma, followed by an inflammatory process in the dental pulp region. Their usual area is the apex of an erupted, nonvital tooth. A tooth negates the diagnosis of inflammatory odontogenic cyst.[17] The concept is that they arise from epithelial rests in the periodontal ligaments.[2] They have a fibrous wall lined by nonkeratinizing stratified squamous epithelium. Within this is a chronic inflammatory infiltrate. The age at occurrence is variable, but most occur in the 20s.[23] The most frequent site is the anterior maxilla, but they also occur in the mandible.[24] They rarely cause any problems and are often diagnosed on routine dental radiographs. An infection results in swelling, pain, and sometimes a sinus into the mouth or out onto the cheek.

On radiologic examination, these are ovoid, radiolucent areas with dense sclerotic margins in relation to the apex of a tooth root.

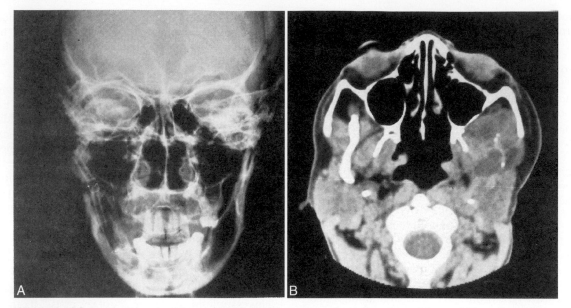

FIGURE 108-1. Keratocyst arising in right mandible and invading infratemporal fossa. *A,* Frontal plain film, right-sided maxillary keratocyst. *B,* Axial CT scan shows the cyst in greater detail on the right side with displacement of the zygomatic arch and temporal area. The cyst is multiloculated. (From Jackson IT, Shaw K: Tumors of the craniofacial skeleton, including the jaws. In McCarthy JG, ed: Plastic Surgery. Philadelphia, WB Saunders, 1990:3336.)

The usual treatment is endodontic observation. If anything untoward occurs (e.g., enlargement), periapical surgical removal is advised.[17] Recurrences are unusual.

RESIDUAL CYST. Failure to remove a root cyst of tooth extraction can result in a residual cyst.[25] If this enlarges, exploration should be performed.

LATERAL PERIODONTAL CYST. These are radicular cysts, lying lateral to the tooth root.[26] These probably occur because of periodontal pocket inflammation. The tooth remains vital. If possible, surgical removal is advised, avoiding injury to the adjacent dental roots.

PARADENTAL CYST. These are similar to radicular cysts and arise in relation to partially erupted third mandibular molars.[27] On radiologic examination, there is an overlying radiolucency near the buccal bifurcation of the third molar. They may arise from enamel epithelium or epithelial rests. Tooth extraction and cyst removal are recommended.

FISSURAL CYSTS

These cysts occur along the lines of embryologic fusion and are related to vital teeth. They are lined with epithelium. The cyst should be excised with tooth preservation.[17] Cysts in the maxilla may be lined by respiratory and squamous epithelium.

NASOPALATINE DUCT CYST. These cysts are common and grow to a large size. Removal is from a palatal approach, with care taken not to damage the vascularity of the incisors.

MEDIAN MAXILLARY PALATAL CYST. This cyst occurs in the midline between the palatal shelves and can involve the nose and maxillary sinus.

GLOBULOMAXILLARY CYST. This cyst occurs between the upper lateral incisor and canine with displacement of the neighboring tooth roots.

MEDIAN MANDIBULAR CYST. This cyst occurs at the symphysis of the mandible.

MANAGEMENT

Most jaw cysts can be enucleated. The mucoperiosteum is elevated, exposing the cyst, and it is removed. Large cysts can weaken the jaw with fracture, damage the inferior alveolar nerve, or enter the maxillary sinus and nasal cavity. A mucoperiosteal flap is elevated, and the histologic type is determined. In a benign cyst, the oral mucosa is sutured to the cyst wall to establish a permanent opening into the cyst, with irrigation; in time, the cyst will gradually become smaller. It is preferable to resect the cyst, but if this is not possible, extensive and complete curettage should be performed. The mucosa is closed over the area. If there is any significant problem, particularly after resection, serial packing is advised.

In large cysts, bone grafting is required; all others will become filled with bone between 6 months and

1 year. The advantages of primary bone grafting include prevention of fracture and maintenance of jaw anatomy.

Odontogenic Tumors

Odontogenic tumors can be benign or malignant. They may be truly epithelial or composed of mixed ectomesenchymal structures. Although most of these lesions are benign, bone destruction and entry into the sinuses may occur.

EPITHELIAL ODONTOGENIC TUMORS

Ameloblastic Tumors

AMELOBLASTOMA (ADAMANTINOMA). This tumor represents 11% of odontogenic tumors.[28] It may originate from dental lamina rests, the enamel organ, basal cells of the oral mucosa, or the epithelial lining of a dentigerous cyst.[29]

On histologic evaluation, the ameloblastic epithelium can be in strands, cords, or nests; there is little connective tissue stroma.[30] Follicular and plexiform varieties have been described.[31] Some can have cysts that are lined with squamous epithelium on microscopic examination.[29] With extensive keratinization, the term *acanthomatous ameloblastoma* has been coined.[29] This must be differentiated from a squamous cell carcinoma on biopsy.

Although it can occur at any age, the most common age is between 20 and 50 years.[31] The mandible is more frequently involved than the maxilla (4:1). The posterior region of both jaws is involved in 80% of tumors. They may be small or large, but the majority are in the 4- to 5-cm range. They grow slowly and are painless in most patients. There may be mobile teeth, malocclusion, ulceration, and ill-fitting dentures. The maxillary antrum can be involved, and there may be nasal obstruction.[32]

On radiologic examination, these tumors are unilocular or expansile multilocular lesions that are usually radiolucent. They may or may not be associated with a tooth (Fig. 108-2). Differentiation from dentigerous cysts may be difficult.[30] They can grow to large sizes with invasion of cancellous bone and sinuses. They are expansile and tend not to grow through cortical bone.

There are three types of ameloblastoma, and each requires a different treatment.[33]

Unicystic Ameloblastoma. This develops in the epithelial wall of a dentigerous cyst in the posterior aspect of the maxilla. Patients are younger than 30 years on most occasions. According to Ellis and Fonseca,[17] it can be treated by enucleation and curettage. When this is adopted, close follow-up is necessary. Unlike for the standard ameloblastoma, this method will result in a low recurrence rate.

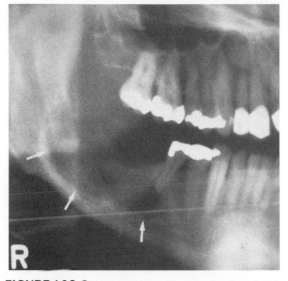

FIGURE 108-2. Ameloblastoma extending from just in front of the angle of the right mandible to the body of the mandible. Its anterior portion lies under the apex of the premolar. (From Jackson IT, Shaw K: Tumors of the craniofacial skeleton, including the jaws. In McCarthy JG, ed: Plastic Surgery. Philadelphia, WB Saunders, 1990:3336.)

Peripheral or Extraosseous Ameloblastoma. This arises from the basal layer of the surface epithelium overlying the tooth-bearing portion of the jaws. On biopsy, it may be difficult to differentiate from a basal cell or squamous cell carcinoma. It has a high recurrence rate, varying from 20% to 25%; thus, it should be resected radically.

Conventional Intraosseous Ameloblastoma. This lesion requires a relatively radical resection. In the mandible, the inferior mandibular margin should be preserved if possible with removal of teeth as required. The soft tissues are closed directly. If the tumor is large, is recurrent, or involves the angle and ramus of the mandible, a partial hemimandibulectomy is indicated. It is wise, if possible, to maintain the condyle and the posterior portion of the ramus. However, there should be no hesitation in carrying out full-thickness en bloc resection that must extend 1 to 2 cm beyond the area of involvement. Reconstruction can be performed with a free bone graft, but vascularized fibula or iliac crest is undoubtedly preferable.

MAXILLARY AMELOBLASTOMA. This is a significant problem and must be excised radically. The eye can usually be preserved, but in some aggressive tumors, it should be removed. Rarely is there intracranial extension, but when it occurs, there should be resection of the base of the anterior fossa or any other involved part of the cranial skeleton. After this, the appropriate reconstruction should be performed (Fig. 108-3).

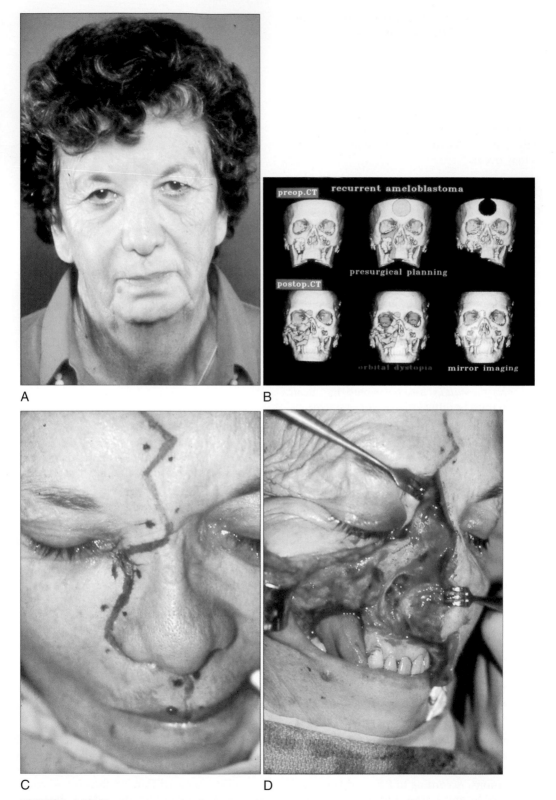

FIGURE 108-3. Recurrent right maxillary ameloblastoma. *A,* Preoperative appearance. *B,* Three-dimensional CT scan to show preoperative and postoperative appearance. *C,* Planned incision. *D,* Maxilla exposed.

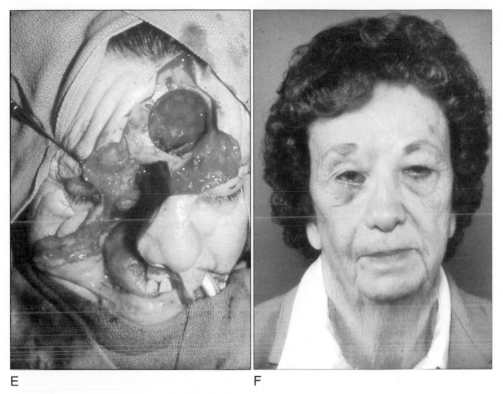

E

F

FIGURE 108-3, cont'd. *E,* Resection of maxilla and floor of anterior cranial fossa. *F.* Postoperative result. (*A, C,* and *E* from Jackson IT, Shaw K: Tumors of the craniofacial skeleton, including the jaws. In McCarthy JG, ed: Plastic Surgery. Philadelphia, WB Saunders, 1990:3336.)

ADENOMATOID ODONTOGENIC TUMOR

Adenomatoid odontogenic tumors are rare and of somewhat unknown origin. They represent approximately 3% of odontogenic tumors.[28] On histologic evaluation, this tumor is a thick-walled, cystic lesion; within this area, there is odontogenic epithelium.[30] It tends to occur in the second decade, and women are affected more than men.[34] The maxilla is involved more than the mandible. It may occur as extraosseous labiogingival swellings that are painless. These tumors are not very large (1 to 3 cm in diameter) and show up as a unilocular translucency around the crown of an impacted tooth. The differentiation from a dentigerous cyst is difficult. The treatment is enucleation and curettage; recurrences are unusual.[35]

CALCIFYING EPITHELIAL ODONTOGENIC TUMOR (PINDBORG TUMOR). Pindborg described this in 1955, and it represents 1% of odontogenic tumors.[28] This tumor probably arises from the enamel organ and occurs in any age group, from children to the elderly.[36] The main site of occurrence is in the molar region of either jaw, frequently in association with unerupted teeth.[28] It can also be found in the gingival area of the anterior mandible.[37] On histologic evaluation, there are collections or sheets of polyhedral epithelial cells with occasional ring-like calcified areas in the center of the fibrous tissue.[30] Very rarely, the epithelial cells are vacuolated and may appear clear on histologic preparation.[38] This tumor presents as a slowly growing, painless lesion; if it grows into the nasal cavity or into the orbit, it may cause airway obstruction or proptosis.[36] On radiologic examination, it is a radiolucent, unilocular lesion related to an impacted tooth. As with other tumors, there can be calcification. It resembles ameloblastoma in its behavior and should be resected with good margins. There is a fairly high recurrence rate of 14% that is probably related to inadequate resection.[36]

SQUAMOUS ODONTOGENIC TUMOR. This rare tumor arises from the rests of Malassez in the periodontic ligaments.[39] The stroma is mature and contains squamous epithelial islands.[30] On radiologic examination, the lesion is translucent in the alveolus and is related to the tooth roots.[40] In the maxilla, it can perforate the cortex and be present in the soft tissue. Excision can be conservative.[41]

AMELOBLASTIC AND ECTOMESENCHYMAL TUMORS

AMELOBLASTIC FIBROMA. This tumor looks histologically like an ameloblastoma with odontogenic epithelial cells and an immature cellular stroma. The cellular stroma runs in cords and islands. It is thought to be the result of a proliferation of ameloblasts.[30] It occurs in patients from 6 months to 42 years; the average age is 14 years.[42] It occurs equally in males and females and makes up 2% of odontogenic tumors.[28] The posterior mandible is most frequently involved, but it can occur in the maxilla.[42] This tumor presents as painless swellings, which may cause problems with dental eruption.[43] Three quarters are associated with unerupted teeth.[44] On radiologic examination, they are multiloculate and their borders are sclerotic. They can be approximately 1 to 8 cm in diameter.[44] Although the cortex is thin, rarely is it perforated. After excision, there is a recurrence rate of 18.3%.[45] Treatment is enucleation and curettage with removal of teeth or tooth buds within the lesion. There may be rapid recurrence, and en bloc resection with the appropriate reconstruction should be performed, depending on whether it is mandible or maxilla.[17]

AMELOBLASTIC FIBRO-ODONTOMA. This is a rare tumor that has features of ameloblastic fibroma with aspects of an odontoma.[30] This tumor occurs in teenagers. With adequate excision, there are usually no recurrences.

ODONTOAMELOBLASTOMA. As the name suggests, this tumor contains enamel and dentin. The stroma is mature fibrous tissue with an ameloblastic component.[30] These are radiolucent lesions containing some radiopacities. Treatment is similar to that of interosseous ameloblastoma, requiring radical resection.[46]

ODONTOMA. This lesion is a hamartoma, and it can be complex or compound.[47] When it is complex, it contains all the dental tissues, but these are not arranged in an organized fashion. In the compound lesion, these tissues are more organized. There are many rudimentary dental structures. This lesion occurs during the second to fourth decades.[48] The complex variety is more common in the posterior mandible, but the compound lesions are more frequent in the anterior maxilla.[42] Odontomas have been reported in the retrotympanic area[49] or in the antrum of the maxilla.[50] The patient will complain of pain and swelling inside the mouth. On radiologic examination, the lesion is radiopaque, but dental structures may be visualized in some patients. Treatment is excision, and recurrence is rare.

ODONTOGENIC FIBROMA. This is a rare tumor that has cords of odontogenic epithelium in what appears to be dysplastic dentin containing calcifications. There may be evidence of unerupted or displaced teeth.[51] When these are resected, recurrence is unusual.

ECTOMESENCHYMAL ODONTOGENIC TUMORS

ODONTOGENIC MYXOMA. This lesion is composed of myxoblasts in a stroma of ground substance that is mucoid and basophilic.[30] Odontogenic myxomas represent 3% of odontogenic tumors.[28] Unfortunately, it tends to recur after conservative treatment, indicating its aggressive behavior.[52] When it involves soft tissue, there should be an extensive resection. It is most frequently seen in the posterior portion of the mandible.[53] The consistency is somewhat gelatinous because of the mucoid matrix; this factor makes excision of this lesion quite difficult. Curettage is a possibility, but recurrence is frequent; therefore, a partial jaw resection with immediate reconstruction is recommended, particularly in larger tumors.[17]

CEMENTOBLASTOMA. This tumor arises from cemental elements and accounts for only 1% of odontogenic tumors.[28] On histologic evaluation, it contains cementoblasts, cementin, and a cellular fibrous stroma.[30] The age of the patients ranges between 10 and 70 years.[54] The lesions occur in the molar region of the mandible. Radiologic examination shows a round radiopaque mass fused to the tooth roots, which may be partially resorbed. It enlarges slowly and can cause facial asymmetry. Pain is present in approximately 50% of patients.[55] The lesion is treated by excision with removal of a portion of the root.[17] The recurrence rate is low.

PERIAPICAL CEMENTAL DYSPLASIA. This lesion makes up 8% of odontogenic tumors.[28] The radiographic appearance is variable; it may be radiolucent, radiopaque, or a mixture of both.[56] It is much more frequent in black patients (70%).[57] One quarter involve the incisor or canine teeth in the lower jaw. These lesions are asymptomatic and are usually an incidental diagnosis or noted when dental radiographs are taken. They do not require treatment.[30]

CEMENTIFYING FIBROMA. This lesion has a cellular fibrous stroma with islands of cementum. Therefore, the radiologic appearance is mixed radiolucent and radiopaque. This lesion accounts for only 2% of odontogenic tumors.[28] It occurs in middle-aged women, usually in the mandible.[58] Growth can be large, up to slightly under 10 cm. Treatment is enucleation, and recurrence is unusual.

MALIGNANT ODONTOGENIC TUMORS

ODONTOGENIC CARCINOMA. This is a rare tumor with a poor prognosis. The 5-year survival rate is in the region of 30% to 40%.[59] These tumors result from malignant change in an intraosseous ameloblastoma. They metastasize by blood vessels and lymphatics, and the patient may aspirate tumor cells.[17,60] Other tumors of this variety are ameloblastic carcinoma and primary interosseous carcinoma. Ameloblastic carcinoma is a poorly differentiated lesion that can arise from an ameloblastoma.[60] Primary interosseous carcinoma is histologically like a standard squamous cell carcinoma. Treatment is wide resection; regional node involvement mandates lymphadenectomy. The usual adjuncts of radiation therapy and chemotherapy may be required.

AMELOBLASTIC FIBROSARCOMA. This is a rare tumor and resembles a low-grade fibrosarcoma. Metastases are rare,[61] but the problem is local spread. On histologic evaluation, the odontogenic epithelial component appears benign, but there is a sarcomatous fibrous stroma. This tumor arises from an ameloblastic fibroma or ameloblastic fibro-odontoma. It can occur at any time during life after the age of 20 years, but around 40 years is the most common time for this to present, and this it does as a painful swelling, sometimes with ulceration.[62] It occurs most frequently in the posterior aspect of the mandible.[63] It should be resected radically to try to prevent local recurrence.[61] In patients with intractable, recurrent disease, chemotherapy is advised because radiation therapy is of no value.[64]

Nonodontogenic Tumors

These tumors arise from bone that is unrelated to development of teeth. They are rare in the jaws compared with long bones.

BENIGN TUMORS

OSTEOMA. Jaw osteomas are relatively uncommon and should not be confused with exostoses, which occur in more than 30% of patients.[65] Osteomas have three distinct patterns: trabecular, compact, and osteoma durum.[66] The durum variety shows both compact and trabecular forms. These tumors are usually discovered on dental radiographs, but they occasionally reach a large size. They are slow growing and may appear in any place on the bone. Most frequently, they are found in the mandibles of young adults, with males being in the 2:1 majority.[67] On radiologic examination, they are well-delineated endosteal sclerotic masses or radiopaque lesions in the subperiosteal region. In Gardner syndrome, which is an inherited condition, there are multiple osteomas together with epidermoid and sebaceous cysts in the skin, supernumerary teeth, and intestinal polyposis. It is the intestinal polyposis that is significant because these polyps may become malignant.[68] Osteomas are treated surgically if they cause symptoms including pain, swelling, mucosal alteration, and difficulty in fitting dentures; if the swelling is considerable, facial asymmetry may result.

They can be removed in a conservative fashion, and recurrence is rare.

OSTEOBLASTOMA. This rare tumor makes up 1% of all primary bone tumors.[69] The majority occur in the long bones, but the jaws can be involved. The male-to-female ratio is 2:1.[70] The tumors occur mostly in the 20s in the tooth-bearing region; the mandible is most frequently involved.[71] They present as a painful, tender swelling with obvious expansion of the jaw. They can be small but can grow to at least 10 cm in diameter. On radiologic examination, there are calcified areas surrounded by a radiolucent zone,[72] but a sunray pattern may occur. Histologic evaluation shows osteoblastic cells and intracellular osteoid material with abundant blood vessels. Surgical excision should be conservative.[16,73]

OSTEOID OSTEOMA. This is a lesion of young adults. It can produce pain, even when it is very small. It grows slowly, rarely becoming more than 1 cm in diameter. There is a central area of bone destruction surrounded by a peripheral zone of cortical bone. There seem to be three stages in this lesion.[74] Initially there is growth of osteoblasts, then an intermediate phase followed by a mature phase. In the mature phase, the osteoid is well mineralized. This can occur in either the maxilla or the mandible.[75] It is usually within the bone but rarely in the subperiosteal area. On radiologic examination, there is a radiolucent central area where bone is being destroyed, and around this is a sclerotic area. The best method of investigation of this tumor is a technetium bone scan.[76] Resection should be conservative, with a small surrounding rim of bone. Recurrence is rare.

BENIGN FIBROUS AND FIBRO-OSSEOUS LESIONS

FIBROUS DYSPLASIA. This lesion is not a neoplasm but it behaves like one. It is a developmental derangement of bone that results from abnormal proliferation of undifferentiated mesenchymal bone-forming cells.[77] There is proliferation of mainly fibroblasts; this produces a dense collagen matrix containing trabeculae of osteoid and bone in a disorganized pattern.[65] Because of this process, the bone mass increases. It may be monostotic or polyostotic; the polyostotic fibrous dysplasia can be part of the Albright syndrome.[78] The other features of this syndrome are endocrine abnormalities (e.g., precocious puberty), café au lait spots, and other extraskeletal abnormalities.

In the head and neck region, its behavior depends on the location. In the cranio-orbital area, it can be aggressive, causing displacement of the globe and compression of the optic nerves. The maxilla and the mandible are involved, the maxilla more frequently than the mandible (Fig. 108-4).[79] It can be monostotic, but

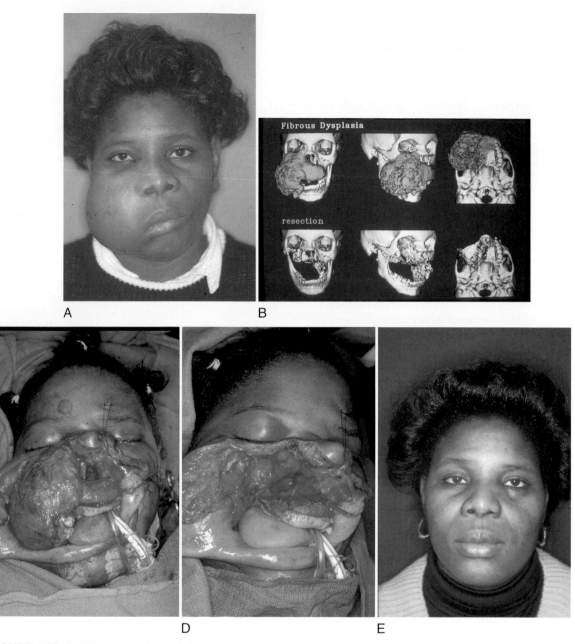

FIGURE 108-4. Fibrous dysplasia of right maxilla. *A,* Preoperative appearance. *B,* Three-dimensional CT scan with preoperative and postoperative views. *C,* Exposure with facial split approach. *D,* Resection of involved maxilla and central alveolus. *E,* Postoperative result.

this is uncommon. It is said to become quiescent after puberty, but this is not usual. This is a condition that may continue to grow for the whole of a patient's life. Most fibrous dysplasia grows slowly; it is frequently unilateral, but it can be bilateral.

The teeth are rarely loosened, but they may be displaced. There can be functional problems, such as blindness due to optic nerve compression and nasal airway obstruction due to growth into the nasal cavity.

Double vision may result from eye displacement, although this frequently does not occur because the lesion slowly displaces the eye; thus, compensation takes place.

Numerous facial deformities can occur, depending on placement of the lesion. It can be associated with pituitary adenomas (Fig. 108-5). The patient will exhibit acromegalic features and is usually tall; visual compromise is possible.

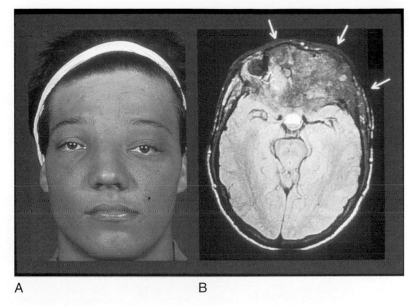

FIGURE 108-5. Albright syndrome. *A,* Fibrous dysplasia causing lateral inferior displacement of left eye. *B,* CT scan showing extensive fibrous dysplasia of orbit together with pituitary adenoma.

A   B

Malignant change is rare (<1%) and can be related to prior radiation therapy.[80] Malignant degeneration should be suspected if the lesion grows rapidly or if there is associated pain. All fibrous dysplasia should be kept under regular review with CT scans to determine any changes in the lesion, its rate of growth, and its involvement of significant areas.

Treatment varies. The lesion may be shaved, but this is not a permanent solution, and there is frequently regrowth. Resection and replacement with noninvolved bone are satisfactory. When noninvolved bone is not available, bone can be autoclaved and used for reconstruction. Bone resection is particularly indicated when there is exorbitism. The use of pamidronate has become popular. This drug is used alone or in conjunction with surgical treatment. It is thought that pamidronate will slow the growth of the condition, although there is no absolute proof of this. It does seem to stop the ingrowth into surrounding uninvolved bone.

Failing vision is treated by decompression of the optic nerve, but this must be done with considerable care by an anterosuperior or temporal approach. There is some question as to whether this approach is in fact prophylactic against decreasing vision (Fig. 108-6). Eye displacement causing double vision should also be treated by excision of the diseased area and by accurate orbital reconstruction. Most patients are operated on for aesthetic reasons to regain facial symmetry. Nasal airway obstruction and dental malocclusion are other reasons for treatment of this condition.[81]

CHERUBISM. This condition, first described by Jones[82] in 1933, is a hereditary form of fibrous dysplasia affecting the maxilla and mandible. Symptoms

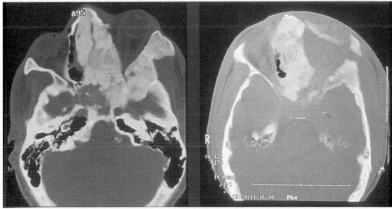

FIGURE 108-6. *A,* Fibrous dysplasia involving nose and left orbit with compression of optic nerve. *B,* Postoperative appearance after resection of fibrous dysplasia and decompression of left optic nerve.

A   B

begin in early childhood and progress through adolescence. Loosening of teeth occurs, together with alveolar bone loss due to the soft, fibrous, dysplastic material that grows into the bone. Both mandible and maxilla are enlarged. There can be an odd rotation of the globe upward with inferior scleral show when there is involvement of the upper portion of the maxilla (Fig. 108-7).

Although this has been treated by observation in the past, effective surgical treatment includes curettage of soft tissue and contouring of abnormal bone in combination with osteotomies as required. These patients should be observed for a long time because there may be spontaneous regression. However, this rarely occurs.

CENTRAL GIANT CELL GRANULOMA. There is some discussion as to whether this is similar to a true giant cell tumor of peripheral bones[83] or a distinct lesion on its own account.[84] It seems this is probably a reactive

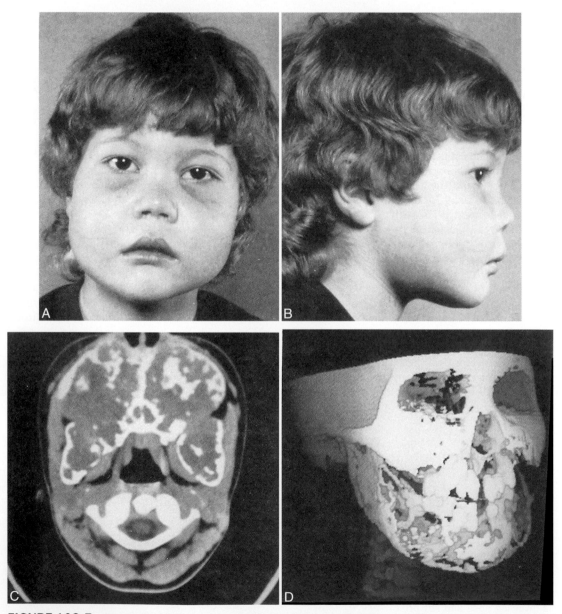

FIGURE 108-7. Fibrous dysplasia causing cherubism. *A* and *B,* Full-face and profile appearance. *C,* Axial CT scan showing extensive involvement of the maxilla. *D,* Three-dimensional CT scan graphically illustrating the involvement of the right orbit, the maxilla, and the mandible. (From Jackson IT, Shaw K: Tumors of the craniofacial skeleton, including the jaws. In McCarthy JG, ed: Plastic Surgery. Philadelphia, WB Saunders, 1990:3336.)

lesion that may result from trauma or inflammation.[85] These tumors are infrequent in the jaws (3.5%)[86] and found mainly in young adults and children, but more commonly in females. The anterior portion of the jaw is more frequently involved than the posterior, and the mandible more often than the maxilla. There may be local, painful swelling, or it may be asymptomatic. Many are discovered only during routine dental examination. Radiologic examination shows unilocular or multilocular radiolucencies with expansion of cortical plates and displacement of teeth.[83]

Histologic evaluation shows fibroblastic connective tissue, vascular tissue, collagen formation, and multinucleated giant cells. There may be hemorrhagic foci. Newly formed bone spicules are often seen. Mitosis in stroma cells is common.[83]

These tumors may be found in hypoparathyroidism. It is recommended that calcium and phosphate serum levels be determined for these patients[87]; if these are raised, the parathyroid adenomas should be excised, not the jaw cysts.

When it comes to removal of the jaw cysts, this procedure can be performed by local excision or curettage; because these lesions are vascular, curettage can produce considerable bleeding. Recurrence is rare.

ANEURYSMAL BONE CYST. These cysts present as rapidly growing, solitary, expansile lesions in patients younger than 20 years.[88] The most frequent areas of occurrence are the vertebral column and the long bones. Causation is unknown, and they account for 1.5% of nonodontogenic jaw cysts.[89] They are local swellings that are painless. There may be associated malocclusion. Occurrence is most frequent in the body of the mandible.

On radiologic examination, this is a unilocular cystic mass, but it may be multilocular with a honeycomb appearance.[90] This cyst frequently erodes the bony cortex. There will be a thin layer of new subperiosteal bone that may not be seen on radiographs but certainly will be encountered at surgery.[91]

The histologic appearance is that of blood-filled spaces lined by compressed fibrous tissue.[72] Multinucleated giant cells can frequently be seen in the wall of the cyst, but the most common cells are fibroblasts.[92]

The treatment of this lesion is removal, and if possible, curettage and cauterization of the tumor bed should be done.[93] If the lesion is less accessible and large, for example, in the ramus of the mandible, en bloc resection may be necessary. Preoperative fine-needle aspiration biopsy should be performed. Removal can be associated with significant bleeding.

An important observation is that radiation therapy is contraindicated. This may induce sarcomatous change.[91,94]

DESMOPLASTIC FIBROMA. This is a benign, locally aggressive bone tumor composed of connective tissue.

Abundant collagen fibers are seen histologically with spindle-shaped fibroblasts. Cells are few, as are mitoses. Difficulty can be encountered in trying to distinguish it from a well-differentiated fibrosarcoma.[95]

This lesion presents as an expanding tumor with little more than swelling.[96] Two thirds of the lesions are in the ramus and the posterior body of the mandible.[97] It is found principally in young adults, but it can occur at any age with a male-to-female ratio of 3:1. It is radiolucent; the bony cortical plates may be thinned and have a honeycombed radiographic appearance. When it is located around the ascending ramus of the mandible, it may penetrate the soft tissue and muscles and cause trismus.[96] This benign tumor is often mistaken for a malignant lesion because of the way it grows and the radiographic appearance. This tumor should be resected en bloc with surrounding normal tissue. Small lesions can be enucleated but should be followed up carefully because there is a high rate of recurrence. The concern is that it may be a fibrosarcoma.[98]

HISTIOCYTOSIS X. The three different clinical lesions in this group present with similar histologic features. They contain many histiocytes that may be present in sheets. There are also eosinophils, plasma cells, lymphocytes, multinucleated giant cells, and foam cells. There may be necrosis.[99] The cause of histiocytosis X is unknown, but there may be a defect in the immunoregulatory mechanisms. The significant cell in this condition is the Langerhans cell, a dendritic histiocyte. With electron microscopy, the presence of Langerhans or Birbeck granules within the cytoplasm of the Langerhans cells confirms the diagnosis.[100] Normal histiocytes do not possess inclusion bodies.

The three types of this condition are eosinophilic granuloma, Hand-Schüller-Christian disease, and Letterer-Siwe syndrome.[101]

Eosinophilic granuloma is a localized form of histiocytosis X; it affects males younger than 20 years twice as often as females of that age.[102] The polyostotic form involves multiple bones, causing symptoms of swelling and pain. Gingival lesions cause a nonspecific erythematous swelling with associated ulceration. Radiographic examination shows unilocular, well-defined radiolucencies. The skull lesions are punched out and multiple. The monostotic form should be treated by vigorous curettage, but long-term follow-up is important.[87] If there is loss of ridge support, the teeth may be mobile and should be removed. Because there is a tendency for other lesions to be present, a radiologic film survey should be carried out. This lesion has a good prognosis.

Hand-Schüller-Christian disease is a chronic disseminated form of histiocytosis X. Classically, there are skull lesions, exophthalmos, and diabetes insipidus in 10% of patients.[103] These findings occur later than with eosinophilic granuloma, occasionally in adults. There may be involvement of liver, spleen, lymph nodes, and bone. The treatment is radiation therapy and local curettage of the bone lesions. Chemotherapy, however, has been used for the extraosseous lesions. Scott and Ellis[87] have quoted a mean survival of 10 to 15 years.

Letterer-Siwe syndrome is an acute disseminated form of histiocytosis X occurring in infants younger than 3 years. Multiple organs are involved. It has a rapid and fatal clinical course. Chemotherapy has limited success.[87]

HEMANGIOMA. Jaw hemangiomas are rare, and they are thought to be hamartomas or developmental malformations rather than true neoplasms. They frequently occur during the second decade of life; the male-to-female ratio is 2:1.[104] The posterior area of the mandible is most frequently involved. The lesions may be discovered incidentally; on dental radiographs, they are seen as multilocular translucencies with a honeycomb appearance.[105] The presentation is frequently by expansion of the buccal cortex; gum bleeding, usually with related mobile teeth; or significant hemorrhage after extraction, gingival biopsy, or tooth eruption. These hemangiomas grow slowly and are painless. On radiologic examination, there may be a sunburst appearance, and this is due to bony trabeculae radiating out from the center. Because the multilocular radiolucent appearance is not absolutely diagnostic, needle aspiration of radiolucent lesions is important. The next step is to carry out carotid angiography. The angiogram will demonstrate the extent of the lesion and the supplying vessels and also illustrate the rate of blood flow and shunt. Vascular mapping is important for choice of treatment.

Vascular lesions are described classically as capillary, cavernous, or mixed, or they may be arteriovenous malformations. Cavernous hemangiomas have large, thin-walled vascular spaces filled with blood, and these are lined by a single layer of endothelial cells. Capillary hemangiomas have multiple capillary channels. This type of classification does not really help in treatment. It is the angiographic study that allows the rate of flow through the lesion to be assessed together with the rate of arteriovenous shunting. Flow is the amount of blood that enters the lesion, and the shunt is the speed by which the blood is transferred from the arterial to the venous system. When the shunt is high, the arterial and venous systems appear on the same radiograph. Hemangiomas are usually low-flow, low-shunt lesions, whereas arteriovenous malformations are high-flow, high-shunt lesions. Normally, low-flow, low-shunt lesions are treated with injections of sclerosing agents such as sodium tetradecyl sulfate (Sotradecol) by direct injection. However, within bone, they are best treated by the method used for treatment of high-flow, high-shunt lesions because there is a risk of severe hemorrhage.

The ideal treatment is preoperative superselective embolization by Gelfoam or sometimes Ivalon; this is followed in 48 hours by resection. Immediate reconstruction can be carried out. It is possible to remove the vascular malformation from the resected segment of bone and use this portion of bone as a tray filled with iliac crest cancellous bone. An alternative approach is microvascular bone reconstruction. Another technique that is becoming much less common is to stabilize the mandible to the maxilla by intermaxillary fixation by placing a spacer on the mandible (e.g., a plate) and delay reconstruction for some time. The external carotid artery should not be tied off, nor should any branch of this artery, because this will simply throw the flow onto the internal carotid system, which may make the lesion unresectable because the supply now comes from the internal carotid. These lesions should be resected after embolization with minimal disturbance of the local vasculature. It may be necessary in the emergency situation, such as a tooth extraction, to tie off the external carotid to gain control of the acute bleed. This is seen when a tooth is extracted in the presence of a previously undiagnosed vascular malformation (Fig. 108-8).[106,107]

Primary Malignant Neoplasms

The malignant odontogenic tumors are discussed earlier in this chapter. The primary malignant neoplasms of the jaw are mainly sarcomas and lymphomas. In the paranasal sinuses, sarcomatous tumors can arise. Rarely, squamous cell carcinoma, basal cell carcinoma, malignant melanoma, and metastatic lesions may be found.

OSTEOSARCOMA. This tumor makes up 20% of primary bone malignant neoplasms[108] but only 6% of jaw malignant neoplasms.[109] It usually occurs during the third or fourth decade of life and is rare in children. The male-to-female ratio is 2:1.[110] Reported causative factors are irradiation, trauma, and preexisting bone disease.[65] Fibrous dysplasia and Paget disease[111] may be precursors of this tumor. In the author's experience, fibrous dysplasia has been associated with an osteogenic sarcoma on only one occasion in more than 100 patients (a middle-aged patient who had previous radiation therapy for the condition as a teenager). It seems likely that radiation exposure was the cause, rather than the fibrous dysplasia.

The lesion usually occurs as a painful swelling, and there may also be numbness; it occurs more frequently in the body of the mandible than in the maxilla.[112] The alveolar ridge is the usual site of occurrence, and there may be gingival ulceration. A large lesion may

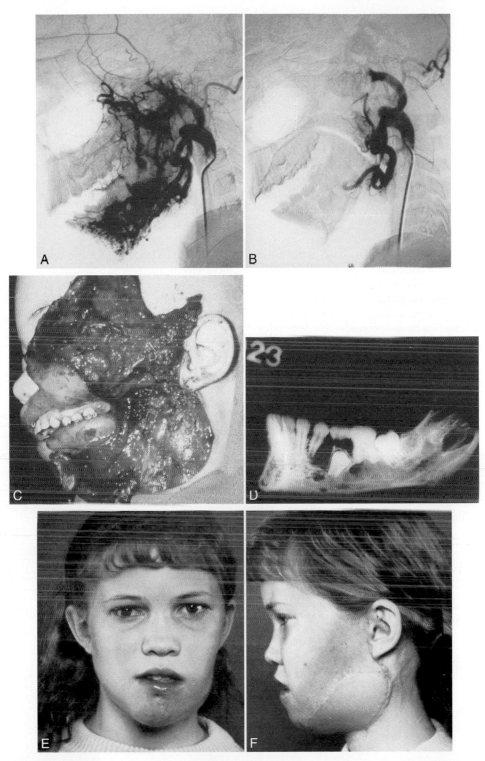

FIGURE 108-8. A patient who presented emergently with massive intraoral bleeding after tooth extraction. *A,* Preoperative angiogram. *B,* Appearance after embolization. *C,* Hemimandibulectomy. *D,* Radiograph of specimen to show involvement with arteriovenous malformation. *E* and *F,* Postoperative result with reconstruction of mandible with free bone graft and free tissue transplantation, which was required because of loss of skin and subcutaneous tissue. (From Jackson IT, Shaw K: Tumors of the craniofacial skeleton, including the jaws. In McCarthy JG, ed: Plastic Surgery. Philadelphia, WB Saunders, 1990:3336.)

cause nasal obstruction and discharge, facial enlargement, and, in maxillary lesions, epistaxis. One in five patients has elevated alkaline phosphatase levels.[113] The radiologic appearance is variable. Some lesions are translucent and fully delineated; others are radiodense and may have a prominent sunburst appearance, and these can also occur in fibrous dysplasia and osteomyelitis. The periodontal membrane space may be widened symmetrically. This is an early finding[109] and is not completely diagnostic, but its presence should suggest osteosarcoma. Rapid growth, pain, and paresthesia are frequent findings. CT scan is the best investigation and gives an excellent view of the lesion. The tumor size and shape can be determined by three-dimensional CT scans (Fig. 108-9).

Histologic evaluation shows a sarcomatous connective tissue stroma producing both osteoid and bone. There are four different subtypes: fibroblastic, chondroblastic, osteoblastic, and telangiectatic.[65]

Surgery is the treatment of choice.[114] A radical resection of bone and surrounding soft tissue is recommended; this resection causes a considerable deformity. Maxillectomy with orbital exenteration is necessary for large maxillary lesions involving the orbit. The skull base can also be involved, and a craniofacial approach through the anterior cranial fossa, and sometimes the middle cranial fossa, is recommended.

Postoperative radiation therapy (4500 cGy) should be given. Preoperative radiation can be helpful in large, unresectable lesions.

When local disease has been controlled, surgical removal of lung metastases improves survival. Chemotherapy is rarely successful in the treatment of metastases.[115] It can safely be said that if the lesion is in a site suitable for surgical resection, the prognosis is good. Inoperable lesions are rarely cured with radiation therapy.[113] The average 5-year survival is 37% for mandibular osteogenic sarcoma and 27% for maxillary lesions.[112]

CHONDROSARCOMA. In the head and neck area, these lesions are 50% as frequent as osteogenic sarcomas. They occur mostly in the nasoseptal region and are composed of fully developed cartilage, being formed from a stroma of sarcoma. It is important to be aware that chondrogenic jaw neoplasms are more often malignant than benign.[116] The histologic differentiation between the two can be difficult.[117] Benign

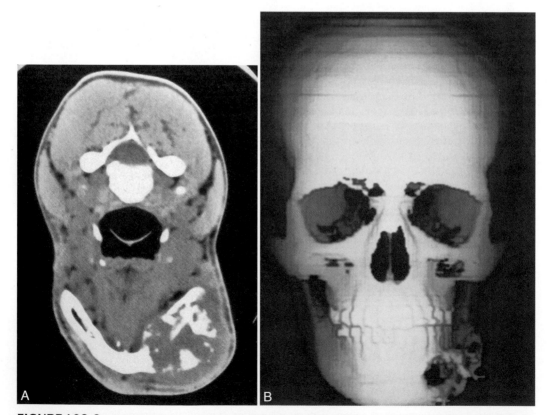

FIGURE 108-9. Osteogenic sarcoma of left mandible. *A,* Axial CT scan to illustrate the extensive destruction of the left mandible. *B,* Three-dimensional image shows this in a more graphic way. (From Jackson IT, Shaw K: Tumors of the craniofacial skeleton, including the jaws. In McCarthy JG, ed: Plastic Surgery. Philadelphia, WB Saunders, 1990:3336.)

lesions can frequently recur after resection; on histologic evaluation, these are often more cellular or have undergone malignant change. There is a theory that chondromas of the head and neck may frequently be incipient chondrosarcomas when they are first diagnosed. Their distribution is the same as that of chondrosarcoma, and it is said that they can be induced by radiation, but the tumor can arise from preexisting Paget disease,[118] fibrous dysplasia,[119] or bone cyst.[120]

There is a wide range of ages at which these occur, from the 20s to the 90s. The symptoms are similar to those of osteogenic sarcoma.

On radiologic examination, they are large, thick-walled, radiolucent areas with central areas of calcification with a cotton-wool appearance; this is due to bone destruction.[65] Cortical destruction is a late occurrence; this causes a fuzzy, shadowy radiologic appearance extending into the surrounding soft tissues. Treatment is radical resection. This is advised for all cartilaginous tumors of the jaws because it is difficult to tell the benign from the malignant (Fig. 108-10).

Radiation therapy is used for unresectable or incompletely removed lesions. Although chemotherapy has been recommended as an adjuvant to surgery or palliation, there is little evidence of its effectiveness.

FIBROSARCOMA. This tumor can be well differentiated, moderately well differentiated, or undifferentiated; the appearance is similar to that of a soft tissue fibrosarcoma.[121] It usually originates in the soft tissue of the face, the paranasal sinus, or the nasopharynx. When it occurs in the mandible or maxilla, it may be endosteal or periosteal. The periosteal lesion has a better prognosis.[66] The condition is radioresistant. Therefore, radical resection should be performed, but the survival rate is only 20% for the endosteal lesion and 50% for the periosteal lesion.[66]

EWING SARCOMA. This tumor is a primary malignant neoplasm of bone and extraskeletal soft tissues. In the head and neck area, it occurs in the first 2 years of life. Metastases are blood-borne; therefore, lungs and bones are frequent sites.[122] The best therapy is radiation (5000 to 5500 cGy).[123] Small mandibular lesions may be excised. Chemotherapy can be an adjunctive treatment.[124] The most frequently used regimen is vincristine, cyclophosphamide, dactinomycin, and doxorubicin hydrochloride. With this combination therapy, the 5-year survival has been reported to be 50%.[125]

MALIGNANT FIBROUS HISTIOCYTOMA. This bone tumor is rare.[126] Electron microscopy shows two cell lines, histiocytic and fibroblastic types. Depending on the differentiation of the neoplastic cells, one or the other may predominate.[127] This tumor presents like other jaw malignant neoplasms; pain and swelling are common.[60,128] The malignant fibrous histiocytoma

occurs during the fourth and fifth decades of life; it invades locally and may metastasize to regional lymph nodes. Wide resection is advised.[129] If there is nodal involvement, a lymph node dissection should be carried out. Radiation is of no value, and the role of chemotherapy is probably minimal.[130] The 5-year survival rate varies from 34.5% to 67%.[131,132]

NON-HODGKIN LYMPHOMA OF BONE. Primary malignant lymphomas make up only 5% of all malignant bone tumors.[72] The most common sites are the maxillary antrum and the mandible. The fifth and sixth decades are the most common time for occurrence. They present with pain followed by a palpable mass, paresthesia, and tooth loosening. Men are involved three times more than women are.[133] There are osteolytic areas with less prominent areas of osteoblastic change radiologically.[87] Unlike with other jaw malignant neoplasms, cortical destruction and soft tissue extension are not commonly seen. The cell type varies, and there may be a nodular or diffuse histologic pattern.[134] The tumor is staged and treated with combined megavoltage radiation and chemotherapy. With early treatment, the prognosis is good. Combined chemotherapy and radiation therapy result in a 5-year survival rate of 70% for patients with stage I disease and 60% in stage II disease.[87]

BURKITT LYMPHOMA. This is a tumor of B lymphocytes seen in African children. There is jaw swelling, abdominal masses, and often paraplegia.[135] It is associated with the Epstein-Barr virus.[136] A nonendemic form of the disease may occur,[66] but jaw lesions are infrequent. In the African tumor, the maxilla is most often involved. However, jaw lesions can be found in all four quadrants. Renal failure due to direct involvement is common. Jaw radiographs show large radiolucent defects with cortical disruption. The tumor grows rapidly, and without early definitive treatment, the outcome is fatal.[136] The lesion responds well to alkylating agents with a 90% remission rate.[87] This tumor can be cured by chemotherapy alone, but in large lesions, surgical debulking is advised before chemotherapy.

ANGIOSARCOMA. This is a rare jaw malignant neoplasm. On microscopic examination, there is neoplastic vascular proliferation within a loose connective tissue stroma. The lesion behaves less aggressively than when it occurs in the soft tissues, and thus the prognosis is much better. It should be treated by radical excision. Well-differentiated lesions have a 5-year survival rate of 95%; but in undifferentiated tumors, the survival rate is 20%.[137]

PRIMARY SALIVARY GLAND TUMORS. These rarely occur in bone, but they can arise from embryonic salivary gland inclusions[138] or from mucous metaplasia of the lining of odontogenic cysts.[139] The majority of

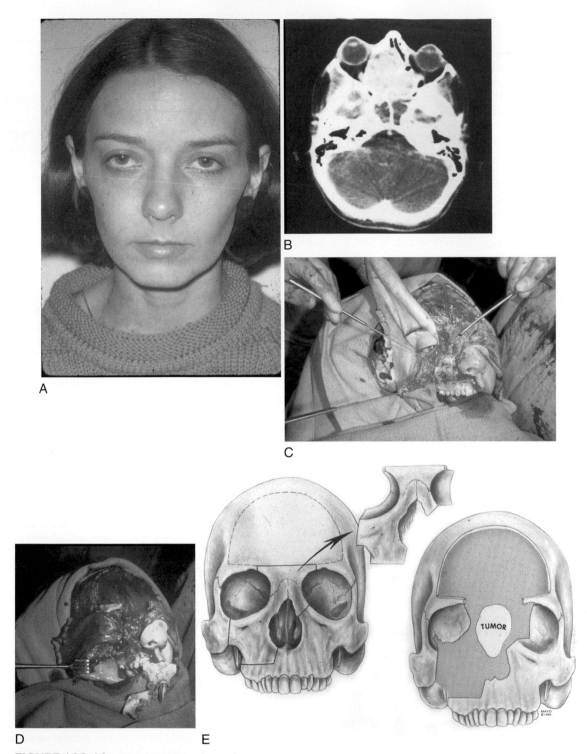

FIGURE 108-10. Chondrosarcoma of anterior central skull base. *A,* Preoperative appearance. *B,* Preoperative axial CT scan showing the anterior skull base mass. *C,* Transfacial transcranial approach. *D,* Removal of frontal nasal maxillary segment for exposure. *E,* Diagram of exposure showing position of tumor.

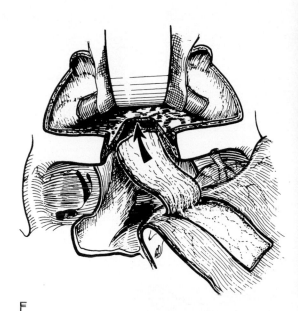

F

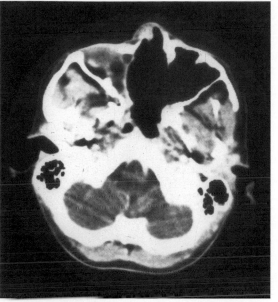

G

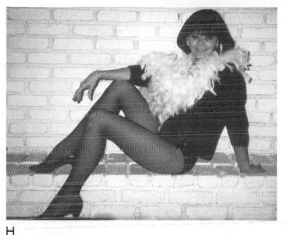

H

FIGURE 108-10, cont'd. *F,* Galeofrontalis myofascial flap to close off anterior cranial fossa from nasal cavity after resection of lesion. *G,* Axial CT scan to illustrate clearance of chondrosarcoma. *H,* The patient tumor free 6 years postoperatively. This has continued for a period of 16 years. (*A, B, C,* and *F* from Jackson IT, Shaw K: Tumors of the craniofacial skeleton, including the jaws. In McCarthy JG, ed: Plastic Surgery. Philadelphia, WB Saunders, 1990:3336.)

these lesions are of the mucoepidermoid type.[140] There is commonly a painless swelling in the posterior aspect of the mandible, and this may be what leads to a quest for treatment. Treatment should be by wide excision. Lesions of the maxilla are best treated by maxillectomy.[141] Although the tumors do not tend to metastasize, they can spread to regional lymph nodes.

TUMORS OF THE NASAL CAVITY AND PARANASAL SINUSES

The paranasal sinuses are lined with respiratory mucosa; this contains pseudostratified columnar ciliated cells, basal cells, and mucous secretory cells (Fig. 108-11). The respiratory mucosa can give rise to squamous cell lesions and salivary gland adenocarcinomas. The lateral nasal wall of the septum, craniad to the superior turbinate, is lined by specialized nonciliated olfactory mucosa with nerve elements; thus, esthesioneuroblastomas occur in this region. Melanomas and teratomas account for the rest of the primary tumors of the sinus area; also, it can be involved secondarily by other tumors, such as sarcomas.

Lymphatic drainage of the frontal, ethmoid, and sphenoid sinuses is transosseous by the ostium of the individual sinus to the lymphatic network of the

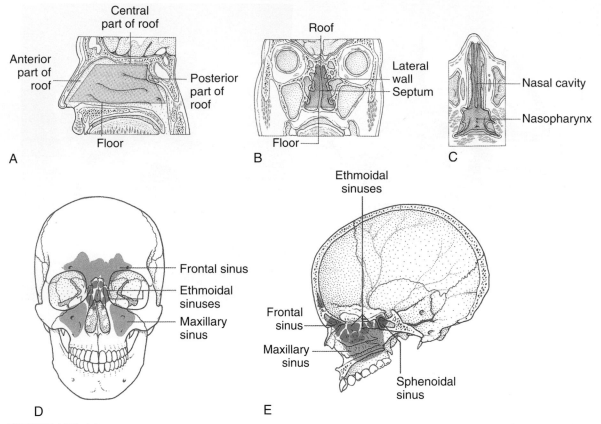

FIGURE 108-11. The nasal cavities, nasopharynx, and location and shape of paranasal sinuses. *A,* Sagittal section. The central part of the roof is parallel to the floor. *B,* Coronal section. Note that the floor is wider than the roof. *C,* Horizontal section. The nasopharynx is wider than the nasal cavity. *D* and *E,* The sinuses have been superimposed on the skull. Illustration *D* shows the anterior view and *E* the medial view. (From Rogers AW: Textbook of Anatomy. Edinburgh, Churchill Livingstone, 1992:82, 83.)

posterior nasal cavity as well as through the meningeal lymphatics. The maxillary sinus drains mainly into the submandibular and upper cervical chains; it also drains to the lymphatics of the posterior nasal cavity and through channels penetrating the nasopharyngeal region to the deep cervical fascia nodes around the carotid and internal jugular veins. The posterior nasal cavity drains to the retropharyngeal nodes and subsequently to the superior deep cervical nodes. The vestibular skin and most anterior nasal mucosa drain to the periparotid and submandibular nodes and then on to the superior deep cervical chain.[142] Most of the malignant neoplasms in this area can affect the retropharyngeal nodes first and thus are surgically inaccessible. Retropharyngeal node involvement means that elective neck dissection will not prophylactically control lymph spread.

Papillomas

These tumors arise from the respiratory mucosa of the nasal cavity and paranasal sinuses. They are

uncommon, unlike the allergic nasal polyp, because they occur in patients in the fifth decade of life. They arise from proliferation of cells from the basement membrane of the mucosa. The overlying epithelium is transitional with a tendency toward squamous cell differentiation. On occasion, multilayered columnar cells may predominate, and the papillomas are then termed cylindrical cell type. This can be confused histologically with a papillary adenocarcinoma.

Papillomas are described according to their area of origin, mainly being lateral wall and septal types. The septal variety is localized and rarely associated with squamous cell carcinoma. The lateral wall type, however, can involve many sites, including the sinuses; it may contain squamous cell carcinoma, which arises as an in situ focus within the papilloma or in the same anatomic area. These papillomas may have one of two patterns, inverted or exophytic. The inverted type is commonly associated with lesions of the lateral wall or the sinuses. This type of lesion grows into the underlying stroma, whereas the exophytic or fungiform type shows surface proliferation, and this is most commonly seen on the nasal septum. If there is excessive keratinization, this is atypical and should raise the question of squamous cell carcinoma. Treatment is by excision of the lesion. Papillomas have a tendency to recur,[143] and if they occur in the lateral wall, squamous cell carcinoma must be considered.

Squamous Cell Carcinoma

This tumor arises from the respiratory mucosa and represents 75% to 90% of malignant neoplasms in this area. It is unusual for it to occur in the nasal cavity; most lesions arise from the turbinates or the nasal septum.[144] In more than one third of patients, there is bone invasion, and 10% exhibit metastases in regional nodes.[144] Resection and irradiation appear to be equally effective therapies for early lesions.

Unfortunately, the paranasal areas are clinically silent, and thus tumor diagnosis is frequently delayed. The majority are moderately well differentiated and are usually keratinizing. Nonkeratinizing and anaplastic carcinomas are in the minority.[145] Although the anaplastic variety can progress more rapidly, the main factor for prognosis is tumor size. Eighty percent of paranasal squamous cell carcinomas arise in the maxillary antrum.[146] The ethmoid sinus is the next most common area, followed by the rare involvement of the frontal and sphenoid sinuses.[147] The signs and symptoms may be related to the oral cavity, nasal cavity, orbit, or nerve involvement. There may be a mass in the palate, erosion of bone, trismus, dental pain, epistaxis, or nasal stuffiness. There may be a nasal mass, exophthalmos, eye dystopia, blindness, facial deformity, pain, paresthesia, or anesthesia in the distribution of the trigeminal nerve or one of its branches. In the early phase, maxillary antral tumors can cause symptoms of chronic sinusitis, but a drainage procedure provides the true diagnosis. There is an increased incidence of maxillary sinus tumors in patients exposed to heavy metals such as nickel.[148] Ninety percent of sinus tumors have invaded through at least one sinus wall at the time of diagnosis and can be radiologically visualized.[144]

Treatment includes surgery and irradiation and yields a 45% 5-year survival rate when the lesion is resectable.[149] Surgery consists of a maxillectomy, sometimes together with the ethmoid sinus and anterior cranial fossa, depending on the extent of tumor spread. Involvement of the cavernous sinus or the trigeminal ganglion, which occurs by infiltration along the first or second division of the trigeminal nerve, usually indicates unresectability. Patients with unresectable lesions treated by irradiation alone have a 5-year survival rate of 12% to 19%.[150]

Nonepidermoid Carcinoma

These tumors arise from glandular elements in the sinus mucosa and ductal epithelium. Adenocarcinomas are most common, and the most common site of origin is the ethmoid region.[144] Adenocarcinomas are papillary, sessile, or alveolar-mucoid. Well-differentiated adenocarcinomas occur but are less frequent. These are usually associated with nasal polyps.[151] They look like gastrointestinal adenocarcinomas histologically. Environmental factors associated with these are wood dust, mustard gas, and isopropanol. Treatment is similar to that recommended for squamous cell carcinoma.

Adenoid cystic carcinomas are similar to the salivary gland lesions; they occur in the paranasal sinuses. Diagnosis is usually delayed; thus, fixation and extension to adjacent structures are present in 75% of patients.[152] Perineural spread is common, occurring along the frontomaxillary division of the trigeminal nerve. Lymphatic spread occurs in 14% of tumors. Blood-borne dissemination is much more common (up to 40%). The lungs and bones are most frequently involved, and hematogenous metastases are usually associated with failure of local control. The treatment is the same as that proposed for squamous cell carcinoma.

Melanoma

Approximately 1% of all melanomas are found in the nasal cavity or paranasal sinuses[153]; 16% are found in blacks.[154] These originate from melanocytes in the mucosa and submucosa of the nasal cavity and paranasal sinuses. They occur most frequently in the anterior part of the nasal septum, the middle and inferior turbinates, and the maxillary antrum.[153] Epistaxis is frequent, followed by nasal obstruction, pain, and soft tissue swelling. If they are amelanotic, they can be misdiagnosed as anaplastic carcinoma or sarcoma. They rarely metastasize to lymph nodes initially.[155] Treatment is radical excision (Fig. 108-12). Ten-year survival ranges from 17% to 38%.[145]

Esthesioneuroblastoma

This rare tumor of the olfactory epithelium occurs in the most superior portion of the nasal cavity, nasal septum, turbinates, ethmoid sinuses, or cribriform plate. It can form exophytic or sessile masses. The age range is extensive, from the first to the ninth decades.[156] It is an aggressive tumor that has symptoms ranging from epistaxis to nasal obstruction, ocular pain, and headaches.[157] Metastases may occur, and the most common sites are the cervical lymph nodes, lungs, and bone. Approximately 50% of patients die of uncontrolled intracranial extension. The most useful preoperative examinations are CT scans and magnetic resonance imaging (MRI). Treatment should be aggressive. When indicated, a combined extracranial and intracranial approach is used with total surgical removal. After radical resection, galeofrontalis

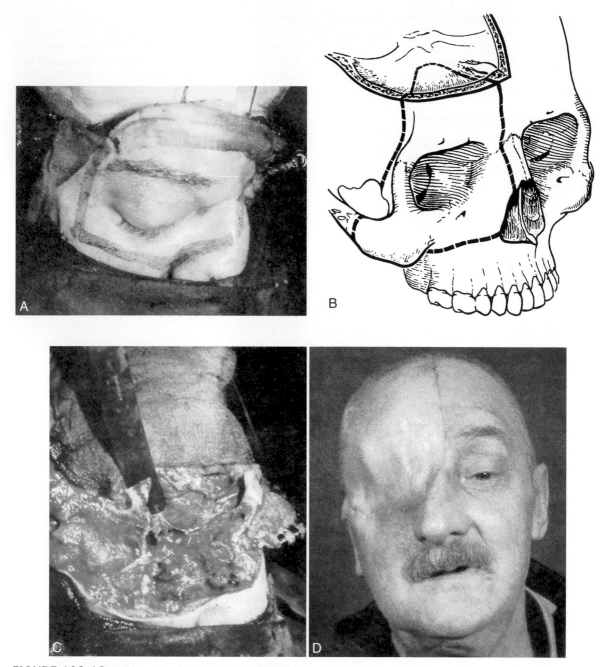

FIGURE 108-12. Melanoma of right orbit. *A,* Planned intracranial and extracranial resection of right orbit, which is filled in its posterior aspect with malignant melanoma. *B,* Planned bone excision. *C,* Resection completed. *D,* Postoperative result at 1 year. (From Jackson IT, Shaw K: Tumors of the craniofacial skeleton, including the jaws. In McCarthy JG, ed: Plastic Surgery. Philadelphia, WB Saunders, 1990:3336.)

myofascial flaps and temporalis muscle flaps are used to separate the oral cavity and the nasopharynx from the extradural space, thus preventing postoperative ascending infection (Fig. 108-13).[157] A full tumoricidal dose of radiation therapy is given postoperatively. Inadequate surgical resection or radiation therapy alone results in a high incidence of recurrence.

Malignant Teratomas

These tumors are extremely rare and characteristically have a combination of epithelial and connective tissue elements, with the prominent feature being the sarcomatous component. The malignant teratoma commonly occurs as a nasal cavity mass,[158] with frequent

322232224232222222232222222

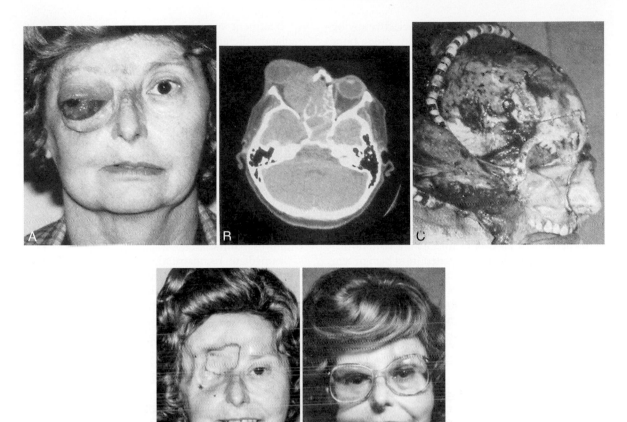

FIGURE 108-13. Esthesioneuroblastoma of right orbit and anterior skull base. *A,* Preoperative appearance with gross proptosis of right eye. *B,* Axial CT scan to illustrate position of the tumor involving the left orbit and the nasal cavity and causing gross protrusion of the right eye. *C,* Tumor resected with frontal craniotomy, superior orbitotomy, and resection of floor of anterior cranial fossa and orbit. *D,* Postoperative appearance with skin graft on dura. *E,* Right orbital area reconstructed with composite prosthesis. (From Jackson IT, Shaw K: Tumors of the craniofacial skeleton, including the jaws. In McCarthy JG, ed: Plastic Surgery. Philadelphia, WB Saunders, 1990:3336.)

involvement of the ethmoid and maxillary sinuses. A wide resection seems to be the only effective treatment.

Metastatic Tumors

Renal tumors are, by far, the most common non–head and neck tumors to metastasize to this area and usually involve the paranasal sinuses.[159] Lung, mammary, and gastrointestinal tract tumors can also metastasize to this area; the maxillary antrum and the nasal cavity are most commonly involved.

The treatment for these tumors depends on their resectability, the histologic features of the primary tumor, and of course the general condition of the patient.

ORBITAL TUMORS

These tumors originate from the orbital contents, from the periorbital skeleton, or by invasion from the structures surrounding the orbit. Only tumors requiring craniofacial surgical resection are reviewed with treatment recommendations.

The most interesting tumors from a surgical standpoint are the neurofibromas. For these tumors, a treatment algorithm can be formulated.

In adults, the majority of orbital cancers are lymphomas, extensive eyelid or sinus tumors, and metastatic lesions.[160] In children, rhabdomyosarcoma is the most frequent orbital malignant neoplasm (up to 75%). The remainder are lymphoid tumors, extraocular retinoblastomas, and metastasizing neuroblastomas.[161]

Orbital tumors are usually diagnosed early because of their presentation, that is, proptosis, alteration of ocular movement, deteriorating vision, eye displacement, headache, and orbital pain. Cicatrizing lesions can lead to enophthalmos.[47] High-resolution CT and MRI scans are useful for diagnosis, as is ultrasonography. In vascular lesions, selective angiography is performed. Aggressive lesions erode bone. Excavation and expansion occur in noninfiltrative tumors.[162] With contrast enhancement, it is often possible to differentiate vascular lesions, mucoceles, and solid tumors.[47] The degree of extension and site of origin can also be determined. This evaluation together with the clinical history can often provide a diagnosis, thus eliminating biopsy. When the diagnosis is unclear, a CT-guided aspiration biopsy can be performed and is of value, but MRI scanning has largely eliminated this for diagnosis.[47]

Lymphoma

Eight percent of all orbital tumors are lymphomas, and these need to be differentiated from benign lymphoid infiltrations, which occur twice as often.[163] The most common type of lymphoma is the lymphocytic variety. This occurs as a palpable mass with or without proptosis, most often during the fifth and sixth decades.[164] Treatment is by radiation therapy.

Rhabdomyosarcoma

This is the most common orbital tumor of childhood (Fig. 108-14).[160] Management and prognosis depend on the site of the tumor. A tumor of intraorbital origin has the best prognosis, probably because the orbital skeleton together with the periorbita acts as a barrier to tumor spread. Biopsy confirms the diagnosis. These tumors can grow rapidly; thus, there should be no delay in diagnosis. Rhabdomyosarcomas frequently metastasize to lungs and bones[161]; regional node involvement also occurs.

Treatment of orbital rhabdomyosarcoma is by radiation therapy and chemotherapy rather than by surgical enucleation.[1,78] It is possible to retain vision, but doses greater than 5000 cGy will preserve useful vision in only 25% of patients. Before the age of 6 years, 4000 to 4500 cGy is given; the older children receive 4500 to 5500 cGy. If the neck is involved, it should be included in the radiation field. Chemotherapy includes actinomycin D, cyclophosphamide, and vincristine. With combined radiation therapy and chemotherapy, there are survival rates of 70%.[165] If the tumor recurs, extensive resection with orbital exenteration should be performed. On some occasions, there will be an alteration of the pathologic process after irradiation, the cell type changing to a chondrosarcoma.

Immediate reconstruction has been performed with microvascular composite tissue transplantation. Free tissue transplantation allows a second tumoricidal dose of radiation therapy.

Other Malignant Tumors

Orbital invasion from surrounding structures, for example, paranasal sinuses and eyelids, accounts for 20% of orbital malignant neoplasms. These are usually squamous cell carcinomas, followed by basal cell carcinomas, sebaceous cell carcinomas, and soft tissue sarcomas.[160] The treatment of these lesions is radical surgery, often with adjuvant local radiation therapy and chemotherapy.

Fifteen percent of orbital neoplasms occur from extensive intraocular retinoblastomas and malignant melanomas.[160] Treatment of these consists of orbital exenteration with or without resection of the orbit.

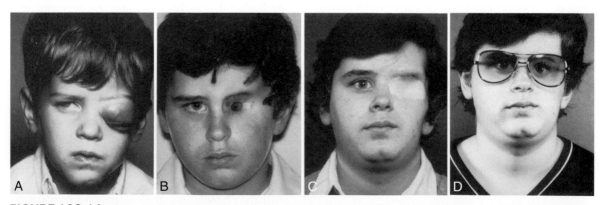

FIGURE 108-14. Recurrent rhabdomyosarcoma after chemotherapy and radiation therapy. *A,* Left recurrent orbital rhabdomyosarcoma. *B,* Postoperative appearance after excision and skin grafting. *C,* Appearance after free pectoralis major musculocutaneous flap application with closure of the defect into the nose and reconstruction of orbit with cranial bone grafts. *D,* Appearance with orbital prosthesis in position. (From Jackson IT, Shaw K: Tumors of the craniofacial skeleton, including the jaws. In McCarthy JG, ed: Plastic Surgery. Philadelphia, WB Saunders, 1990:3336.)

Surgery is followed by adjuvant radiation therapy and chemotherapy (Fig. 108-15).

Hemangiopericytomas are aggressive vascular orbital tumors and produce the signs of a mass lesion, often with pain. More than 75% of these tumors originate from the superior orbit.[166] These tumors should be radically resected (Fig. 108-16).

Malignant optic nerve gliomas are rare, and they occur almost exclusively in adults. They should be resected. Tumors involving the skull base or those located superior and posterior require a transcranial approach. Schwannomas, fibrous dysplasia, and neurofibromas of the orbit are not malignant, but they frequently require a craniofacial approach for adequate exposure and resection.

LACRIMAL GLAND TUMORS

The adenoid cystic carcinoma is the most common lacrimal gland malignant tumor, followed by adenocarcinoma, malignant mixed tumors, and mucoepidermoid carcinoma.[160] These tumors may occur at any age and act as mass orbital lesions. They also cause pain from perineural invasion. They generally have a poor prognosis.[167] The recommended treatment is en bloc intracranial and extracranial radical resection. Radiation therapy is not a useful adjuvant.

Metastatic Neoplasms

Five percent of solid orbital masses are metastatic.[163] In adults, they are usually from the breast or the lung.[168] In children, the metastases are from abdominal or thoracic neuroblastomas. Management is determined by the primary tumor. Surgery is not usually indicated, but if there is severe pain, this should be considered.

SOFT TISSUE SARCOMAS OF HEAD AND NECK

These tumors are rare. They are seen frequently in the facial skeleton and the skull base. It is fortunate that craniofacial surgery for deformity has allowed the development of approaches that are helpful in gaining access to many of these tumors.

Sarcomas in this region occur less frequently than in any other body areas. Although adult sarcomas are different from those in children, the management is similar. After the diagnosis is established by biopsy, treatment includes surgery, radiation therapy, and chemotherapy. If surgery is chosen, this treatment provides the best chance of success. Local recurrence is usually due to inadequate resection, and in the past, this has been a frequent cause of treatment failure. Access to this area was previously much less developed than it is today. As with all tumors, when they are treated surgically, the first procedure is the best in terms of success. Nodal dissection is carried out only when there is clinical evidence of involvement. If the vascular anatomy is being displayed (e.g., in the neck), the draining nodes can be removed, whether they are involved or not. Radiation therapy is given preoperatively, intraoperatively, or postoperatively. Chemotherapy has been useful in the treatment of rhabdomyosarcoma; it is also of value in the treatment of other sarcomas.[169] Preoperative chemotherapy and radiation therapy may be used to reduce the size of large sarcomas and of tumors that are difficult to approach surgically, a situation that was common in the past but is rare nowadays.

Preoperative examination includes plain radiography of the skull and facial bones, high-resolution axial and coronal CT scans of the skull and facial bones, and, when indicated, MRI scans. In some orbital tumors, ultrasonic scanning can be helpful; radioactive scanning of the brain, skeleton, liver, and spleen is performed, if indicated. Other investigations can include fine-needle aspiration of the tumor, bone marrow aspiration and biopsy, and lumbar puncture.

Rhabdomyosarcoma

This is a common tumor of the head and neck in children. The management depends on the site of origin. In 1972, the Intergroup Rhabdomyosarcoma Study was established to evaluate treatment modalities. Three groups were identified, depending on the tumor's anatomic location: the eyelid and orbit; parameningeal; and other. Tumors in the orbit were found to have the best prognosis. Parameningeal tumors (middle ear, mastoid, ear canal, nasal cavity, paranasal sinuses, nasopharynx, and infratemporal fossa) had an increased risk for meningeal extension and thus a poor prognosis. Lesions in other locations were intermediate in prognosis.

Orbital rhabdomyosarcoma is discussed previously. Parameningeal lesions frequently have bone or meningeal involvement; central nervous system treatment, either craniospinal axis irradiation or intrathecal chemotherapy, may be of benefit. Treatment of the remainder of the rhabdomyosarcomas is surgical excision with resection of as much tumor as possible without causing a mutilating defect. Residual tumor is treated by radiation therapy or chemotherapy. Neck dissection should be performed for clinically abnormal nodes. The radiation dose is a total of 4000 to 4500 cGy in children younger than 6 years; older children receive 4500 to 5500 cGy. The chemotherapy regimen is usually vincristine, actinomycin D, and cyclophosphamide.

Rhabdomyosarcomas should be staged on the basis of postsurgical findings: group I, completely resected without residual tumor; group II, resected with histologic evidence of microscopic residual tumor; group

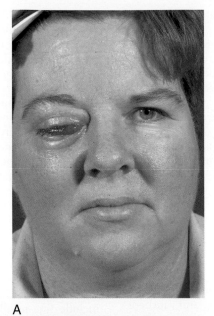

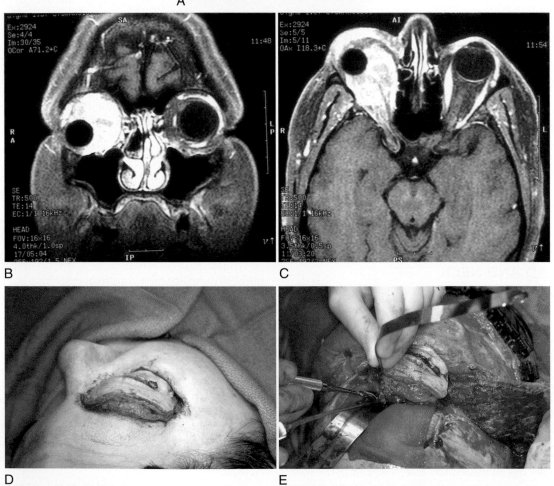

FIGURE 108–15. Orbital malignant melanoma. *A,* Patient with melanoma of right orbit with chemosis and moderate exophthalmos. *B* and *C,* Coronal and axial CT scans. *D,* External resection of orbital contents. *E,* Through a frontal craniotomy, intracranial resection of orbital contents.

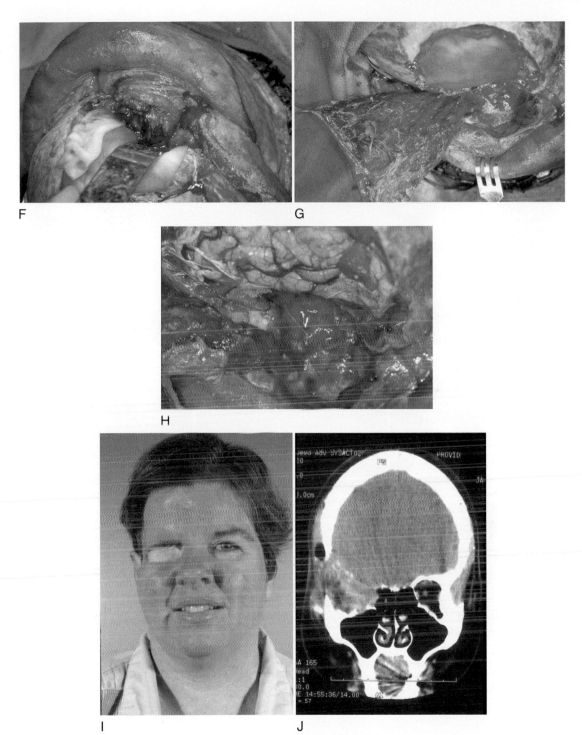

FIGURE 108-15, cont'd. *F,* Resection completed. *G* and *H,* Right temporalis muscle placed into the postoperative defect. *I,* Postoperative result. *J,* Coronal CT scan showing the resection of the tumor and the placement of the temporalis muscle.

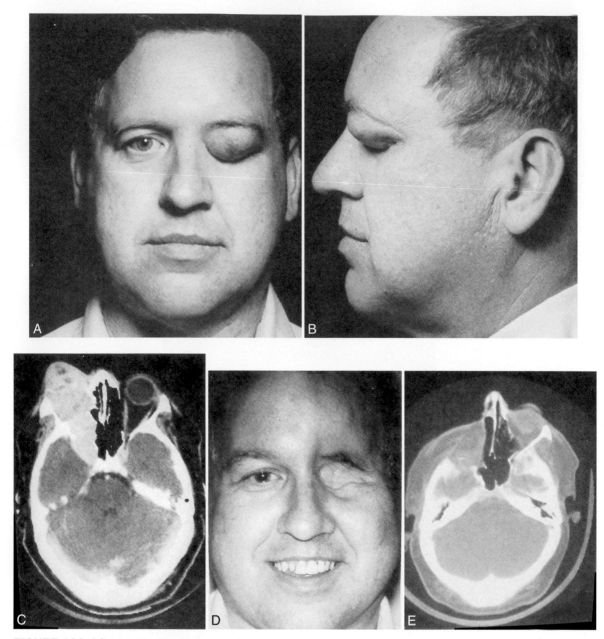

FIGURE 108-16. *A* and *B,* Hemangiopericytoma of left orbit. *C,* Axial CT scan to show extensive involvement of left orbit. *D,* After resection of hemangiopericytoma with reconstruction with left temporalis muscle and split-thickness skin graft. *E,* Axial CT scan to show postoperative appearance. (From Jackson IT, Shaw K: Tumors of the craniofacial skeleton, including the jaws. In McCarthy JG, ed: Plastic Surgery. Philadelphia, WB Saunders, 1990:3336.)

III, gross residual tumor; and group IV, documented metastasis. Except for group I lesions, triple chemotherapy and radiation therapy are given according to a strict protocol. In group IV, doxorubicin (Adriamycin) can be added. With this treatment, there has been a significant improvement in survival rates. However, in patients having parameningeal tumors or distant metastases, the prognosis is poor.

Fibrosarcoma

This is the most common soft tissue sarcoma in adults[170] and the second most common in children. The recommended treatment is radical surgery. Radiation therapy and chemotherapy are not curative but can be used in recurrent or metastatic disease.[171] The prognosis is excellent in the infantile fibrosarcoma (i.e., younger than 5 years), with 5-year survival rates of 80% or greater.

Neuroblastoma

This uncommon head and neck tumor may be congenital. Metastases are frequent and should be looked for carefully before therapy is begun. Staging of the disease is important.[172] In stage I and stage II, complete excision results in 90% survival in patients younger than 1 year. In stage II with residual tumor and stage III, postoperative irradiation can achieve satisfactory results.[173] Older patients and those with stage IV disease have uniformly poor prognosis. Patients younger than 1 year with stage IV lesions again have a good survival rate, probably because of activation of the immune system. Metastases are treated with chemotherapy.

Neurofibrosarcoma (Malignant Schwannoma)

This neoplasm is rare. It may arise independently or as part of von Recklinghausen disease. Twelve percent of neurofibrosarcomas occur in the head and neck region. It is difficult to determine the exact incidence because of institutional differences in classification.[174] There can be malignant change in neurofibromatosis, but the true incidence is not known because of poor follow-up. TNM staging and histologic grading of the malignancy correlate well with outcome; the 5-year survival rate for stage I tumors is 80%, whereas it is less than 20% for stage III tumors. Treatment is radical excision. If the nerve from which the tumor arises is found, it should be removed and the remainder cut and examined by frozen section intraoperatively to rule out any further tumor infiltration. The spread is usually blood-borne, and therefore neck dissection is rarely indicated. Adjuvant radiation therapy has not been evaluated in a prospective fashion, but it does seem to decrease local recurrence. Adjuvant chemotherapy may be useful because many patients die of systemic disease.

Malignant Fibrous Histiocytoma

This tumor is rare, and that of the jaws is discussed earlier. It is treated by wide local excision. The place of regional node dissection is not established; but in small groups of patients with clinically involved nodes, satisfactory results have been reported. Adjuvant chemotherapy may decrease the recurrence rate. The prognosis is influenced by the depth of invasion, size, and histologic grade of the tumor. Five-year survival is reported to be 65%.[174]

Hemangiopericytoma

This tumor is rare; only 1% occur in the head and neck area. These tumors are usually benign, but there is a malignant variety; histologic differentiation is difficult. They usually occur in the sixth to seventh decades with equal male and female prevalence. Local excision is performed for benign histiotypes, radical excision for malignant ones (see Fig. 108-16). Neck dissection is performed for clinically involved nodes. Radiation may be used in large doses, but chemotherapy is of doubtful value. The recurrence rates have decreased with more aggressive surgery. In tumors that show much mitotic activity with necrosis and bleeding into the tumor, the 10-year survival rate is only 29%. However, with a low rate of mitosis and little tissue necrosis, the 10-year survival rate is 80%. There can be metastases 10 years or more after primary excision.

Liposarcoma

Head and neck liposarcomas are rare (2% to 6%).[174 176] The recommended treatment is radical excision. The tumors are radiosensitive, but this treatment does not produce cure. Chemotherapy and radiation therapy are used for recurrences or incompletely resected tumors. Chemotherapy alone is not a useful treatment. The 5-year survival is above 80% for myxoid types and well-differentiated tumors but 50% for round cell and pleomorphic varieties.[176]

In patients younger than 18 years, the tumor is rare. There may be recurrence after incomplete excision. Even with complete removal, a proportion will recur. However, 80% survival has been reported on a minimum of 18 months of follow-up.[177]

Synovial Cell Sarcoma

Only 1% of these occur in the head and neck region; they require wide excision. They are only moderately sensitive to radiation therapy and chemotherapy; these are used as adjuvant treatments. Prognosis depends on the size and grade of the tumor; the larger the tumor and the higher the grade, the worse is the prognosis. The overall 5-year survival rate has been reported to be 47%.

Leiomyosarcoma

This tumor is rare in the head and neck region. Wide excision followed by chemotherapy and possibly radiation therapy is recommended. With good resection, survival is relatively good.

Desmoplastic Melanoma

Desmoplastic melanoma is a cutaneous lesion that is characterized histologically by spindle cell morphology with the associated production of fibrous connective tissue.[178] It is locally aggressive and has a poor prognosis. It may occur in a nevus that has an underlying subcutaneous portion. In the head and neck area, the incidence is 7%, and the patients are usually older. It can penetrate locally, involving bone, muscle, and nerve. Even with satisfactory excision, it may recur. Lymph node involvement is late but is not uncommon. Blood-borne spread is frequent. Mortality approaches 100% at 10 years.[178] These tumors should be treated by wide local resection with careful follow-up. Biopsy specimens should be obtained of any areas of swelling or induration. Reconstruction is performed only for functional reasons. If possible, closure alone is done to allow close follow-up. Involved lymph nodes should be removed (Fig. 108-17).

SURGICAL TREATMENT OF JAW AND CRANIOFACIAL SKELETON TUMORS

Surgical management can range from the straightforward, for example, segmental mandibulectomy or maxillectomy, to the exceedingly complex when the cranial base or the infratemporal fossa is involved. Even with sophisticated imaging, unlike in many other areas, the surgical resection may become much more complex than anticipated. The development and application of craniofacial surgical techniques have increased the ability to totally remove tumors that in the past would have been considered unresectable; thus, the incidence of local recurrence has decreased.

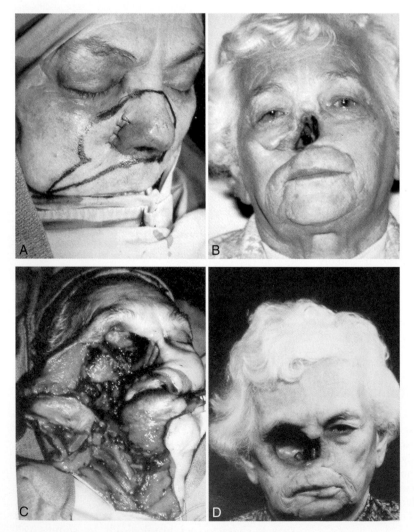

FIGURE 108-17. *A,* Desmoplastic melanoma involving the tip of the nose, medial aspect of right cheek, and nasolabial region. Biopsy was previously performed. *B,* After resection, there was recurrence at 6 months. *C,* Radical resection of orbit, maxilla, base of the middle cranial fossa, and infratemporal fossa together with a modified radical neck dissection by a mandibular swing. *D,* Postoperative appearance at 6 months. The patient survived for 3 years. (From Jackson IT, Shaw K: Tumors of the craniofacial skeleton, including the jaws. In McCarthy JG, ed: Plastic Surgery. Philadelphia, WB Saunders, 1990: 3336.)

Reconstruction has radically changed as a result of microsurgery. Plastic surgeons have had a great influence on these developments.

Tumors of the Mandible

The tumors of the mandible can be divided into those that grow slowly and are somewhat limited and those that are locally aggressive. The second group are frankly malignant. In benign, slow-growing lesions of limited size, the treatment is local resection. This is done through an intraoral approach, elevating a buccal or lingual mucoperiosteal flap, which is related to the position of the tumor. The mandibular cortex is removed, the tumor is enucleated or curetted, and the base is cauterized. If there has not been a previous biopsy, the benign nature of the tumor should be ascertained by frozen section. The mucoperiosteal flap is then sutured back into position.

The tumors that are locally aggressive or frankly malignant will require extensive resections. The four types of surgical procedures include marginal resection, segmental resection, hemimandibulectomy with condylar preservation, and hemimandibulectomy with disarticulation. With extensive mandibular involvement, a subtotal mandibulectomy may be indicated. Tumor perforation of the mandibular cortex requires the resection of a generous margin of soft tissue.

ANESTHETIC REQUIREMENTS

In most instances, the patient will require tracheal intubation. With symphyseal involvement and the possibility of tongue instability after resection, a prophylactic tracheostomy should be established. Hypotensive anesthesia can provide reduction of blood loss and consequently more accurate dissection.

SURGERY

The size and location of the tumor will determine whether the approach should be intraoral or extraoral. If the tumor is located posteriorly or if it is large, a lip split will provide optimal exposure. The next consideration is whether a simultaneous neck dissection is indicated. The upper incision of the Hayes-Martin approach or the McPhee approach will allow access to the mandible. If a lip-splitting incision is used, this can be vertical to the transverse lip crease and then curve around the chin soft tissue, ending in the center of the submental area, where it continues into the upper neck dissection incision. The segment of mandible to be excised is now exposed, usually with a cuff of soft tissue. A tooth should be extracted at the osteotomy site. If at all possible in hemimandibulectomies, the condyles should be preserved because this will greatly improve the functional rehabilitation. In all mandibular

resections for malignant disease, the proximal end of the inferior dental nerve should be sampled and subjected to frozen section. A positive biopsy result will necessitate a more extensive procedure, or it may be an indication of unresectability.

Mandibular Disarticulation

In this procedure, the lip is split and the neck is incised inferior to the lower border of the mandible. This approach allows a flap of lip and cheek soft tissue to be retracted laterally, and the position and the size of the tumor can be seen. The soft tissue is now dissected from the mandible, leaving the periosteum in place. Invasion of the cortex by the tumor necessitates that a second layer of soft tissue be retained over the tumor region, and a frozen section specimen is taken in that area from the cheek side just to ensure that tumor removal has been complete. The masseter is divided, as is the periosteum, and the remainder of the dissection on the external aspect of the mandible is subperiosteal. The mandibular notch is identified; should there be a tooth in the projected area of resection anteriorly, this is removed. The mandible is then cut with a microsagittal saw; if this is not available, a reciprocating saw or a side-cutting burr can be used. The mandible is retracted laterally, and all attachments to the floor of the mouth are divided. Posteromedially, the dissection continues parallel to the mandible with detachment of the mylohyoid muscle and division of the pterygomandibular ligament. This allows the temporalis muscle to be divided just above the coronoid. The jaw specimen can now be swung outward and downward, freeing the coronoid process from beneath the zygomatic arch. Any extensive invasion in this area will necessitate removal of the zygomatic arch. The pterygoid muscles are now divided. The insertion of the external pterygoid muscle is cut through, and the joint capsule is opened; following this maneuver, all other attached soft tissues are removed. There may be considerable bleeding, but this can easily be dealt with because exposure is now excellent. There is a little collection of pterygoid veins around this area together with the maxillary artery. If either of these is damaged, bleeding can be considerable.

Mandibular Reconstruction

Reconstruction is either immediate or delayed. The reasons to delay reconstruction are prolonged operating time; concerns about wound healing; and a large, aggressive tumor, causing doubts in the mind of the operator about recurrence in spite of negative frozen sections. A space-occupying appliance should be inserted to prevent postoperative segmental collapse. Kirschner wires are not advisable because they can allow telescoping and shortening in the mandibular body region. A premade condylar ramus and body prosthesis is excellent. It is securely fixed to the remainder of the mandible anteriorly with screws, and then the condyle is seated into the condylar fossa. Intraoral soft tissue defects should be replaced with a free vascularized flap of appropriate dimensions or a regional musculocutaneous flap; pectoralis major is the flap of choice, although platysmal, sternocleidomastoid, and trapezius flaps can be used.

There are some segmental resections that may not require reconstruction; a unilateral resection of the ramus and a posterior portion of the body is such an example. In this situation, immediate reconstruction may result in significant trismus. Extensive soft tissue resection in this region requires primary replacement to avoid mandibular shift, which can occur from contracture of the residual soft tissues. Again, free tissue transplantation or a regional flap should replace the resected soft tissue.

It is obvious that immediate mandibular reconstruction is ideal, if it is possible, especially when satisfactory tumor excision has been achieved and the patient's status is good; thus, extended operating time need not be a consideration. The initial question is whether a nonvascularized bone graft is adequate or whether vascularization is necessary. The vascularization procedure is favored when there is inadequate residual soft tissue cover requiring a soft tissue flap, when there has been previous irradiation, or with the consideration of early postsurgical irradiation.

There are two forms of vascularized bone reconstruction, pedicled flaps and microvascular complete tissue transplantation (free flap). Free tissue transplantation is favored when there is inadequate residual soft tissue cover, previous tumor irradiation, or planned irradiation after resection. The bone reconstruction can be carried out with pedicled flaps or free microvascular transfers. The pedicled flaps include the pectoralis major with a rib,[179-181] the sternomastoid muscle with a portion of the clavicle,[182] the serratus anterior with a rib, and the trapezius with the spine of scapula.[183,184] Only the last two are consistently reliable. The trapezius flap may not be possible because of division of the transverse cervical vessels in the neck dissection. Other disadvantages to these flaps are donor site morbidity and flap bulk.

Several microvascular osseous transfers, with or without soft tissue, include rib,[185] iliac crest,[186] fibula, scapula, and metatarsal. These can be tailored to the required replacement; they provide good contour and allow early osseointegration. This approach is generally the reconstruction of choice, and those flaps are described in detail elsewhere in this book.

Maxillary Tumors

Benign maxillary tumors, when they are low and small, can be resected with or without teeth, depending on the patient's dental situation, and the defect can be allowed to heal spontaneously. If bone is involved and there seems the possibility of a palatal fistula, local flaps from the palate or from the buccal sulcus can be used to close most defects. This approach is particularly easy in the edentulous patient. However, it is advisable that a two-flap closure be provided whenever possible. In the palate, closure is accomplished by use of a local flap followed by a tongue flap. The tongue flap is left in position for 2 to 3 weeks and then divided. Tumors in other areas can be dealt with by a buccal sulcus incision with removal of the tumor, usually within the maxillary antrum, and direct closure of the upper buccal sulcus.

Should there be a resection of a nonmalignant tumor involving the floor of the orbit, as long as the periosteum on the orbital floor is not disturbed, no reconstructive surgery is necessary apart from the insertion of a mold made from Stent (dental compound) carrying a split-thickness skin graft. If the periosteum is taken, a small flat bone graft harvested from an available donor site should be inserted with small plates and screws for stabilization. The graft should be covered with vascularized tissue, such as a small free flap (e.g., rectus abdominis), with or without skin. An alternative is the medial plate of the ileum with its periosteum. The tissue should be covered with mucosa fairly quickly.

MALIGNANT LESIONS

In malignant lesions, it is the position and the extension of the tumor that dictate the extent of maxillary resection, which in turn has a significant influence on the type of reconstruction used. In highly malignant lesions with any question of the possibility of recurrence, a cautious approach to reconstruction is advised. A prosthesis used in this area after split-thickness skin grafting allows clear inspection of the residual area of tumor resection, and recurrences can be recognized early. Failure to carry out this surveillance can lead to serious consequences, such as loss of an eye or intracranial extension. Therefore, radical resection and careful follow-up with good exposure are recommended. Free tissue transplantation should not be used if at all possible.

Malignant neoplasms can extend into the nasal cavity, the nasopharynx, the oral cavity and alveolus, the orbit, the soft tissues of the face, the infratemporal fossa, the paranasal sinuses, and the base of the skull. Some, ultimately, extend into the intracranial cavity.

In low-grade malignant and benign lesions of the lateral nasal wall, for example, the inverted papilloma,[149] a medial maxillectomy can be performed. The skin approach is through a Weber-Fergusson incision, which allows a broad, laterally based cheek flap to be elevated. An alternative is to leave the upper lip intact and expose the area through a lateral rhinotomy incision with a Caldwell-Luc exposure to approach the tumor. These two approaches allow access to the medial portion of the maxilla. After exposure of the medial maxilla and after the floor and the medial orbital walls are exposed subperiosteally, the orbital contents can be retracted. In this way, there is exposure that allows osteotomies to be performed, with removal of the medial orbital wall and the ethmoid sinuses en bloc. If necessary, the medial canthal ligament attachment, nasal mucosa, and any overlying involved skin can be included, although if it seems possible on preoperative examination, the cutaneous resection alone can be used as an entry to achieve the whole resection. In some patients, the tumor may be so extensive that a decision is made to perform a more extensive subtotal maxillectomy or even a total maxillectomy. In addition, it may be necessary to combine this approach with a coronal flap exposure to resect any superior extension, which could include removal of the floor of the anterior cranial fossa and cribriform plate.

Although it is usually possible to make an accurate preoperative forecast of what is required to be removed by three-dimensional CT scans and MRI scans, this is not always so. The patient should be informed that it may be necessary to remove part or all of the orbital contents, and this includes the eye. Frozen section examination will be used to help make these decisions. It is in this junctional area that total resection may become a much more extensive procedure than was first appreciated. The inferior extension may require resection of the lower maxilla and palate and, if necessary, removal of the orbital contents; the best reconstruction of that area, once it is thought that complete resection has been obtained, is to place a skin graft into the cavity and hold it in place with petrolatum gauze and a sponge pack. If the palate has been resected, it is held in place with a dental obturator. If there is an extension out onto the face, the cavity can be packed from the facial defect. Any reconstruction of this type of lesion is left until there is absolute proof of total tumor resection. In some patients, depending on the pathologic behavior of the tumor and the completeness of excision, the whole area may be reconstructed with free tissue transplantation with later secondary reconstruction as required. If the eye is retained, the Lockwood suspensory ligament should be kept intact to prevent globe dystopia and diplopia. However, resection of the periorbita will inevitably cause eye displacement, which can be ameliorated by an intraoral prosthesis that fits high into the cavity and suspends the orbital contents. Again, at some time in the future, total reconstruction may be performed.

In this area, probably the biggest and most frequent error is to underestimate the aggressiveness of the tumor and consequently to underresect it. Failure to completely resect the tumor is usually the result of reluctance to produce a large defect resulting in a significant cosmetic deformity. In malignant tumors, appearance should come second in decision-making; but if possible, the basic foundation for secondary reconstruction should be maintained. This situation is considered further in the next section on tumors of the skull base.

Tumors of the Skull Base

The skull base may be involved by tumor from above or from below. Frequently, intracranial lesions exit through one of the skull base foramina to become extracranial. In the past, surgical removal was often incomplete; but with the recent cooperation between plastic surgery, otorhinolaryngology, and neurosurgery, total resection is frequently possible, although this does not necessarily mean cure of the tumor. In all of these patients, careful and regular long-term follow-up is required.

Advances such as the endoscopic and the navigational techniques used by otorhinolaryngology and neurosurgery, together with microsurgical reconstructions and sophisticated radiologic investigations, allow more complete excision of these lesions and better possibilities for reconstruction and cure.

Before surgery, CT scans, MRI scans, and carotid angiograms are obtained, as indicated. In some patients, three-dimensional reformatting may be helpful. MRI scans can frequently supply more accurate information about the extent of soft tissue infiltration in difficult areas, such as the infratemporal and temporal fossae. Extensive and vascular tumors require carotid angiography to indicate the vascular pattern of the tumor or displacement of major vessels. When a tumor is vascular (e.g., a vascular malformation), a neurofibroma, or a meningioma, it can be embolized immediately before surgery; this reduces the intraoperative bleeding and makes surgery less difficult. The excisional surgery must be performed within 2 to 5 days to make the best use of the embolization. Careful consideration of all the radiologic investigations and occasionally a craniotomy may be necessary before a tumor is considered to be totally inoperable.

ANATOMY OF THE SKULL BASE

There have been various classifications of skull base anatomy, but one that is useful from a practical point of view is to divide the skull into the anterior area, which is the anterior cranial fossa, and the posterior area, which consists of the remainder of the base. The posterior area is divided into three further segments: the anterior is the segment between the greater wing of the sphenoid and the anterior margin of the petrous bone; the central is the petrous bone itself; and the posterior is the segment between the posterior margin

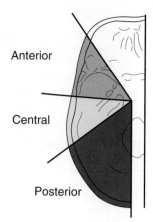

Anterior

Central

Posterior

FIGURE 108-18. The posterior area of the skull base can conveniently be divided into three segments—anterior, central, and posterior. This is convenient to describe tumor position. (From Jackson IT, Shaw K: Tumors of the craniofacial skeleton, including the jaws. In McCarthy JG, ed. Plastic Surgery. Philadelphia, WB Saunders, 1990:3336.)

of the petrous bone and the posterior border of the posterior fossa (Fig. 108-18).[157] These areas contain foramina through which tumors enter or leave the cranium. In the anterior cranial fossa area, the foramina lie in the cribriform plate. In the posterior area of the anterior segment, there are the optic nerve foramen, the foramen rotundum for the maxillary nerve, the foramen ovale for the mandibular nerve, the foramen lacerum for the internal carotid artery, the foramen spinosum for the middle meningeal artery, and the vidian canal for the deep petrosal and greater superficial petrosal nerves. In the central segment within the petrous bone, there are the internal carotid canal, the facial nerve canal and its foramen, and the interior auditory meatus. The posterior segment contains the jugular foramen with the internal jugular vein and the foramen magnum. The intracranial exit of long foramina may not lie in the same position as the extracranial end, and this is important, particularly in relation to the carotid canal.

ANTERIOR SKULL BASE

Tumors involving the frontal bone, frontal ethmoid sinuses, medial canthus, orbit, orbital contents, or nasopharynx can directly invade the anterior cranial fossa.[187] Indirect involvement by skin, maxilla, or muscle tumors can occur, usually through the ethmoid sinuses or the orbit. Tumors arising from the brain or meninges can also involve the skull base. Any suggestion of tumors arising in these areas should be confirmed or refuted by CT scans, although the MRI scan is better for vascular tumors.

Nonmalignant Tumors

Fibrous dysplasia is a good example of a nonmalignant tumor that requires fronto-orbital resection.[188] This condition can cause eye displacement, proptosis, diplopia, deteriorating vision, and blindness. Blindness appears to be due to nerve compression from narrowing of the optic nerve canal. The condition progresses through adolescence, and growth stops at different times in different patients. There is no uniformity of progression in this condition.

With incomplete resection, there may or may not be recurrence. Recurrence seems to depend on the particular tumor's behavior or characteristics. Malignant change may occur, but this is rare unless there has been prior irradiation. If possible, treatment should be total resection with immediate reconstruction. Three-dimensional reformatting of CT scans is helpful in both resection and reconstruction.

Resection is undertaken with a bicoronal flap being elevated in the frontal area (Fig. 108-19). The orbit and the nasal skeleton are exposed until healthy bone is identified. It may be necessary to extend this dissection into the temporal region intracranially and extracranially. The orbital contents are dissected in the subperiosteal plane. A craniotomy is performed to expose and assess the intracranial situation, and all involved bone is discarded. All orbital, nasal, and skull base areas are resected, if possible. The optic nerve canal is carefully unroofed in its entirety together with the medial and lateral walls to decompress the optic nerve. It must be understood that it may not be possible to totally remove the involved skull base area. With experience, complete tumor extirpation becomes feasible. Should there be any worry about malignant change, which is usually associated with prior irradiation, frozen sections are recommended.

If the central skull base is resected and there is an opening into the sinuses or into the nasopharynx, which is common for all skull base tumors, the galeofrontalis myofascial flap[189] is elevated from the undersurface of the coronal flap and brought down into the anterior cranial fossa. Drill holes are made laterally around the area of basal resection, and these are used to suture the galeofrontalis myofascial flap into position. This can be done in a virtually watertight fashion with an overlap of the flap on the bone intracranially. An attempt should be made to block out every connection between the nasopharynx and the intracranial contents. The galeofrontalis myofascial flap is based on the supraorbital and supratrochlear vessels and is exceedingly robust. When it has been placed and sutured securely, there have been no ascending intracranial infections because the brain holds the correct overlapping position. Once this has been accomplished, all bone defects are reconstructed with split skull grafts of healthy skull; these are held in place with either metal plates or, in children, resorbable

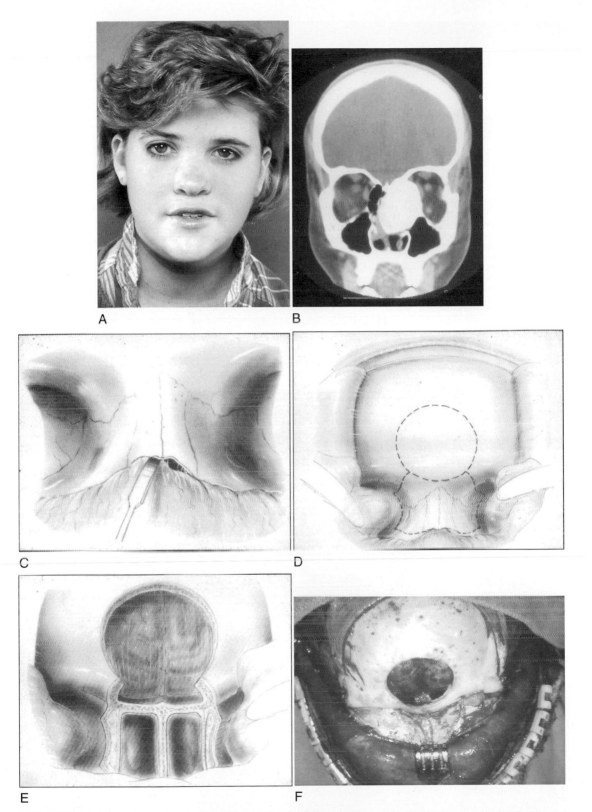

FIGURE 108-19. Fibrous dysplasia of the left frontoethmoid area. *A,* Preoperative appearance. *B,* Coronal CT scan to illustrate extent of the fibrous dysplasia. *C,* Coronal flap has been taken down, subperiosteal dissection of the anterior aspect of the nasal cavity. *D,* Dotted lines show the area of the planned osteotomies. *E,* Frontonasal segment removed. *F,* Limited frontal craniotomy.   *Continued*

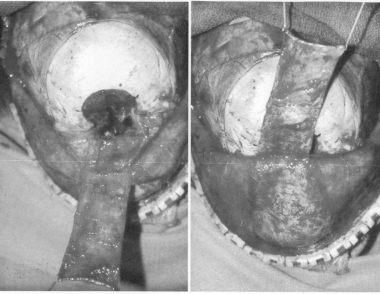

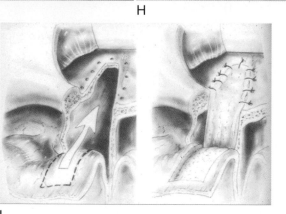

FIGURE 108-19, cont'd. *G* and *H,* After resection of anterior skull base area and illustrating the length of the galeofrontalis musculofascial flap. *I,* Diagram to illustrate how the flap is sutured in such a way that it is watertight. *J,* Insertion and stabilization of flap. *K,* Long-term postoperative result. (*A, B,* and *K* from Jackson IT, Shaw K: Tumors of the craniofacial skeleton, including the jaws. In McCarthy JG, ed: Plastic Surgery. Philadelphia, WB Saunders, 1990: 3336.)

plates. It has been reported that if the involved skull is placed in the sterilizing unit in the operating room and heated to 270°F for 5 minutes, this will result in destruction of the fibrous dysplastic process, and this bone may then be used for reconstruction. However, if it is treated at too high a temperature, the bone becomes soft and unusable. Certainly, it has been the author's experience in a significant number of patients that bone treated in this way does not undergo further dysplastic change.

Malignant Tumors

Malignant tumors may be intracranial or extracranial, but the extracranial tumors may require an intracranial approach. These tumors can recur in spite of surgical treatment, radiation therapy, or chemotherapy. It is advised that reconstruction be limited to the absolute essentials after radical resection because a more sophisticated reconstruction might mask later recurrence and further treatment may be delayed. Also, the patient may be reluctant to undergo additional surgery. Loss of future reconstructive options is unfortunate if there is a recurrence.

The main concerns in reconstruction after craniofacial resection are cover of vital structures and separation of the oronasopharynx from the extradural space. If it is not possible to completely resect a lesion and there is a considerable defect, the best option might be to provide immediate reconstruction with a microvascular free flap followed by a tumoricidal dose of radiation therapy. This treatment plan will allow the patient to have some hope of cure, and if no cure is available, the patient may have as reasonable a quality of life as can be provided.

Orbital Tumors

The orbit may be involved by tumors that arise from its contents, its architecture, or structures outside of it. Tumors outside of the orbit may arise in the anterior and middle cranial fossae; the frontal, ethmoid, and maxillary sinuses; the nose; and the temporal and infratemporal fossae. Indirect invasion occurs when tumors such as meningioma escape from the middle cranial fossa by way of a cranial base foramen. It is advisable to consider these anterior cranial fossa tumors until proven otherwise. This will lead to a more effective assessment and treatment. Encroachment on the skull base seen on high-resolution CT scans and MRI scans is an indication for a transcranial approach.

There are several options for the treatment of orbital tumors (Figs. 108-20 to 108-24 and Table 108-3).[190] Exposure orbitotomy involves removal of a portion of the orbit to gain access for resection of the lesion. With this accomplished and with reconstruction of any residual bone defect, the removed portion of orbit is reinserted. This approach can be used for benign tumors, such as neurofibromas, schwannomas, heman-

TABLE 108-3 ✦ PROCEDURES USED IN THE TREATMENT OF ORBITAL TUMORS

Exposure osteotomy consisting of orbitectomy and segment replacement (see Fig. 108-20)
Partial orbitectomy with preservation of the orbital contents without reconstruction
Partial orbitectomy with resection of the orbital contents without reconstruction (see Fig. 108-21)
Partial orbitectomy with resection of the orbital contents with orbital reconstruction (see Fig. 108-23)
Total transcranial orbitectomy with preservation of the orbital contents with reconstruction (see Fig. 108-22)
Total transcranial orbitectomy with resection of the orbital contents with reconstruction by free tissue transplantation[100] (see Fig. 108-24)

giomas, some meningiomas, and nonspecific granulomas involving the superior half of the orbit, particularly if they lie behind the meridian of the globe. This approach should not be used in malignant tumors, for which exenteration is the treatment of choice.

In all orbitectomies, a bicoronal flap approach is mandatory. After this, the orbital contents are dissected subperiosteally, the frontal pericranium and temporalis are elevated, and a total frontal or hemifrontal craniotomy is performed by the neurosurgeon, leaving the supraorbital area intact. The frontal lobe is gently elevated from the orbital roof. The orbital contents are then dissected from the roof and protected with a malleable retractor. In fact, a spoon of an adequate size is the most suitable for this maneuver. With use of a power drill, the supraorbital rim is cut medially and laterally. This extends as far down the lateral wall as is necessary for exposure. The orbital roof is cut around as extensively as necessary; the block of supraorbital rim, roof, and, if necessary, lateral orbital wall is removed. This approach gives excellent exposure to the orbital contents. The frontal lobe is now retracted, an incision is made through the periorbita, and the orbital tissues are retracted to expose the tumor under direct vision. The tumor can then be directly removed atraumatically. Bleeding points are coagulated, and the periorbita can be loosely closed but should be left open if there is tightness. The orbitectomy segment is replaced and fixed in position with resorbable or metal plates and screws; wires may also be used.

For deeper lateral tumors, which may extend into the subcranial area, the exposure osteotomy consists of the lateral orbital rim with or without the wall, orbital floor, and a portion of the maxilla. The segments are removed, and good exposure of the tumor is obtained. If the tumor involves the orbital wall, whether it is the lateral orbital wall, the floor, the anterior cranial fossa, or the nasal area, a radical resection of the whole area, including bone, is performed, taking

Text continued on p. 134

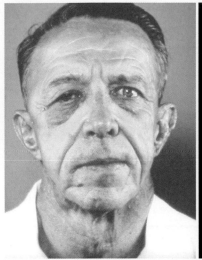

A

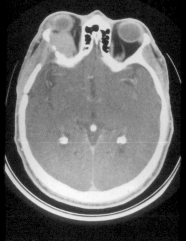

B

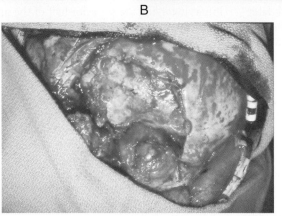

C

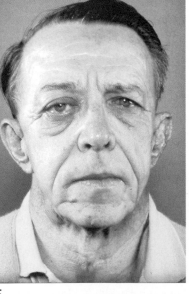

D

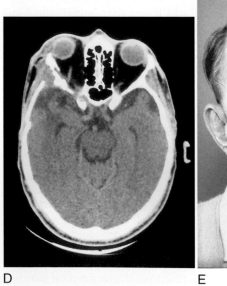

E

FIGURE 108-20. Meningioma of left orbit. *A,* Preoperative appearance. *B,* Axial CT scan to show the extent of the lesion. *C,* Transcranial resection of meningioma. *D,* Postoperative CT scan, lateral orbital wall reconstructed with cranial bone graft. *E,* Postoperative result.

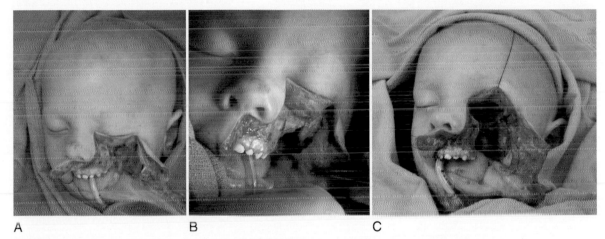

A   B   C

FIGURE 108-21. Partial orbitectomy with resection of orbital contents without reconstruction in a child with rhabdomyosarcoma of left maxilla. *A*, Exposure through a Weber-Fergusson approach. *B*, Hemimaxillectomy and complete excision. *C*, Hemimaxillectomy and resection of left orbit.

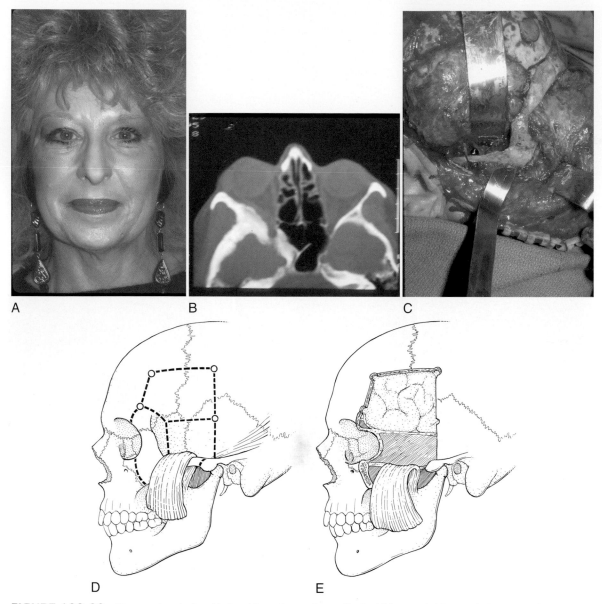

FIGURE 108-22. Fibrous dysplasia of left orbit and anterior wall of middle cranial fossa. *A,* Preoperative appearance. *B,* Preoperative axial CT scan. *C,* Exposure with plan to remove lateral orbital wall, lateral portion of superior orbital rim, and zygoma. *D,* Diagram to show the osteotomies of zygomatic arch, orbit, and temporal area; the temporalis muscle is then turned down. *E,* Diagram of exposure once bone has been removed.

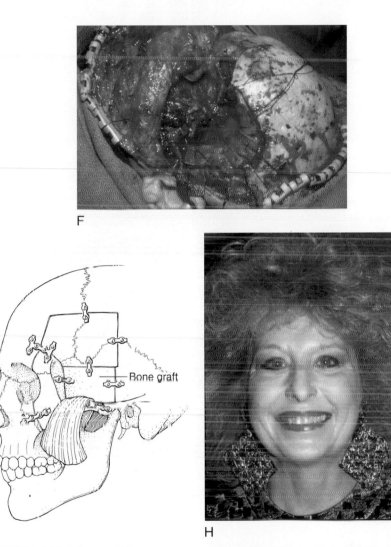

FIGURE 108-22, cont'd. *F,* After resection, temporalis muscle being placed back in position. *G,* Diagram of reconstruction. *H,* Postoperative result at 1 year.

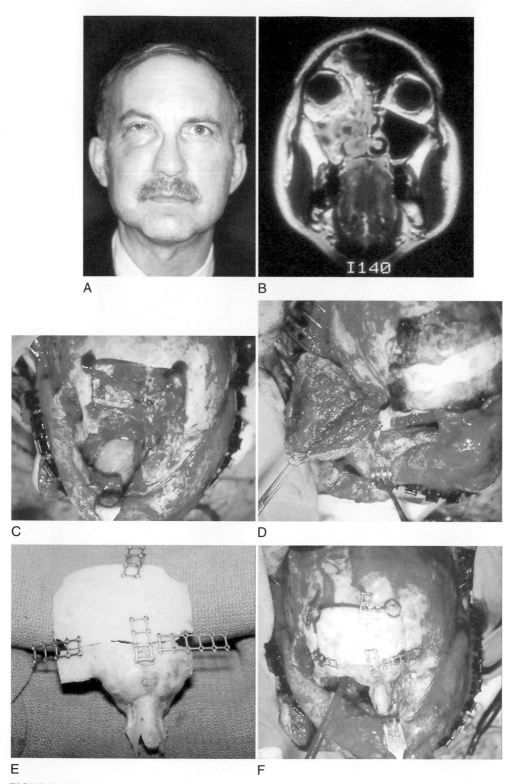

FIGURE 108-23. Removal of orbit, resection of orbital contents. *A,* The patient presented with swelling of right cheek and displacement of right eye. *B,* Coronal CT scan to show the distribution of the lesion, which turned out to be a squamous cell carcinoma. *C,* Radical resection of right frontal area, orbit, maxilla, and palate. *D,* Temporalis muscle elevated. *E,* The removed frontal and nasal bone. *F,* Replacement of the frontonasal bone.

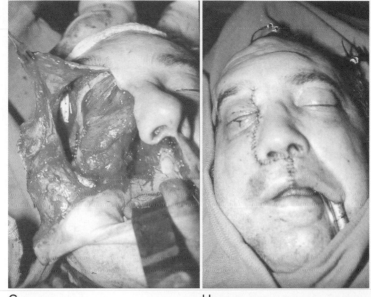

G   H

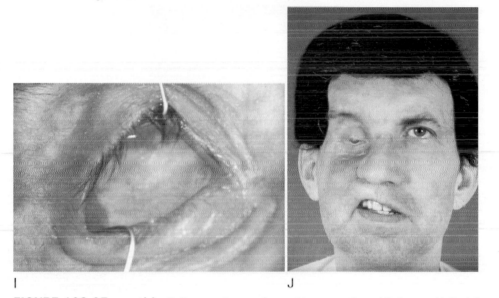

I   J

FIGURE 108-23, cont'd. *G,* Temporalis muscle used to cover the orbital area. *H,* Facial skin and periorbital closure. *I,* Reconstructed socket with split-thickness skin graft. *J,* Post-operative result. Further reconstructive surgery is planned.

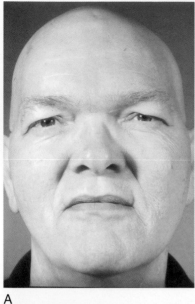

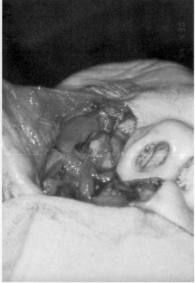

FIGURE 108-24. *A,* Adenoid cystic carcinoma of right orbit. *B* and *C,* Total orbital resection. *D,* Postoperative appearance after reconstruction with rectus abdominis free tissue transplantation.

whatever is necessary to remove the tumor. If there is any suggestion of involvement of the eye in any area, the eye is removed en bloc with any involved orbital bone segments. Reconstruction is then carried out by replacing whatever segments are not involved and by using cranial bone grafts to replace missing segments.

If the involvement is extensive in and around the orbit or if the behavior of the tumor is aggressive, there should be total resection of the orbit and its contents. A procedure that is similar to a hypertelorism correction is then used, consisting of a box osteotomy that cuts around all four walls of the orbit as far back as possible. Bone resection begins with the retraction of the brain. A cut is now made across the orbital roof, down the lateral wall, across the floor of the orbit, and across the front of the maxilla below the infraorbital nerve, then vertically up the medial wall, going far enough posteriorly to include the ethmoid sinuses. When the orbital bones are removed together with the tumor, there is a defect into the nasopharynx, and this is sealed off with a galeofrontalis myofascial flap. Skin closure can be obtained with skin graft, scalp rotation, forehead transposition flap, or distant flap such as pectoralis major or deltopectoral flap; but in most instances, microvascular composite tissue transplantation is most satisfactory as long as it has been confirmed by frozen section that resection of the original tumor is complete. Again, if there is any doubt, reconstruction is delayed.

Penetrating Midface Tumors

These tumors are now uncommon, but patients continue to present with this problem. It is important to have a clear concept of how these must be resected to give the patient some chance of cure with the possibility of later reconstruction.

The tumors involved are recurrent, aggressive basal cell carcinomas or squamous cell carcinomas. Less frequently, they may be adenoid cystic carcinoma, mucoepidermoid carcinoma, adenocarcinoma, sarcoma, or esthesioneuroblastoma.[191] In the past, inadequate resection has been the main problem; thus, Mohs micrographic resection, radiation therapy, and chemotherapy have all been employed. It is important to approach the resection of these tumors with the plan of good exposure, radical resection with clear margins, and a safe reconstructive method that may not be aesthetically satisfactory but should ensure rapid healing with a good local blood supply. If these requirements can be supplied, the possibility of effective radiation treatment becomes much more of a reality. It is often necessary to remove the nose or its remnants, the medial portions of the orbits, sometimes the orbital contents unilaterally or even bilaterally, the maxilla, the palate, a varying amount of the nasopharynx, the base of the anterior cranial fossa, the overlying dura, the frontal bone, and the frontal ethmoid and sphenoid sinuses.

If the tumor does not involve the nasal skeleton or the frontal bone, an exposure osteotomy technique is used.[190] The bicoronal flap is used to expose the area. On occasion, the direct approach may be used for exposure, the soft tissue excision giving enough space to allow the bone osteotomies to be carried out. In other patients, a face-splitting procedure, or a combination of any of these, may be used (Fig. 108-25). With the required area of skull exposed, a frontal craniotomy or a trephine craniotomy can be carried out. The frontal craniotomy is preferred because it allows a good assessment of the dura and the ability to retract the frontal lobes to see how far back the tumor extends. If there is extensive involvement of the posterior wall of the sphenoid sinus with penetration into the cavernous sinus, this is an indication of inoperability.

Adequate resection in most patients will involve removal of the central part of the skull base and, if necessary, the medial walls of the orbit; the resection is controlled by frozen section. If the dura is removed, this must be replaced, preferably with fascia lata or stored dura, but stored dura should be avoided if possible because of unreliability. This closure must be done carefully. The graft is placed on the inside of the dura as an overlap and sutured in that position to produce watertight closure and to prevent ascending infection into the subdural area. Infection must be avoided at all costs; this can result in meningitis with a loss of any nonvascularized bone, which in turn may lead to an overwhelming infection that may cause death of the patient. A two-layered closure is preferable and is obtained in various ways by use of a midline forehead flap, an extended glabellar flap, or a galeofrontalis musculofascial flap.[189] Elevation of the galeofrontalis musculofascial flap, which is very malleable, is based on the supraorbital vessels; it is then secured in an overlapping fashion to the edge of the bone defect in the floor of the anterior cranial fossa by drill holes and sutures (see Fig. 108-19). A single flap is usually satisfactory, but two flaps can be sutured together to close a wider defect. If necessary, this can be skin grafted on the nasal side. An alternative is to insert a free flap that will also ensure a satisfactory seal and rapid healing.[82]

If it has been necessary to remove the nose or the orbit and its contents, long-term reconstruction with a prosthesis is strongly advised. First, a prosthesis allows inspection of the area of resection and early detection of recurrences. Second, the prosthesis can be stabilized by osseointegration. Third, the quality of prostheses has been improved, resulting in acceptable rehabilitation.[107]

Free tissue transplantation has made this type of surgery much safer because it can be used at the primary resection; if infection occurs because of intracranial dead space or connection down into the nasopharynx, it is used as a secondary technique to deal with this situation.[192] These patients require a careful follow-up because, in the past, there was a high rate of recurrence. The patients are examined routinely every 3 months with a flexible endoscope, when indicated, or with a dental mirror, and they have at least annual CT scans. Biopsies of any suspicious area should be undertaken without delay; if the biopsy result is positive, and if it is possible, another aggressive resection should be performed.

ETHMOID CARCINOMA. Tumors arising in and invading the ethmoid sinuses are also considered anterior cranial base tumors. The bicoronal approach is used with a limited craniotomy. To obtain better exposure, the frontal glabellar area together with the nasal bones is often removed en bloc (Fig. 108-26). This makes it easier to perform total resection with wide margins. With retraction of the frontal lobes, the roof of the ethmoid sinuses is clearly exposed, and osteotomies can be made around this. The nose and the medial orbital walls are exposed subperiosteally,

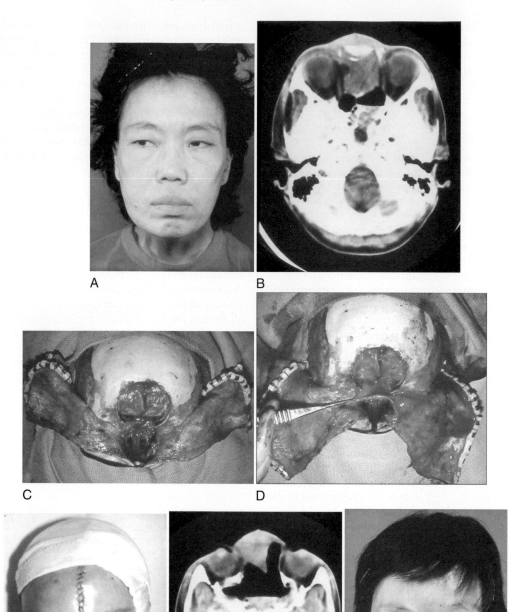

FIGURE 108-25. Recurrent squamous cell carcinoma of anterior skull base. *A,* Preoperative appearance. *B,* Axial CT scan showing tumor. *C,* Approach by coronal flap and face split with removal of frontonasal region. *D,* Reconstruction of skull base with galeofrontalis myofascial flap. *E,* Immediate postoperative result. *F,* Axial CT scan shows good clearance of tumor. *G,* Postoperative result. (From Jackson IT, Shaw K: Tumors of the craniofacial skeleton, including the jaws. In McCarthy JG, ed: Plastic Surgery. Philadelphia, WB Saunders, 1990:3336.)

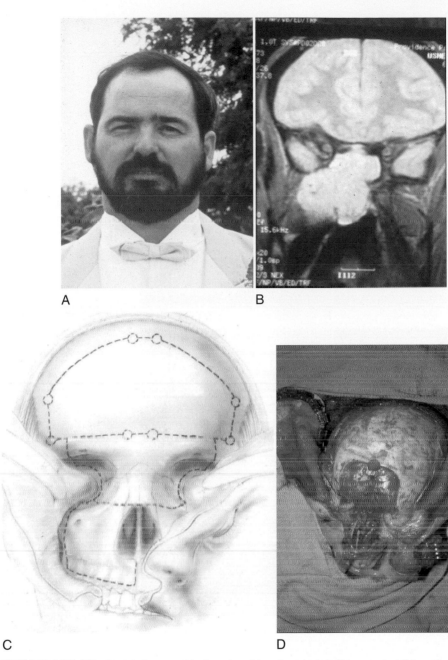

FIGURE 108-26. Facial disassembly for ethmoid and central skull base adenoid cystic carcinoma. *A,* Preoperative appearance. *B,* Preoperative coronal CT scan. *C,* Diagram showing
planned facial disarticulation. *D,* Soft tissue approach. The nose has been divided vertically and
swung laterally on the left flap. Frontal craniotomy has been performed.   *Continued*

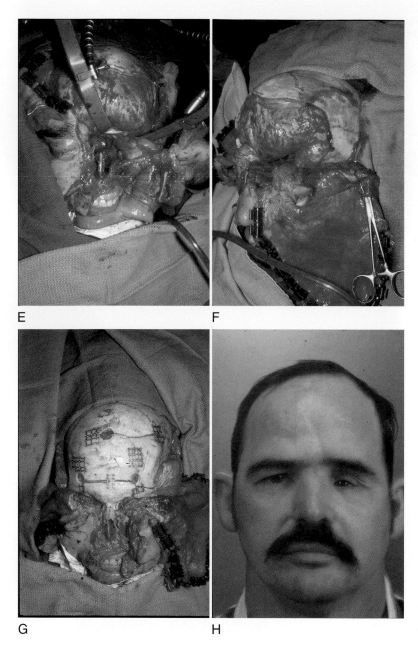

FIGURE 108-26, cont'd. *E,* Skull base resection. *F,* Exposure of cavernous sinus for resection of tumor. *G,* Reconstruction. *H,* Postoperative result. The patient remains alive at 10 years but has recurrent tumor.

and the extracranial resection is performed as required, depending on the position of the tumor and the extent to which it invades neighboring tissues. Thus, the nasal bone and the involved side, together with the medial wall of the orbit and the base of the skull directly above this, can be excised en bloc. When indicated, this incision can also include the overlying skin, the nasal septum, and the orbital contents. Should there be extension down into the maxillary area, a partial or total maxillectomy is included. If it is necessary to have greater exposure in this area, a Weber-Fergusson incision can be made. This incision, on certain occasions,

will continue onto a mid-vertical forehead incision. With such an approach, a wide exposure of the facial skeleton is obtained. A partial maxillectomy, a total maxillectomy, a partial orbitectomy, or a total orbitectomy with the orbital contents can be carried out with only moderate blood loss. This is reserved for patients with advanced disease in which there is a hope of cure (see Figs. 108-23 and 108-26).

In such tumors, which are frequently highly malignant and infiltrative, it is prudent to simply close off the aerodigestive tract from the intracranial contents with a galeofrontalis myofascial flap sutured to drill holes in the skull base as described earlier, followed by reconstruction at a later date if possible. If indicated, and this could be to have a more secure prevention of ascending infection or to cover replaced, nonvascularized bone, microvascular composite tissue transplantation (free flap) may bring a source of good blood supply into these regions.

Reconstruction should be undertaken with an external prosthesis. If the total maxilla has been taken, prosthetic dental rehabilitation will be necessary. Definitive reconstruction with the patient's own tissue should be undertaken at 12 to 18 months postoperatively, provided the area remains tumor free. If the patient does not want treatment by this complex approach, prosthesis wearing continues.

MIDFACE SARCOMAS. Chondrosarcoma and osteogenic sarcoma can arise in the nasal septum and the surrounding nasal area. They can rapidly involve the anterior skull base, frequently in the posterior region, and will then extend intracranially. The usual presentation is that of nasal congestion with a mass that is easily seen in the nasal cavity, with either the nasal speculum or the nasendoscope. The investigations are CT and MRI scans and a biopsy of the mass.

The preferred approach is through a bicoronal flap; when indicated, this is accompanied by a face-splitting incision. It is preferable not to extend the paranasal lip-splitting incision into the forehead unless this is absolutely necessary. The bicoronal flap is elevated by lifting the pericranium, and this continues down over the nasal bones and medial aspect of both orbits and also onto the front of the maxilla. An incision is made in the upper buccal sulcus, either unilaterally or bilaterally, depending on the position of the tumor. This approach allows a wide dissection of the anterior aspects of the maxilla and upper alveolus. In many patients, the infraorbital nerve can be kept intact. If a wider exposure is indicated, the conjunctiva can be divided, and the lids are then included in the flap and the whole of the orbit is exposed. The eye must be protected with ointment to prevent injury. A limited craniotomy allows exposure to the anterior cranial fossa with visualization of intracranial involvement. With extensive posteriorly located tumors, the glabellar area, the nasal skeleton, the medial orbital wall, and as much of the inferior orbital rim as is needed can be osteotomized as a single segment. The lower portion of this segment may be bilateral; all the segments mentioned can be removed. With this extensive exposure, it is possible to carry out an en bloc resection of the medial orbital walls, nasal septum, anterior cranial fossa, and ethmoid and sphenoid sinuses. The bone blocks that have been removed and are uninvolved with tumor will be placed back in position; but before this, two galeofrontalis myofascial flaps are raised—one to cover any portions of the osteotomy

exposed into the nose, the other to separate the anterior cranial fossa from the nasopharynx. This vascularized tissue prevents the development of complications related to intracranial and extracranial connections. If it is not available, a thin free tissue transplantation, such as the radial forearm flap, may be indicated.[192] However, it is usually possible to obtain local tissue to deal with this situation. A skin graft can be placed into the cavity and held in place with iodoform gauze. This can later be removed through the nostril. All osteotomy sites are put back in position and stabilized with plates and screws, which may be metal or resorbable. The facial flap is returned to its position, and the bicoronal flap is closed.

The areas where recurrence is possible can be monitored by regular nasendoscopy, CT scan, or MRI scan. Biopsy of any suspicious area should be done because early detection of recurrence may mean the difference between life and death of the patient.

POSTERIOR AREA OF THE SKULL BASE

The posterior area is considered in three segments. The concept of three segments represents an artificial division, but it does help in terms of surgical planning (see Fig. 108-18).

Anterior Segment of Posterior Area

NONMALIGNANT TUMORS. These are neurofibroma and fibrous dysplasia.

Neurofibroma. The orbital neurofibroma without skeletal involvement occurs far back in the orbit, which is, in effect, the anterior wall of the middle cranial fossa. It will cause proptosis. In most patients, there is a defect in the greater wing of the sphenoid to a varying degree. There may also be a defect between the orbit and the middle cranial fossa, allowing herniation of the temporal lobe. When this occurs, pulsating exophthalmos results.[187] The orbital walls are expanded; this also means depression of the floor. There is a resulting hypoplasia of the zygomatic arch, which may be considerably elongated by the pressure of the lesion from the temporal fossa. Another feature of the condition is an arachnoid cyst of the temporal lobe. When the eyelids are infiltrated in patients with severe neurofibroma, they become nonfunctional. If the bone defect is in the inferior portion of the greater wing of the sphenoid, there is a connection into the temporal fossa. This may result in enophthalmos; in this situation, there will be no pulsation.

There is a more extensive variety of neurofibroma in which there is generalized unilateral facial involvement. The orbit is infiltrated, there is proptosis, and there is enlargement of the cheek area. This type of tumor is frequently associated with the other generalized stigmata of neurofibromatosis. This situation presents a considerable challenge in terms of resection, reconstruction, and the possibility of recurrence, which is high. To plan surgery, it is convenient to divide the orbital involvement into three categories. The simplest is orbital soft tissue involvement, and the eye is functional. In the second group, there is involvement of both soft tissue and bone, and again the eye is functional. In the third group, there is more extensive orbital soft tissue and bone involvement, but the eye is nonfunctional. The investigations most useful, apart from clinical examination, are facial bone radiographs; but most times, only a CT scan is taken and almost always converted into three-dimensional representation to allow more accurate surgical treatment planning. An MRI scan can be added for complete soft tissue assessment.

Group 1. When there is only soft tissue involvement and the eye is functional, depending on the position of the lesion, it can be approached through either an upper or lower eyelid incision and, on many occasions, can be dissected out and removed. This will result in the eye going back into its normal position. This procedure is not usually prejudicial to vision.

Group 2 (Fig. 108-27). In the presence of a seeing eye with soft tissue and bone involvement, the orbit should be approached with a bicoronal flap. The orbital contents are dissected subperiosteally, as is the temporalis muscle, which is taken down to the zygomatic arch. Orbital osteotomies are performed transversely through the superior portion of the lateral orbital rim, then vertically down the lateral orbital wall, horizontally across the maxilla, preferably above the infraorbital nerve foramen, and vertically upward through the medial part of the infraorbital rim, leaving the lacrimal drainage system intact. The

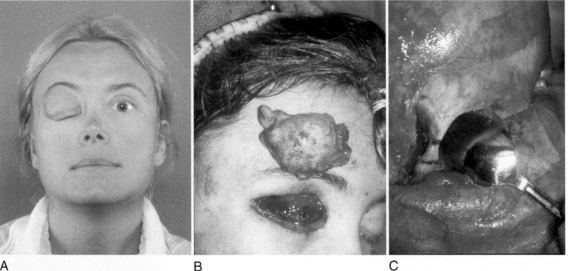

A   B   C

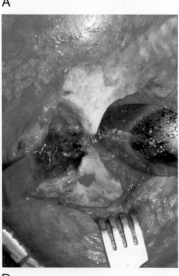

D

FIGURE 108-27. Group 2 neurofibroma of right orbit with seeing eye. *A,* Preoperative appearance. *B,* Tumor removed through a supraorbital approach. *C,* Osteotomy of orbit planned. The lateral orbital rim is exposed. *D,* Osteotomy performed.

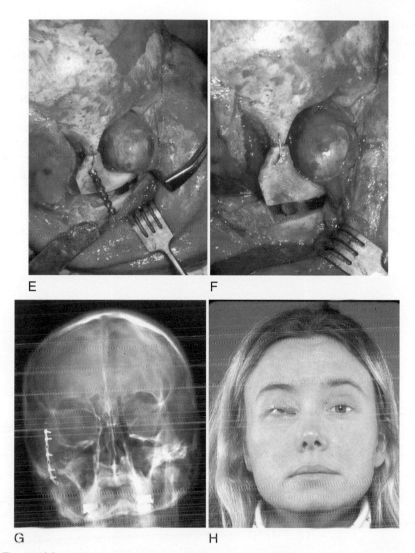

FIGURE 108-27, cont'd. *E,* The osteotomized segment has been moved upward to reduce orbital volume. *F,* Stabilization of segment. *G,* Anteroposterior skull view to show the symmetry of the orbits. *H,* Early postoperative result. (*A, B,* and *H* from Jackson IT, Shaw K: Tumors of the craniofacial skeleton, including the jaws. In McCarthy JG, ed: Plastic Surgery. Philadelphia, WB Saunders, 1990;3336.)

zygomatic arch is divided anteriorly, and the bone block can be removed or swung laterally on the temporal soft tissue. This osteotomy gives wide exposure of the orbital contents. It also allows examination of the posterior area of the orbit; any defect in the posterior orbital wall can be exposed and its magnitude assessed.

Again, the periorbita is incised, and the tumor is dissected out. It is usually possible to do this without significant damage to the normal orbital anatomy. This having been done, the defect in the posterior aspect of the orbit is reconstructed with a split calvarial bone graft. It is possible to use metal mesh, which can easily be contoured to provide a normally positioned posterior orbital wall. An adjustment of the lateral orbital

wall needs to be made because this has been displaced by the expanding intraorbital tumor. This has usually been preplanned with the reformatted three-dimensional CT scan. Once this has been done and the orbital segment is replaced and stabilized with wires and miniplates, the orbital volume should be correct. It is important in performing this type of procedure or any other procedure that involves removal of the lateral orbital wall to replace the temporalis muscle in position and relocate it on the lateral orbital rim and also to the skull. This is done by making drill holes in the lateral orbital rim and drill holes on the temporal crest in the skull. The muscle is reattached with 3-0 silk sutures. At the lateral canthal ligament position, two drill holes are made and a wire is placed through them to secure the ligament in its correct position. The bicoronal flap is closed over suction drainage.

Group 3 (Fig. 108-28). In this group, in addition to the soft tissue and bone involvement, there is a blind eye. The deformity of these patients can be considerable. Typically, many operations have been carried out without acceptance of the inevitability of exenteration. Retention of a blind eye that may be of the wrong size and of poor appearance is an error. It is better to remove the blind eye, reconstruct the socket, and use an osseointegrated prosthesis.

The skin involvement in the temporal area is outlined and excised. The temporal fascia is the deep boundary of the abnormality; rarely, it may be involved, and it should be resected. The eyelids in these patients

are usually significantly involved and certainly contribute greatly to the abnormality. Therefore, again, a radical approach is taken. An incision is made along the rim of the lid superior to the lashes on the upper lid and inferior to them on the lower lid. The skin is dissected off the underlying subcutaneous tissue; this continues to the margins of the bony orbit and includes a resection of the medial and lateral canthal areas. Next, a total orbital exenteration is performed. In most of these patients, the eye is very much enlarged and, as stated earlier, is abnormal in appearance and does not have function. Frequently, there is herniation of the temporal lobe through the posterior orbital wall. The lobe is reduced back into the temporal fossa, and the bone defect is reconstructed

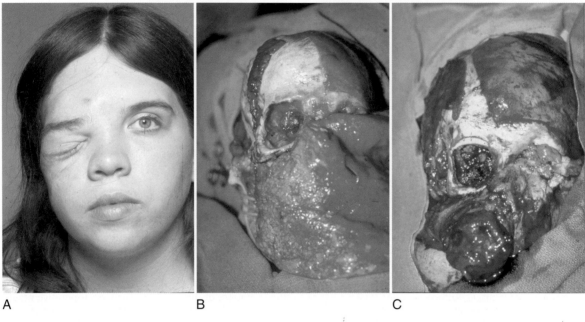

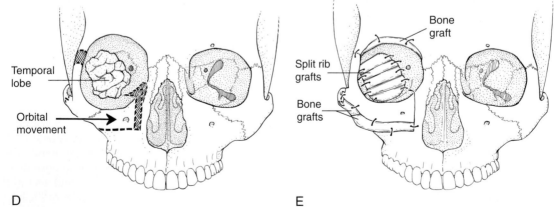

FIGURE 108-28. Group 3 neurofibroma. *A,* Right neurofibromatosis showing involvement of skin. The right eye was previously removed. *B,* Coronal flap turned down to show the expanded egg-shaped orbit. *C,* Reconstruction of orbit by reduction osteotomies, split rib grafts, and iliac crest bone graft. *D,* Posterior orbital resection and osteotomy for orbital movement. *E,* Position of bone grafts in posterior and inferior orbit.

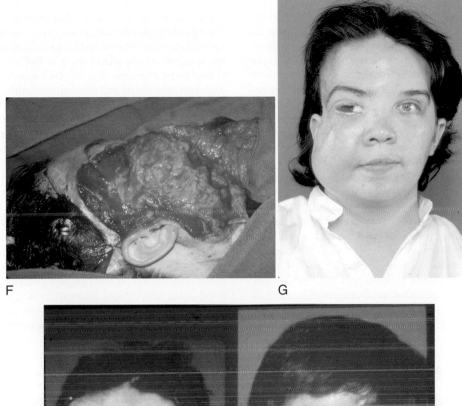

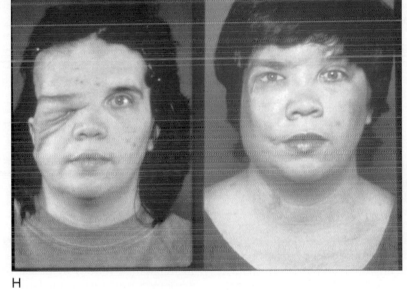

FIGURE 108-28, cont'd. *F,* Free tissue transplantation to right cheek. *G,* Postoperative result with increased bulk of right cheek. *H,* Preoperative appearance and postoperative result with prosthetic eye in place.

with split cranial bone grafts. These are plated in position to give a secure posterior boundary to the orbit.

With use of measurements obtained by manipulation of the three-dimensional images, osteotomies are performed to reduce both the orbital volume and the circumference of the orbital rim. The osteotomies are then stabilized with wire that can be manipulated in such a way to make it easier to be covered with the

thin skin flaps that will be used for the reconstruction. In many patients, it is necessary to augment the supraorbital, lateral orbital, infraorbital, and malar areas with bone grafts. In the temporal area, the excess skin has been radically excised with the underlying neurofibroma. This skin is now advanced upward, and with it the stretched lower eyelid skin is introduced into the orbit. The upper eyelid skin is also placed in the orbit, and any excess is trimmed. These two portions of skin are sutured together, as is the skin in the temporal area. The orbit is now carefully packed with petrolatum gauze, and a pressure dressing is applied. It is most important that the eyelid skin adhere to the orbital bone. Later reconstruction will be with a composite eye and eyelid prosthesis mounted on Branemark implants. If necessary, an eyebrow can be included, but it is usually not possible to maintain the eyebrow in its correct position. A well-designed pair of glasses will cover the junction between the prosthesis and the surrounding normal skin.

In patients with extensive intracranial disease, it may be considered safer to carry out the neurosurgical resection as a separate initial procedure with bone grafting of the posterior orbital wall defect. After the intracranial resection, if there is severe involvement of the temporal area and in the eyelids, the procedure described previously should be performed. In some patients, it is possible to maintain the eyelids. The eyelids should be adjusted in an open position and an eye prosthesis placed into the orbital cavity.

Although there are many methods of treatment for this condition, there is no doubt that the method described here gives, by far, the best results. However, it does require some significant and correct decision-making, and it is necessary to spend time discussing this in great detail with the patient and the parents, if the patient is a child, so that they can understand exactly what has been planned and why. Having other patients' photographs with a similar condition treated in this way is most helpful and allows the parents to make an informed decision for their child.

Fibrous Dysplasia. This condition can involve any area of the craniofacial skeleton. This tumor will result in facial deformity with possible dental malocclusion in all dimensions, nasal airway obstruction, frontonasal deformity, and orbital deformity. When it occurs in the posterior area of the orbit or any other area of the orbital walls, there can be displacement of the eye; most frequently, this is proptosis. Involvement of the optic nerve canal can lead to blindness, and progressive symptomatic narrowing may be the indication for surgery. More frequently, surgery is undertaken to correct the deformity or, in the midface area, to realign the occlusion and, in some patients, to open the nasal airway.

A bicoronal flap is used and the frontal supraorbital area is exposed. The temporal area will be displayed by elevation of the temporalis muscle. The orbital contents are dissected out until all the areas of fibrous dysplasia are exposed. The intracranial exposure is achieved by a standard frontal craniotomy with a temporal craniotomy, depending on the extent of the tumor and the area to be resected. If the orbit and the frontal or temporal cranium are mainly involved, these areas can be excised and reconstructed with cranial bone grafts from an unaffected area of the skull. If necessary, iliac crest bone or, less frequently, rib may supply the reconstruction where there is not enough uninvolved bone available. The affected bone can be fashioned into the shape and size required, autoclaved, and used to reconstruct the defect.[193]

If the optic nerve canal is narrowed, the frontal lobe is retracted, and the optic nerve is exposed posteriorly; decompression is performed from posterior to anterior. This dissection must be performed with care by use of a combination of a small, sharp dissector and fine rongeurs to break off the roof and walls of the orbit, whenever possible. This continues until only the floor of the optic nerve canal is left intact throughout the full extent of the canal.

It is possible to make a lateral approach to the orbit, taking off the sphenoid wing. This approach is a little more difficult but, again, can give good exposure and good optic nerve canal decompression. It should be understood that decompression will probably not improve vision in any way, but it may prevent a further deterioration of vision. There has been much discussion about this portion of the operation and the indications for doing it. Significant narrowing of the canal on CT scan does justify release, but again, this is on the basis of considerable experience with this problem. Certainly, if there appears to be deterioration of vision, this is a definite indication for the operation, but it will not bring back lost vision. Obviously, the patient really has to understand the possibility of blindness resulting from such a decompression, since this has been reported.[194]

SUPERIOR AND LOW INFRATEMPORAL TUMORS. The terms used for these tumors identify their site of extension or origin. The importance of the classification is that it aids in the decision as to which surgical approach to use.

Superior Infratemporal Tumors. Tumors of the superior portion of the infratemporal fossa may be meningiomas, fibrous dysplasia, or neurofibromas. They frequently involve the lateral wall of the orbit, resulting in a decrease of orbital volume with proptosis of the globe, dystopia, and visual problems such as diplopia. This occurs through invasion of the posterior or lateral wall but can also result from invasion through the superior orbital fissure.

CT and MRI scans are recommended for operative planning; in some tumors, carotid angiography will give information as to the vascularity of the tumors, their main supply, and also their position in relation to local vessels. If there is significant vascularity (e.g., some meningiomas or true vascular malformations), embolization should be considered before the surgical procedure.

Meningiomas represent 14% to 18% of all primary intracranial tumors; the male-to-female ratio is 1:3 or 1:4. The average age at occurrence is 45 years. In 20% of intracranial meningiomas, there is an extracranial extension, and this extension is along anatomic pathways. In the orbit, the tumor may enter through the optic nerve canal or the superior orbital fissure. The nasopharynx and nasal cavity may be involved by tumor erosion through the cribriform plate. The paranasal sinuses and the pterygoid area are infiltrated through the floor of the middle cranial fossa. The cranial vault is involved by direct penetration of the skull, or there may be extension through cranial suture lines; ultimately, the scalp will be involved.

Although intracranial meningiomas have, in the past, been considered somewhat locally contained tumors, there are many patients with an extracranial spread. This indicates a variety of tumor that is more aggressive, the so-called invading meningioma. The surgical approach is that previously described. The bicoronal flap allows exposure of the temporal fossa, the orbits, and the upper maxilla. If the tumor is more extensive and a maxillectomy is required, the facial soft tissues are lifted off the maxilla through a paranasal lip-splitting incision with a buccal mucosal extension posteriorly on the involved side. This approach allows a maxillectomy to be performed, if required. All of this will have been determined before the procedure.

Intracranial access is gained through a frontotemporal craniotomy with removal of whatever part of the orbit, zygoma, and maxilla is necessary. If possible, an en bloc resection is performed, removing the tumor and its extensions into any surrounding tissue. Dural tears are repaired, and if necessary, dural defects can be reconstructed with fascia lata, galea, or allografts such as AlloDerm. As with all of these procedures, any communication with the nasopharynx or the frontal sinus is closed off with a galeofrontalis myofascial flap. This is absolutely essential to prevent ascending infection. If there is a large defect that requires volume reconstruction, microvascular composite tissue transplantation should be performed. The muscle most frequently used is the rectus abdominis, although there are other muscles available that are less debilitating to the patient (e.g., latissimus dorsi, vastus lateralis).

Reconstruction of bone defects is performed with split cranial bone, whenever possible, but iliac crest or rib might be necessary on some occasions.

Additional procedures that might be necessary are orbital exenteration when the orbit is extensively involved and occasionally maxillectomy.

There are occasions when complete resection is not possible because of the inevitable neurologic complications. This situation is commonly encountered in recurrent lesions. In these patients, it is worthwhile to carry out debulking procedures to improve any future symptoms the patient may have. One should also be prepared to observe the patient carefully and to reoperate should there be an indication of tumor regrowth.

Low Infratemporal Tumors. The main tumors in this area are meningiomas; neurofibromas; and invasive extracranial tumors, including squamous cell carcinoma, adenocarcinoma, adenoid cystic carcinoma, neglected basal cell carcinomas, and various types of sarcoma (Fig. 108-29). These tumors may arise from the orbit, the maxilla, the tonsil area, the parotid, and the retromaxillary region, or there may be invasion of skin tumors, particularly after radiation therapy. If left long enough, extracranial tumors may invade the cranial cavity. Tumors of this area can cause proptosis and tonsillar, retromandibular, and temporal swelling. There can be dysphagia, dyspnea, or visual complications. Involvement of the trigeminal nerve will result in anesthesia or, more rarely, hyperesthesia. Facial weakness indicates facial nerve invasion.

Once again, CT and MRI scans are essential in planning surgery. An angiogram is always worthwhile for assessment of changes in normal vascular anatomy, the vascularity of the tumor, and cerebral cross-flow. This is essential if there is any suggestion of internal carotid involvement.

The approach to these tumors should be designed in such a way that a total en bloc resection will be possible. This approach is similar to that described for superior infratemporal fossa tumors. A hemicoronal or more frequently a bicoronal incision will be used that continues down into the neck, passing in front of the ear. The neck incision may be limited, or it may be taken down to the clavicle, depending on what needs to be done in the neck area. The flap is composed of the scalp, the frontal area, the temporal region, the cheek, and the neck. It has a wide base anteriorly and gives excellent exposure to the frontotemporal region, the orbit, the lateral face, and the neck. The type of craniotomy is determined by the position of the tumor. It may be simply frontotemporal or more extensive. The temporal lobe is elevated until the tumor comes into view, and resectability can be assessed at this time. This approach will allow the extent of tumor invasion to be assessed; it also allows the trigeminal ganglion to be exposed in Meckel cave and, if necessary, biopsy specimens to be obtained. If the result is positive, one is probably dealing with an unresectable tumor, and local irradiation by implants should be instituted. However, one may decide to perform some tumor debulking. Alternatively, it may be preferable to avoid major resection and adjuvant treatment for the patient to have a good quality of life for however few months remain.

If resection is feasible, it is wise to begin with an upper neck dissection to identify the vascular anatomy in the upper neck and in the base of the skull. If nodes

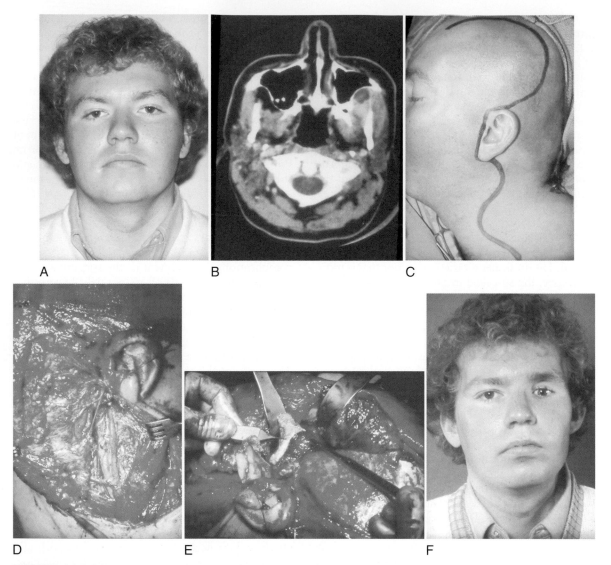

FIGURE 108-29. Infratemporal fossa tumor. *A,* The patient presented with proptosis of left eye. *B,* Axial CT scan showing adenoid cystic carcinoma of infratemporal fossa region. *C,* Approach through an extended skin incision and intracranial-extracranial approach to temporal region. *D,* Parotidectomy with preservation of facial nerve. *E,* Removal of zygomatic arch and temporal craniotomy for exposure and resection of tumor. *F,* Postoperative result at 1 year. (*A* to *D* and *F* from Jackson IT, Shaw K: Tumors of the craniofacial skeleton, including the jaws. In McCarthy JG, ed: Plastic Surgery. Philadelphia, WB Saunders, 1990:3336.)

are present, a full neck dissection is performed to remove all nodes. The ascending ramus of the mandible is removed if it is essential for exposure to the infratemporal fossa. A temporal craniotomy allows the intracranial and extracranial position of the tumor to be assessed. The temporal lobe is elevated, and the skull is resected until the involved foramen or area of skull is located.

With the exposure provided by this approach, the location of the tumor can be accurately assessed. There are two structures that are of importance, the carotid artery and the styloid process. The styloid process is

a key structure in this dissection. Lateral to the styloid process, the dissection can be performed safely without too much concern; whereas medially, one encounters the internal carotid artery. The tumor is now dissected from above and below as completely as possible, with removal of whatever bone or soft tissue is indicated. Use of the operating microscope is essential for portions of this procedure. Nonmalignant tumors require bone removal for exposure. In malignant lesions, the resection of bone and other structures is absolutely indicated for total resection of tumor. Should the cavernous sinus be involved, the tumor is probably noncurable. If the orbit is invaded, an orbital osteotomy is performed, and if necessary, the orbital contents are removed. Should there be extension into the maxilla and if this is of significant size, it is recommended that an anterior approach by a Weber-Fergusson incision be performed. In this way, the required maxillary resection can be undertaken. Any invasion of the ethmoid sinuses is reason to resect this region completely. The reconstruction is performed according to the completeness of excision. If it is thought that excision is complete and the defect is significant, transplantation of a free vascularized muscle flap is indicated. If there has been resection of skin, then skin will be added to this flap. On occasion, if the tumor resection is subtotal and subsequent radiation therapy is indicated, vascularized tissue is recommended.

On some occasions, a decision may be made to simply close the skin, institute drainage, and accept the deformity. This approach is rarely indicated, but it might be chosen for medical reasons, when radiation is the treatment of choice, or when the tumor is completely inoperable and only a partial resection has been performed.

When the lesion lies at the skull base but does not involve the skull base or any surrounding structures (e.g., an isolated neural tumor), a mandibular swing procedure (Fig. 108-30) is the indicated approach because an intracranial resection will not be necessary.[195,196] Routine tracheostomy has been advocated but is not always necessary.[197,198] This procedure can be combined with an intracranial approach rather than removing the ascending ramus of the mandible, and this approach is certainly acceptable when there is no involvement of the temporomandibular area. An incision is made in a step fashion on the lower lip, and an osteotomy is performed through the mandible between the lateral incisor and the canine. This osteotomy is anterior to the emergence of the mandibular nerve.

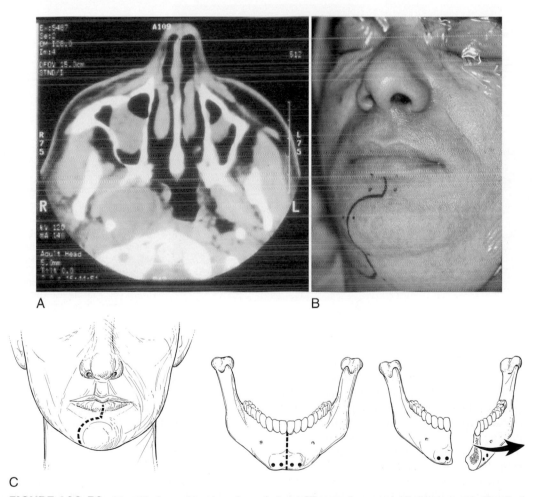

FIGURE 108-30. Mandibular swing procedure. *A,* Axial CT scan shows a right-sided mass in the skull base area at the level of the jugular foramen. *B,* Design of skin incision. *C,* Diagram to show the mandibular swing procedure.   *Continued*

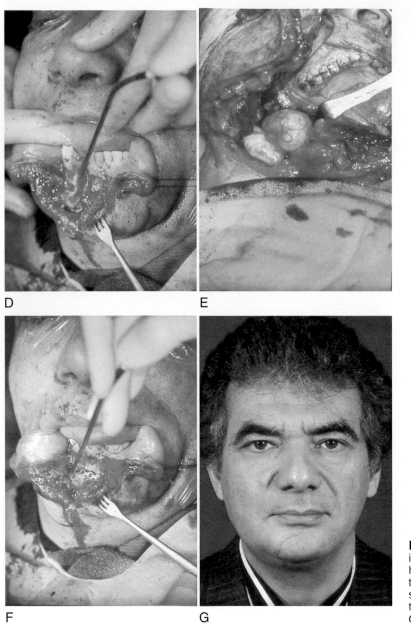

FIGURE 108-30, cont'd. *D,* The incision has been made; the mandible has been osteotomized and is about to be swung laterally. *E,* Good exposure of the skull base showing the tumor. *F,* Plating of the mandible. *G,* Postoperative result.

The floor of the mouth is incised medial to the mandible, avoiding the medially placed lingual nerve. This incision is carried up to the temporomandibular joint region, the hemimandible is swung laterally, and the dissection proceeds from there up to the base of the skull. The external carotid artery is tied off, and the internal carotid is dissected medially up to its entry through the base of the skull, gradually isolating the tumor site. Resectability is now confirmed on the basis of both radiologic studies and tumor exposure. One cannot be absolutely sure of resectability until this region is reached. The tumor is now separated off the

skull base and resected.[199] The mucosal incision is closed; the mandible is put back into position with one or two mandibular reconstruction plates. One plate is placed inferior and one more superior, avoiding the tooth roots. The lip incision is then closed, as is the incision in the neck.

Central Segment of the Posterior Area

The tumors that present in this region are basal cell and squamous cell carcinomas of the external ear growing medially to involve the petrous bone. Other lesions are advanced primary but more frequently recurrent malignant parotid tumors and squamous cell carcinomas arising in the middle ear. Glomus tumors and other entities are not discussed in this chapter; these now tend to be handled by neuro-otologists.

The procedure of a partial petrosectomy is an extracranial one. When indicated, the external ear is resected, and the external portion of the petrous bone that underlies this is removed. The facial nerve is located and preserved. Skin cover is frequently required and can best be supplied by a temporal muscle transposition and the application of a split-thickness skin graft. Should anything more sophisticated be necessary to obtain tumor resection, it should probably be performed at a later date. The patient should make an informed decision after being told what is involved.

More extensive tumors will be resected by a subtotal or total petrosectomy.[200] The skin incision, as described previously, is indicated by the size and position of the tumor if this is a skin lesion. In cancers of the middle ear, however, the ear may be left attached to the anterior flap, and the external canal is transected.

Through a temporal craniotomy, the temporal lobe is lifted and the tumor is inspected intracranially. A decision is now made as to whether resection is feasible, which involves obtaining clearance anteriorly and posteriorly but also medially, which is the danger zone because of the internal carotid anatomy and the brainstem. If enough exposure and clearance can be obtained, anterior, posterior, and medial osteotomies are made and the tumor is removed. In tumors that have extended far medially, total resection is frequently not possible. The neuro-otologists using the microscope hold out some hope for such patients. Microvascular composite tissue transplantation for coverage is often indicated.

Posterior Segment of the Posterior Area

The role of plastic surgery in these areas relates to incision on the scalp for exposure (particularly if prior scar exists), dissection of the posterior neck area, and provision of cover with local scalp rotation flaps or free tissue transplantation (microvascular composite tissue transplantation) when wound closure with local flaps is not feasible. This allows the neurosurgeon to concentrate on tumor resection without the worry of closing the defect.

CLIVAL TUMORS. The main clival tumor that involves the plastic surgeon is the chordoma or the more aggressive tumor, the chondrosarcoma. The chordoma arises from notochord remnants; the chondrosarcoma originates from the unossified chondrocranium. Approaches that can be used are the extended subfrontal, the extended subfrontal subtemporal-infratemporal, the frontotemporal transcavernous sinus, and the facial translocation, but they are complex and time-consuming. The unilateral

maxillary swing approach provides adequate exposure for resection and so far has been complication free. The maxillary swing approach is subcranial and causes minimal anatomic and functional disturbance (Fig. 108-31).

With use of orotracheal intubation, an incision is made from the glabellar area curving down to the lateral side of the nose and continuing around the alar base to the base of the columella and down through the center of the lip. The center of the alveolus is incised to between the incisors; the incision continues into the center of the hard palate and ends at the anterior soft palate. With a thin, straight osteotome, the palate is split back to the soft palate. A lower subciliary incision is made to the lateral canthus. The inferior and medial periorbita are elevated from the floor and medial wall of the orbit. A horizontal osteotomy is made on the medial orbital wall superiorly, below the lacrimal duct, which is followed by a vertical osteotomy on the medial wall. The orbital floor periorbita is now elevated; a transverse osteotomy is made on the floor, avoiding the infraorbital nerve, and this cut continues up the lateral wall to a point below the lateral canthal ligament, where a horizontal osteotomy is performed on the lateral orbital wall. The zygomatic arch is now osteotomized. The final separation of the hemi-Le Fort III is completed by an osteotomy behind the maxillary osteotomy with a curved osteotome. The hemimaxilla is mobilized with maxillary mobilizing forceps and is rotated laterally to expose the skull base. The nasal mucosa is incised and dissected off the skull base, and the septum is dislocated to the contralateral side, again with an osteotome. The dissection is made back to the clivus, and the floor is drilled out. Using the microscope, the neurosurgeon can dissect and remove the tumor. At the end of the procedure, muscle can be placed in the surgical defect; the mucosa is closed. The maxilla is returned to its position and plated, first on the alveolus and then on the lateral orbital wall. The arch can be plated for extra security. The buccal mucosa and face are sutured. On occasion, sutures are required in the palatal mucosa.

Radiation-Induced Tumors

It is not uncommon to find that children who have had treatment of retinoblastoma by radiation therapy will present with a new tumor at a later date. Surgery alone is not particularly successful in these patients, and another dose of radiation therapy cannot be given. In this instance, further resection can be performed. If a free flap is inserted into the area, the radiation therapist can treat the resected area with another dose of radiation directed through the free flap region where there is now adequate blood flow. The approach has been effective in carefully selected patients (Fig. 108-32).

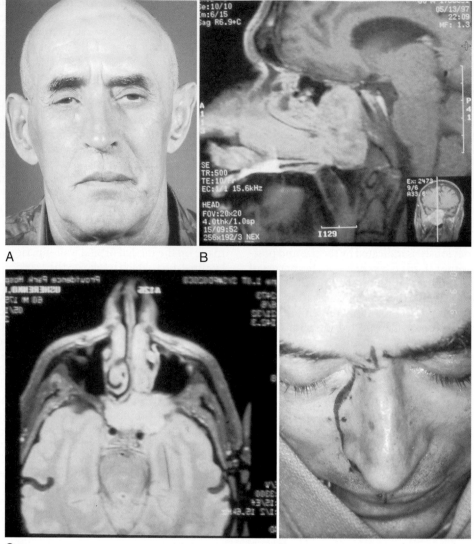

FIGURE 108-31. Maxillary swing procedure for clival exposure. *A,* The patient presented with headache and airway obstruction. *B* and *C,* Lateral and axial CT scans to show large clival tumor. *D,* Planned skin excision in paranasal area and lip splitting.

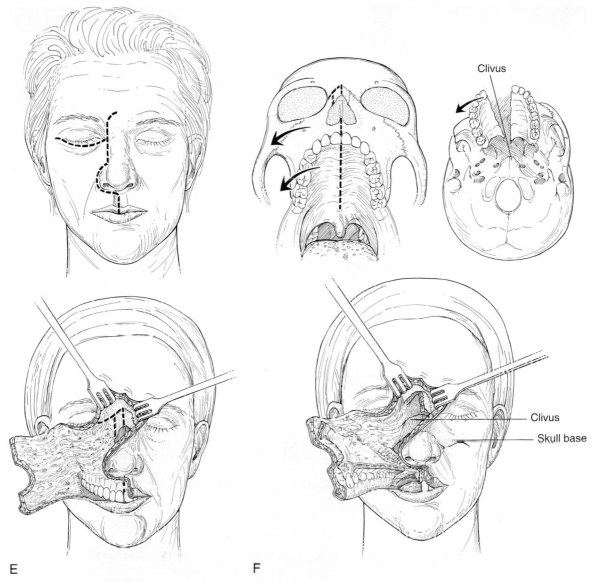

E   F

FIGURE 108-31, cont'd. *F,* Diagram of the soft tissue approach. *F,* Diagram of the maxillary osteotomy with the palatal split, which allows good exposure of the clivus.   *Continued*

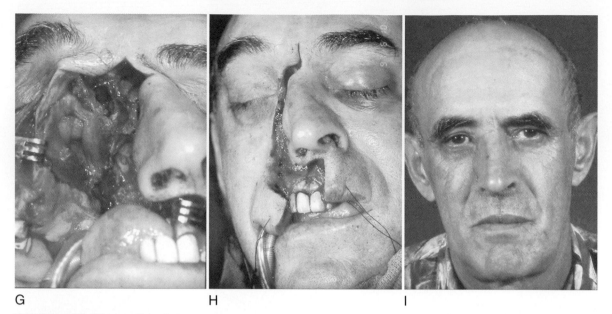

G   H   I

FIGURE 108-31, cont'd. *G,* Skull base exposure for resection of clival tumor. *H,* Maxilla placed back in position. *I,* Postoperative result at 2 years.

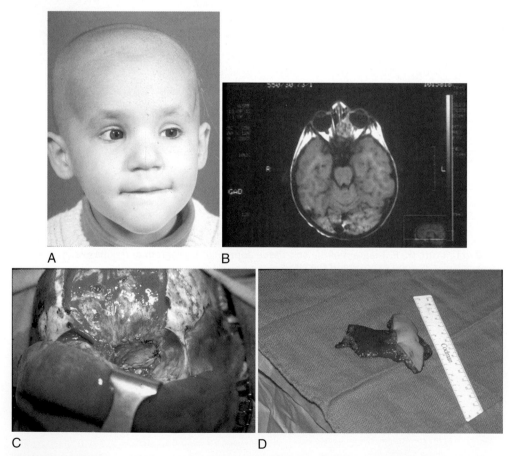

A   B

C   D

FIGURE 108-32. *A,* Patient who underwent radiation therapy for retinoblastoma. *B,* Axial CT scan shows a new lesion in the area of irradiation. This proved to be a chondrosarcoma. *C,* Exploration of the area revealed bone involvement in addition to involvement of the dura and the left frontal lobe. Radical resection was performed. *D,* Rectus abdominis free flap harvested.

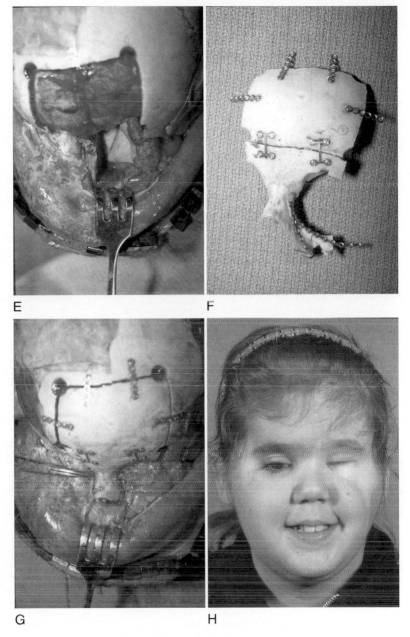

FIGURE 108-32, cont'd. *E,* Rectus abdominis free flap placed in the area of the socket overlying the fascia lata graft to replace dura. *F,* Reconstruction of the removed segments. *G,* The bone reconstruction placed back in position. *H,* The patient 5 years after postoperative radiation treatment.

General Comment

In most of the approaches using osteotomies that have been discussed, it is not unusual to perform the bone cuts and the bone shifts that are convenient for the particular exposure required. For this, the term *exposure by facial disassembly* can be conveniently employed. It is this concept, freedom from rigid boundaries and anatomic terms, that has allowed the development of newer and safer methods of exposure. This adaptability has helped establish an "as required" approach, much to the patient's benefit.

CONCLUSION

The head and neck area is a source of varied and challenging tumors. In the past, these were unresectable or not reconstructable, or both. With the help of sophisticated imaging, better surgical approaches, the operating microscope, microvascular composite tissue transplantation, interspecialty cooperation (e.g., neurosurgery, neuro-otology, radiation oncology, and medical oncology), and most of all experience, what seemed impossible is now possible. Plastic surgeons have become head and neck and skull base surgeons.

New frontiers have been opened and crossed. Challenges remain, but as technology improves in terms of sophisticated guidance systems, more precise and effective radiation treatment, and new chemotherapeutic agents together with earlier diagnosis, the outlook for previously incurable conditions continues to improve.

REFERENCES

1. Reichart PA, Ries P: Consideration on the classification of odontogenic tumours. Int J Oral Surg 1983;12:323.
2. Shear M: Cysts of the Oral Region, 2nd ed. Boston, Wright-PSG, 1983.
3. Stanley HR Jr, Krogh HW, Pannkuk E: Age changes in the epithelial components of follicles (dental sacs) associated with impacted third molars. Oral Surg Oral Med Oral Pathol 1965;19:128.
4. Baden E, Moskow BS, Moskow R: Odontogenic gingival epithelial hamartoma. J Oral Surg 1968;26:702.
5. Browne RM: The pathogenesis of odontogenic cysts: a review. J Oral Pathol 1975;4:31.
6. Cataldo E, Berkman MD: Cysts of the oral mucosa in newborns. Am J Dis Child 1968;116:44.
7. Stout FW, Lunin M, Calonius PEB: A study of epithelial remnants in the maxilla. Abstracts of the 46th General Meeting of the International Association for Dental Research, San Francisco, March 1968. Abstracts 419, 420, 421.
8. Moreillon MC, Schroeder HE: Numerical frequency of epithelial abnormalities, particularly microkeratocysts in the developing human oral mucosa. Oral Surg Oral Med Oral Pathol 1982;53:44.
9. Wysocki GP, Brannon RB, Gardner GD, Sapp P: Histogenesis of the lateral periodontal cyst and the gingival cyst of the adult. Oral Surg Oral Med Oral Pathol 1980;50:327.
10. Buchner A, Hjansen LS: The histomorphologic spectrum of the gingival cyst in the adult. Oral Surg Oral Med Oral Pathol 1979;48:532.
11. Grand NG, Marwah AS: Pigmented gingival cyst. Oral Surg Oral Med Oral Pathol 1964;17:635.
12. Struthers P, Shear M: Root resorption by ameloblastomas and cysts of the jaws. Int J Oral Surg 1976;5:128.
13. Dachi SF, Howell FV: A survey of 3,874 routine full mouth radiographs. II. A study of impacted teeth. Oral Surg Oral Med Oral Pathol 1961;14:1165.
14. Brannon RB: The odontogenic keratocyst. Part I. Oral Surg Oral Med Oral Pathol 1976;42:54.
15. Gorlin RJ, Goltz RW: Multiple nevoid basal cell epithelium, jaw cysts, and bifid rib: a syndrome. N Engl J Med 1960;269:908.
16. Shafer WG, Hine MK, Levy BM, eds: A Textbook of Oral Pathology, 4th ed. Philadelphia, WB Saunders, 1983.
17. Ellis E III, Fonseca RJ: The management of odontogenic cysts and tumors. In Thawley SE, Panje WR, eds: Comprehensive Management of Head and Neck Tumors. Philadelphia, WB Saunders, 1987:1483.
18. Moskow BS, Siegel K, Zegarelli EV, et al: Gingival and lateral periodontal cysts. J Periodontol 1970;41:249.
19. Altini M, Farman AG: The calcifying odontogenic cyst. Eight new cases and a review of the literature. Oral Surg Oral Med Oral Pathol 1975;40:751.
20. Gorlin RJ, Pindborg JJ, Clausen FP, Vickers RA: The calcifying odontogenic cyst—a possible analogue of the cutaneous calcifying epithelioma of Malherbe. Oral Surg Oral Med Oral Pathol 1962;15:1235.
21. Freedman PD, Lumerman H, Gee JK: Calcifying odontogenic cyst. Oral Surg Oral Med Oral Pathol 1975;40:93.
22. Browne RM: Metaplasia and degeneration in odontogenic cysts in man. J Oral Pathol 1972;1:145.

23. Bhaskar SN: Oral surgery—oral pathology conference No. 17, Walter Reed Army Medical Center. Periapical lesions—types, incidence, and clinical features. Oral Surg Oral Med Oral Pathol 1966;21:657.
24. LaLonde ER, Luebke RG: The frequency and distribution of periapical cysts and granulomas. Oral Surg Oral Med Oral Pathol 1968;25:861.
25. Weine FS, Silverglade LB: Residual cysts masquerading as periapical lesions: three case reports. J Am Dent Assoc 1983;106:833.
26. Standish SM, Shafer WG: The lateral periodontal cyst. J Periodontol 1958;29:27.
27. Craig GT: The paradental cyst. A specific inflammation odontogenic cyst. Br Dent J 1976;141:9.
28. Regezi JA, Kerr DA, Courtney RM: Odontogenic tumors: analysis of 706 cases. J Oral Surg 1978;36:771.
29. Gorlin RJ: Odontogenic tumors. In Gorlin RJ, Goldman HM, eds: Thoma's Oral Pathology, 6th ed. St. Louis, CV Mosby, 1970.
30. McDaniel RK: Odontogenic cysts and tumors. In Thawley SE, Panje WR, eds: Comprehensive Management of Head and Neck Tumors. Philadelphia, WB Saunders, 1987:1446.
31. Small IA, Waldron CA: Ameloblastomas of the jaws. Oral Surg Oral Med Oral Pathol 1955;8:281.
32. Mehlisch DR, Dahlin DC, Masson JK: Ameloblastoma: a clinicopathologic report. J Oral Surg 1972;30:9.
33. Gardner DG, Pecak AM: The treatment of ameloblastoma based on pathologic and anatomic principles. Cancer 1980;46:2514.
34. Giansanti JS, Someren A, Waldron CA: Odontogenic adenomatoid tumor (adenoameloblastoma): survey of three cases. Oral Surg Oral Med Oral Pathol 1970;30:69.
35. Courtney RM, Kerr DA: The odontogenic adenomatoid tumor. A comprehensive study of twenty new cases. Oral Surg Oral Med Oral Pathol 1975;39:424.
36. Franklin CD, Pindborg JJ: The calcifying epithelial odontogenic tumor: a review and analysis of 113 cases. Oral Surg Oral Med Oral Pathol 1976;42:753.
37. Wertheimer FW, Zielinski RJ, Wesley RK: Extraosseous calcifying epithelial odontogenic tumor (Pindborg tumor). Int J Oral Surg 1977;6:266.
38. Anderson HC, Kim B, Minkowitz S: Calcifying epithelial odontogenic tumor of Pindborg. An electron microscopic study. Cancer 1969;24:585.
39. Swan RH, McDaniel RK: Squamous odontogenic proliferation with probable origin from the rests of Malassez (early squamous odontogenic tumor?). J Periodontol 1983;54:493.
40. Pullon PA, Shafer WG, Elzay RP, et al: Squamous odontogenic tumor. Report of six cases of a previously undescribed lesion. Oral Surg Oral Med Oral Pathol 1975;40:616.
41. Goldblatt LI, Brannon RB, Ellis GL: Squamous odontogenic tumor. Report of five cases and review of the literature. Oral Surg Oral Med Oral Pathol 1982;54:187.
42. Slootweg PJ: An analysis of the interrelationship of the mixed odontogenic tumors—ameloblastic fibroma, ameloblastic fibro-odontoma, and the odontomas. Oral Surg Oral Med Oral Pathol 1981;51:266.
43. Nilsen R, Magnusson BC: Ameloblastic fibroma. Int J Oral Surg 1979;8:370.
44. Trodahl JN: Ameloblastic fibroma. A survey of cases from the Armed Forces Institute of Pathology. Oral Surg Oral Med Oral Pathol 1972;33:547.
45. Zallen RD, Preskar MH, McClary SA: Ameloblastic fibroma. J Oral Maxillofac Surg 1982;40:513.
46. LaBriola J, Steiner M, Bernstein ML, et al: Odontoameloblastoma. J Oral Surg 1980;38:139.
47. Pindborg JJ, Kramer IRH, Torloni H: Histological Typing of Odontogenic Tumors, Jaw Cysts, and Allied Lesions. Geneva, World Health Organization, 1971:15.

48. Budnick SD: Compound and complex odontomas. Oral Surg Oral Med Oral Pathol 1976;42:501.
49. McClatchey KD, Hakimi M, Batsakis JG: Retrotympanic odontoma. Am J Surg Pathol 1981;5:401.
50. Mendelsohn DB, Hertzanu Y, Glass RB, et al: Giant complex odontoma of the maxillary antrum. S Afr Med J 1983;63:704.
51. Dahl EC, Wolfson SH, Haugen JC: Central odontogenic fibroma: a review of recent literature. J Oral Surg 1981;39:120.
52. Killey HC, Kay LW: Fibromyxomata of the jaws. Br J Oral Surg 1965;2:124.
53. Gorlin RJ, Chaudhry AP, Pindborg JJ: Odontogenic tumors: classification, histopathology and clinical behavior in man and domesticated animals. Cancer 1961;14:73.
54. Farman AG, Kohler WW, Nortje CJ, Van Wyk CW: Cementoblastoma: report of a case. J Oral Surg 1979;37:198.
55. Corio RL, Crawford BE, Schaberg SJ: Benign cementoblastoma. Oral Surg Oral Med Oral Pathol 1976;42:524.
56. Hamner JE III, Scofield HH, Cornyn J: Benign fibro-osseous jaw lesions of periodontal membrane origin. Cancer 1968;22:861.
57. Zegarelli EV, Kutscher AH, Napoli N, et al: The cementoma—a study of 230 patients with 435 cementomas. Oral Surg Oral Med Oral Pathol 1964;17:219.
58. Waldron CA, Giasanti JS: Benign fibro-osseous lesions of the jaws: a clinical-radiologic-histologic review of sixty-five cases. II. Benign fibro-osseous lesions of periodontal ligament origin. Oral Surg Oral Med Oral Pathol 1973;35:340.
59. Shear M: Primary intra alveolar epidermoid carcinoma of the jaw. J Pathol 1969;97:645.
60. Slootweg PJ, Muller H: Malignant ameloblastoma or ameloblastic carcinoma. Oral Surg Oral Med Oral Pathol 1984;57:168.
61. Howell RM, Burkes EJ Jr: Malignant transformation of ameloblastic fibro-odontoma to ameloblastic fibrosarcoma. Oral Surg Oral Med Oral Pathol 1977;43:391.
62. Leider AS, Nelson JF, Trodahl NJ: Ameloblastic fibrosarcoma of the jaws. Oral Surg Oral Med Oral Pathol 1972;33:559.
63. Adekeye EO, Edwards MB, Goubran GF: Ameloblastic fibrosarcoma. Oral Surg Oral Med Oral Pathol 1978;46:254.
64. Goldstein G, Parker FP, Hugh GS: Ameloblastic sarcoma: pathogenesis and treatment with chemotherapy. Cancer 1976;37:1673.
65. Greer RO Jr, Rohrer MD, Young SK: Nonodontogenic tumors, clinical evaluation and pathology. In Thawley SE, Panje WR, eds: Comprehensive Management of Head and Neck Tumors. Philadelphia, WB Saunders, 1987:1510.
66. Batsakis JG, ed: Tumors of the Head and Neck. Clinical and Pathological Considerations, 2nd ed. Baltimore, Williams & Wilkins, 1979.
67. Hallberg OE, Bagley JW: Origin and treatment of osteomas of the paranasal sinuses. Arch Otolaryngol 1950;51:750.
68. Shiffman MA: Familial multiple polyposis associated with soft and hard tissue tumors. JAMA 1962;182:514.
69. McLeod RA, Dahlin DC, Beabout JW: The spectrum of osteoblastoma. Am J Roentgenol 1976;126:321.
70. Greer RO Jr, Mierau GW, Favara BF: Tumors of the Head and Neck in Children. New York, Praeger, 1983:125.
71. Smith RA, Hansen LS, Resnick D, Chan W: Comparison of the osteoblastoma in gnathic and extragnathic sites. Oral Surg Oral Med Oral Pathol 1982;54:285.
72. Dahlin DC, ed: Bone Tumors. General Aspects and Data in 6,221 Cases, 3rd ed. Springfield, Ill, Charles C Thomas, 1978.
73. Lichtenstein L: Benign osteoblastoma: a category of osteoid and bone forming tumors other than classical osteoid osteoma which may be mistaken for giant cell tumor or osteogenic sarcoma. Cancer 1956;9:1044.
74. Jaffe HL: Osteoid-osteoma. A benign osteoblastic tumor composed of osteoid and atypical bone. Arch Surg 1935;31:709.
75. Farman AG, Nortje CJ, Grotepass F: Periosteal benign osteoblastoma of the mandible: report of a case and review of the literature pertaining to benign osteoblastic neoplasms of the jaws. Br J Oral Surg 1976;14:12.
76. Marsh BW, Bonfiglio M, Brady LP, Enneking WF: Benign osteoblastoma: range of manifestations. J Bone Joint Surg Am 1975;57:1.
77. Lichtenstein L: Diseases of Bone and Joints, 2nd ed. St. Louis, CV Mosby, 1975.
78. Albright F, Butler AM, Hampton AO, et al: Syndrome characterized by osteitis fibrosa disseminata, areas of pigmentation and endocrine dysfunction, with precocious puberty in females: report of five cases. N Engl J Med 1937;16:727.
79. Eversole LR, Sabes WR, Rovin S: Fibrous dysplasia: a nosologic problem in the diagnosis of fibro-osseous lesions of the jaws. J Oral Pathol 1972;1:189.
80. Gross CW, Montgomery WW: Fibrous dysplasia and malignant degeneration. Arch Otolaryngol 1967;85:653.
81. Jackson IT, Bone HG, Jaju H: Fibrous dysplasia. In Ward Booth P, Schendel SA, Hausamen JE, eds: Maxillofacial Surgery, vol 2. London, Churchill Livingstone, 1999:889-904.
82. Jones WA: Familial multilocular cystic disease of the jaws. Am J Cancer 1933;17:946.
83. Waldron CA, Shafer WG: The central giant cell reparative granuloma of the jaws. An analysis of 38 cases. Am J Clin Pathol 1966;45:437.
84. Jaffe HL: Giant-cell reparative granuloma, traumatic bone cyst, and fibrous (fibro-osseous) dysplasia of the jawbones. Oral Surg 1953;6:159.
85. Hirschl S, Katz A: Giant cell reparative granuloma outside the jaw bone: diagnostic criteria and review of the literature with the first case described in the temporal bone. Hum Pathol 1974;5:171.
86. Austin LT Jr, Dahlin DC, Royer RO: Giant cell reparative granuloma and related conditions affecting the jawbones. Oral Surg Oral Med Oral Pathol 1959;12:1285.
87. Scott RF, Ellis E III: Surgical treatment of nonodontogenic tumors. In Thawley SE, Panje WR, eds: Comprehensive Management of Head and Neck Tumors. Philadelphia, WB Saunders, 1987:1559.
88. Biesecker JL, Marcove RC, Huvos AG, Mike V: Aneurysmal bone cysts. A clinicopathologic study of 66 cases. Cancer 1970;26:615.
89. El Deeb M, Sedano HO, Waite DE: Aneurysmal bone cyst of the jaws. Report of a case associated with fibrous dysplasia and review of the literature [review]. Int J Oral Surg 1980;9:301.
90. Lichtenstein L: Aneurysmal bone cyst. A pathological entity commonly mistaken for giant-cell tumor and occasionally hemangioma and osteogenic sarcoma. Cancer 1950;3:279.
91. Tillman BP, Dahlin DC, Lipscomb PR, Stewart JR: Aneurysmal bone cyst: an analysis of ninety-five cases. Mayo Clin Proc 1968;43:478.
92. Steiner GC, Kantor EB: Ultrastructure of aneurysmal bone cyst. Cancer 1977;40:2967.
93. Lovely FW: Recurrent aneurysmal bone cyst of the mandible. J Oral Maxillofac Surg 1983;41:192.
94. Daugherty JW, Eversole LR: Aneurysmal bone cyst of the mandible: report of case. J Oral Surg 1971;29:737.
95. Stout AP: Fibrosarcoma in infants and children. Cancer 1962;15:1028.
96. Hinds EC, Kent JN, Fechner RE: Desmoplastic fibroma of the mandible: report of case. J Oral Surg 1969;27:271.
97. Freedman PD, Cardo VA, Kerpel SM, Lumerman H: Desmoplastic fibroma (fibromatosis) of the jawbones. Oral Surg Oral Med Oral Pathol 1978;46:386.
98. Masson JK, Soule DH: Desmoid tumors of the head and neck. Am J Surg 1966;12:615.

99. Oberman HA: Idiopathic histiocytosis: a clinicopathologic study of 40 cases and review of the literature on eosinophilic granuloma of bone, Hand-Schüller-Christian disease and Letterer-Siwe disease. Pediatrics 1961;28:307.

100. Newton WA Jr, Hamoudi AB: Histiocytosis: a histologic classification with clinical correlation. Perspect Pediatr Pathol 1973;1:251.

101. Lichtenstein L: Histiocytosis X. Integration of eosinophilic granuloma of bone, "Letterer-Siwe disease," and "Schüller-Christian disease," as related manifestations of a single nosologic entity. Arch Pathol 1953;56:84.

102. Huvos AG, ed: Bone Tumors: Diagnosis, Treatment, and Prognosis. Philadelphia, WB Saunders, 1979.

103. Nolph MB, Luikin GA: Histiocytosis X. Otolaryngol Clin North Am 1982;15:635.

104. Lund BA, Dahlin DC: Hemangiomas of the mandible and maxilla. J Oral Surg 1964;22:234.

105. Worth HM, Stoneman DW: Radiology of vascular abnormalities in and about the jaws. Dent Radiogr Photogr 1979;62:1.

106. Forbes G, Earnest F IV, Jackson IT, et al: Therapeutic embolization angiography for extra-axial lesions in the head. Mayo Clin Proc 1986;61:427.

107. Jackson IT, French DJ, Tolman DE: A system of osseointegrated implants and its application to dental and facial rehabilitation. Eur J Plast Surg 1988;11:1.

108. Coley B: Neoplasms of Bone. New York, Paul B. Hoeber, 1960:298.

109. Garrington GE, Scofield HH, Cornyn J, Hooker SP: Osteosarcoma of the jaws. Analysis of 56 cases. Cancer 1967;26:377.

110. Finkelstein JB: Osteosarcoma of the jaw bones. Radiol Clin North Am 1970;8:425.

111. Slow IN, Friedman EW: Osteogenic sarcoma arising in a preexisting fibrous dysplasia: report of a case. J Oral Surg 1971;29:126.

112. Curtis ML, Elmore JS, Sotereanos GC: Osteosarcoma of the jaws: report of case with review of the literature. J Oral Surg 1974;32:125.

113. Caron AS, Hajdu SI, Strong EW: Osteogenic sarcoma of the facial and cranial bones: a review of forty-three cases. Am J Surg 1971;112:719.

114. Russ JE, Jesse RH: Management of osteosarcoma of the maxilla and mandible. Am J Surg 1980;140:572.

115. de Fries HO, Kornblut AD: Malignant disease of the osseous adnexae: osteogenic sarcoma of the jaws. Otolaryngol Clin North Am 1979;12:129.

116. Chaudhry AP, Robinovitch MR, Mitchell DF, Vickers RA: Chondrogenic tumors of the jaws. Am J Surg 1961;102:403.

117. Miles AC: Chondrosarcoma of the maxilla. Br Dent J 1950;88:257.

118. Thompson AD, Turner-Warwick RT: Skeletal sarcomata and giant cell tumor. J Bone Joint Surg Br 1955;37:266.

119. Feintuch TA: Chondrosarcoma arising in a cartilaginous area of previously irradiated fibrous dysplasia. Cancer 1973;31:877.

120. Grabias S, Mankin JH: Chondrosarcoma arising in histologically proved unicameral bone cyst. A case report. J Bone Joint Surg Am 1974;56:1501.

121. Conley J, Stout AP, Healey WV: Clinicopathologic analysis of 84 patients with an original diagnosis of fibrosarcoma of the head and neck. Am J Surg 1967;114:564.

122. Telles NC, Rabson AS, Pomeroy TC: Ewing's sarcoma: an autopsy study. Cancer 1978;41:2321.

123. Potdar GG: Ewing's tumors of the jaws. Oral Surg Oral Med Oral Pathol 1970;29:505.

124. Pomeroy TC, Johnson RE: Combined modality therapy of Ewing's sarcoma. Cancer 1975;35:36.

125. Nesbit ME Jr, Perez CA, Tefft M, et al: Multimodal therapy for the management of primary, non-metastatic Ewing's sarcoma of bone: an Intergroup Study. Natl Cancer Inst Monogr 1981;56:255.

126. Dahlin DC, Unni KK, Matsuno T: Malignant (fibrous) histiocytoma of bone—fact or fancy? Cancer 1977;39:1508.

127. Fu Y, Gabbiani G, Kay GI, Lattes R: Malignant soft tissue tumors of probable histiocytic origin (malignant fibrous histiocytomas): general considerations and electron microscopic and tissue culture studies. Cancer 1975;35:176.

128. Webber WB, Wienke EC: Malignant fibrous histiocytoma of the mandible. Case report. Plast Reconstr Surg 1977;60:629.

129. Weiss SW, Enzinger FM: Malignant fibrous histiocytoma: an analysis of 200 cases. Cancer 1978;41:2250.

130. Weiner M, Sedlis M, Johnston AD, et al: Adjuvant chemotherapy of malignant fibrous histiocytoma of bone. Cancer 1983;51:25.

131. Huvos AG: Primary malignant fibrous histiocytoma of bone: clinicopathologic study of 18 patients. N Y State J Med 1976;76:552.

132. Ghandur-Mnaymneh L, Zych G, Mnaymneh W: Primary malignant fibrous histiocytoma of bone: report of six cases with ultrastructural study and analysis of the literature. Cancer 1982;49:698.

133. Boston HC Jr, Dahlin DC, Ivins JC, Cupps RE: Malignant lymphoma (so-called reticulum cell sarcoma) of bone. Cancer 1974;34:1131.

134. Rappaport H: Tumors of the Hematopoietic System. Atlas of Tumor Pathology, Section 3, Fascicle 8. Washington, DC, Armed Forces Institute of Pathology, 1966.

135. Burkitt DP: A sarcoma involving the jaws of African children. Br J Surg 1958;46:218.

136. Ziegler JL: Burkitt's lymphoma [review]. N Engl J Med 1981;305:735.

137. Wold LE, Unni KK, Beabout JW, et al: Hemangioendothelial sarcoma of bone. Am J Surg Pathol 1982;6:59.

138. Bhaskar SN: Central mucoepidermoid tumors of the mandible. Report of two cases. Cancer 1963;16:721.

139. Marano PD, Hartman KS: Central mucoepidermoid carcinoma arising in a maxillary odontogenic cyst. J Oral Surg 1974;32:915.

140. Browand BC, Waldron CA: Central mucoepidermoid tumors of the jaws. Report of nine cases and review of the literature. Oral Surg Oral Med Oral Pathol 1975;40:631.

141. Smith RL, Dahlin DC, Waite DE: Mucoepidermoid carcinomas of the jawbones. J Oral Surg 1968;26:387.

142. Moss-Salentijn L: Anatomy and embryology. In Blitzer A, Lawson W, Friedman WH, eds: Surgery of the Paranasal Sinuses. Philadelphia, WB Saunders, 1985.

143. Hyams VJ: Papillomas of the nasal cavity and paranasal sinuses. A clinicopathologic study of 315 cases. Ann Otol Rhinol Laryngol 1971;80:192.

144. Batsakis JG: The pathology of head and neck tumors: nasal cavity and paranasal sinuses, part 5. Head Neck Surg 1980;2:410.

145. Batsakis JG: Pathology of tumors of the nasal cavity and paranasal sinuses. In Thawley SE, Panje WR, eds: Comprehensive Management of Head and Neck Tumors. Philadelphia, WB Saunders, 1999:522.

146. Frazell EL, Lewis JS: Cancer of the nasal cavity and accessory sinuses: a report of the management of 416 patients. Cancer 1963;16:1293.

147. Robin PE, Powell DJ, Stansbie JM: Carcinoma of the nasal cavity and paranasal sinuses: incidence and presentation of different histological types. Clin Otolaryngol 1979;4:431.

148. Pedersen E, Hogetveit AC, Andersen A: Cancer of respiratory organs among workers at a nickel refinery in Norway. Int J Cancer 1973;12:32.

149. Rice DH, Stanley RB Jr: Surgical therapy of nasal cavity, ethmoid sinus, and maxillary sinus tumors. In Thawley SE, Panje WR, eds: Comprehensive Management of Head and Neck Tumors. Philadelphia, WB Saunders, 1999:368.

150. Hamberger CA, Martensson G, Sjorgren HA: Treatment of Malignant Tumors of the Paranasal Sinuses in Cancer of the Head and Neck. International Workshop on Cancer of the Head and Neck. Washington, DC, Butterworth, 1967.

151. Heffner DK, Hyams VJ, Hauck KW, Lingeman C: Low-grade adenocarcinoma of the nasal cavity and paranasal sinuses. Cancer 1982;50:312.

152. Spiro RH, Huvos AG, Strong EW: Adenoid cystic carcinoma of salivary origin: a clinicopathologic study of 242 cases. Am J Surg 1974;128:512.

153. Batsakis JG, Regezi JA, Solomon AR, Rice DH: The pathology of head and neck tumors: mucosal melanomas, part 13. Head Neck Surg 1982;4:404.

154. Holdcraft J, Gallagher JC: Malignant melanomas of the nasal and paranasal sinus mucosa. Ann Otol Rhinol Laryngol 1969;78:5.

155. Shah JP, Huvos AG, Strong EW: Mucosal melanomas of the head and neck. Am J Surg 1977;134:531.

156. Silva EG, Butler JJ, Mackay B, Goepfert H: Neuroblastomas and neuroendocrine carcinomas of the nasal cavity. Cancer 1982;50:2388.

157. Jackson IT: Craniofacial approach to tumors of the head and neck. Clin Plast Surg 1985;12:375.

158. Heffner DK, Hyams VJ: Teratocarcinosarcoma (malignant teratoma?) of the nasal cavity and paranasal sinuses. A clinicopathologic study of 20 cases. Cancer 1984;53:2140.

159. Batsakis JG: Pathology consultation. Nasal (schneiderian) papillomas. Ann Otol Rhinol Laryngol 1981;90:190.

160. Dutton JJ, Anderson RL: Treatment of tumors of the eye, orbit and lacrimal apparatus. In Thawley SE, Panje WR, eds: Comprehensive Management of Head and Neck Tumors. Philadelphia, WB Saunders, 1999.

161. Porterfield JT, Zimmerman LE: Rhabdomyosarcoma of the orbit: a clinicopathologic study of 55 cases. Virchows Arch Pathol Anat 1962;335:329.

162. Rootman J, Allen LH: Clinical evaluation and pathology of tumors of the eye, orbit and lacrimal apparatus. In Thawley SE, Panje WR, eds: Comprehensive Management of Head and Neck Tumors. Philadelphia, WB Saunders, 1999.

163. Henderson JW, ed: Orbital Tumors, 2nd ed. New York, BC Decker, 1980.

164. Knowles DM II, Jakobiec FA: Orbital lymphoid neoplasms. A clinicopathologic study of 60 patients. Cancer 1980;46:576.

165. Maurer HM, Moon T, Donaldson M, et al: The Intergroup Rhabdomyosarcoma Study: a preliminary report. Cancer 1977;40:2015.

166. Croxatto JO, Font RL: Hemangiopericytoma of the orbit: a clinicopathologic study of 30 cases. Hum Pathol 1982;13:210.

167. Font RL, Gamel JW: Epithelial tumors of the lacrimal gland: an analysis of 265 cases. In Jakobiec FA, ed: Ocular and Adnexal Tumors. Birmingham, Ala, Aesculapius, 1978.

168. Font RL, Ferry AP: Carcinoma metastatic to the eye and orbit. III. A clinicopathologic study of 28 cases metastatic to the orbit. Cancer 1976;38:1326.

169. Glenn J, Kinsella T, Glatsein E, et al: A randomized prospective trial of adjuvant chemotherapy in adults with soft tissue sarcomas of the head and neck, breast, and trunk. Cancer 1985;55:1206.

170. Greager JA, Patel NK, Briele HA, et al: Soft tissue sarcomas of the adult head and neck. Cancer 1985;56:820.

171. Das Gupta TK: Tumors of the Soft Tissue. New York, Appleton & Lange, 1983.

172. Evans AE, D'Angio GJ, Randolf J: A proposed staging for children with neuroblastoma. Cancer 1971;27:374.

173. Breslow N, McCann B: Statistical estimation of prognosis for children with neuroblastoma. Cancer Res 1971;31:2098.

174. Enzinger FM, Weiss SW: Soft Tissue Tumors. St Louis, CV Mosby, 1983.

175. Spittle MF, Newton KA, Mackenzie DH: Liposarcoma: a review of 60 cases. Br J Cancer 1970;24:696.

176. Barnes L: Tumors and tumor-like lesions of the soft tissues. In Barnes L, ed: Surgical Pathology of the Head and Neck. New York, Marcel Dekker, 1985;809.

177. Saunders JR, Jacques DA, Casterline PF, et al: Liposarcoma of the head and neck: a review of the literature and addition of four cases. Br J Cancer 1979;43:162.

178. Constanzo C, Jackson IT, McEwan C, Self JM: Desmoplastic malignant melanoma: an aggressive tumor. Eur J Plast Surg 1987;9:137.

179. Cuono CB, Ariyan S: Immediate reconstruction of a composite mandibular defect with a regional osteomusculocutaneous flap. Plast Reconstr Surg 1980;65:477.

180. Little JW III, McCullough DT, Lyons JR: The lateral pectoral composite flap in one-stage reconstruction of the irradiated mandible. Plast Reconstr Surg 1983;71:326.

181. Lam KH, Wei WI, Sui KF: The pectoralis major costomyocutaneous flap for mandibular reconstruction. Plast Reconstr Surg 1984;73:904.

182. Siemssen SO, Kirkby B, O'Connor TP: Immediate reconstruction of a resected segment of the lower jaw, using a compound flap of clavicle and sternocleidomastoid muscle. Plast Reconstr Surg 1978;61:724.

183. Panje W, Cutting C: Trapezius osteomyocutaneous island flap for reconstruction of the anterior floor of the mouth and the mandible. Head Neck Surg 1980;3:66.

184. Guillamondegui OM, Larson DL: The lateral trapezius musculocutaneous flap: its use in head and neck reconstruction. Plast Reconstr Surg 1981;67:143.

185. Serafin D, Villareal-Rios A, Georgiade N: Rib-containing free flap to reconstruct mandibular defects. Br J Plast Surg 1977;30:263.

186. Taylor GI: Reconstruction of the mandible with free composite iliac bone grafts. Ann Plast Surg 1982;9:361.

187. Jackson IT, Marsh WR: Anterior cranial fossa tumors. Ann Plast Surg 1983;11:479.

188. Jackson IT, Hide TAH, Gomuwka PK, et al: Treatment of cranio-orbital fibrous dysplasia. J Maxillofac Surg 1982;10:138.

189. Jackson IT, Adham MN, Marsh WR: Use of the galeal frontalis myofascial flap in craniofacial surgery. Plast Reconstr Surg 1986;77:905.

190. Jackson IT, Marsh WR, Bite U, Hide TAH: Craniofacial osteotomies to facilitate skull base tumor resection. Br J Plast Surg 1986;39:153.

191. Jackson IT, Somers P, Marsh WR: Esthesioneuroblastoma: treatment of skull-base recurrence. Plast Reconstr Surg 1985;76:195.

192. Fisher J, Jackson IT: Microvascular surgery as an adjunct to craniomaxillofacial reconstruction. Br J Plast Surg 1989;42:146.

193. Lauritzen C, Alberius P, Santanelli F, et al: Repositioning of craniofacial tumorous bone after autoclaving. Scand J Plast Reconstr Surg Hand Surg 1991;25:161.

194. Edelstein C, Goldberg RA, Rubino G: Unilateral blindness after ipsilateral prophylactic transcranial optic canal decompression for fibrous dysplasia. Am J Ophthalmol 1998;126:469-471.

195. Spiro RH, Gerold FP, Strong EW: Mandibular swing approach for oral and oropharyngeal tumors. Head Neck Surg 1981;2:371.

196. Biller HF, Shugar JM, Krespi YP: A new technique for wide-field exposure of the base of the skull. Arch Otolaryngol 1981;107:698.

197. Shaha AR: Mandibulotomy and mandibulectomy in difficult tumors of the base of the tongue and oropharynx. Semin Surg Oncol 1991;7:25.

198. Sardi A, Walters PJ: Modified mandibular swing procedure for resection of carcinoma of the oropharynx. Head Neck 1991;13:394.

199. Ammirati M, Ma J, Cheatham ML, et al: The mandibular swing-transcervical approach to the skull base: anatomical study. J Neurosurg 1993;78:673.

200. Jackson IT, Hide TAH: A systematic approach to tumors of the base of the skull. J Maxillofac Surg 1982;10:92.

Tumors of the Lips, Oral Cavity, and Oropharynx

DAVID L. LARSON, MD

SCOPE OF THE PROBLEM

Cancer of the head and neck is relatively uncommon compared with other tumor locations, but it can have a major impact on patients. It often affects patients' self-perception, their interaction with others, and such basic functions as speech, deglutition, and breathing. Tumors of the lips, oral cavity, and oropharynx are intimately associated with these functions. It is vitally important that the surgeon appreciate the anatomy of the head and neck, the varieties of tumors and their metastatic patterns of spread, the ablative techniques, the adjunctive treatments, and the potential need for reconstruction.

IDENTIFICATION OF THE PROBLEM

Head and neck cancer accounts for 5% of newly diagnosed invasive malignant neoplasms in the United States each year or about 60,000 cases. About half of these cases involve the oral cavity. Approximately 9500 people die annually of oral cavity cancer; between 40% and 50% of these deaths are due to local and regional disease, with the remainder due to metastatic disease. Two thirds of the deaths occur in men and the remainder in women.[1] Many of these deaths are preventable because early detection and appropriate treatment are associated with a high rate of cure.

Alcohol and tobacco (which appear to act synergistically) act as local irritants on the mucosa and are associated with most of the cancers of the lips, oral cavity, and oropharynx in the United States.[2] This is in contrast to other countries, such as India, where the widespread use of betel nut chewing and *chutta* (placing the lighted end of the cigarette within the mouth) accounts for 35% of all cancers. Regardless, a history of smoking (cigars, cigarettes, or a pipe) or the use of smokeless tobacco (chewing tobacco or snuff) should alert the clinician to the possibility of a tumor of the aerodigestive tract. Other factors that should raise suspicion include poor oral hygiene, ill-fitting dentures, and lichen planus.

It has also been suggested that oral malignant neoplasms develop as a consequence of immune incompetence or a failure of host defense mechanisms. This is particularly true with the ever-increasing use of immunosuppression related to transplantation of major organs such as kidney, liver, pancreas, and heart. These patients frequently develop cancers of the skin but are also susceptible to oral squamous cell cancers. When they occur in this setting, patients should always receive surgery, saving radiation for appropriate indications noted later. The patient with acquired immunodeficiency syndrome is also immunosuppressed, but oral manifestations of this problem are most frequently infectious rather than neoplastic in nature; the same cautions for oral cancers noted before apply in this setting as well.

Anecdotal evidence for this is found in relatively young patients (<30 years) and elderly women (>70 years) who have never smoked or ingested alcohol, yet in whom the same tumors develop as in those who have abused these substances. Another clinical setting that might suggest a systemic defect as a cause of oral cancer is "field cancerization," in which multiple primary tumors occur either synchronously or asynchronously in the same patient.[3] Of course, it is commonly known that individuals who have one cancer of the aerodigestive tract (head and neck, lung, esophagus) are at a greater risk for a second cancer, particularly if they continue the social habits that produced the first.

DESCRIPTION OF COMPONENT PARTS

Premalignant Lesions

Certain lesions of the oral mucosa tend to undergo malignant change, although they are benign initially. These include leukoplakia, erythroplakia, and lichen planus. Traditionally, leukoplakia, or white patch, is frequently a cause for great concern among primary care physicians and dentists. However, when noted clinically, it is most often clinically or pathologically unrelated to any other disease process and will undergo malignant change in only 5% of cases.[4] Regardless, once it is observed, leukoplakia should be monitored by both the clinician and the patient and should undergo biopsy only if it changes in character, seems to be invasive, or becomes painful. Biopsy usually shows epithelial hyperplasia, but patients with dysplasia tend to have the highest rate of malignant transformation.

Erythroplakia, on the other hand, is less common and much more aggressive, having a propensity to develop malignant change in more than 90% of patients. Many times, carcinoma in situ can be found at the initial diagnosis of erythroplakia.[5] As with leukoplakia, there is rarely an apparent etiologic factor associated with its appearance. Biopsy is indicated at presentation.

Lichen planus rarely undergoes malignant change. Patients with this disease, particularly the erosive form, should undergo regular long-term follow-up.

Malignant Lesions

SQUAMOUS CELL CARCINOMA

By far the most common type of cancer of the lip, oral cavity, and oropharynx (Fig. 109-1) is squamous cell carcinoma, which accounts for more than 90% of cancers in these areas. Squamous cell carcinoma grows along mucosal surfaces and infiltrates deeper structures in a fairly predictable pattern—so much so that the surgeon would do well to think in terms of these patterns in the initial evaluation and on subsequent follow-up visits. Other histologic types seen in the head and neck include primary tumors of the minor salivary glands, lymphoma, sarcoma, and melanoma; these tumors are so uncommon that they are mentioned only for the sake of completeness and are noted as appropriate later in the chapter.

Most squamous carcinomas of the upper aerodigestive tract present as an ulcer that does not heal and will frequently produce blood-tinged sputum. The lesion may or may not be associated with local pain. This is in contrast to a primary tumor of the minor salivary glands (e.g., adenocarcinoma), which is initially submucosal and ulcerates only in its later stages. Once the squamous carcinoma establishes itself, its growth is steady and unresponsive to local medicinal measures (e.g., antibiotics, mouthwash). As the tumor grows, it can spread along tissue planes of muscle, fascia, and nerves, all of which produce symptoms that can potentially divert the clinician's attention from the tumor (e.g., ear pain, headache, toothache).

LOCAL EXTENSION

Squamous cell carcinoma usually presents in one of three ways: superficial exophytic, infiltrating, and ulcerating-fungating. The exophytic variant tends to be infiltrating, spreading along the mucosal surface; the ulcerating variety invades early, producing an "iceberg" effect. Ulcerating, fungating tumors metastasize earlier than the exophytic tumor does.

REGIONAL METASTASIS

Lymphatic spread of the tumor usually takes place after the primary tumor is readily identifiable. The time frame of presentation of pathologically suspicious lymph nodes in the neck is frequently related to the aggressiveness of the primary tumor, its size, and differentiation. However, tumor size is not necessarily directly related to regional metastases; the most obvious example of this is the patient with a biopsy-proven squamous cell carcinoma in the neck with no apparent primary tumor ("unknown primary"). The pattern of regional dissemination of lymphatics from oral and oropharyngeal cancers has been well documented.[6,7]

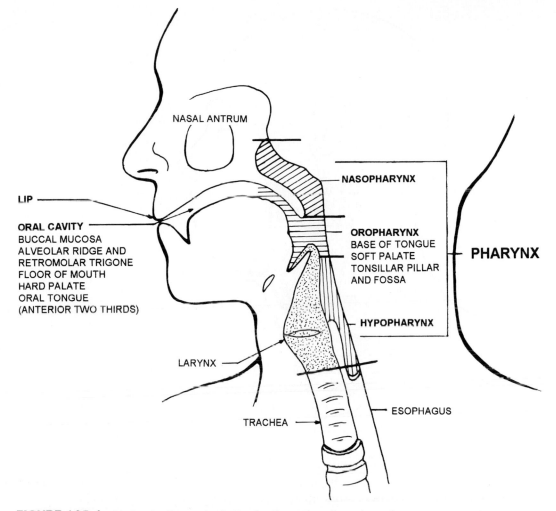

FIGURE 109-1. Anatomic sites and subsites for the oral cavity and oropharynx.

A common method of identifying the cervical lymphatics is shown in Figure 109-2. Oral cavity cancers initially drain into the submental and supraomohyoid lymph nodes (zone I) and then to the upper deep jugular chain (zones II and III). Bilateral nodal involvement is commonly seen in patients with large tumors that cross the midline and those originating from the midline (e.g., floor of the mouth). Although the incidence of cervical metastases in T1 and T2 tumors is between 10% and 20%, as the tumor increases in size and aggressiveness (T3 and T4), there is an incidence of greater than 50% of disease in the nodes. When neck nodes are involved with disease, the survival rate plunges to half of what it would be otherwise. The location of the primary tumor will, to some extent, dictate the treatment of the neck. For example, an invasive T1 or T2 tumor of the mobile tongue will develop metastases to the neck nodes much earlier than will a similarly staged tumor of the lip. This predilection for nodal disease is discussed in more detail as the anatomic sites are noted.

In the oropharynx cancers, the primary drainage site is to the jugulodigastric (level II) lymph nodes in the upper deep jugular chain.[8] The retropharyngeal and parapharyngeal nodes also drain the tonsil, soft palate, pharyngeal walls, and base of the tongue. The larger the primary tumor, the greater the chance of lymph node metastases. Tumors close to the midline demonstrate an increased propensity for bilateral lymphadenopathy.

DISTANT METASTASIS

It is highly unusual for a primary, untreated cancer of the lip, oral cavity, or oropharynx to present with a metastatic lesion below the clavicle. In fact, when such a lesion is suspected in the initial work-up, the chances are great that it will, in fact, be a second primary cancer.

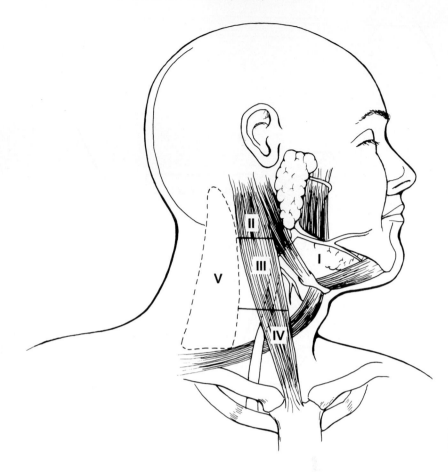

FIGURE 109-2. Level designation for cervical lymphatics of the neck.

The most common site for this to occur is the lung. This "distant disease" finding requires a work-up as though it were a primary tumor, because that is commonly the case. The importance of distinguishing between the two cannot be overstated; for example, treatment of two synchronous primary tumors carries a better prognosis than does treatment of a primary tumor with a distant metastasis.

As the treatment of the primary and regional disease becomes more predictable and higher cure rates occur, there is a greater incidence of distant disease that is fatal in most patients. Interestingly, during the last 50 years, the number of people with cancer of the oral cavity who die has remained the same. However, rather than dying of recurrent local and regional disease, they died of distant disease that occurs below the clavicles.

After a primary tumor has received some type of definitive treatment (e.g., surgery or surgery plus radiation therapy), the chance for distant disease increases significantly. Therefore, a suspicious lesion of the lung, brain, bone, or liver, although requiring a biopsy for the diagnosis to be confirmed, may be assumed to be a metastatic lesion rather than a second primary lesion. The reason for this difference between untreated and treated lesions and distant disease findings is thought to be related to the alteration of lymphatic drainage that occurs after surgery or radiation. Regardless, proven distant metastasis carries a grave prognosis.

Verrucous Carcinoma

Pathologically considered a low-grade variant of squamous cell carcinoma, verrucous carcinoma has unique characteristics that deserve special mention for the clinician. These include the fact that it classically occurs in the buccal mucosa of older women who do not have social history of smoking and alcohol ingestion. Verrucous carcinoma is exophytic and nonaggressive and never metastasizes to lymph nodes or other sites. Once the proper diagnosis is made, it should be treated with surgery since it is radioresistant. Because there are no preventable predisposing factors, it will often recur in the same patient, not as a local failure but as a second or even a third primary tumor. The key to appropriate treatment of this disease is to make sure of the diagnosis by biopsy. Even then, it is key to do serial sections of the primary tumor to make sure that there are no areas of more infiltrative disease. These patients require frequent follow-up, just as those with more invasive disease do.

Minor Salivary Gland Neoplasms

Tumors occur in the minor salivary glands of both the hard and soft palate and the lips. These glands are ubiquitous throughout the oral cavity. When a tumor does develop in a minor salivary gland, it is usually a firm, painless, submucosal mass. These neoplasms are often initially seen in the dentist's office, and the patient will usually arrive in the head and neck surgeon's office with a pathologic diagnosis already established. Differentiation between benign and malignant tumors cannot be made clinically, but statistically, more than two thirds of the tumors are malignant. The most common malignant gland tumor within the oral cavity is the adenoid cystic carcinoma, followed by the mucoepidermoid carcinoma and then adenocarcinoma. Definitive treatment of these tumors is individualized according to the aggressiveness of the tumor, its size, location, and prior treatment.

SURGICAL ANATOMY

Lip

The lip starts at the vermilion border of the skin and usually includes that portion of the lip that comes into contact with the opposing lip. The upper and lower lips join laterally at the commissures of the mouth.

Oral Cavity

The oral cavity (Fig. 109-3) extends from the vermilion border (white roll) of the lips to the junction of the hard and soft palate superiorly and to the line of the circumvallate papillae of the tongue below. The lateral margin on each side is the anterior tonsillar pillar formed by the palatoglossus muscle. Embryologically, these areas correspond to the contributions of the ectoderm contained in the first and second branchial arches.

BUCCAL MUCOSA

This area includes the epithelial lining of the inner surface of the lips and the oral surface of the cheeks to the line of attachment of mucosa superiorly and inferiorly at the alveolar ridge of the upper and lower jaws. Its posterior limit is the attachment at the retromolar trigone (pterygomandibular raphe).

ALVEOLAR RIDGE

This structure is composed of a matched set of upper (maxillary) and lower (mandibular) osseous alveolar processes that support dentition with its overlying mucosal (gingiva) layer. It extends from the buccal gutter to the line of free mucosa of the floor of the mouth and ascends posteriorly to the ascending ramus of the mandible.

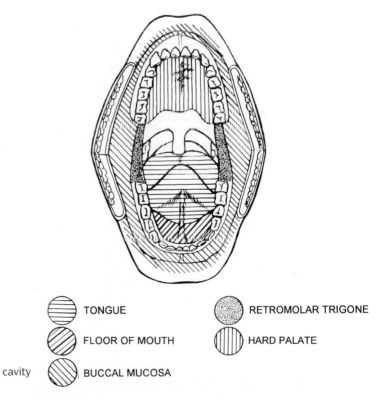

TONGUE

FLOOR OF MOUTH

BUCCAL MUCOSA

RETROMOLAR TRIGONE

HARD PALATE

FIGURE 109-3. Topography of the oral cavity (anterior view).

RETROMOLAR TRIGONE

This portion of the mouth corresponds to the area posterior to the last mandibular molar tooth to its apex superiorly at the tuberosity of the maxilla. Its lateral and medial limits, respectively, are the buccal mucosa and the anterior tonsillar pillar.

FLOOR OF THE MOUTH

The floor of the mouth is a semilunar area that extends from the inner surface of the lower alveolar ridge to the ventral (undersurface) surface of the tongue. The posterior border is the base of the anterior tonsillar pillar. Surface anatomy is separated into halves on either side of the frenulum of the tongue; each side provides the ducts of the respective submaxillary gland, which lies in a submucosal plane. The mucosa covers the muscle sling of tongue muscles, including the genioglossus, mylohyoid, and geniohyoid muscles.

HARD PALATE

This is a similar semilunar area that extends from the upper alveolus anteriorly and laterally to its junction with the soft palate posteriorly. The mucosa of the hard palate covers the palatine process of the maxillary bones.

ORAL TONGUE

The anterior two thirds of the tongue is that portion that is freely mobile (easily examined by patient and clinician alike) and extends posteriorly to the circumvallate papillae and inferiorly on each side to the junction with the floor of the mouth. It is composed of four areas: tip, lateral borders, dorsum, and undersurface. The muscular portion of the tongue has distinct planes, separated in the midline by the septum linguae. The extrinsic muscles of the tongue include the genioglossus, hyoglossus, styloglossus, and palatoglossus.

Oropharynx

The oropharynx (Figs. 109-4 and 109-5) is located between the posterior edge of the hard palate and the base of the tongue just above the epiglottis.

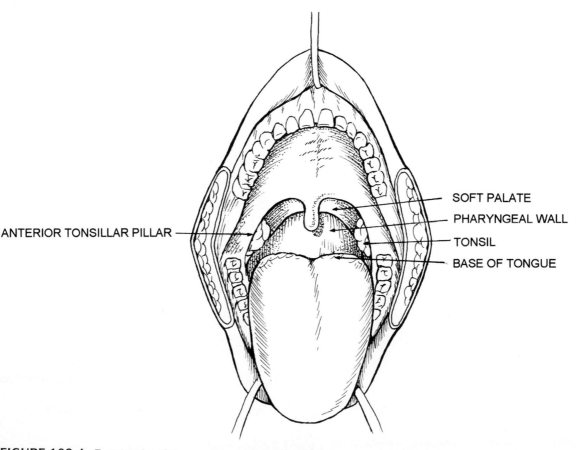

FIGURE 109-4. Topography of the oropharynx (anterior view).

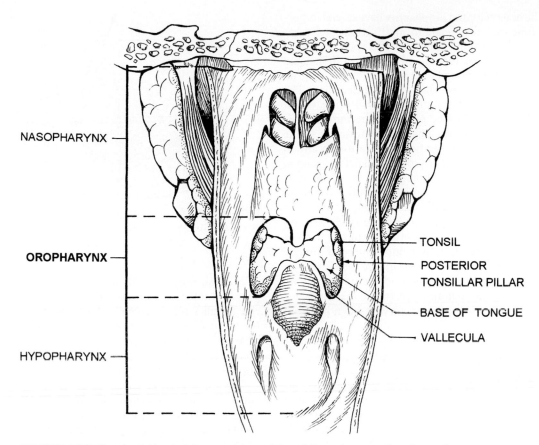

FIGURE 109-5. Topography of the oropharynx (viewed from the posterior pharynx).

BASE OF TONGUE

The posterior third of the tongue constitutes the base of the tongue. This is the portion that extends posteriorly from the circumvallate papillae to the base of the epiglottis (vallecula). Laterally, it extends to the glossopalatine sulcus. It is composed of the same muscles as the anterior two thirds of the tongue.

SOFT PALATE

Posterior to the hard palate is the soft palate, which includes the uvula and generally distinguishes the oral cavity from the oropharynx and both of these structures from the nasopharynx. It is contiguous with the tonsillar pillars laterally and forms the roof of the oropharynx and the floor of the nasopharynx.

TONSILLAR PILLAR AND FOSSA

The tonsil and its accompanying anterior and posterior pillars have an almond-shaped depression between them, which, in adults, may contain tonsillar tissue. The tonsil is located on the lateral wall of the oropharynx. The pillars of the tonsil contain the palatoglossus and palatopharyngeus muscles and converge superiorly to join the soft palate. At the foot of the tonsil is the base of the tongue, which is an important determinant for documenting extension of disease of a tonsil primary tumor. The anterior tonsillar pillar is also a valuable landmark for determining extension of a primary tumor of the retromolar trigone. If the anterior pillar is violated by a primary tumor of this area, it implies more aggressive disease, thereby affecting treatment options.

PHARYNGEAL WALLS

The pharyngeal wall extends from the posterior tonsillar pillars laterally and across the posterior wall. Superiorly, it starts at the inferior aspect of the nasopharynx; inferiorly, it goes to the level of the vallecula or base of the tongue and continues into the lateral aspect of the piriform sinus of the larynx. The pharyngeal constrictor muscle constitutes the framework of the pharyngeal wall. The nerve supply is from cranial nerves IX and X. The pharyngeal wall is rich in lymphatics, receiving drainage pathways from both sides of the pharynx equally.

The oral cavity and oropharynx have several important functions that relate to mastication, oral competence, deglutition, and articulated speech. Each of the anatomic structures identified has a designated function. Mastication of food depends on the integrity of the alveolar ridges, which support dentition. The tongue initiates the oral phase of swallowing, which propels the bolus of food posteriorly to the oropharynx, at which point the pharyngeal muscles assume control. If there is a significant alteration in any of these structures related to a congenital defect, trauma, or tumor, the normal function of these areas is altered. For instance, if tongue mobility is altered or its volume significantly diminished, there will be difficulty in swallowing. If there is loss of cheek or lip function, the patient may drool and be unable to chew effectively. Articulation is compromised if tongue mobility or mass is lost. It is therefore incumbent on the reconstructive surgeon to understand the importance of restoring anatomic structure to maintain continued function once the primary problem has been corrected.

Metastatic Patterns of Oral and Oropharyngeal Cancers

Squamous cell carcinoma of the oral cavity and oropharynx can spread by direct extension, involving contiguous areas; by tracking along nerves and spreading proximally to the central nervous system; or through vascular invasion, extending to regional nodes or distant sites.

The specific anatomy of each of the component structures of the oral cavity and oropharynx plays an important role in the extension of disease involving that area. Squamous cell carcinoma extends along mucosal surfaces and can extend into deeper structures. Tumors of the buccal mucosa commonly spread along the surface plane but may penetrate underlying muscle and present on the cheek skin. Lesions of the alveolar ridge may take the path of least resistance and extend into the jaw bone through the socket of a recently extracted tooth.[9,10] Once tongue cancers penetrate the musculature, they may spread along the intermuscular planes and make assessment of the tumor a difficult task.

Tumors of the floor of the mouth may extend inferiorly and involve the muscular diaphragm and the soft tissue of the submental skin (Fig. 109-6).

Tumors of the tongue, in particular, may invade the hypoglossal and lingual nerves, causing restriction of motion and local pain. In such a setting, the surgeon should not attempt transoral resection of the tumor. Rather, the surgeon should approach the oral cavity through the neck, identifying the tumor mass and involved nerves proximally and then tracing the nerve distally to the area of tumor involvement.

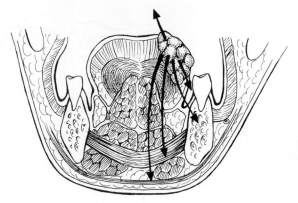

FIGURE 109-6. Coronal section through mouth demonstrating patterns of spread of a cancer of the tongue.

Interestingly, unless there is massive involvement, primary tumors of the oral cavity rarely cross the anterior tonsillar pillar, which is the posterior border of the oral cavity. For instance, a tumor of the retromolar trigone will extend preferentially along the lateral floor of mouth and tongue before extending into the tonsillar fossa and lateral pharyngeal wall.

When a tumor of the floor of the mouth or tongue abuts or seems to invade the mandible, it causes a significant problem for the clinician in properly evaluating and treating the mandible. Obviously, the surgeon should preserve as much normal tissue as possible but not compromise the oncologic principles of appropriate resection. In the early years of the 20th century, there was a belief that oral cancers involved the lymphatics of the neck by spreading through the lymphatics of the mandible. This thinking required segmental or full-thickness resection of the mandible. In the early 1970s, it was shown that such involvement occurred only if there was direct invasion of the periosteum. It was this finding that led to procedures known as marginal resection of the mandible.[11] At times, it is necessary to take this margin of tissue when there is uncertainty about invasion of the tumor. The best indicator of tumor invasion is a good clinical examination and plain (Panorex) films of the mandible.

Tumors of the oropharynx spread by direct extension to contiguous structures of that area. A tumor of the posterior pharyngeal wall can extend laterally, superiorly toward the nasopharynx, or inferiorly to the mucosa behind the cricoid region of the larynx. It can also penetrate deeply into the musculature of the neck and produce local pain in that area. Tumors of the lateral pharyngeal walls can invade the tonsil and extend into the base of the tongue, just as primary cancers of the tonsil are capable of doing. Tumors that originate in the oropharynx have relatively few symptoms, causing only discomfort or dysphagia until they are large.

An interesting thing about the metastatic patterns of spread of primary tumors of the oral cavity and oropharynx is that in general, these tumors respect each other's anatomic boundaries until they become large (T4). It is the anterior tonsillar pillar that separates these two anatomic areas.

CLINICAL EVALUATION

Physical Examination

Patients with cancer of the oral cavity or oropharynx may present with an ulcer or mass, pain, or even referred otalgia. The most common complaint is a painless mass that has persisted for a variable time. It is not unusual for even large lesions to be described as being present for only a few days or weeks. Other symptoms might include a loose tooth, nonhealing oral sore, blood-tinged sputum, halitosis, or an ill-fitting denture. Later complaints may include difficulty in chewing or swallowing, trismus, neck pain, or altered speech and breathing. Some patients may have a mass in the neck as the presenting sign of an oral or oropharyngeal primary tumor. A social history that includes alcohol and tobacco abuse is common, although not always elicited.

The clinical examination, which is always performed by digital palpation with a gloved hand, includes defining the site of origin, extent of the tumor, and degree of infiltration. When available, a flexible laryngoscope is useful, particularly for clinicians not comfortable with the mirror examination. A diagram in the patient's chart with line drawings is always helpful to later examiners. In tongue cancers, it is particularly important to assess tongue mobility. Any impairment of motion might signify deep invasion of the tumor or nerve involvement. Mandibular invasion is difficult to determine by clinical examination unless the tumor is firmly adherent to the jaw or actual bone invasion is seen on plain film. Mental nerve invasion of a lip cancer can be elicited by identification of anesthesia of the lip and then confirmed with a plain (Panorex) film demonstrating a widened mental foramen.

After examination of the primary tumor, the neck must be clinically examined. The author finds that this is best performed with the patient sitting in a chair and the clinician standing behind the patient to systematically palpate each nodal group in a bimanual fashion. This allows a comparison between both sides of the neck and an accurate appraisal of suspicious masses. Again, the results of this are documented by written word and line drawing in the patient's chart.

Biopsy

The easiest way to perform a biopsy of a suspected tumor of the oral cavity or oropharynx is simply to take a piece of tissue with a punch forceps after the tissue has been infiltrated with a small amount of anesthetic. The biopsy specimen should include a portion of the tumor that does not contain an excessive amount of necrosis. This will allow the pathologist to evaluate not only the depth (thickness) of the tumor but also the tumor-host interface. It is important not to remove all of the tumor tissue with the biopsy specimen, but rather just enough to establish a diagnosis. This is of particular importance if the physician performing the biopsy will not be the treating physician. The appearance of the tumor (exophytic, infiltrative, ulcerative) offers valuable clues to the invasiveness of the disease and may determine the need for adjunctive therapy. Fine-needle aspiration is a valuable tool that has application in the evaluation of the neck in case there is doubt about a mass. It does not alter later therapy and is usually accurate. The routine biopsy findings of the common tumors of the lip, tongue, and oropharynx can easily be interpreted by frozen section because of their characteristic morphology.

Examination Under Anesthesia

Examination under anesthesia is probably not necessary before general anesthesia associated with the definitive surgery. It includes panendoscopy of the nasopharynx, oropharynx, hypopharynx, and larynx to eliminate the possibility of a second primary tumor.[12]

TNM Classification and Staging

The American Joint Committee on Cancer has developed the TNM system.[13] As is true for cancer elsewhere in the body, this staging system is routinely used for cancers of the oral cavity and oropharynx (Table 109-1). It is important to stage the cancer correctly when the patient is initially seen because the treatment plan (e.g., surgery versus radiation, with or without neck lymph node dissection) is based on the documentation of the first treating surgeon to examine the patient. The initial staging can also have significant impact on the prognosis and subsequent frequency of follow-up. Contrary to cancer staging in some other areas of the body, the clinical staging of the primary tumor and the neck is a classification assigned to the patient during the entire course of his or her disease. There is no "pathologic" staging in head and neck cancer.

The tumor stage describes the greatest dimension of the tumor: T1 indicates size less than 2 cm; T2, between 2 and 4 cm; and T3, larger than 4 cm. The T4 designation denotes tumor invasion of the adjacent structures; this might extend from the bone to the soft tissues of the face and neck. One thing that the clinician must keep in mind is that the TNM classification addresses only two dimensions of a three-dimensional

TABLE 109-1 ✦ STAGING FOR CANCER OF THE OROPHARYNX AND ORAL CAVITY (INCLUDING THE LIP), WITH 5-YEAR SURVIVAL RATES BY STAGE

Primary Tumor (T)

TX	Primary tumor cannot be assessed
T0	No evidence of primary tumor
Tis	Carcinoma in situ
T1	Tumor 2 cm or less in greatest dimension
T2	Tumor more than 2 cm but not more than 4 cm in greatest dimension
T3	Tumor more than 4 cm in greatest dimension
T4	(lip) Tumor invades adjacent structures (e.g., through cortical bone, tongue, skin of neck)
T4	(oropharynx and oral cavity) Tumor invades adjacent structures (e.g., through cortical bone, soft tissues of neck, deep [extrinsic] muscle of tongue)

Regional Lymph Nodes (N)

NX	Regional lymph nodes cannot be assessed
N0	No regional lymph node metastasis
N1	Metastasis in a single ipsilateral lymph node, 3 cm or less in greatest dimension
N2	Metastasis in a single ipsilateral lymph node, more than 3 cm but not more than 6 cm in greatest dimension; or in multiple ipsilateral lymph nodes, none more than 6 cm in greatest dimension; or in bilateral or contralateral lymph nodes, none more than 6 cm in greatest dimension
N2a	Metastasis in a single ipsilateral lymph node more than 3 cm but not more than 6 cm in greatest dimension
N2b	Metastasis in multiple ipsilateral lymph nodes, none more than 6 cm in greatest dimension
N2c	Metastasis in bilateral or contralateral lymph nodes, none more than 6 cm in greatest dimension
N3	Metastasis in a lymph node more than 6 cm in greatest dimension

Distant Metastasis (M)

MX	Presence of distant metastasis cannot be assessed
M0	No distant metastasis
M1	Distant metastasis

Stage Grouping		*Approximate 5-Year Survival Rate (%)*
0	Tis, N0, M0	99%
I	T1, N0, M0	90%-92%
II	T2, N0, M0	75%-85%
III	T3, N0, M0	
	T1, N1, M0	
	T2, N1, M0	50%
	T3, N1, M0	
IV	T4, N0, M0	
	T4, N1, M0	
	Any T, N2, M0	25%-35%
	Any T, N3, M0	
	Any T, any N, M1	

Adapted from American Joint Committee on Cancer: Manual for Staging of Cancer, 5th ed. Philadelphia, Lippincott-Raven, 1997.

tumor. There is no allowance made in the classification for depth of invasion (superficial versus deeply invasive). For this reason, a relatively small T2 cancer of the tongue may be deeply invasive and may therefore be treated with adjunctive radiation therapy after surgery because it would act like a T3 tumor. On the other hand, an exophytic tumor on the tongue that might be 3 cm in diameter would also be classified as a T2 tumor but would not possess the invasive characteristics that dictate adjunctive radiation therapy.

The nodal staging is as follows: N1 denotes an ipsilateral lymph node with metastases less than 3 cm in greatest dimension; N2, 3 to 6 cm; and N3, greater than 6 cm. The latter N (N2 and N3) stages denote significant disease and are stage IV cancer.

As can be seen in Table 109-1, it would seem that there are two staging systems—the TNM and the stage groupings. Most surgeons use the TNM classification in referring to a patient. The stage groupings are commonly used by chemotherapists, who consider stage I

(T1 N0 tumors) and stage II (T2 N0 tumors) early disease (not normally treated with chemotherapy) and stage III (any T3 tumor or any that is associated with N+ disease) and stage IV (large tumors >4 cm and N2+ disease) candidates for adjunctive chemotherapy. As noted earlier, distant disease is uncommon at presentation. In general, the survival rate of patients with locally advanced (stage III or stage IV) disease is less than half that of patients with early-stage disease.

DIAGNOSTIC STUDIES
Radiologic Studies

A chest radiograph is typically sufficient radiologic work-up for cancers of the lip, tongue, and oropharynx. This is ordered primarily to look for a second primary tumor in the lung because most of these patients have a significant history of tobacco abuse. For tumors of the floor of the mouth, a plain film (Panorex) with occlusal views to see the lingual aspect of the anterior mandible is also obtained. The plain film can also help in identifying a widened mental foramen that would suggest nerve extension of a lip cancer in association with anesthesia of the lip. A computed tomographic scan is indicated only for evaluation of an extensive cancer and is nondiagnostic for evaluation of the neck. On some occasions, there might be need to use magnetic resonance imaging, with gadolinium enhancement to view the invasion of the posterior portion of the tongue by a large, invasive tumor. In certain circumstances, the magnetic resonance imaging and computed tomographic studies can complement each other in attempting to evaluate bone and soft tissue involvement. Other adjunctive studies (e.g., esophagography, ultrasonography) depend on the patient's symptoms or an unusual physical finding. In general, almost all the information of relevance can be obtained from an adequate clinical evaluation and an examination with the patient under anesthesia.

Laboratory Studies

The only studies that are essential for the initial work-up of a patient with head and neck cancer are a complete blood cell count, liver function studies, and any other chemistry panels that would be indicated by the patient's general health.

APPROPRIATE CONSULTATION

Today, the concept of multispecialty care is apparent in the treatment of head and neck cancer.[14] In general, this health care team is headed by the ablative surgeon but, importantly, includes the reconstructive surgeon, who generally will perform a complex reconstruction beyond the capabilities of the cancer surgeon. This is in direct contrast to the head and neck surgeon of the 1980s and earlier who "did it all." With the universal availability of microsurgery in community hospitals and medical centers alike, most large resections are reconstructed immediately with a form of free tissue transfer of bone and soft tissue. This reconstruction is usually performed by a separate surgical team and frequently takes longer than the ablative procedure. Musculocutaneous flaps and regional, pedicled flaps for reconstruction of complex defects of the bone and soft tissue today are not considered state of the art.

Other members of the multidisciplinary team include the dentist, the radiotherapist, frequently the chemotherapist, and the social support team (social worker and visiting home nurse). It is also important to have the functional support team of a speech pathologist and a swallowing therapist see the patient preoperatively to orient the patient about problems and solutions that may be initiated by the treatment.

TREATMENT
Treatment Goals

The following discussion of the treatment of head and neck cancer deals with patients who have "resectable disease." There is another class of patients who may be considered to have "unresectable disease." Although there may be some who might quibble with this definition, unresectable tumors are those that cannot be removed without imposing unacceptable morbidity and those that occur in patients whose constitutional state precludes an operation (even if the cancer is readily resectable with few sequelae). By use of this definition, when the surgeon thinks that all gross tumor cannot be removed or is certain that local control will not be achieved after an operation (even with the addition of radiotherapy), the patient's tumor is termed unresectable. Tumors that involve the cervical plexus, brachial plexus, deep neck muscles, and carotid artery might be termed unresectable, and palliative measures might be considered. The most common clinical setting in which these unresectable tumors are found is in recurrent disease after definitive surgery and radiation. Even in circumstances in which no treatment has been initiated and a large mass involves the carotid artery (N3), a decision to resect the common carotid artery requires balancing the benefit with the risk of morbidity.

In considering a prolonged, complex ablation and reconstruction, it is always wise to meet with the anesthesia team before the day of surgery to inform them of the intentions of the surgical team. When intraoral ablation and reconstruction are performed, a tracheotomy is commonly used because it eliminates the

TABLE 109-2 ✦ RADIOTHERAPY FOR CANCER OF THE LIP

Definitive RT	Primary and gross adenopathy: ≥66 Gy (2.0 Gy/day) External beam RT ≥ 50 Gy + brachytherapy *or* brachytherapy alone Neck Low-risk nodal stations: ≥50 Gy (2.0 Gy/day)
Adjuvant RT	Primary: ≥60 Gy (2.0 Gy/day) Neck High-risk nodal stations: ≥60 Gy (2.0 Gy/day) Low-risk nodal stations: ≥50 Gy (2.0 Gy/day)

presence of an endotracheal tube in the surgical field, but it also offers better control of the airway—both during and after the surgery. The author prefers to do this procedure under local anesthesia at the beginning of the surgery, but it can also be performed over a temporarily placed endotracheal tube. For smaller, less complicated tumors, particularly those of the floor of mouth or mobile tongue, a well-placed nasotracheal tube is useful. In this setting, the patient can generally be extubated in the operating room to ensure a controlled airway. A tracheotomy should be considered if there is any suspicion of compromised airway during or after surgery.

Management Approaches

A number of options are available to treat cancer of the oral cavity and oropharynx: surgery alone, radiation therapy alone, or surgery combined with postoperative radiation therapy. The modality employed depends clearly on the staging of the tumor, the physiologic and emotional status of the patient, and the patient's preference. In the hands of most head and neck surgeons, all cancers of the oral cavity and lip should be treated with surgery and postoperative radiation as an adjunct when there are poor prognostic indicators.[15] These might include multiple levels of positive lymph nodes, extracapsular extension of the cancer in a lymph node, deep invasion of the primary tumor, neural and vascular invasion, tumor margins less than 5 mm, and the need to take multiple layers of frozen section before a "clear" margin is obtained.[16] In the oropharynx, the most favorable group (T1-3, N0) is treated with radiation for cure,[17-19] and those with a larger tumor burden are treated with a combination of surgery and radiation.[20] Many of the patients in the

latter group are entered into protocols that include adjunctive chemotherapy.[21]

Planned preoperative radiation therapy is no longer popular. The primary reason is that initial surgery removes the gross disease and identifies areas of suspected microscopic seeding so that larger, more directed doses of radiation can be provided after ablative surgery.

SURGICAL APPROACHES

Lip Cancer

Tumors of the lip commonly occur in the lower lip and are located between the midline and lateral commissure. Upper lip tumors are frequently closer to the midline. As conspicuous as these lesions might be, most lip cancers are 1 to 2 cm in size when finally diagnosed and require a full-thickness resection of the skin, muscle, and underlying mucosa to facilitate an aesthetic closure. At times, these tumors are associated with leukoplakia and also may require a lip shave of the premalignant tissue. Rarely are regional lymph nodes involved with lip cancer, but if they are present, an appropriate neck dissection should be carried out (Fig. 109-7 and Table 109-2).

Oral Cavity

Resections of the floor of mouth, buccal mucosa, tongue, and mandible can be performed by one of four approaches: transoral, mandible sparing (pull-through), mandibulotomy, or composite resection (including the mandible and associated neck dissection). Factors that might influence the approach include the size, location, and invasive characteristics of the tumor; mandible invasion (or suspicion thereof); need for neck dissection; and prior treatment (surgery or radiation therapy) (Fig. 109-8 and Table 109-3).

Text continued on p. 177

TABLE 109-3 ✦ RADIOTHERAPY FOR CANCER OF THE ORAL CAVITY

Definitive RT	Primary and gross adenopathy: ≥70 Gy (2.0 Gy/day) External beam RT ≥50 Gy ± brachytherapy Neck Low-risk nodal stations: ≥50 Gy (2.0 Gy/day)
Adjuvant RT	Primary: ≥60 Gy (2.0 Gy/day) Neck High-risk nodal stations: ≥60 Gy (2.0 Gy/day) Low-risk nodal stations: ≥50 Gy (2.0 Gy/day)

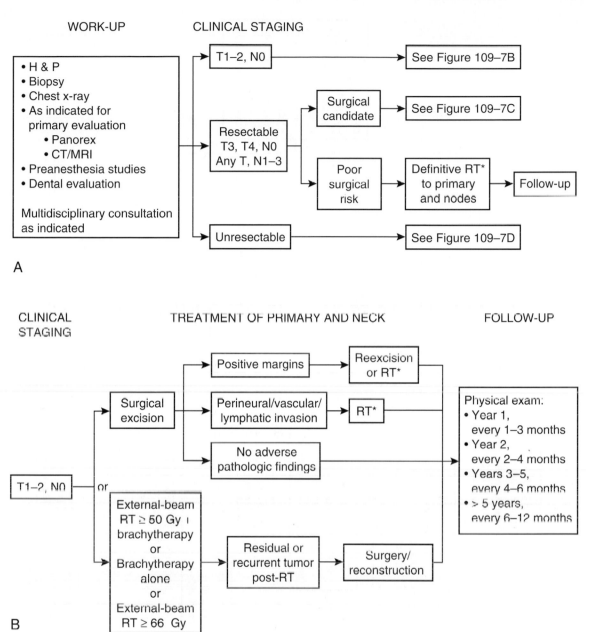

FIGURE 109-7. *A–D,* NCCN Practice Guidelines: Treatment algorithm for cancer of the lip. *See Table 109-2. †The various single-agent chemotherapy regimens have not been compared in randomized trials. Therefore, no optimal standard regimen is defined. Single-agent cisplatin (100 mg/m² days 1, 22, and 43) is effective and relatively easy to administer. Combination chemotherapy regimens are more toxic and have not been directly compared to single-agent regimens. ‡Cisplatin 100 mg/m² day 1 + 5FU 1000 mg/m²/24 hr continuous IV infusion for 120 hours for 3 cycles. Note: All recommendations are category 2A unless otherwise indicated. Clinical Trials: NCCN believes that the best management of any cancer patient is in a clinical trial. Participation in clinical trials is especially encouraged. (Version 1.2004, 01/14/04 © 2004 National Comprehensive Cancer Network, Inc. All rights reserved. See disclaimer at end of chapter.)   *Continued*

TREATMENT OF PRIMARY AND NECK

CLINICAL STAGING:
RESECTABLE T3, T4, N0; Any T, N1–3

FOLLOW-UP

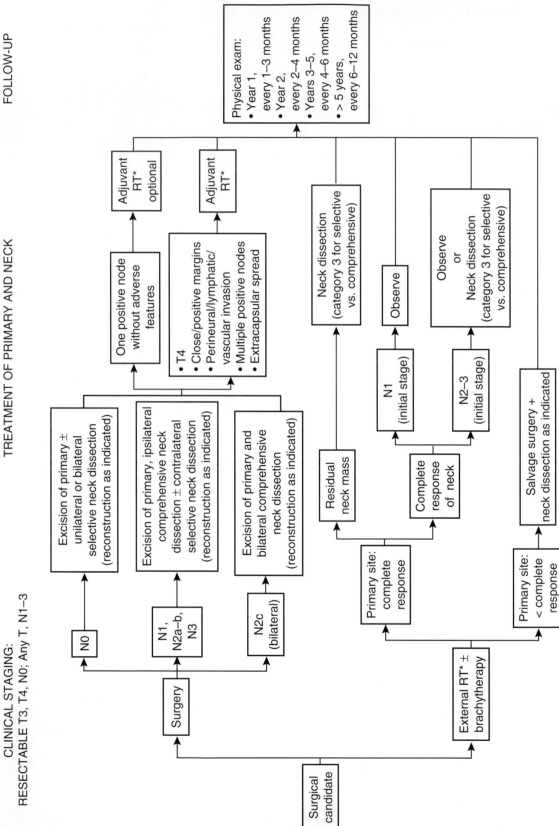

C

FIGURE 109-7, cont'd.

DIAGNOSIS   TREATMENT OF HEAD AND NECK CANCER

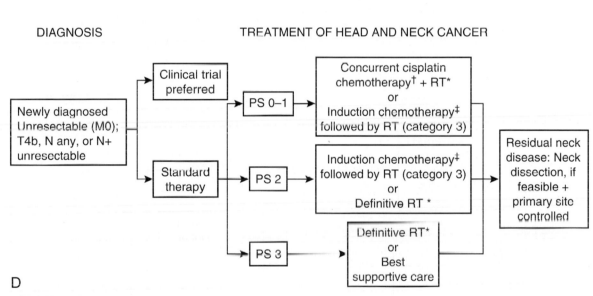

D
FIGURE 109-7, cont'd.

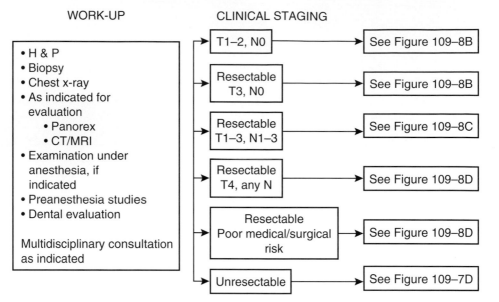

A

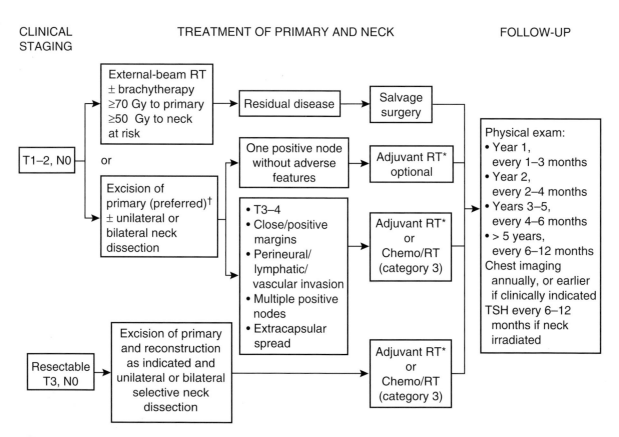

B

FIGURE 109-8. *A–D,* NCCN Practice Guidelines: Treatment algorithm for cancer of the oral cavity: buccal mucosa, floor of the mouth, anterior tongue, alveolar ridge, retromolar trigone, and hard palate. *See Table 109-3. †Excluding buccal mucosa. Note: All recommendations are category 2A unless otherwise indicated. Clinical Trials: NCCN believes that the best management of any cancer patient is in a clinical trial. Participation in clinical trials is especially encouraged. (Version 1.2004, 01/14/04 © 2004 National Comprehensive Cancer Network, Inc. All rights reserved. See disclaimer at end of chapter.)

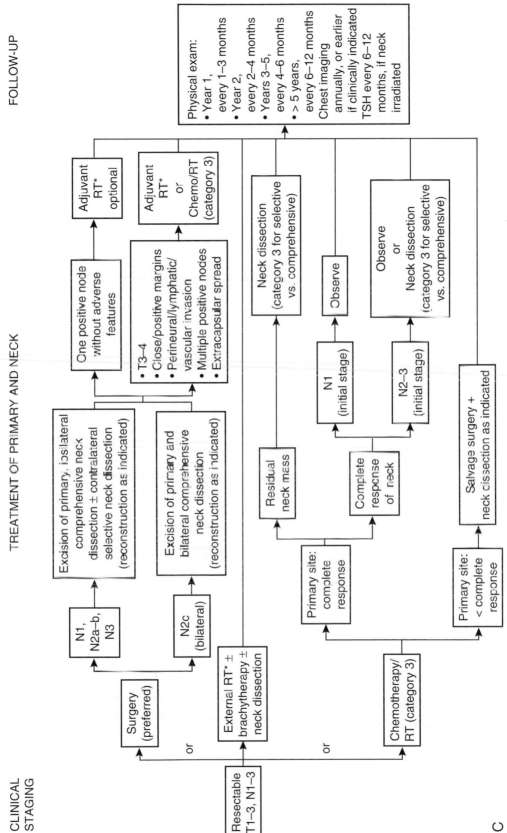

FOLLOW-UP

Physical exam:
• Year 1,
  every 1–3 months
• Year 2,
  every 2–4 months
• Years 3–5,
  every 4–6 months
• > 5 years,
  every 6–12 months
Chest imaging
annually, or earlier
if clinically indicated
TSH every 6–12
months, if neck
irradiated

Adjuvant
RT*
optional

Adjuvant
RT*
or
Chemo/RT
(category 3)

One positive node
without adverse
features

• T3-4
• Close/positive margins
• Perineural/lymphatic/
  vascular invasion
• Multiple positive nodes
• Extracapsular spread

Neck dissection
(category 3 for selective
vs. comprehensive)

Observe

Observe
or
Neck dissection
(category 3 for selective
vs. comprehensive)

Excision of primary, ipsilateral
comprehensive neck
dissection ± contralateral
selective neck dissection
(reconstruction as indicated)

Excision of primary and
bilateral comprehensive
neck dissection
(reconstruction as indicated)

Residual
neck mass

Complete
response
of neck

N1
(initial stage)

N2-3
(initial stage)

Salvage surgery +
neck dissection as indicated

N1,
N2a–b,
N3

N2c
(bilateral)

Primary site:
complete response

Primary site:
< complete
response

Surgery
(preferred)

External RT* ±
brachytherapy ±
neck dissection

Chemotherapy/
RT (category 3)

or

or

Resectable
T1–3, N1–3

C

FIGURE 109-8, cont'd.

Continued

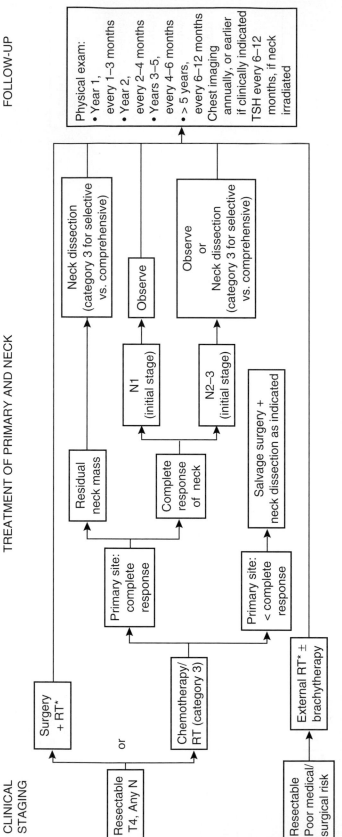

CLINICAL
STAGING

TREATMENT OF PRIMARY AND NECK

FOLLOW-UP

Resectable
T4, Any N

Surgery
+ RT*

or

Chemotherapy/
RT (category 3)

Primary site:
complete
response

Residual
neck mass

Complete
response
of neck

Neck dissection
(category 3 for selective
vs. comprehensive)

Observe

N1
(initial stage)

N2–3
(initial stage)

Observe
or
Neck dissection
(category 3 for selective
vs. comprehensive)

Resectable
Poor medical/
surgical risk

External RT* ±
brachytherapy

Primary site:
< complete
response

Salvage surgery +
neck dissection as indicated

Physical exam:
• Year 1,
  every 1–3 months
• Year 2,
  every 2–4 months
• Years 3–5,
  every 4–6 months
• > 5 years,
  every 6–12 months
Chest imaging
annually, or earlier
if clinically indicated
TSH every 6–12
months, if neck
irradiated

D

FIGURE 109-8, cont'd.

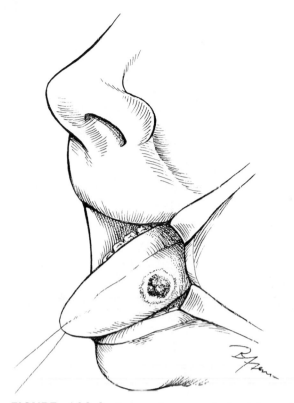

FIGURE 109-9. Transoral approach to intraoral resection.

TRANSORAL RESECTION. Transoral resection (Fig. 109-9) is reserved for smaller lesions that are easily accessible. Tumors removed through the transoral approach are usually anterior, superficial, and well-circumscribed lesions of the floor of the mouth, the mobile (anterior two thirds) tongue, the buccal mucosa, or the palate. This includes all T1 and early, exophytic T2 cancers. If the tumor involves the submandibular duct or ducts, reconstruction is usually not attempted, nor is it necessary. In these early lesions, a discontinuous neck dissection is easily accomplished if the primary tumor dictates. Interestingly, resection of small tumors of the floor of the mouth can be left to heal secondarily, with little morbidity. If the wound is larger, a split-skin graft, with a bolster for 5 days, suffices. Defects of less than one third of the tongue can be closed primarily, with little long-term morbidity of speech or swallowing.

A variation of the transoral resection is resection of the upper half of the mandible as a marginal resection (Fig. 109-10). This is usually performed when there is no obvious clinical tumor involvement of the mandible. Reconstruction is accomplished with a split-thickness skin graft placed on the cancellous bone surface of the remaining mandible.

PULL-THROUGH PROCEDURE. The pull-through procedure is ideal for moderate-sized cancers of the anterior and lateral floor of mouth areas, particularly if the mandible is not involved or a margin of mandible has been removed as a deep margin. This approach has the distinct advantage of maintaining the contour of the mandible while the primary tumor is excised in continuity with the neck specimen. Reconstruction is usually accomplished with a free tissue transfer.

MANDIBULOTOMY. Patients with a large tumor of the posterior oral cavity or oropharynx are best suited for mandibulotomy (Fig. 109-11) when the tumor does not involve the mandible. Also called a mandibular swing, mandibulotomy involves dividing the mandible just lateral to the midline (anterior to the mental foramen), thereby preserving sensation to the lip. Once the tumor is resected and reconstruction is performed (e.g., skin graft; musculocutaneous, regional, or free flap), the mandible is returned to its original position and plated in place. This approach can be used for patients regardless of dentition. Another advantage of this method is that the portion of the mandible that has been divided is out of the field of postoperative radiation therapy. The mandibulotomy is the most common approach for resection of tumors of the retromolar trigone, base of the tongue, tonsil, and lateral pharyngeal wall.

Of course, it is the surgeon's choice to apply either the pull-through procedure or the mandibulotomy. The pull-through procedure preserves the continuity of the mandible but is technically more difficult and is indicated in smaller tumors that approach, but do not involve, the mandible; mandibulotomy (used in large tumors that lay close to the jaw) violates the mandible but provides an unfettered view of the tumor and subsequent reconstruction.

COMPOSITE RESECTION WITH MANDIBULECTOMY. When the mandible is obviously involved with cancer, it must be removed as a full-thickness, segmental resection. When late-stage disease such as this is treated, there is almost always a soft tissue deficit, and restoration of both bone and soft tissue is necessary. This may often require a free tissue transfer (and at times two transfers) to be performed immediately after the ablative surgery. The composite resection (Fig. 109-12) is usually performed when the tumor invades the lateral or anterior arch of the mandible. If the tumor is within the lateral portion of the mandible distal to the angle of the mandible, there is no indication to remove the ramus of the mandible and its attendant musculature. Preservation of this important structure, including the coronoid, greatly aids autologous mandible reconstruction and thereby facilitates a more rapid recovery. If the tumor involves the ramus, such as a primary tumor of the retromolar trigone, that structure must be removed. Even in this circumstance, however, the

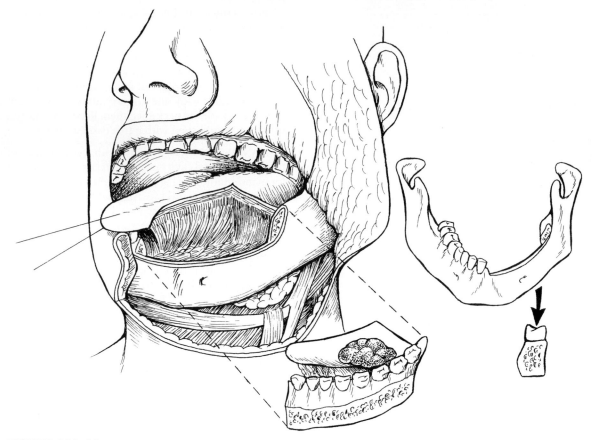

FIGURE 109-10. Marginal resection approach of removal of lateral floor of mouth tumor. This may be performed by splitting the lip (as shown) or by a transoral approach.

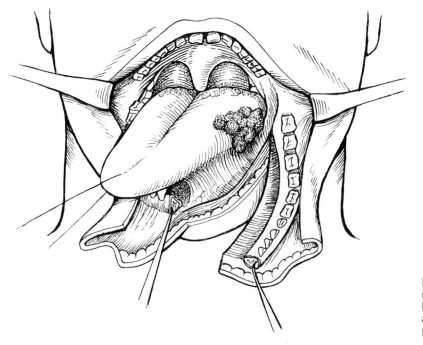

FIGURE 109-11. Dividing the mandible anteriorly between the lateral incisor teeth allows wide access to the posterior tongue and pharynx.

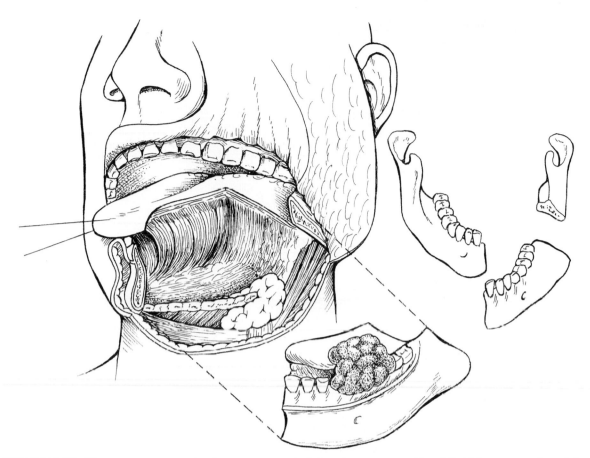

FIGURE 109-12. Composite resection includes removal of the primary tumor with a full-thickness resection of the mandible and the nodal contents of the neck.

condyle and many times the posterior edge of the ramus can be preserved without compromise of oncologic principles. The condyle, with or without the posterior piece of ramus, can act as a source of fixation for later reconstruction. In resection of the retromolar trigone, the pterygoid fossa and associated muscles (medial and lateral pterygoid) are violated and thereby no longer provide countertraction to the same muscle on the contralateral side. This will result in significant jaw deviation if it is not reconstructed immediately.

The reconstructions of the mandible, whether anterior arch, lateral segment, or ramus, should always be performed immediately, if at all possible. Surgical rehabilitation is always more predictable and supportive of the patient when it is done immediately, rather than "waiting for the cancer to recur" and dealing with the predictable contracture and deviation that will occur in the remaining jaw when the delayed reconstructive pathway is used.

Oropharynx

Tumors of the oropharynx are generally removed by mandibulotomy for posterior pharyngeal lesions, and reconstruction is accomplished with regional or distant tissue. Those of the soft palate can be resected through a transoral approach as described earlier (Fig. 109-13 and Table 109-4).

MANAGEMENT OF THE NECK LYMPH NODES

Concomitant with the management of any cancer of the oral cavity or oropharynx is making a decision of how to manage the regional lymph nodes. Obviously, if the neck has nodes that are palpable (positive for cancer) in the first or second echelon of drainage of the primary tumor, a neck dissection is required. Usually, this would be a classic radical neck dissection. When the neck has no palpable nodes that are suggestive of cancer (N0), but there is still a high (>15%) likelihood of the presence of microscopic disease on the basis of the location of the primary tumor, a less radical operation can be performed. Some term this a modified radical neck dissection, in which the sternomastoid muscle, jugular vein, and spinal accessory nerve are preserved.[22]

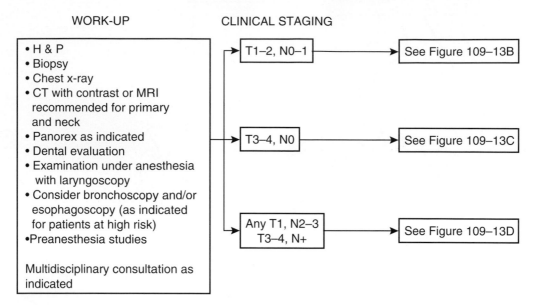

WORK-UP

CLINICAL STAGING

- H & P
- Biopsy
- Chest x-ray
- CT with contrast or MRI recommended for primary and neck
- Panorex as indicated
- Dental evaluation
- Examination under anesthesia with laryngoscopy
- Consider bronchoscopy and/or esophagoscopy (as indicated for patients at high risk)
- Preanesthesia studies

Multidisciplinary consultation as indicated

T1–2, N0–1 → See Figure 109–13B

T3–4, N0 → See Figure 109–13C

Any T1, N2–3
T3–4, N+ → See Figure 109–13D

A

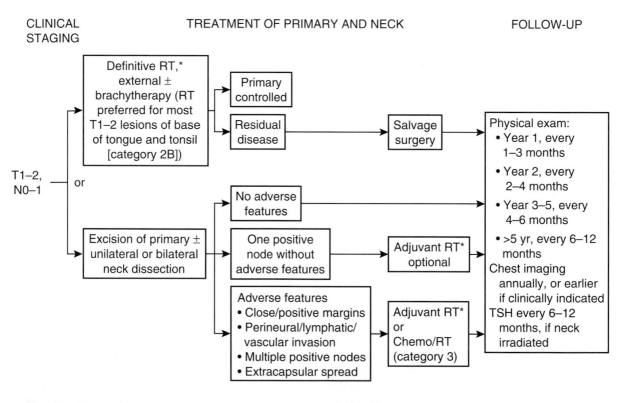

CLINICAL STAGING

TREATMENT OF PRIMARY AND NECK

FOLLOW-UP

T1–2, N0–1

or

Definitive RT,* external ± brachytherapy (RT preferred for most T1–2 lesions of base of tongue and tonsil [category 2B])

Primary controlled

Residual disease → Salvage surgery

Excision of primary ± unilateral or bilateral neck dissection

No adverse features

One positive node without adverse features → Adjuvant RT* optional

Adverse features
- Close/positive margins
- Perineural/lymphatic/ vascular invasion
- Multiple positive nodes
- Extracapsular spread

→ Adjuvant RT* or Chemo/RT (category 3)

Physical exam:
- Year 1, every 1–3 months
- Year 2, every 2–4 months
- Year 3–5, every 4–6 months
- >5 yr, every 6–12 months

Chest imaging annually, or earlier if clinically indicated

TSH every 6–12 months, if neck irradiated

B

FIGURE 109-13. *A–D*, NCCN Practice Guidelines: Treatment algorithm for cancer of the oropharynx: base of tongue, tonsil, posterior pharyngeal wall, and soft palate. *See Table 109-4. Note: All recommendations are category 2A unless otherwise indicated. Clinical Trials: NCCN believes that the best management of any cancer patient is in a clinical trial. Participation in clinical trials is especially encouraged. (Version 1.2004, 01/14/04 © 2004 National Comprehensive Cancer Network, Inc. All rights reserved. See disclaimer at end of chapter.)

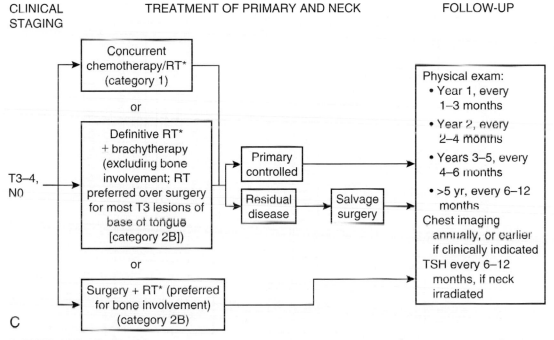

CLINICAL STAGING   TREATMENT OF PRIMARY AND NECK   FOLLOW-UP

FIGURE 109-13, cont'd.   *Continued*

182

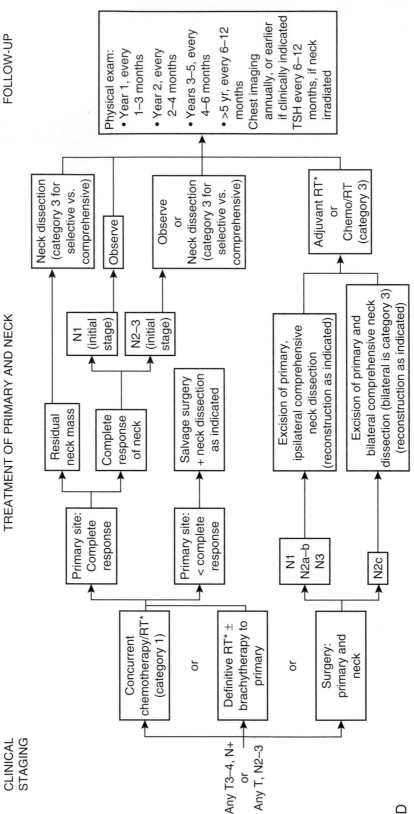

TREATMENT OF PRIMARY AND NECK

CLINICAL STAGING

FOLLOW-UP

Any T3–4, N+
or
Any T, N2–3

Concurrent chemotherapy/RT*
(category 1)

or

Definitive RT* ± brachytherapy to primary

Primary site: Complete response

Residual neck mass

Complete response of neck

Neck dissection (category 3 for selective vs. comprehensive)

Observe

Primary site: < complete response

Salvage surgery + neck dissection as indicated

N1 (initial stage)

N2–3 (initial stage)

Observe
or
Neck dissection (category 3 for selective vs. comprehensive)

Surgery: primary and neck

N1
N2a–b
N3

N2c

Excision of primary, ipsilateral comprehensive neck dissection (reconstruction as indicated)

Excision of primary and bilateral comprehensive neck dissection (bilateral is category 3) (reconstruction as indicated)

Adjuvant RT*
or
Chemo/RT
(category 3)

Physical exam:
• Year 1, every 1–3 months
• Year 2, every 2–4 months
• Years 3–5, every 4–6 months
• >5 yr, every 6–12 months
Chest imaging annually, or earlier if clinically indicated
TSH every 6–12 months, if neck irradiated

D

FIGURE 109-13, cont'd.

TABLE 109-4 ✦ RADIOTHERAPY FOR CANCER OF THE OROPHARYNX

Chemoradiation	Conventional fractionation: ≥70 Gy (2.0 Gy/day)
Definitive RT (alone)	T1-2, N0 Conventional fractionation: ≥70 Gy (2.0 Gy/day) ± brachytherapy
	Selected T2, T3-4, N1-3 Altered fractionation (preferred): Concomitant boost accelerated RT: 72 Gy/6 weeks (1.8 Gy/fraction, large field; 1.5 Gy boost as second daily fraction during last 12 treatment days) Hyperfractionation: 81.6 Gy/7 weeks (1.2 Gy/fraction BID)
Adjuvant RT	Primary: ≥60 Gy (2.0 Gy/day) Neck High-risk nodal stations: >60 Gy (2.0 Gy/day) Low-risk nodal stations: ≥50 Gy (2.0 Gy/day)

Version 1. 2004, 01/14/04 © 2004 National Comprehensive Cancer Network, Inc. All rights reserved. These guidelines and this illustration may not be reproduced in any form without the express written permission of NCCN. See disclaimer at end of chapter.)

The National Comprehensive Cancer Network (NCCN), a consortium of university cancer centers, has published the thoughts of a head and neck panel who prefer to consider cervical lymph node dissections either "comprehensive" or "selective."[23] By use of their definition, a comprehensive neck dissection is one that removes all lymph node groups that would be included in a classic neck dissection. Whether the sternomastoid muscle, jugular vein, and accessory nerve are preserved does not affect whether the dissection is comprehensive. Selective neck dissections have evolved on the basis of an understanding of the common pathways for spread of head and neck cancers to regional nodes (Fig. 109-14). The supraomohyoid neck dissection is designed to remove the nodal echelons most commonly associated with metastasis from the oral cavity. It includes nodes found above the omohyoid muscle (levels I, II, and III and the superior parts of level V). In a similar way, the lateral neck dissection removes the nodes most commonly involved with cancers of the pharynx, oropharynx, and larynx (nodes in levels II, III, and IV). When there is no clinical involvement of nodes from a squamous cancer in the head and neck, nodal spread beyond the confines of an appropriate selective neck dissection is less that 10% of the time.[24]

Patients with superficial T1 cancers and an N0 neck will not receive a prophylactic neck dissection because these tumors will rarely (<10%) spread to regional nodes. Those with an invasive T1 or T2 oral cavity cancer should receive a supraomohyoid neck dissection, thereby providing both a therapeutic and a staging function. Those with T3 or T4 cancers should receive a full comprehensive neck dissection on the ipsilateral side and, in selected cases (when the midline is crossed by the primary), a supraomohyoid selective neck dissection. The spinal accessory nerve can usually be preserved in all elective neck dissections. Dissection of only the submaxillary triangle for an oral cavity cancer is not effective treatment, nor does it provide accurate staging because the cancer in many of these patients will develop a "skip" area and progress directly to level III nodes.

Radiotherapy

The administration of radiation therapy for the treatment of cancer of the head and neck is an extremely complex process and should be accomplished only by a special team that consists of a radiation oncologist, physiatrist, dosimetrist, and radiation technologist. In addition, modern radiotherapy equipment must be employed. The anatomic location, tumor histology findings, and clinical circumstances will dictate the use of radiation as a primary therapy or adjuvant treatment to surgery or chemotherapy.

In general, in an area that has not received surgery (such as an N0 neck), subclinical microscopic cancer requires that 4500 to 5000 cGy of radiation be administered during 5 or 6 weeks. This dose will offer the

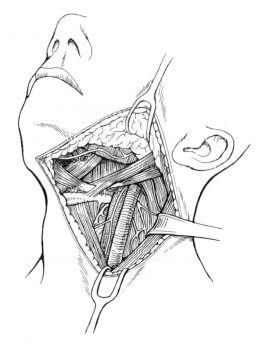

FIGURE 109-14. In a comprehensive neck dissection in an N0 neck, the functional structures (sternomastoid muscle, eleventh cranial nerve, and internal jugular vein) are preserved.

probability of tumor control in more than 90% of cases; early tumors (e.g., T1) require 6600 cGy, and larger lesions (e.g., T2 and T3) may require up to 7000 cGy.

When radiation therapy is given in the postoperative setting, the dose is based on tumor stage and histologic and surgical findings after tumor resection. Because of the interruption of normal vasculature, scarring, and relative hypoxia in the tumor bed after surgery, higher doses of radiation are required (6500 cGy during $6^1/_2$ weeks) to decrease the chances of local and regional failure.[25]

The fractionation, or frequency, with which radiation therapy is administered may vary as well. In most radiation oncology units, the treatments are delivered once a day, 5 days a week, at 180 to 200 cGy/fraction. External radiation doses that exceed 7500 cGy at conventional fractionation will invariably lead to complications and unacceptable morbidity.

There are other dose schemes for administering radiation, such as hyperfractionation (smaller doses two or three times a day) and hypofractionation (one larger dose every 2 or 3 days). These approaches have been evaluated in hopes of being able to administer larger doses of radiation while decreasing the morbidity of a large dose. The biologic basis for use of multiple fractions daily is that a large, consistent difference in the repair capacity of late- and early-responding tissues exists.[26,27] At this point, hyperfractionation is considered experimental, and there is no definitive treatment apart from the conventional dose.

Another method of delivering radiation therapy is brachytherapy. In this technique, artificially produced radioisotopes are placed in implants that are put directly into tumor-bearing tissue. This can be used as a definitive treatment of early superficial lesions with an expectation of good control and preservation of function.[28] In combination with external beam radiation, described earlier in this chapter, excellent results have been obtained but long-term morbidity can be a problem, particularly 10 years or more after treatment.[29]

MANAGEMENT OF THE LOCAL RECURRENCE

Part of the management of tumors of the oral cavity is the local recurrence, that is, a tumor that occurs in the previously treated anatomic area within 2 years of the initial, definitive treatment. If it occurs later than in that time frame, there is a good chance that it is a second primary tumor. This is more of an academic question, however, because the surgeon must deal with the same issues that surround the local recurrence. Whether a local recurrence or a second primary, the tumor will more than likely be a squamous cell carcinoma of varying grade.

There is no particular predisposition to a local recurrence; it can occur in any clinical setting, regardless of size or location of the primary in the head and neck. It is most important for the surgeon always to be mindful that a local recurrence can develop and not hesitate to perform biopsy of any area of suspicion. A symptom as subtle as local pain or restriction of movement of the tongue, with no objective signs, should be closely observed. Regardless, there is probably no indication for "random" biopsies to disprove local recurrence. If there is a recurrence in this setting, the symptoms will persist and a lesion will eventually present itself for biopsy. More frequently, the patient will present with a concern about a nodule in the oral cavity or neck. When this occurs, the biopsy can be performed in the office under local anesthesia. If the result of this biopsy proves negative, the surgeon should continue to observe the patient closely, recognizing that the biopsy specimen might have been inadequate or a general anesthetic might be required for thorough examination and biopsy of the suspected lesion.

Once the result of biopsy is proved to be positive, a complete work-up must be carried out to identify any regional or distant disease. If there is distant disease, systemic therapy must be considered, and treatment of the local recurrence must be tempered by its size, location, and use as a local monitor of the response to the chemotherapy. This decision must obviously be individualized to each patient. More than likely, there will not be any other disease identified, and then decisions must be made about management of the patient's local problem.

The ideal management of any local recurrence in the oral cavity is always surgical resection. If the patient has not had radiation and the recurrence is small, local resection with clear margins is the ideal, thereby avoiding radiation therapy. If, on the other hand, surgical resection can be performed but there are specific tumor factors that dictate radiation, and it has not been given previously, it should be administered as an adjunct to the surgery that has resected gross disease.

The most likely scenario is the patient who has received radiation in the initial treatment, and radiation, of course, cannot be used a second time—even with brachytherapy. The tissues will not withstand a second assault with radiation; if radiation is used, a chronic, nonhealing wound will result. This circumstance leaves surgery as the only alternative for recurrence in a radiated field. In this setting, the surgeon must consider the disability (and practicality) of a wide resection. This, obviously, requires a frank discussion with the patient and the patient's family about the expectations of surgical intervention. At times, even the application of the most sophisticated reconstruction will leave the patient with a significant deformity or disability.

There is little indication for chemotherapy in the management of local recurrence; but it should be considered an adjunct for both local and systemic disease.

In summary, a local recurrence should always be treated by surgical resection of gross disease with expectations of getting clear margins. If those are obtained, no more treatment is indicated. If there is a question about the margins and no radiation has previously been administered, adjunctive radiation therapy should be administered. Radiation or chemotherapy without surgical removal of the gross disease is usually doomed to failure.

PRINCIPLES OF RECONSTRUCTION

The obvious advantages to immediate reconstruction of a defect after ablation of a tumor have been recognized for more than 3 decades and are still valid today. Although these principles have been applied for many years, the techniques currently used in reconstruction have changed dramatically—use of dermal grafts, forehead flaps, and delayed flaps has moved more to multiple simultaneous free tissue transfer and customization of compound free flaps for the special tissue requirements of a particular defect.

The basic principles of reconstruction of the oral cavity and oropharynx include the following:

- Use tissue in any repair that does not compromise or limit the ablative surgery.
- Immediate reconstruction is the norm. There are few if any clinical circumstances that dictate delayed reconstruction, particularly now that most large cancers of the oral cavity and oropharynx are treated by both an ablative team and a reconstructive surgical team.
- The reconstruction should not add to the morbidity of the ablative surgery.
- Every attempt to replace "like tissue with like tissue" should be made with use of the patient's own soft tissue and bone. With the advent and widespread availability of microvascular surgery techniques and a wide variety of donor sites, this principle can be followed in most cases.
- Adapt the reconstruction to the needs of the patient.

OUTCOMES AND ECONOMIC ISSUES

As is true in other areas of surgery, cancer of the upper aerodigestive tract presents many potential opportunities for outcomes and economics research. As noted from the discussion of the numerous treatment options available, it is obvious that experienced clinicians will approach a given problem differently—be it a specific treatment modality or reconstructive option. In addition, many interventions and reconstructions are costly, and in certain settings, given the prognosis of the patient, the associated benefits have been questioned.[30]

One problem in performing outcomes research in patients with head and neck cancer rests in the tumors' clinical heterogeneity and the variability of their prognostic behaviors, making it tempting for clinicians and inexperienced researchers to combine into groups tumors that actually have little in common.[31] Other factors that affect comparison of data include concomitant medical problems, second primary cancers that are so common among these patients, elderly age, alcoholism, and other psychosocial problems. Poor compliance can also hamper the evaluation or treatment and affect reported outcomes. Compliance is an important issue in patients with these tumors; many have a history of alcoholism with its attendant social, psychological, and economic consequences. These comorbid factors, which do complicate the management of these patients, must be included in valid outcomes studies.[32-34]

Traditional factors that have been considered in outcomes studies, such as TNM stage, patient performance status, type of procedure, use of radiation therapy, local control, patient survival, and therapeutic toxicity, are an adequate start; but other variables, such as those noted in the preceding paragraph, must be considered to sharpen the data. The current outcomes and economics literature has a relatively limited number of reports applicable to cancers of the oral cavity and oropharynx.

Weymueller and Goepfert[35] have made recommendations for standardized results reporting for studies of head and neck cancer. They suggest that even in the face of traditional endpoints, there is little uniformity that is understandable or that would facilitate comparison between studies. The focus of the article is a plea to clinical researchers to report more specific and directed information on disease status, survival, patterns of recurrence, and cause of death.

Physiologic tests of speech and swallowing can provide a standardized, reproducible way to assess outcomes in patients with head and neck cancer. These measures are often integrated with psychometric assessments. In 1994, Pauloski and colleagues[36] used a standard protocol—testing speech and swallowing capability—to assess 38 patients undergoing surgical treatment of cancer of the oral cavity and oropharynx. There were preoperative measurements, and a series of postoperative studies were performed the first year after treatment. They found that improvements in both speech and swallowing plateaued by 3 months. Interestingly, 70% of the postoperative rehabilitative effort occurred during the first month.

The medical literature frequently refers to a treatment's being *cost-effective*, when, in fact, the data are primarily cost-identification analyses.[37] Few studies attempt to quantitate anything but the direct medical costs, and those are generally related to hospital charges, which usually do not reflect true cost.

Helmus and associates[38] reported on the feasibility of performing certain head and neck cancer procedures in the outpatient setting and compared those costs with the same procedures for inpatients. They reviewed the results of 200 consecutive same-day procedures during a 5-year period for parotidectomy, submandibular gland resection, miscellaneous neck procedures, transoral resection of oral cavity lesions (T1), and a variety of benign congenital lesions. Three fourths of the procedures took less than 2 hours, and 82% of the patients were discharged the same day as planned; 33 required an overnight stay. The most common reason for a required stay was a surgical start after 1 PM. The authors estimated that on the basis of the cumulative 164 successful same-day discharges, $23,000 was saved in bed charges alone.

Blair and coworkers[39] assessed the economic impact of prophylactic antibiotics in head and neck procedures. They performed a retrospective review of 192 patients who, between 1976 and 1989, received a neck dissection without exposure to the upper aerodigestive tract. Although the groups were matched for other factors (e.g., tracheotomy, prior radiation therapy, use of flap reconstruction, neck nodal stage), wound infections were three times more common in those patients who did not receive antibiotics. They then assessed cost by use of hospital charges and determined that the infection resulted in an added cost of $36,030. The charges for the prophylactic antibiotics ranged from $14,660 (clindamycin) to $46,600 (cefoperazone) per 100 patients, depending on the drug used. Their conclusion was that withholding perioperative antibiotics might not decrease overall hospital cost in this setting.

Microsurgical reconstruction is commonly used for reconstruction of major soft tissue and bone defects of the oral cavity. Miller and colleagues[40] reviewed the experience at M. D. Anderson Cancer Center in 39 consecutive free tissue transfers performed on 36 patients during a 4-year period. The complication rate leading to prolonged hospitalization was 28%. A survey of 24 of the 36 patients found that all were satisfied with their result, and most had returned to their preoperative levels of social productivity. The only cost information provided in this report was that of hospital-based direct costs. Obviously, the data provided in this report were "soft," and conclusions could only be inferred rather than deduced.

There must be an ongoing effort to further refine and improve existing outcomes research methods. Simple measures such as developing guidelines (e.g., the NCCN guidelines noted earlier) would change the physician's behavior and, it is hoped, provide definitions and communication between researchers that can provide uniformity to information reported.[23,41]

Head and neck oncology obviously provides many opportunities as well as challenges for outcomes and economic investigators. Much of this is driven by the health care system that has evolved during the 1990s and will continue to be demanded by the limited funds available for an expanding and aging population in the coming years. We would do well to place greater emphasis on uniformity of data reporting to justify expenses related to care of the patient with cancer of the upper aerodigestive tract and its associated reconstruction.

DISCLAIMER

REFERENCES

1. Parker SL, Tang T, Bolden S, et al: Cancer statistics. CA Cancer J Clin 1997;47:5.
2. Rothman K, Keller A: The effect of joint exposure to alcohol and tobacco on risk of cancer of the mouth and pharynx. J Chronic Dis 1972;25:711.
3. Slaughter DP, Southwick HW, Smejkal W: "Field cancerization" in oral stratified squamous epithelium. Clinical implications of multicentric origin. Cancer 1953;6:963.
4. Waldron CA, Shafer WG: Leukoplakia revisited: a clinicopathologic study of 3256 oral leukoplakias. Cancer 1975;36:1386.
5. Mashberg A, Samit AM: Early diagnoses of asymptomatic oral and oropharyngeal cancers. CA Cancer J Clin 1995;45:328.

6. Shah JP: Patterns of cervical lymph node metastases from squamous carcinoma of the upper aerodigestive tract. Am J Surg 1990;160:405.

7. Lindberg RD: Distribution of cervical lymph node metastasis from squamous cell carcinoma of the upper respiratory and digestive tract. Cancer 1972;29:1446.

8. Candela FC, Kothari K, Shah JP: Patterns of cervical node metastases from squamous carcinoma of the oropharynx and hypopharynx. Head Neck 1990;12:197.

9. McGregor AD, MacDonald DG: Patterns of spread of squamous cell carcinoma within the mandible. Head Neck 1989;11:457.

10. McGregor AD, MacDonald DG: Patterns of spread of squamous cell carcinoma to the ramus of the mandible. Head Neck 1993;15:440.

11. Larson DL, Sanger JR: Management of the mandible in oral cancer. Semin Surg Oncol 1995;11:190.

12. Leipzig B, Zellmer JE, Klug D: The role of endoscopy in evaluating patients with head and neck cancer. Arch Otolaryngol 1985;111:589.

13. American Joint Committee on Cancer: Manual for Staging of Cancer, 4th ed. Philadelphia, JB Lippincott, 1992.

14. Harrison LB, Sessions RB, Hong WK, eds: Head and Neck Cancer: A Multidisciplinary Approach. Philadelphia, Lippincott-Raven, 1999.

15. Johnson JT, Barnes EL, Myers EL, et al: The extracapsular spread of tumors in cervical node metastasis. Arch Otolaryngol 1981;107:725.

16. Looser KG, Shah JP, Strong EW: The significance of "positive margins" in surgically resected epidermoid cancer. Head Neck 1978;1:107.

17. Amdur RJ, Mendenhall WM, Parson JT, et al: Carcinoma of the soft palate treated with irradiation: analysis of results and complications. Radiother Oncol 1987;9:185.

18. Pernot M, Malissard L, Taghian A: Velotonsillar squamous cell carcinoma: 277 cases treated by combined external irradiation and brachytherapy—results according to extension, localization, and dose rate. Int J Radiat Oncol Phys 1992;23:715.

19. Remmler D, Medina JE, Byers RM, et al: Treatment of choice for squamous carcinoma of the tonsillar fossa. Head Neck 1985;7:206.

20. Perez CA, Purdy JA, Breaux SR, et al: Carcinoma of the tonsillar fossa: a nonrandomized comparison of preoperative radiation and surgery or irradiation alone: Long-term results. Cancer 1982;50:2314.

21. Merlano M, Vitale V, Rosso R, et al: Treatment of advanced squamous cell carcinoma of the head and neck with alternating chemotherapy and radiotherapy. N Engl J Med 1992;327:1115.

22. Shah JP, Andersen PE: The impact of patterns of neck metastases on modifications of neck dissection. Ann Surg Oncol 1994;1:521.

23. Forastiere A, Goepfert H, Gothnet D, et al: NCCN practice guidelines for head and neck cancer. National Comprehensive Cancer Network. Oncology (Huntingt) 1998;12:39.

24. Byers R, Clayman M, McGill MD, et al: Selective neck dissections for squamous cell carcinoma of the upper aerodigestive tract: patterns of regional failure. Head Neck 1999;21:499.

25. Parson JT: Time-dose-volume relationships in radiation therapy. In Million RR, Cassisi NJ, eds: Management of Head and Neck Cancer: A Multidisciplinary Approach, 2nd ed. Philadelphia, JB Lippincott, 1994:203-243.

26. Thames HD, Wither HR, Peters LJ, et al: Changes in early and late radiation responses with altered dose fractionation: implications for dose-survival relationships. Int J Radiat Biol Phys 1982;8:219.

27. Horiot JC, Fur RL, N'Guyen T, et al: Hyperfractionation vs conventional fractionation in oropharyngeal carcinoma: final analysis of a randomized trial of the EORTC Cooperative Group of Radiotherapy. Radiother Oncol 1992;25:231.

28. Puthawala AA, Syed NAM, Neblett D, et al: The role of afterloading iridium 192 implant in the management of carcinoma of the tongue. Int J Radiat Oncol Biol Phys 1981;7:407.

29. Larson DL, Lindberg R, Jesse R: Major complications of radiotherapy in cancer of the oral cavity and oropharynx. A 10-year retrospective study. Am J Surg 1983;146:531.

30. Benninger MS, Enrique RR, Nichols RD: Symptom directed selective endoscopy and cost containment for evaluation of head and neck cancer. Head Neck 1993;15:532.

31. Jacobs C: The internist in the management of head and neck cancer. Ann Intern Med 1990;113:771.

32. Greenfield S, Apolone G: The importance of coexistent disease in the occurrence of postoperative complications and one-year recovery in patients undergoing total hip replacement: comorbidity and outcomes after hip replacement. Med Care 1993;31:141.

33. Charlston ME, Pompei P, Ales HL, et al: A new method of classifying prognostic comorbidity in longitudinal studies: development and validation. J Chronic Dis 1987;40:373.

34. Kaplan MH, Feinstein AR: The importance of classifying comorbidity in evaluating the outcome of diabetes mellitus. J Chronic Dis 1974;27:387.

35. Weymueller EA, Goepfert H: Uniformity of results reporting in head and neck cancer. Head Neck 1991;13:275.

36. Pauloski BR, Logemenn JA, Rademaker AW, et al: Speech and swallowing function after oral and oropharyngeal resections: one-year follow-up. Head Neck 1994;16:313.

37. Winn RJ: Current status of practice guidelines in oncology. Oncology (Huntingt) 1995;9:601.

38. Helmus C, Grin M, Westfall R: Same day stay head and neck surgery. Laryngoscope 1992;102:1331.

39. Blair EA, Johnson JT, Wagner RL, et al: Cost analysis of antibiotic prophylaxis in clean head and neck surgery. Arch Otolaryngol Head Neck Surg 1995;121:269.

40. Miller MJ, Swartz WM, Miller RH, et al: Cost analysis of microsurgical reconstruction in the head and neck. J Surg Oncol 1991;46:230.

41. Greco PJ, Eisenberg JM: Changing physicians' practices. N Engl J Med 1993;329:1271.

110

Tumors of the Mandible

GREGORY L. BORAH, MD, DMD ✦ SHAHID R. AZIZ, MD, DMD

Identification, diagnosis, and treatment of lesions of the mandible are essential components of plastic and maxillofacial surgery. Tumors of the mandible comprise a large and complex series of pathologic entities that the World Health Organization has categorized into cysts or true tumors and then further classified as odontogenic (dental in origin) or nonodontogenic. These lesions are often found incidentally on routine dental radiographs; conversely, these lesions may present with specific symptoms. This chapter reviews lesions of the mandible potentially encountered by the surgeon, with an emphasis on clinical, radiographic, and histopathologic aspects of each coupled with differential diagnosis and treatment (Table 110-1).

Before any discussion of this topic, a basic review of dental tissue anatomy and development is necessary. The tooth is composed of a crown and root; the outer layer of the crown is composed of enamel, an extremely hard, calcified material. Below the enamel is dentin, which makes up most of the crown and root. It is a calcified organic matrix similar to bone. Within the root, under the dentin, is the dental pulp, where the nerve of each tooth is contained. The outer layer of the root is covered in cementum, an amorphous calcified substance that allows the periodontal ligament to attach; the periodontal ligament is basically a fibrous attachment between the surrounding alveolar bone and the tooth root. The tissues of the teeth are derived from two embryologic sources. The enamel is of epithelial (ectodermal) origin; the dentin, cementum, pulp (nerve), and periodontal ligament are of mesenchymal (mesodermal) origin. Tooth development commences at the sixth week of fetal life, at which time an epithelial (ectodermal) proliferation termed dental lamina develops in each of the four quadrants of the future oral cavity. These laminae then mature into enamel organs, one for each primary and permanent tooth. Adjacent to each enamel organ, the mesenchyme proliferates into a mass known as the dental papilla. The enamel organ surrounds the dental papilla, and its cells differentiate into ameloblasts, which later synthesize enamel. The developing ameloblasts stimulate the dental papillary cells to differentiate into odontoblasts, which later synthesize dentin. As this combination enamel organ-dental papilla (now known as a tooth bud) matures, it becomes surrounded by another mesenchymal proliferation, the dental follicle (dental sac), which later matures into the periodontal ligament and cementum. As the tooth bud develops, more and more enamel and dentin are laid down by ameloblasts and odontoblasts, respectively, and the crown and root of the tooth begin to take shape. The enamel organ later breaks up along the developing root; its remnants are known as the epithelial rests of Malassez. The dental papilla eventually shrinks to become the dental pulp. Once they are fully developed, the primary and permanent teeth erupt into the oral cavity at varying times of the first 10 years of life.

CYSTS OF THE MANDIBLE

The World Health Organization loosely classifies cystic neoplasms of the mandible into three groups: odontogenic cysts (which are subclassified into developmental and inflammatory), nonodontogenic cysts, and pseudocysts. A true cyst is simply defined as an epithelium-lined pathologic space. The mandible has a much higher rate of cystic development compared with the rest of the skeleton, primarily because of the

TABLE 110-1 ✦ CLASSIFICATION OF MANDIBULAR CYSTS AND TUMORS

Cystic Neoplasms

Odontogenic Cysts

Developmental
  Gingival cysts
    Newborn
    Adult
  Lateral periodontal cysts
  Dentigerous (follicular) cysts
    Eruption cyst
  Odontogenic keratocysts
    Nevoid basal cell carcinoma syndrome
  Calcifying odontogenic cyst (Gorlin cyst)
  Glandular odontogenic cyst
Inflammatory
  Radicular (periapical) cyst
  Residual cyst
  Paradental cyst

Nonodontogenic Cysts

Median mandibular cyst

Pseudocysts

Aneurysmal bone cyst
Traumatic bone cyst
Static bone cyst
Focal osteoporotic bone marrow defect

Odontogenic Tumors: Benign

Tumors of odontogenic epithelium without odontogenic
    ectomesenchyme
  Ameloblastoma
  Malignant ameloblastoma/ameloblastic carcinoma
  Pindborg tumor (calcifying epithelial odontogenic
    tumor)
  Squamous odontogenic tumor
  Clear cell odontogenic tumor
Tumors of odontogenic epithelium with odontogenic
    ectomesenchyme
  Ameloblastic fibroma
  Odontoameloblastoma
  Odontoma
  Ameloblastic fibro-odontoma
  Ameloblastic fibrosarcoma
  Adenomatoid odontogenic tumor
Tumors of odontogenic ectomesenchyme with or
    without odontogenic epithelium
  Odontogenic myxoma
  Cementoblastoma
  Cementifying fibroma
  Odontogenic fibroma
    Central
    Granular cell
    Peripheral

Odontogenic Tumors: Malignant

Odontogenic carcinoma
  Malignant ameloblastoma
  Primary intraosseous carcinoma
Odontogenic sarcoma
  Ameloblastic fibrosarcoma
  Ameloblastic fibrodentinosarcoma
  Odontogenic carcinosarcoma

Nonodontogenic Tumors

Benign osseous tumors
  Osteoma
  Osteoblastoma
  Osteoid osteoma
  Tori/exostoses
Benign fibrous and fibro-osseous tumors
  Fibrous dysplasia
  Cherubism
  Central giant cell granuloma
  Ossifying fibroma
  Histiocytosis (Langerhans cell disease)
  Chondroma
  Coronoid hyperplasia
  Chondromyxoid fibroma
  Desmoplastic fibroma
  Cemento-osseous dysplasia
    Peripheral cemental dysplasia
    Focal cemento-osseous dysplasia
    Florid osseous dysplasia
Vascular lesions
  Vascular malformations
  Hemangiomas
Neurogenic tumors
  Schwannoma
  Neuroma
  Neurofibroma

Primary Nonodontogenic Malignant Tumors of the Mandible

Osteosarcoma
  Juxtacortical
    Parosteal
    Periosteal
Chondrosarcoma
  Mesenchymal
Fibrosarcoma of bone
Ewing sarcoma
Burkitt lymphoma
Plasma cell neoplasia
  Multiple myeloma
  Solitary plasmacytoma of bone

Metastases to Mandible

uniqueness of the odontogenic epithelium found within it. Those cysts found in the mandible vary greatly in histologic features, frequency, behavior, and treatment.

Odontogenic Cysts

Odontogenic cysts are derived either from the odontogenic epithelium that is present before tooth development or from remnants of odontogenic epithelium that remain after tooth formation is complete. Odontogenic cysts are subclassified into developmental or inflammatory. Developmental cysts include gingival cysts, dentigerous cysts, odontogenic keratocysts, lateral periodontal cysts, calcified odontogenic cysts, and glandular odontogenic cysts. Inflammatory cysts include radicular, paradental, and residual cysts.[1,2]

GINGIVAL CYSTS. Gingival cysts are divided into gingival cysts of the newborn and adult. Gingival cysts of the newborn appear as multiple nodules along the alveolar ridge of the mandible in neonates. They are thought to be derived from fragments of dental lamina that proliferate in the alveolar ridge and from small keratinized cysts. On histologic evaluation, these cysts are lined by a thin epithelium; they typically rupture or spontaneously involute before 3 months of age, therefore not requiring treatment.

A gingival cyst of the adult is a rare mandibular lesion and is considered to be the soft tissue counterpart of the lateral periodontal cyst. It is derived from the dental lamina. Clinically, 60% to 75% of cases appear in the facial-buccal aspect to the canine or premolar region of the mandible, often in patients in the fifth to sixth decade, with a slightly higher incidence in women. These cysts are painless, dome-like firm swellings about 0.5 cm in diameter, often with a blue-gray color. On histologic evaluation, gingival cysts of the adult contain an epithelial lining with a thin layer of keratinized or nonkeratinized squamous epithelium. Differential diagnosis includes fibroma, pyogenic granuloma, parulis, and peripheral giant cell granuloma. Treatment is typically surgical excision without recurrence.[3,4]

LATERAL PERIODONTAL CYST. The lateral periodontal cyst is a nonkeratinized developmental odontogenic cyst that occurs lateral to the root of a tooth. These lesions make up less than 3% of lined jaw cysts. The origin of the lateral periodontal cyst is unclear; however, it is hypothesized to originate from a proliferation of rests of the dental lamina that lie within the bone (unlike the gingival cyst of the adult, which arises from rests in the soft tissue of the oral cavity). Clinically, the lateral periodontal cyst is asymptomatic, associated with vital teeth, and most commonly diagnosed as an incidental finding on routine dental radiographic examination. It is most commonly found in

association with either the mandibular canine or the premolar teeth. There is a significant male predilection, with a male-to-female ratio of 2 : 1; the lateral periodontal cyst is usually seen in patients older than 30 years (mean age at occurrence, 50 years). It typically appears as painless, small, bluish soft tissue swellings in the interdental papilla of the gingiva. Conversely, it may not be clinically apparent. On radiographic examination, the lateral periodontal cyst appears as a well-circumscribed unilocular radiolucency lateral to the roots of teeth; as it enlarges, this cyst can rarely cause divergence of tooth roots. On histologic evaluation, the lateral periodontal cyst is lined by a thin nonkeratinized squamous epithelium; clusters of glycogen-rich clear epithelial cells may be noted in the cyst lining. Differential diagnosis includes odontogenic keratocyst, myxoma, glandular odontogenic cyst, and ameloblastoma. Definitive diagnosis is made histologically because the clinical findings of lateral periodontal cyst are identical to those of other mandibular cysts. Treatment usually involves local excision (conservative enucleation). Recurrence is rare.[5,6]

Botryoid Odontogenic Cyst. On occasion, lateral periodontal cysts may be multilocular; this is known as the botryoid odontogenic cyst. On radiographic examination, a multilocular radiolucency is noted lateral to tooth roots. Histologic evaluation of these lesions shows a grape-like cluster of small individual cysts. Botryoid cysts are considered to result from cystic degeneration and subsequent fusion of adjacent foci of dental lamina rests. Treatment consists of enucleation.

DENTIGEROUS CYSTS. The dentigerous cyst is a fluid-filled space of variable size located between the crown of an impacted or unerupted tooth and the epithelial lining of the pericoronal dental follicle. It is the most common developmental odontogenic cyst, making up 20% of all mandibular cysts. It occurs most often around impacted mandibular third molars of adolescents and young adults; however, dentigerous cysts may be found around any impacted or unerupted tooth at any age. The dentigerous cyst encloses the impacted tooth's crown and is attached to the tooth at the cementum-enamel junction. The cyst forms when fluid accumulates between reduced enamel epithelium and the tooth crown.

Dentigerous cysts most commonly affect patients between the ages of 10 and 30 years, with a slight male predilection; in addition, they occur more commonly in white individuals than in other ethnic groups. Because they are typically asymptomatic, dentigerous cysts are usually diagnosed on routine dental radiographs. Although typically small in size, these cysts can enlarge, causing bone expansion or pathologic fracture. As the dentigerous cyst increases in size, the risk for subsequent infection increases as well; when infected, these cysts become painful, with associated erythema and swelling. Dentigerous cysts can also, in contact with adjacent tooth roots, cause root resorption.[7]

On radiographic examination, the dentigerous cyst is typically a well-defined unilocular radiolucency associated with the crown of an impacted or unerupted tooth. These cysts can be classified on the basis of their radiographic presentation as central, lateral, or circumferential. Central dentigerous cysts surround the crown of the tooth and are the most common type. The lateral variant grows alongside the root of the tooth and partially surrounds the crown of the tooth; mesioangular impacted third molars usually display this radiographic appearance. Circumferential dentigerous cysts surround both the crown and root of the affected tooth. On histologic evaluation, dentigerous cysts may or may not display inflammation. If it is not inflamed, the dentigerous cyst reveals a fibrous connective tissue wall containing glycosaminoglycan ground substance. The epithelial lining consists of two to four layers of cuboidal epithelial cells. In the inflamed type, the fibrous wall is more collagenized with a variable infiltration of chronic inflammatory cells. The epithelial lining shows hyperplasia with the development of rete ridges and squamous features. A keratinized surface is sometimes seen. Differential diagnosis includes odontogenic keratocyst, ameloblastoma, adenomatoid odontogenic tumor, and ameloblastic fibroma (Fig. 110-1).[8]

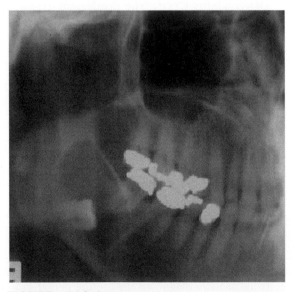

FIGURE 110-1. Well-circumscribed radiolucency associated with an impacted lower right third molar. Differential diagnosis includes odontogenic cyst versus odontogenic tumor. Biopsy revealed this lesion to be consistent with a dentigerous cyst.

The diagnosis of dentigerous cyst is based on a combination of radiographic and histologic features. The usual treatment is careful enucleation of the cyst together with removal of the unerupted or impacted tooth. If eruption of the involved tooth is feasible, enucleation alone is performed. Larger dentigerous cysts may also be treated by marsupialization, which allows decompression of the cyst. The cyst can then be excised at a later date with a less extensive surgical procedure.[9]

Provided that complete excision of the dentigerous cyst is performed, prognosis is excellent and recurrence rare. Untreated dentigerous cysts rarely undergo transformation into ameloblastoma, squamous cell carcinoma, or intraosseous mucoepidermoid carcinoma.

Eruption Cyst. The eruption cyst is a dentigerous cyst that results from fluid accumulation within the follicular space of an erupting tooth. Clinically, an eruption cyst is a soft translucent swelling in the gingiva overlying an unerupted tooth (deciduous or permanent). Most commonly, these cysts occur in children younger than 10 years. Trauma to the area may result in bloody accumulation into the cyst, causing the swelling to appear purple-brown. This is referred to as an eruption hematoma. Treatment is not usually required because the cyst spontaneously ruptures as the tooth erupts. However, if this does not occur, marsupialization of the cyst is recommended.

ODONTOGENIC KERATOCYSTS. Odontogenic keratocysts are developmental odontogenic cysts that arise from the remnants of the dental lamina. What makes odontogenic keratocysts different from other mandibular cysts is that these cysts show a high frequency of recurrence. Odontogenic keratocysts make up 10% to 12% of all developmental odontogenic cysts.[10]

Odontogenic keratocysts can be found in any age range; however, the majority of cases occur between the ages of 10 and 40 years; males are more commonly affected than are females. Whereas odontogenic keratocysts occur in either jaw, there is a 3:1 preference for the mandible compared with the maxilla. The posterior body and ascending ramus of the mandible are most commonly affected. The odontogenic keratocyst presents radiographically as a well-circumscribed unilocular radiolucency with radiopaque margins. Larger lesions are often multilocular. Up to 40% of odontogenic keratocysts are associated with the crown of an unerupted tooth, mimicking the radiographic appearance of a dentigerous cyst. Approximately 50% of mandibular odontogenic keratocysts cause buccal plate expansion of the mandible but rarely lingual plate involvement.[11]

Small odontogenic keratocysts are asymptomatic and found only during routine dental radiographic examination. Larger odontogenic keratocysts may also be asymptomatic or may cause pain, swelling, or bone expansion. Definitive diagnosis is based on biopsy findings. On histologic evaluation, the epithelial lining is thin, usually 8 to 10 cells thick, made up primarily of parakeratinized stratified squamous epithelium with a palisading basal layer of columnar or cuboidal hyperchromatic cells. There is often some adherence of the cyst to the surrounding connective tissue stroma. Five percent of odontogenic keratocysts present with an orthokeratinized epithelium. Compared with parakeratinized odontogenic keratocysts, orthokeratinized cysts are less aggressive and have a much lower recurrence rate. Therefore, it is important to verify which variant of odontogenic keratocyst is being treated from a prognostic standpoint.[12]

Differential diagnosis often depends on the position of the odontogenic keratocyst in association with adjacent teeth. An odontogenic keratocyst surrounding an unerupted tooth may resemble a dentigerous cyst; on the lateral aspect of a tooth root, it may resemble a lateral periodontal cyst on radiographic examination; finally, if it occurs at the apices of teeth, it resembles the radiographic appearance of a radicular cyst (however, unlike with a radicular cyst, the associated teeth are vital). Other differential diagnoses include ameloblastoma, calcified odontogenic cyst, and adenomatoid odontogenic tumor.

The treatment of most odontogenic keratocysts is standard enucleation and curettage. Complete removal of the cyst is essential to minimize the recurrence risk. This can pose a challenge to the clinician because some odontogenic keratocysts adhere to the surrounding tissue. Some surgeons therefore prefer to treat odontogenic keratocysts more aggressively by either a peripheral ostectomy or resection of cyst, surrounding bone, and any associated teeth. Odontogenic keratocysts, compared with other odontogenic cysts, have a much higher recurrence rate after treatment, ranging from 5% to 62% in different studies. Why recurrence develops is unclear; it may potentially be secondary to residual odontogenic keratocyst tissue after treatment, or a new odontogenic keratocyst may develop de novo. Although most recur within 5 years of initial treatment, recurrence is possible at any time after surgery. Therefore, long-term clinical and radiographic follow-up is warranted. In patients with multiple odontogenic keratocysts, it is necessary to rule out nevoid basal cell carcinoma syndrome (Gorlin syndrome), which occurs in 7% of patients with multiple odontogenic keratocysts. Inherited as an autosomal dominant trait with a high penetrance, the genetic basis for this syndrome is associated with chromosome 9, located at q22.3. Nevoid basal cell carcinoma syndrome clinically comprises bifid ribs, vertebral abnormalities, and multiple basal cell skin carcinomas in addition to the multiple odontogenic keratocysts. There is also palmar and plantar pitting

and dermal calcinosis. Facial abnormalities including prognathism, hypertelorism, and dystopia canthorum may be noted. Uncommon neurologic findings are also rarely noted: medulloblastoma, calcified falx cerebri or falx cerebelli, and dysgenesis of the corpus callosum (Fig. 110-2).

GLANDULAR ODONTOGENIC CYST. The glandular odontogenic cyst (sialo-odontogenic cyst) is an exceptionally rare cyst first described in 1987. The glandular odontogenic cyst is an entity sharing features of odontogenic cysts and also mucin-producing salivary gland tumors. This lesion is typically found in the anterior mandible with associated pain and expansion as the only symptoms. Whereas the glandular odontogenic cyst can occur at any age, its incidence peaks in the fifth decade of life. It occurs equally in both sexes. This lesion is noted radiographically to be a uniloculated or multiloculated well-circumscribed radiolucency with a wide variation in size. Some enlarge to the point of eroding through the cortical plate. On histopathologic study, this lesion resembles both the lateral periodontal cyst and the salivary gland tumor mucoepidermoid carcinoma. The glandular odontogenic cyst is lined by stratified squamous nonkeratinized epithelium, usually cuboidal with cilia. Pools of mucin and clear cells are often scattered throughout. Treatment includes peripheral curettage or marginal excision. Long-term follow-up is necessary because up to 25% recur.[13-15]

CALCIFIED ODONTOGENIC CYST (GORLIN CYST). Calcified odontogenic cyst (Gorlin cyst) is an uncommon developmental odontogenic lesion that resembles a true cyst but has the aggressive behavior of a neoplasm, giving the description "ghost cell neoplasm." In addition, calcified odontogenic cysts are often associated with odontomas, adenomatoid odontogenic tumors, or ameloblastomas. The calcified odontogenic cyst is thought to arise from odontogenic epithelial remnants within the gingiva. Clinically, this cyst is typically an intraosseous lesion, but up to 20% can occur in the oral soft tissues. Approximately 65% of calcified odontogenic cysts are found in the canine and incisor region of the maxilla and mandible. This lesion can occur at any age (mean age, 35 years). Calcified odontogenic cyst also has a female predilection. It may present radiographically as a unilocular or multilocular well-circumscribed radiolucency, often with focal areas of radiopaque calcification in the lumen.[16] On histopathologic evaluation, most calcified odontogenic cysts present as a cyst contained in a fibrous capsule with a lining of odontogenic epithelium 4 to 10 cells thick. The basal cell layer is often cuboidal or columnar. The characteristic histologic feature is ghost cells—anuclear epithelial cells that retain the outline of the cell membrane. Ghost cells are thought to arise from either coagulative necrosis

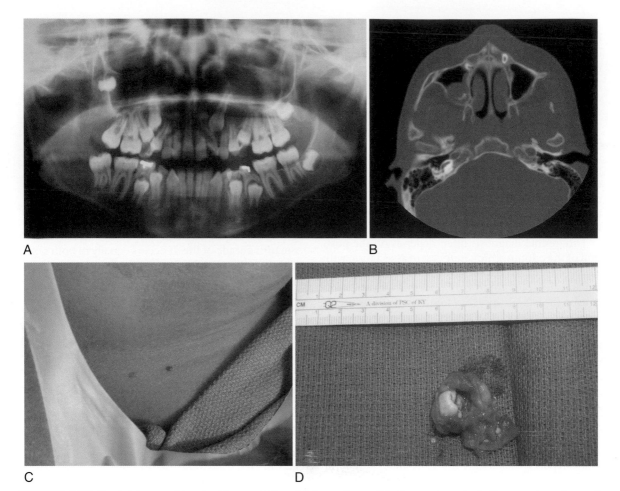

FIGURE 110-2. A 14-year-old girl with nevoid basal cell syndrome (Gorlin syndrome). *A,* Panoramic radiograph demonstrating an impacted upper right third molar in the maxillary sinus with a cyst associated with it. *B,* Axial computed tomogram of lesion. *C,* Basal cell carcinomas on neck. *D,* Tooth removed from sinus with keratocyst attached.

of epithelial cells or aberrant keratinization of odontogenic epithelium.[17]

Differential diagnosis depends on the age of the lesion. Newly developed calcified odontogenic cysts are usually radiolucent only, therefore resembling dentigerous cysts and ameloblastomas on radiographic evaluation. In later stages, there is some radiopacity in the lumen of the calcified odontogenic cyst, mimicking the appearance of an odontoma, calcifying epithelial odontogenic tumor, or adenomatoid odontogenic tumor. Calcified odontogenic cyst has the potential to undergo malignant transformation into odontogenic ghost cell carcinoma; as a result, treatment is usually aggressive excision of the lesion because of its unpredictable behavior. Recurrences are rare.[18]

INFLAMMATORY ODONTOGENIC CYSTS

RADICULAR CYSTS. Radicular cysts are the most common cysts of the jaws. They are inflammatory

odontogenic cysts, the end result of the necrosis of the dental pulp, usually from infection. Originating as dental caries (localized infection of the crown of a tooth), this infection slowly spreads apically with necrosis of the dental pulp, rendering the tooth nonvital. As the degradation products of the necrotic pulp travel through the apex of the nonvital tooth, a focus of chronically inflamed fibrous tissue develops, termed a periapical dental granuloma. This granuloma in turn gives rise to the radicular cyst. The inflammation within the granuloma is thought to stimulate the residual odontogenic epithelium in the apex of the tooth, creating the epithelial lining of the radicular cyst. Within the cyst cavity are fluid and cellular debris; as tooth necrosis continues, the osmotic pressure of the cyst lumen increases, causing enlargement of the cyst with resorption of adjacent bone.[19]

Radicular cysts are usually found between the third and sixth decades of life; men are more commonly affected than are women. By definition, they are found in association with a nonvital tooth. Because the dental pulp of the tooth has degenerated, radicular cysts are typically asymptomatic. If the cyst reaches a large size, periapical swelling is seen as well as mobility of adjacent teeth as surrounding bone is resorbed. The radicular cyst averages 1.5 cm in diameter, although it can become larger.

These cysts appear radiographically as well-circumscribed radiolucent lesions at the apex of a nonvital tooth; they are usually round to ovoid. On histologic evaluation, the radicular cyst is lined by nonkeratinized stratified squamous epithelium of variable thickness. In the lumen of the cyst is found cellular debris as well as inflammatory blood cells, polymorphic nuclear cells, and macrophages; dystrophic calcification, cholesterol clefts, and hemosiderin pigmentation may also be found.

Treatment of radicular cysts is initially conservative nonsurgical endodontic therapy, which removes the inflammatory stimulus that causes the cyst. If this fails to resolve the periapical radiolucency in 4 to 6 months, more aggressive surgical endodontic treatment may be considered, such as resection of the apex of the tooth and cyst (apicoectomy and cystectomy). If, in turn, this treatment fails to resolve the radicular cyst, extraction of the tooth with subsequent curettage of the periapical cyst is the definitive therapy. If the nonvital tooth is extracted but the associated radicular cyst is left untouched, a residual cyst develops. Residual cysts have the potential of expanding and causing surrounding bone destruction. Treatment is identical to that of the radicular cyst—curettage. With proper therapy, the cyst does not recur.[20]

PARADENTAL CYST. The paradental cyst represents a cystic change of the rests of Malassez caused by inflammation around the crowns of erupting mandibular molars. It typically arises in the buccal aspect of a vital molar tooth in an area of inflammation, commonly the bifurcation or trifurcation of the roots. On radiographic examination, it is a well circumscribed radiolucency. Clinically, the paradental cyst occurs in adolescents around the time the mandibular molar teeth erupt (6 to 12 years of age); symptoms include pain, localized swelling, and drainage of pus from an associated periodontal pocket. On histopathologic evaluation, the paradental cyst contains nonkeratinized stratified squamous epithelium surrounded by inflammatory connective tissue. Surgical excision (enucleation and thorough curettage) is the treatment of choice.[21,22]

Nonodontogenic Cysts

Whereas there are multiple cysts not of dental origin in the maxilla, the mandible has only one questionable entity that falls into this category, the median

mandibular cyst. At one time, this lesion was thought to be a fissural cyst in the symphysis of the mandible that arose from epithelial entrapment during fusion of the halves of the mandible in embryologic development. However, it is now known that the mandible develops as a single mesenchymal unit with a central isthmus at midline. Therefore, the median mandibular cyst is not fissural in origin; its true origin remains unknown, although the current thinking is leaning toward an odontogenic source. The median mandibular cyst is clinically asymptomatic and incidentally noted on routine dental films. The median mandibular cyst appears radiographically as a midline lucency apical to the central incisors. On histologic evaluation, the epithelium is stratified squamous. Treatment is enucleation (Fig. 110-3).[23]

Pseudocysts

Pseudocysts comprise a group of lesions that resemble true cysts; however, because they lack an epithelial lining, these lesions are considered false cysts. There are four pseudocysts that are found in the mandible: aneurysmal bone cyst, simple (traumatic) bone cyst, static bone cyst, and focal osteoporotic bone marrow defect.

ANEURYSMAL BONE CYST. The aneurysmal bone cyst is a benign lesion of bone; approximately 5% arise in the maxillofacial skeleton. This lesion is composed of a septated blood-filled cavity containing a fibrous connective tissue lining. The etiology and pathogenesis are unclear; however, the aneurysmal bone cyst is thought to be a reactive process. There is controversy as to whether this lesion arises de novo or is secondary to a vascular "accident" in a preexisting intrabone lesion, such as fibrous dysplasia or ossifying fibroma. The majority of aneurysmal bone cysts occur in patients younger than 30 years; incidence peaks in the second decade of life. There is a slight female predilection. In the mandible, 40% occur in the body, 30% in the ramus, 9% at the angle, 9% at the symphysis, and 2% at the condyle. Pain is sometimes associated, and a firm pulsatile swelling is frequently noted. Approximately 20% of aneurysmal bone cysts are associated with bone disease elsewhere in the body (central giant cell tumor, osteoblastoma, fibrous dysplasia).[24-26]

On radiographic examination, aneurysmal bone cyst appears as a unilocular or multilocular radiolucent lesion associated with cortical bone expansion and thinning. It is characterized histopathologically as a blood-filled space surrounded by fibroblastic tissue. Within this fibrous tissue are multinucleated giant cells and trabeculae of osteoid and woven bone. Differential diagnosis includes odontogenic keratocyst, central giant cell granuloma, and ameloblastic fibroma. Traditional treatment involves curettage; however, this

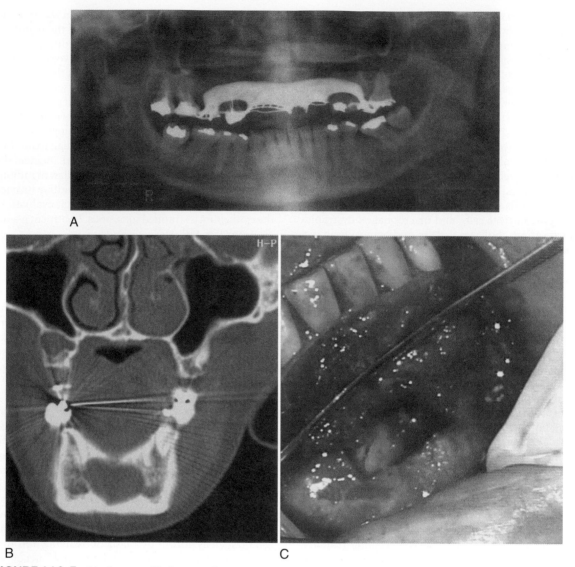

FIGURE 110-3. Median mandibular cyst. *A,* Panoramic radiograph. *B,* Coronal computed tomographic view. *C,* Intraoperative view of surgical site.

is associated with a 20% to 60% recurrence rate. Therefore, excision with supplemental cryotherapy is preferred, with an 8% recurrence rate.

SIMPLE BONE CYST. The simple bone cyst, also known as the traumatic bone cyst, is an intrabone dead space. Although uncommon in the mandible, it occurs frequently in the long bones. Its cause is unproven; however, it is assumed to be associated with a traumatic event to the affected bone. It is hypothesized that a traumatically induced hematoma develops within an intramedullary portion of bone; in lieu of resolving and allowing bone replacement, the hematoma creates an empty bone cavity. The simple bone cyst most commonly develops in teenagers, and it may arise in any portion of the mandible; it is

typically unilateral but can occur bilaterally. There is a slight male predilection. Swelling occasionally occurs; however, simple bone cysts tend to be painless. A well-circumscribed radiolucency with scalloped borders is seen radiographically. Differential diagnosis includes lateral periodontal cyst, central giant cell granuloma, and ameloblastic fibroma. Treatment is usually limited to opening of the cavity and allowing bleeding within it, with subsequent closure of the overlying gingiva. The resulting blood clot usually resolves by bone repair, filling in the dead space.[27,28]

STATIC BONE CYST. Static bone cyst is an anatomic landmark on the facial (buccal) aspect of the angle of the mandible, where the ramus and body meet. This developmental depression is thought to be due to entrapment of the submandibular salivary gland during mandibular development. It is a painless lesion, typically found on panoramic film of the mandible. On radiographic examination, static bone cyst is a well-circumscribed oval radiolucency inferior to the inferior alveolar nerve canal. No treatment is required.

FOCAL OSTEOPOROTIC BONE MARROW DEFECT. The final mandibular pseudocyst is the focal osteoporotic bone marrow defect, a localized radiolucency in the posterior mandible. It has a significant female predilection (70% are found in women). Its pathogenesis is uncertain; however, because this defect occurs in areas of extracted teeth, it is thought to be related to abnormal bone healing in the extraction site. Biopsy is required for definitive diagnosis; no treatment is required.[29]

ODONTOGENIC TUMORS

Odontogenic tumors encompass a diverse spectrum of lesions, including malformations, hamartomas, and neoplasms. The World Health Organization divides odontogenic tumors into benign and malignant. Benign tumors are further subdivided on the basis of the histologic tissue of origin (epithelial, mesenchymal, or both). Malignant tumors obviously require aggressive surgical intervention coupled with radiation therapy and chemotherapy. Benign tumors are surgically important from both a physical and neoplastic standpoint. These tumors often enlarge to the point that they interfere with function or cause unsatisfactory aesthetics. In addition, some have the potential to undergo malignant transformation.[30,31]

Odontogenic tumors are often asymptomatic, discovered incidentally. Therefore, proper imaging and biopsy (incisional, excisional, or frozen section) are required for definitive diagnosis. Imaging modalities include basic dental radiography (periapical, occlusal, and orthopantomographic), computed tomography, and magnetic resonance imaging. From these studies, a differential diagnosis may be developed and a treatment plan formed. The goals of surgical management of odontogenic tumors are the eradication of the lesion, preservation of normal tissue, and restoration of function. On the basis of the biopsy diagnosis, surgical intervention ranges from conservative excision (curettage and enucleation) to radical ablation with reconstruction. Ideally, surgical treatment maintains the aforementioned goals and minimizes the risk of recurrence. A properly planned resection-reconstruction is preferred to multiple smaller surgeries.[32-34]

Benign Odontogenic Tumors

Odontogenic tumors originate from epithelium and mesenchyme, which are part of the tooth-forming apparatus. Benign odontogenic tumors are often clinically asymptomatic; however, they can cause jaw expansion, movement of teeth, and bone loss. They are a diverse group of lesions, each with unique characteristics. Benign odontogenic tumors are classified on the basis of their tissue of origin and are divided into three classes: tumors of odontogenic epithelium only, tumors of odontogenic ectomesenchyme only, and tumors containing both ectomesenchyme and odontogenic epithelium.

TUMORS OF ODONTOGENIC EPITHELIUM ONLY

AMELOBLASTOMAS. Ameloblastomas are benign, locally aggressive tumors whose importance lies in their potential to grow to enormous size with resulting bone deformity. Ameloblastomas originate from epithelium within the jaws that is involved with the formation of teeth: enamel organ, odontogenic rests of Malassez, reduced enamel epithelium, and odontogenic cyst lining. Ameloblastomas occur in adults (mean age, 40 years). They are most commonly found in the molar-ramus region of the mandible. There is no gender predilection. Ameloblastomas are usually asymptomatic and found on routine dental radiographs; however, they may also present with jaw expansion. On radiographic examination, ameloblastomas can be either unilocular or multilocular with well-circumscribed margins. Their slow-growing nature may cause movement of tooth roots or root resorption.[35]

Ameloblastomas are typically differentiated into unicystic intraosseous, multilocular (solid) intraosseous (80% to 90% of all ameloblastomas), and peripheral.[36] The solid subtype is considered the most aggressive of the three and subsequently requires more aggressive treatment. It also has a higher recurrence rate (50% to 90%) if it is treated by curettage alone. There are several histologic patterns in solid ameloblastomas. Some display a single pattern; others display multiple patterns in the same lesion. The most common pattern is the follicular type, which is composed of islands of tumor cells that mimic the normal dental follicle. The plexiform pattern consists of long cords of odontogenic epithelium bound by columnar or cuboidal ameloblastic-like cells. In the acanthomatous pattern, squamous metaplasia and keratin formation arise within the ameloblastoma. In the granular cell pattern, the ameloblastic epithelial cells transform into cells filled with eosinophilic granules, giving rise to a "granular cell ameloblastoma" considered to be a more aggressive variant. The desmoplastic variant of ameloblastoma contains small islands and cords of odontogenic epithelium in a densely collagenized stroma. This form occurs most commonly in the anterior jaw and, unlike other ameloblastomas, has a mixed radiolucent and radiopaque appearance; as a result, it is often mistaken for a fibro-osseous lesion. The basaloid variant is the least common type; these lesions are composed of nests of uniform basaloid cells.

Differential diagnosis of the solid ameloblastoma is based on age, location, and radiographic features. The differential diagnosis includes odontogenic tumors, cysts, and benign nonodontogenic lesions (central giant cell granuloma, ossifying fibroma) (Fig. 110-4).[37,38]

Unicystic ameloblastoma makes up about 15% of all ameloblastomas. The etiology is uncertain, but it is thought to arise either de novo or as a neoplastic transformation of an existing odontogenic cyst. Clinically, unicystic ameloblastomas are seen in younger patients preoperatively compared with the solid variant; diagnosis often occurs in the second to third decade of life. These lesions are usually asymptomatic and found in the posterior mandible. On radiographic examination, unicystic ameloblastomas are well-circumscribed radiolucencies. Because they often occur in the posterior mandible adjacent to impacted third molars, unicystic ameloblastomas often resemble dentigerous cysts on radiographic examination.

There are three histopathologic types of unicystic ameloblastoma: luminal, intraluminal, and mural. The luminal unicystic ameloblastoma is confined to the luminal surface of the cyst. It consists of a fibrous cyst wall with an ameloblastic epithelial lining. The intraluminal ameloblastoma is a variant in which one or more nodules of ameloblastoma project from cystic lining into the lumen of the cyst. In the third variant, the mural ameloblastoma, the fibrous wall of the cyst is infiltrated by typical follicular or plexiform ameloblastoma.

The third and final class of ameloblastoma is the peripheral ameloblastoma, which accounts for 1% of all ameloblastomas. It is thought to be caused by odontogenic epithelial rests beneath the oral mucosa. Peripheral ameloblastoma presents clinically as a painless nonulcerated sessile or pedunculated mass of the alveolar gingiva in the incisor-premolar region. There is a predilection for both white individuals and men; the average age at diagnosis is 50 years. The highest frequency of occurrence is in the fifth to sixth decade. Any histologic pattern of solid ameloblastoma can be noted in the peripheral variant, but the most common is the acanthomatous pattern. The peripheral ameloblastoma is not aggressive. It typically remains in the gingiva without invasion of underlying bone. Treatment is limited to local surgical excision. Recurrence rates approach 8%.

Basic management of all ameloblastomas is based on the potential for malignant change and the significant localized damage of hard tissues as the tumor enlarges. The goal of treatment is the total removal of the tumor to minimize recurrence. Curettage and enucleation are associated with recurrence (solid, 55% to 100%; unicystic, 18% to 25%; peripheral, 8%). Therefore, resection is often preferred. After resection, safe margins are 2 cm for treatment of solid ameloblastomas and about 1 to 1.5 cm for unicystic and peripheral ameloblastomas. The inferior alveolar nerve should be sacrificed if it is involved in the lesion. Immediate reconstruction can be performed only if there are documented clean margins. If this is not immediately feasible, reconstruction should wait until surgically negative margins are verified.

Because the presentation of unicystic ameloblastoma is typically identical to that of an odontogenic cyst, treatment is identical: enucleation initially, with the specimen sent for biopsy. If the pathologic examination reveals unicystic ameloblastoma limited to the

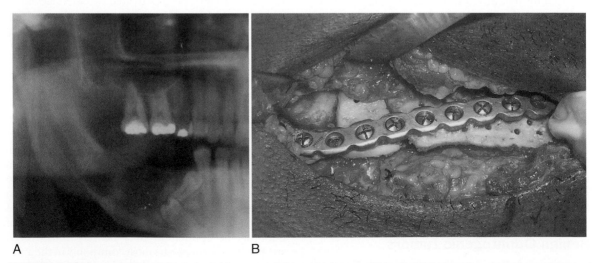

A   B

FIGURE 110-4. *A,* Radiograph of ameloblastoma, right posterior mandible. *B,* Intraoperative view of resection and reconstruction of mandibular defect with posterior iliac crest bone graft.

lumen of the cyst, the initial enucleation is satisfactory. However, if the tumor extends into or beyond the cystic wall, more aggressive treatment is required to minimize recurrence, usually peripheral ostectomy. Recurrence is significantly less for unicystic ameloblastoma than for its multicystic counterpart after enucleation.

Less than 1% of ameloblastomas undergo malignant change with subsequent metastases. These lesions have been noted clinically in patients between 4 and 75 years of age, with a peak incidence during the third to fourth decade of life. Metastases from ameloblastomas are most often found in the lungs and to a lesser extent in the cervical lymph nodes. Spread to vertebrae and viscera has also been documented. Malignant transformation of ameloblastomas is divided into two groups: malignant ameloblastomas, in which the primary and metastatic lesions are well differentiated and histologically resemble multicystic ameloblastoma; and ameloblastic carcinoma, which is less well differentiated. On radiographic examination, both types are poorly defined radiolucencies with evidence of cortical destruction. Prognosis is poor.[39,40]

CALCIFYING EPITHELIAL ODONTOGENIC TUMOR (PINDBORG TUMOR). Calcifying epithelial odontogenic tumor (Pindborg tumor) is a rare benign lesion that represents less than 1% of all odontogenic tumors. It is most often found in patients between 30 and 50 years of age, equally between both sexes. Calcifying epithelial odontogenic tumor most commonly occurs in the posterior mandible and presents as a painless, slowly growing swelling. On radiographic examination, the tumor shows a unilocular or multilocular radiolucent defect with scalloped margins. On occasion, there may be calcified foci within the tumor, giving it a mixed radiolucent and opaque appearance. The multilocular variant has a honeycombed pattern. Commonly, calcifying epithelial odontogenic tumors are associated with impacted mandibular third molars. On histologic evaluation, calcifying epithelial odontogenic tumor has distinct islands, strands, or sheets of polyhedral epithelial cells in a fibrous stroma, often with varying amounts of amyloid. These epithelial cells contain nuclei that vary in size and shape. Some nuclei are huge and may be multinucleated. Differential diagnosis includes dentigerous cysts, odontogenic keratocysts, ameloblastomas, and odontogenic myxoma. If the calcifying epithelial odontogenic tumor appears as a mixed radiolucent and opaque lesion, differential diagnosis includes calcified odontogenic cyst, adenomatoid odontogenic tumor, and ossifying fibroma. Treatment includes local resection; recurrence rates are around 15%.[41-43]

SQUAMOUS ODONTOGENIC TUMOR. Squamous odontogenic tumor is a rare, benign, locally invasive odontogenic neoplasm that arises from the neoplastic transformation of the epithelial rests of Malassez. The tumor appears to originate from within the periodontal ligament associated with the lateral root surface of an erupted tooth. The mean age at occurrence is 37 years; however, this neoplasm can occur at any age. There is no gender or race predilection. The tumor can occur in either jaw equally. Clinically, there may be alveolar bone loss with mobility of teeth. Squamous odontogenic tumor appears radiographically as a small triangular radiolucent defect lateral to the roots of teeth that is often mistaken for vertical periodontal bone loss. On histologic evaluation, squamous odontogenic tumor consists of squamous epithelium in a fibrous connective tissue stroma. Treatment includes conservative local excision or curettage. Recurrence is rare.[44,45]

CLEAR CELL ODONTOGENIC TUMOR. Clear cell odontogenic tumor is a rare, potentially malignant jaw tumor that is odontogenic in origin. Most cases are diagnosed in women (4:1 female-to-male ratio) after the fifth decade of life, and patients usually complain of pain and bone swelling; however, clear cell odontogenic tumor can be asymptomatic. Rarely, clear cell odontogenic tumor may present as sudden, rapid jaw enlargement with soft tissue extension. The anterior mandible is the most common site of occurrence. The clear cell odontogenic tumor presents radiographically as a radiolucent unilocular or multilocular lesion with poorly defined borders; adjacent tooth root resorption may be noted. Clear cell odontogenic tumor has a variable histologic appearance. Some consist of varying sized nests of epithelial cells with a clear eosinophilic cytoplasm; thin strands of hyalinized connective tissue separate the clear cell nests. Another pattern displays cords of hyperchromatic basaloid epithelial cells in a fibrous stroma. These cords contain clear cells. Metastasis to lungs and regional lymph nodes may occur. Clear cell odontogenic tumors are aggressive, with invasion of adjacent structures. Therefore, equally aggressive surgery is indicated. Involved neural tissue should be resected as well. Pulmonary or lymphatic metastasis may occur. Follow-up is essential.[46-48]

TUMORS OF ODONTOGENIC EPITHELIUM WITH ODONTOGENIC ECTOMESENCHYME

These are a group of mixed odontogenic tumors composed of odontogenic epithelium in a cellular ectomesenchyme. They vary from non-neoplastic lesions to true neoplasms.

AMELOBLASTIC FIBROMA. Ameloblastic fibroma is a true benign mixed tumor in which the epithelial and mesenchymal tissues are both neoplastic. These lesions occur in younger patients; diagnosis is typically made before the age of 20 years, with a slight male predilection. Ameloblastic fibromas are usually asymptomatic, causing painless swelling of jaws, unless they are large; 70% occur in the posterior mandible. On radiographic examination, these lesions can be either unilocular or multilocular radiolucencies with well-defined sclerotic margins; 50% are associated with an unerupted tooth, resembling a dentigerous cyst.

On histologic evaluation, ameloblastic fibroma is composed of cell-rich mesenchymal tissue consistent with dental papilla with odontogenic epithelium mixed in. A connective tissue capsule is frequently present. Differential diagnosis includes ameloblastoma, odontogenic myxoma, odontogenic keratocyst, central giant cell granuloma, and histiocytosis. Treatment is generally conservative local excision; however, there is a 20% recurrence rate. Larger lesions (7 to 8 cm) require resection. There may be cause for more aggressive treatment of all ameloblastic fibromas because up to 45% of ameloblastic fibrosarcomas arise from incompletely treated ameloblastic fibromas.

Ameloblastic Fibro-odontoma. Ameloblastic fibro-odontoma is similar to ameloblastic fibroma; however, it also contains enamel and dentin. Some believe that this lesion represents a developing odontoma. Ameloblastic fibro-odontoma can grow to enormous size, causing significant bone destruction. Clinically, ameloblastic fibro-odontoma occurs in children and is typically diagnosed by 10 years of age. It is asymptomatic and found on routine dental radiographs. As it enlarges, painless mandibular swelling may occur. On radiographic examination, ameloblastic fibro-odontoma is a well-circumscribed unilocular radiolucency containing multiple radiopacities. An erupting tooth is often associated. Ameloblastic fibro-odontoma is histologically identical to ameloblastic fibroma. Differential diagnosis includes calcifying epithelial odontogenic tumor, calcified odontogenic cyst, and odontoma. Treatment is conservative curettage and enucleation with virtually no recurrence.[49,50]

Adenomatoid Odontogenic Tumor. Adenomatoid odontogenic tumor represents 3% to 7% of all odontogenic tumors and is derived from enamel organ epithelium. It is a benign, nonaggressive tumor primarily found in patients younger than 20 years, with a slight female predilection. It usually occurs in the anterior jaws, in the maxilla more often than in the mandible. Adenomatoid odontogenic tumors are typically small (<3 cm), asymptomatic, and discovered on routine dental radiography. On radiographic examination, adenomatoid odontogenic tumor is a well-circumscribed, pear-shaped radiolucency that often occurs in association with an unerupted canine tooth or between the roots of incisors. It often contains fine "snowflake" opacities within the radiolucency. On histologic evaluation, adenomatoid odontogenic tumor

is contained in a fibrous capsule with a semisolid center. It contains spindle-shaped epithelial cells that form sheets, strands, or whorled masses of cells in a fibrous stroma. The characteristic histologic feature of adenomatoid odontogenic tumor is a tubular duct-like structure that consists of a central space surrounded by a layer of columnar or cuboidal epithelial cells. Differential diagnosis includes dentigerous cyst, calcified odontogenic cyst, and calcifying epithelial odontogenic tumor. Because adenomatoid odontogenic tumor is a benign lesion, treatment is surgical enucleation.[51-53]

Odontoameloblastoma. Odontoameloblastoma is an extremely rare odontogenic tumor that contains a mixture of ameloblastic and odontoma-like elements. It occurs in the posterior mandible of patients usually younger than 20 years, with a male predilection. Odontoameloblastoma is typically asymptomatic, although it can cause pain, delayed eruption of permanent teeth, or expansion of bone. It is a well-circumscribed radiolucent process containing radiopacities consistent with tooth structure. The epithelium histologically resembles the follicular pattern of the solid ameloblastoma with adjacent dental tissue resembling a compound or complex odontoma. Treatment is local curettage and enucleation; however, recurrences have been noted, and given its ameloblastic component, more aggressive treatment may be indicated in those lesions that are histologically primarily ameloblastic.

Odontoma. Odontomas are the most common type of odontogenic tumor and are considered developmental anomalies, hamartomas, and not true neoplasms. Fully developed odontomas consist of enamel, dentin, pulp, and cementum. There are two types: compound odontomas, which are composed of multiple tooth-like structures; and complex odontomas, consisting of an unruly mass of enamel and dentin. Odontomas are usually detected clinically before the age of 20 years. They are asymptomatic, discovered on routine dental radiographs. Typically small in size, they rarely enlarge or cause jaw expansion. Compound odontomas present radiographically as a collection of tooth-like structures of varying size and shape surrounded by a narrow radiolucent zone. Complex odontomas present as a calcified mass with the radiodensity of tooth structure that is also surrounded by a radiolucent rim. Odontomas are often associated with an unerupted tooth, the lesion preventing eruption. On histologic evaluation, compound odontomas resemble teeth; mature enamel, dentin, and pulp are noted. Complex odontomas consist of tubular dentin with an enclosed enamel matrix. Differential diagnosis of complex odontomas includes osteoma, periapical cemental dysplasia, ossifying fibroma, and cementoblastoma. Compound odontomas are diagnostic radiographically. Treatment is indicated only if the odontoma is blocking tooth eruption or its diagnosis (radiographically) is uncertain. Removal consists of enucleation without recurrence (Fig. 110-5).[54,55]

TUMORS OF ODONTOGENIC ECTOMESENCHYME WITH OR WITHOUT ODONTOGENIC EPITHELIUM

These odontogenic tumors are primarily composed of odontogenic mesenchyme and may or may not have odontogenic epithelium.

ODONTOGENIC FIBROMA. Odontogenic fibromas are rare benign connective tissue tumors found both intraosseously (central odontogenic fibroma) and in the soft tissues (peripheral odontogenic fibroma). Central odontogenic fibroma has a wide age range of occurrence (14 to 70 years, with a mean of 37 years). Females are more commonly affected, and there is a preference for the maxilla greater than for the mandible. When it arises in the mandible, the tumor occurs typically posterior to the first molar. Most are asymptomatic, discovered on dental radiographs; however, there may be associated bone enlargement and root resorption causing pain. On radiographic examination, central odontogenic fibroma is a multilocular radiolucency with well-defined borders. There may be adjacent tooth root resorption or divergence. On histologic evaluation, odontogenic fibromas consist of bundles of cellular fibrous connective tissue with collagen fibers interlacing these bundles. Odontogenic epithelium is noted throughout the lesion.

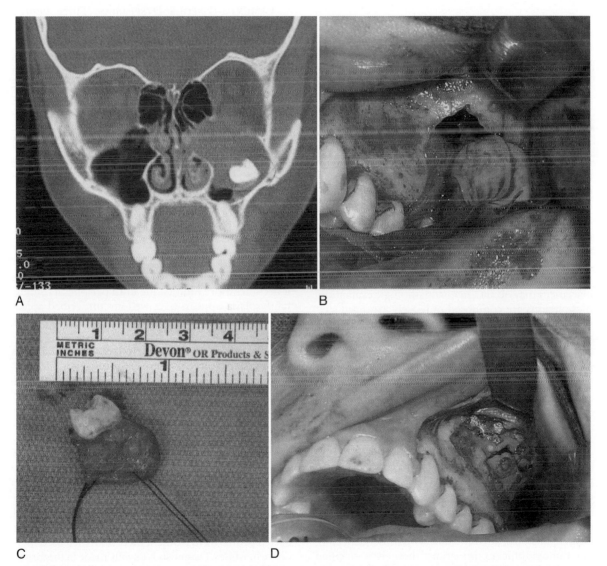

FIGURE 110-5. Odontoma. *A,* Coronal computed tomographic scan of odontoma in right maxillary sinus. *B,* Surgical removal. *C,* Specimen. *D,* Surgical defect repaired with bone graft and secured with resorbable mesh.

Often, its borders merge with surrounding bone. Treatment includes enucleation. If there is neural involvement, attempts should be made to preserve the nerve. Involved teeth should be extracted.[56,57]

Granular Cell Odontogenic Fibroma. Granular cell odontogenic fibroma is an extremely rare benign lesion that occurs in the molar region of the mandible. Most cases occur after the age of 40 years. Typically, granular cell odontogenic fibroma is asymptomatic. This lesion appears radiographically as a well-circumscribed radiolucency. On histologic evaluation, granular cell odontogenic fibroma is composed of large eosinophilic granular cells similar to the granular cell variant of the ameloblastoma. Scattered among the granular cells is odontogenic epithelium. Treatment is limited to curettage, without recurrence.

Peripheral Odontogenic Fibroma. Peripheral odontogenic fibroma is considered to be the soft tissue counterpart of odontogenic fibroma. It arises primarily in the facial aspect of the anterior mandibular gingiva. It appears clinically as a firm, sessile, slowly growing mass covered by normal gingival mucosa. There is no bone involvement. Treatment consists of local excision.

ODONTOGENIC MYXOMA. Odontogenic myxomas are benign, slow-growing tumors that arise from odontogenic ectomesenchyme. They are found primarily in the younger patient, commonly between the ages of 25 and 30 years, in women more often than in men. Odontogenic myxomas are clinically asymptomatic or may present as a painless expansion of the jaw. On radiographic examination, odontogenic myxomas are either unilocular or multilocular radiolucencies with scalloped margins. Tooth root resorption or displacement may occur. On histopathologic evaluation, these lesions are composed of loosely arranged stellate, spindle-shaped, and round cells in a myxoid stroma with minimal collagen. Differential diagnosis includes ameloblastoma, ameloblastic fibroma, odontogenic fibroma, and desmoplastic fibroma. Myxomas often infiltrate into the surrounding bone, so local curettage often results in recurrence (recurrence rate of 25%); surgical excision is the treatment of choice (Fig. 110-6).[58-60]

CEMENTOBLASTOMA. Cementoblastoma is a rare benign neoplasm of cementoblastic origin. It occurs in the second to third decade of life, usually before 25 years of age.[61] It is primarily found in the mandibular molar region. Cementoblastomas are associated with roots of teeth. They are slow growing and may cause local expansion of adjacent bone with subsequent pain. On radiographic examination, there is a calcified mass (radiopaque) associated with the root of a tooth surrounded by a thin radiolucent ring. On histopathologic evaluation, cementoblastoma is composed of sheets of mineralized cementum-like material with prominent basophilic reversal lines. Multinucleated giant cells are often present. Intervening well-vascularized soft tissue contains cementoblasts and cementoclasts.

Diagnosis is based on the classic radiographic appearance; however, differential diagnosis can include odontoma, osteoblastoma, and hypercementosis. Because of the intimate association of the cementoblastoma with a tooth root, surgical extraction of the affected tooth is the most common treatment. However, it is reasonable to attempt amputation of the associated root with subsequent endodontic treatment of the involved tooth, coupled with excision of the cementoblastoma.[62-65]

CEMENTO-OSSEOUS DYSPLASIAS. Three benign disease processes of the mandible involving the production of cementum and bone are termed cemento-osseous dysplasias. These are peripheral cemental dysplasia, focal cemento-osseous dysplasia, and florid osseous dysplasia.

Peripheral cemental dysplasia is a reactive process of periapical bone and cementum of anterior mandibular teeth. Peripheral cemental dysplasia is typically associated with multiple vital teeth. There is a significant female predilection (14:1) and a higher incidence in blacks. Peripheral cemental dysplasia is usually diagnosed around the fourth or fifth decade of life during routine dental radiography. This is clinically a benign and asymptomatic process; it appears initially on radiographs as a radiolucency around the apices of the mandibular incisor roots. Differential diagnosis at this point includes periapical granuloma and periapical cyst. As the lesion matures over time, it becomes more radiopaque until peripheral cemental dysplasia appears as a well-circumscribed apical opacity with a radiolucent rim. Lesions are usually less than 1.0 cm in diameter. On histologic evaluation, multiple fragments of moderately cellular, collagenous tissue in bone-cementum matrices containing cementoblasts and odontoblasts are noted. Differential diagnosis of peripheral cemental dysplasia in its early stage includes ossifying fibroma and periapical granuloma and cyst. Differential diagnosis for late-stage peripheral cemental dysplasia includes odontoma, osteoblastoma, and focal sclerosing osteomyelitis. Treatment of peripheral cemental dysplasia is limited to periodic observation.[66]

Focal cemento-osseous dysplasia is a disease thought to lie in the spectrum between peripheral cemental dysplasia and focal osseous dysplasia. It occurs primarily in women; there is an increased incidence in whites. Diagnosis is usually made in the fourth to fifth decade of life as an incidental finding on routine dental films. Focal cemento-osseous dysplasia occurs

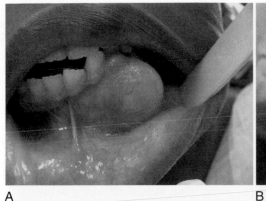

A

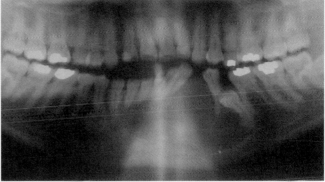

B

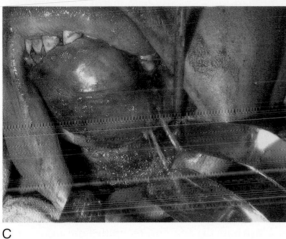

C

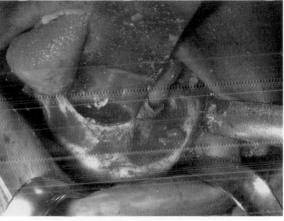

D

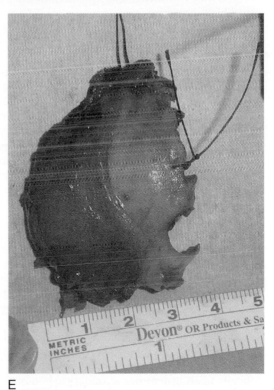

E

FIGURE 110-6. Myxoma. *A,* Large mass in the left anterior mandible that has been growing for several years. *B,* Panoramic radiograph of mass. *C,* Intraoperative exposure of mass; note that two branches of the mental nerve are dissected free before resection to maintain nerve function postoperatively. *D,* Residual mandible after resection. *E,* Specimen.

as an asymptomatic solitary lesion in the posterior mandible. On radiographic examination, there is a mixed radiolucent and radiopaque presentation, usually less than 1.5 cm in diameter. It resembles peripheral cemental dysplasia histologically. Treatment is observation.[67]

A more generalized type of peripheral cemental dysplasia, florid osseous dysplasia, involves most of the mandibular dentition. It affects black women between the ages of 25 and 60 years. Florid osseous dysplasia appears radiographically as diffuse radiopaque masses associated with the apices of multiple mandibular teeth. On histologic evaluation, it is a mixture of benign fibrous tissue, bone, and cementum. Differential diagnosis for florid osseous dysplasia includes diffuse sclerosing osteomyelitis and Paget disease. Manipulation of florid osseous dysplasia (biopsy, extraction of associated teeth) causes an increased risk of development of osteomyelitis. As for peripheral cemental dysplasia, treatment is limited to observation.[68]

CEMENTIFYING FIBROMA. Cementifying fibroma is a well-circumscribed lesion composed of cementum. It usually occurs in adults about 40 years of age but has a wide age range with a female predilection. Usually asymptomatic, it can cause tooth movement. It has a variable radiographic appearance of mixed radiolucent and opaque. Differential diagnosis includes cementoblastoma, ossifying fibroma, and chronic osteomyelitis. Treatment includes enucleation or excision, which is curative.

Malignant Odontogenic Tumors

Malignant odontogenic tumors can be divided into three categories: odontogenic carcinoma, odontogenic sarcoma, and odontogenic carcinosarcoma. Intraosseous jaw carcinomas are collectively known as odontogenic carcinomas because their tissue of origin is odontogenic epithelium. Odontogenic carcinomas can arise from benign odontogenic tumors, de novo from odontogenic residue, or from odontogenic cysts. The literature notes that 1% to 2% of all oral cavity cancer arises from odontogenic cysts.

Whereas odontogenic carcinomas can occur at any age, they are typically seen in the older patients (older than 60 years), and there is a distinct prevalence in men (2:1). However, the frequency of odontogenic carcinoma is increasing in women, primarily because of the increasing frequency of risk factors in women (smoking, alcohol). The posterior mandible is the most common site of occurrence.

The most common complaint is pain and swelling; however, a significant minority of patients are asymptomatic. The presenting complaint may often be difficulty wearing dentures secondary to bone expansion. Paresthesia is an ominous sign of malignant disease. Differential diagnosis is based on histopathologic study. On radiographic examination, odontogenic carcinomas are radiolucent and usually resemble the lesion they arise from (odontogenic cyst, ameloblastoma). The borders are often ragged. Most odontogenic carcinomas on histopathologic study are found to have well-differentiated squamous cell carcinoma. Treatment is obviously aggressive from local block excision to radical resection, with or without radiotherapy and chemotherapy. There is a 50% 5-year survival rate after treatment.

ODONTOGENIC CARCINOMA. The only documented odontogenic carcinoma arising de novo is the primary intraosseous carcinoma. It is a squamous cell carcinoma arising in either jaw, having an initial connection with the oral mucosa, and presumably develops from residues of the odontogenic epithelium. It affects men more often than women and the mandible more often than the maxilla. The prognosis is poor with a 2-year survival rate of 40%.

ODONTOGENIC SARCOMA. Odontogenic sarcomas are a second group of odontogenic malignant neoplasms. Sarcomas are malignant neoplasms originating from mesenchymal or embryonic connective tissue. This group includes ameloblastic fibrosarcoma; ameloblastic fibrodentinosarcoma (fibro-odontosarcoma), which contains dysplastic dentin and enamel; and odontogenic carcinosarcoma, a rare neoplasm in which both the odontogenic epithelium and ectomesenchyme have undergone malignant change.

Ameloblastic fibrosarcoma is the malignant version of ameloblastic fibroma. More than 45% develop as a recurrence of ameloblastic fibroma or rarely fibroodontoma. There is a 2:1 male-to-female ratio in ameloblastic fibrosarcoma, and it occurs more commonly in younger patients (mean age, 26 years). Most of these lesions (75%) occur in the mandible. Symptoms include pain, swelling, and paresthesia. Mobility of teeth may also be noted. On radiographic examination, ameloblastic fibrosarcoma is an ill-defined radiolucent lesion with associated lytic destruction of surrounding bone. On histologic evaluation, ameloblastic fibrosarcoma contains odontogenic epithelium identical to ameloblastic fibroma and is benign. The mesenchymal portion, however, is highly cellular and hyperchromic and displays pleomorphic cells with prominent mitoses. Treatment involves radical surgical excision because of the locally aggressive nature. Metastasis rarely occurs. Mortality rate of 23% is associated with uncontrolled local disease. Long-term follow-up is required.[69-71]

NONODONTOGENIC TUMORS

Nonodontogenic tumors are tumors of the jaws that originate from nondental tissue. They are classified as osseous versus fibrous and fibro-osseous. Benign osseous lesions include osteomas, osteoblastomas, osteoid osteoma, and exostoses.

OSTEOMA. Osteomas are benign tumors of compact or cancellous bone. Those that arise on the surface of bone are termed periosteal osteomas; those that develop centrally within medullary bone are endosteal osteomas. They are unique to the medullary bones of the craniofacial complex. Osteomas are commonly diagnosed in the second to third decade of life, in men more commonly than in women, and are asymptomatic. The etiology is unknown. Periosteal osteomas are slow-growing masses on the surface of the jaws. They have been documented in the mandibular condyle, causing gradual change in occlusion and deviation of the chin toward the unaffected side.

Endosteal osteomas can become large, resulting in facial deformity, or may develop in the paranasal sinuses, resulting in sinusitis. They present radiologically as circumscribed sclerotic radiopaque masses. There are two histologic types: compact osteomas, composed of normal-appearing bone with small marrow spaces; and cancellous osteomas, composed of lamellar trabeculae with abundant marrow spaces. Osteoblastic activity is prominent. Differential diagnosis includes exostoses of the jaws, odontomas, osteoid osteomas, and osteoblastomas. Treatment is based on cosmesis or the prevalence of symptoms. Osteomas that cause facial asymmetry, malocclusion, pain, and swelling are routinely treated by surgical conservative excision. Those that are small or asymptomatic do not require treatment but should be periodically observed. Osteomas do not recur.[72,73]

Osteomas are typically solitary in nature. However, multiple osteomas indicate the diagnosis of Gardner syndrome. Gardner syndrome is an autosomal dominant disorder characterized by fibromas of the skin, epidermal cysts, impacted supernumerary dentition, odontomas, intestinal polyposis, and, as noted, multiple osteomas. The associated gene is located on the small region of the long arm of chromosome 5. Multiple osteomas associated with this syndrome are commonly found in the mandibular angle. Investigation and diagnosis of Gardner syndrome are essential because the intestinal polyposis often undergoes malignant transformation into colorectal carcinoma.[74,75]

OSTEOBLASTOMA. Osteoblastoma is an uncommon primary lesion of bone occurring in the mandible. Although benign, its rapid onset and associated pain often give the clinician the impression of malignancy. The etiology is unclear; however, it is thought to be a reactive process in bone. Although osteoblastoma occurs primarily in the vertebrae and long bones, the mandible is the most commonly affected bone in the craniofacial complex. Most cases occur in the second decade of life with a male-to-female ratio of 2:1. The presenting complaint is pain, often severe, in the area of the lesion. There may be localized swelling and bone expansion with mobility of associated teeth. On radiographic examination, osteoblastoma is a mixed radiolucent and radiopaque lesion. It has variable presentation histopathologically. Irregular trabeculae of osteoid and bone are seen within a vascular stroma. There are osteoblasts and multinucleated giant cells throughout the stroma. Differential diagnosis includes cementoblastoma, ossifying fibroma, fibrous dysplasia, and osteosarcoma. Surgical excision is the treatment of choice. Recurrence is rare. A subgroup of osteoblastoma termed aggressive osteoblastoma is characterized by a locally aggressive behavior coupled with atypical histologic features. These lesions usually occur in older patients with associated severe pain as the primary complaint. Again, aggressive surgical excision is warranted.[76,77]

OSTEOID OSTEOMA. Osteoid osteoma is considered to be an entity closely related to osteoblastoma. Some oral pathologists consider the two to be the same entity, only differing in size of occurrence and radiographic appearance. The etiology of osteoid osteoma, like that of osteoblastoma, is unclear, but it is thought to be a reactive process. This tumor occurs in the second to third decade of life with a male predominance. It most commonly occurs in the long bones and rarely in the mandible. Osteoid osteoma presents clinically with pain that increases at night and is relieved by nonsteroidal anti-inflammatory drugs (pain associated with osteoblastoma is never relieved solely by nonsteroidal anti-inflammatory drugs). There may or may not be associated swelling. The classic radiographic appearance is a small radiolucency surrounded by a ring of sclerotic bone. Osteoid osteoma never exceeds 2 cm in diameter (osteoblastomas are usually larger than 2 cm). It resembles osteoblastoma histologically and shares a common differential diagnosis. Treatment includes conservative surgical excision.

EXOSTOSES. Exostoses are localized bone protuberances that arise from the cortical plate. These lesions have minimal clinical significance; they are nonneoplastic and usually asymptomatic. Their clinical significance arises when their presence is an impediment to dental prosthesis placement and function, necessitating their removal. The etiology of bony oral exostosis is obscure; however, it is thought to be both genetic and environmental in origin. In the mandible, the most common exostosis is the torus mandibularis, which develops along the lingual aspect of the anterior mandible, usually lingual to the premolars; 90% are bilateral. These tumors have a preference for the black race, and their incidence in the United States ranges from 6% to 12% of the population.[78]

Most mandibular tori present as firm solitary nodules on the lingual aspect of the mandible; however, not uncommonly, mandibular tori can have multiple nodules. On radiographic examination, mandibular tori are radiopacities that are often superimposed on the roots of teeth on periapical dental films. These lesions consist histologically of cortical lamellar bone. No treatment is required unless there is difficulty associated with a mandibular denture.[79]

Other mandibular exostoses include buccal exostoses, which occur on the mandibular alveolar ridge, and reactive subpontine exostosis, which develops on the alveolar crest of the mandible lying directly under the pontic of a mandibular bridge.

Benign Fibrous and Fibro-osseous Lesions

Fibro-osseous lesions of the jaws are a diverse group of lesions characterized by replacement of normal bone with fibrous tissue. These lesions include fibrous dysplasia, cemento-osseous dysplasia, and ossifying fibroma.

FIBROUS DYSPLASIA. Fibrous dysplasia is a condition in which normal medullary bone is gradually replaced by fibrous connective tissue. There is arrest of bone development in the woven bone stage with failure to mature to lamellar bone. The resulting fibroosseous tissue is poorly structured. The etiology is unknown; however, it is thought to result from altered mesenchymal cell activity or a defect in the control of bone cell activity. Fibrous dysplasia occurs in two forms, monostotic (limited to one bone) and polyostotic (multiple bones); 80% of fibrous dysplasia is monostotic; 3% of the polyostotic form has associated cutaneous pigmented lesions (café au lait spots) and hyperfunction of endocrine glands, known as McCune-Albright syndrome. Cutaneous melanotic pigmentation coupled with polyostotic fibrous dysplasia is termed Jaffe-Lichtenstein syndrome. The mandible is commonly affected in monostotic fibrous dysplasia, which is typically diagnosed in the first to second decade of life. The most common clinical finding is a painless, unilateral swelling of the affected area caused by expansion of the buccal plate of the mandible as the lesion enlarges. Teeth involved remain vital and immobile; however, as jaw expansion develops, teeth may become displaced, causing a malocclusion and facial asymmetry.

On radiographic examination, fibrous dysplasia has a ground-glass radiopaque appearance due to disorganized, poorly calcified bone trabeculae. Its borders are poorly defined and tend to blend into adjacent bone. There may be superior displacement of the mandibular canal. Histopathologic evaluation of fibrous dysplasia reveals irregularly shaped trabeculae of immature woven bone in a fibrous stroma. There is a cellular proliferation of uniform spindled fibroblasts. Consistent with its radiographic findings, the margins of the lesion blend in with normal bone, making it difficult to distinguish the lesion's borders. Differential diagnosis includes ossifying fibroma and Paget disease. After an initial period of rapid growth, fibrous dysplasia stabilizes, typically with the onset of puberty. Small lesions require no treatment. If mandibular expansion has occurred, resulting facial asymmetry is corrected by osseous recontouring, and any malocclusion is treated orthodontically. Once the mandibular lesion is diagnosed as fibrous dysplasia, a skeletal survey must be conducted to determine whether the polyostotic form is present. Treatment must only be undertaken once fibrous dysplasia has completed its rapid growth phase. Less than 1% of polyostotic fibrous dysplasia undergoes malignant transformation (Fig. 110-7).[68]

OSSIFYING FIBROMA. Ossifying fibroma is a benign, slow-growing expansile lesion closely resembling cementifying fibroma. It develops from undifferentiated cells of the periodontal ligament. It contains varying amounts of calcified tissue resembling bone, cementum, or both. Usually asymptomatic, ossifying fibroma arises in tooth-bearing regions of the jaws, primarily in the mandibular premolar region. Ossifying fibroma can occur at any age but most commonly develops during the third to fourth decade of life. There is a female predilection (5 : 1). Most are small; however, if it is left unchecked, this lesion may significantly enlarge and produce thinning of the buccal, lingual, and cortical plates, causing facial asymmetry.

Ossifying fibroma is a well-circumscribed unilocular lesion radiographically. Early on, it is radiolucent; however, as calcified material is deposited within the tumor, ossifying fibroma gradually becomes a mixed lucent and opaque lesion. The adjacent roots of teeth are often displaced; rarely, there is root resorption. On histopathologic evaluation, ossifying fibroma is composed of fibrous tissue stroma with varying amounts of cellularity and calcified material. Irregular trabeculae of woven immature bone are present, and there are varying degrees of vascularity. Osteoblasts are occasionally noted. Differential diagnosis includes fibrous dysplasia, osteoblastoma, and osteoid osteoma. As ossifying fibroma has the potential to enlarge, causing facial asymmetry. Treatment is recommended and consists of surgical enucleation. Recurrence is rare (Fig. 110-8).[80,81]

DESMOPLASTIC FIBROMA. Desmoplastic fibroma is a benign, locally aggressive lesion of the bone that is most often found in bones of the pelvis and long bones; it is rarely noted in the posterior mandible. The etiology in unknown. Cases of desmoplastic fibroma in the mandible typically arise in individuals younger than

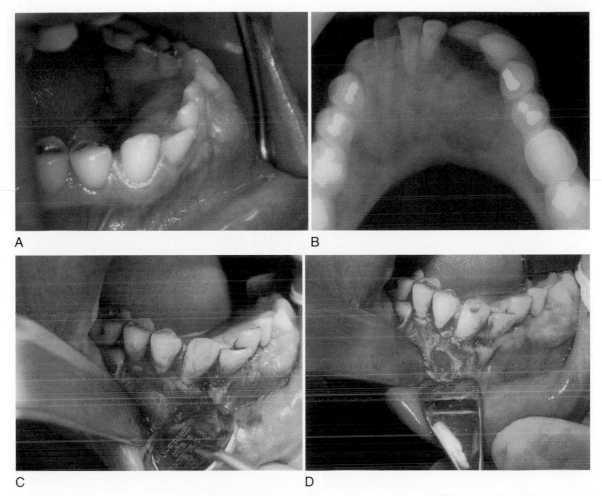

A

B

C

D

FIGURE 110-7. Fibrous dysplasia of anterior mandible. *A,* Presenting clinical examination. *B,* Mandibular occlusal radiograph. *C,* Intraoperative exposure of right parasymphyseal region. *D,* Area after shave.

30 years. The mandibular body-ramus area is most commonly affected. A slowly progressive asymptomatic swelling of the jaws is noted clinically; soft tissue extension results in a palpable gingival mass. Desmoplastic fibroma can cause bone expansion with subsequent destruction. It appears radiographically as a multilocular radiolucency with well-circumscribed borders. On histologic evaluation, desmoplastic fibroma contains dense collagenous tissue with elongated fibroblasts. Differential diagnosis includes odontogenic cysts, odontogenic tumors, and fibromas. Treatment by curettage results in a recurrence rate of 30%; therefore, surgical resection is preferred.[82,83]

CHONDROMA. Chondroma is a benign tumor of mature cartilage. The etiology is unknown, and it rarely occurs in the mandible. Chondroma presents as a painless, slowly progressive swelling usually found in the mandibular symphysis and to a lesser extent in the body, condyle, and coronoid process. The lesion appears radiographically as an irregular radiolucency. Root resorption of adjacent teeth is seen. On histopathologic evaluation, chondromas consist of well-defined mature hyaline cartilage. Differential diagnosis includes chondrosarcoma. Surgical excision (excisional biopsy) is the treatment of choice because chondromas and the malignant chondrosarcomas are clinically and radiographically indistinguishable.[84,85]

CHONDROMYXOID FIBROMA. Chondromyxoid fibroma is a rare benign neoplasm usually found in the long bones and to a much lesser extent in the mandible. Age at occurrence ranges from 10 to 67 years. When it occurs in the mandible, the presenting complaint is pain in the area of the lesion. A radiolucent well-circumscribed defect with sclerotic borders is noted radiographically. On histologic evaluation, chondromyxoid fibroma consists of areas of spindle-shaped cells with abundant myxoid or chondroid intracellular substance. Treatment is curettage.

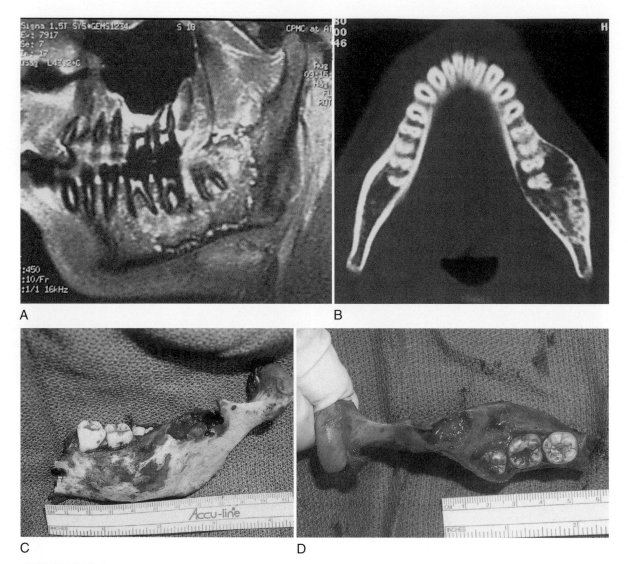

FIGURE 110-8. Ossifying fibroma. *A,* Magnetic resonance image of left posterior mandible demonstrating soft tissue mass in mandible. *B,* Computed tomographic scan of left posterior mandible. *C* and *D,* Resected specimen.

CENTRAL GIANT CELL GRANULOMA. Central giant cell granuloma is a benign lesion unique to the maxilla and mandible. The etiology is unknown; however, it is thought either to arise as a developmental anomaly or to represent repair of an intraosseous hemorrhage. It presents at any age and is typically asymptomatic, diagnosed on routine dental films. Rarely, a more aggressive form of this lesion arises, causing pain, and bone expansion may occur with or without paresthesia of the inferior alveolar nerve. The expansion may be so significant (>10 cm) that bone perforation occurs with associated root resorption of adjacent teeth. There is a female predilection. Mandibular lesions usually involve the symphysis-parasymphyseal area. Central giant cell granuloma appears radiographically as a solitary, well-circumscribed, multilocular radiolucency. Differential diagnosis includes ameloblastoma, odontogenic myxoma, odontogenic keratocyst, and aneurysmal bone cyst. On histopathologic evaluation, central giant cell granuloma is composed of a proliferation of spindled fibroblasts in a vascular collagen stroma. Also within the stroma are macrophages, red blood cells, and multinucleated giant cells. Foci of osteoid may also be noted. Treatment of the more common nonaggressive type includes curettage, with a recurrence rate of 15% to 25%. Aggressive central giant cell granulomas may require aggressive curettage with associated removal of the peripheral bone margins. Because the histologic appearance of central giant cell granuloma often resembles the brown tumor of hyperparathyroidism, it is prudent to check the serum levels of calcium, phosphate, and parathyroid hormone to rule out primary or secondary hyper-parathyroidism.[86-88]

CHERUBISM. Cherubism is a rare benign hereditary mandibular condition usually diagnosed in children by the age of 5 years. It is named after the characteristic facial appearance of afflicted individuals: bilateral posterior mandibular swellings, which give the patient the appearance of a "cherub" (little angel). Cherubism occurs as an autosomal dominant disorder, with 100% penetrance in males and 75% in females; there is a 2:1 male predominance. Its cause is thought to be a mesenchymal alteration during the development of the mandible as a result of reduced oxygenation due to perivascular fibrosis. A painless bone expansion in the region of the mandibular angle is noted clinically as the initial manifestation. This expansion can range from mild to so severe that the masticatory, speech, and swallowing functions are impaired. The posterior mandible is typically involved. In severe cases, the whole mandible is affected. Intraoral hard nontender swellings are also noted. There may be a premature exfoliation of the primary dentition; the bone expansion may also displace the developing permanent tooth bud, causing ectopic eruption of permanent teeth and in turn creating a significant malocclusion later in life. Submandibular and cervical lymphadenopathy is often noted at the time of diagnosis, but it is unclear why this occurs.[89,90]

Cherubism is characterized radiographically by multilocular, well-defined radiolucencies in the posterior mandible. The borders are distinct and deviled by bone trabeculae. These lesions histologically resemble central giant cell granulomas; a highly vascular fibrous stroma is noted containing fibroblasts and multinucleated giant cells. Red blood cells may also be present. A unique histologic feature of cherubism is eosinophilic perivascular cuffing of collagen surrounding capillaries. Diagnosis is based on clinical symptoms and family history. Differential diagnosis includes odontogenic keratocyst and hyperparathyroidism. After an initial period of rapid bone expansion, cherubism is self-limited, and spontaneous regression begins at puberty. Surgical intervention is questionable; some studies have shown excellent results after excision of lesions, whereas others have noted pronounced recurrence after curettage. Orthodontic therapy may be required to resolve any associated malocclusion.

LANGERHANS CELL DISEASE. Langerhans cell disease is a condition in which there is a proliferation of cells exhibiting phenotypic characteristics of Langerhans cells (histiocytes). Formerly known as histiocytosis X, it comprises a group of similar diseases: eosinophilic granuloma, Hand-Schüller-Christian disease, and Letterer-Siwe disease.

Eosinophilic granuloma is the mildest form of histiocytosis X. Clinically, there are solitary or multiple bone lesions throughout the body. The mandible is often involved. There is a predilection for males, and peak incidence is in the third decade of life. Typically asymptomatic, it may manifest symptoms of pain or swelling in the mandible accompanied by generalized malaise. On radiographic examination, eosinophilic granuloma of the mandible is a well-circumscribed osteolytic lesion that may appear punched out.

Hand-Schüller-Christian disease is the disseminated chronic disease involving bone, skin, and viscera. It occurs primarily in children 10 years of age or younger, with a male predilection of 2:1. Clinically, there is a classic triad of associated symptoms: calvarial defects, exophthalmos, and diabetes insipidus. Mandibular lesions appear radiographically as irregular radiolucent defects. Affected teeth often appear to be "floating in space" because of destruction of alveolar bone. This is a slowly progressing variant of Langerhans cell disease, with a mortality rate of 60%.[91,92]

Letterer-Siwe disease is the most lethal, acute disseminated form of histiocytosis X. In addition to bone involvement, there are cutaneous, visceral, and bone marrow lesions as well. It is generally fatal and occurs in infants younger than 1 year. Radiographic mandibular findings include small rounded radiolucencies with well-defined borders.

The etiology of Langerhans cell disease is obscure; however, it is hypothesized that Langerhans cells undergo neoplastic transformation. Another hypothesis is that Langerhans cell disease is the result of an immune response to a viral antigen challenge, specifically human herpesvirus 6. A third hypothesis is that Langerhans cell disease arises from a defect in the cell-mediated immune system, specifically the normal cellular regulatory mechanisms, allowing uncontrolled proliferation of Langerhans cells.

Mandibular lesions occur in 10% to 20% of Langerhans cell disease. These lesions may be asymptomatic or associated with pain and swelling. Alveolar bone involvement causes tooth mobility. On histopathologic evaluation, Langerhans cell disease shows a diffuse infiltration of large, pale-staining mononuclear cells. Plasma cells, lymphocytes, and multinucleated cells are often seen. Diagnosis usually requires electron microscopy to detect cytoplasmic Birbeck granules unique to Langerhans cells. Treatment of mandibular bone lesions is by curettage. If recurrence does not develop 1 year after treatment, prognosis for recovery is good. Systemic treatment of disseminated disease involves multiple chemotherapeutic agents.

CORONOID HYPERPLASIA. Coronoid hyperplasia is a rare condition that restricts mandibular motion. The etiology is unknown, although it is thought to be associated with trauma to the affected area. Coronoid hyperplasia is classically bilateral, rarely unilateral; there is a male predilection, and diagnosis occurs around puberty. Clinically, there is a gradual decrease in range of motion of the mandible. Enlarged, elongated coronoid processes are noted radiographically. Treatment involves surgical excision of the hyperplastic coronoid processes with postoperative physical therapy.

Vascular Lesions

Vascular lesions of the mandible include hemangiomas and vascular malformations.

HEMANGIOMAS. Hemangiomas of bone are benign tumors composed of capillary, cavernous, or venous blood vessels. The mandible is a common location for occurrence, typically in individuals 10 to 20 years of age and more commonly in females. Hemangiomas of the mandible are typically asymptomatic; however, pain, mandibular swelling, or mobility of adjacent teeth may be noted. A bruit or pulsation may be appreciated on physical examination. Deeper tumors may require the assistance of computed tomography or magnetic resonance imaging for diagnosis.[93]

On radiographic examination, most mandibular hemangiomas show a multilocular radiolucency. The major risk associated with bone hemangiomas is sudden hemorrhage of larger tumors. If a hemangioma is suspected or cannot be ruled out, needle aspiration of the lesion is indicated for confirmation. Treatment of mandibular hemangiomas that are asymptomatic and found incidentally is often limited to observation. If the tumor causes impairment of function, treatment modalities include cryotherapy, radiation, embolization, steroid treatment, sclerosing agents, and interferon alfa therapy. Smaller lesions may be treated with surgical curettage.[94]

VASCULAR MALFORMATIONS. Vascular malformations of the mandible are typically present at birth but not often clinically evident until later in childhood. A minority are secondary to trauma. These are vascular lesions in which there is a direct communication between arterial and venous blood supply, bypassing the capillary network. They are subdivided into low-flow and high-flow lesions on the basis of angiographic findings. Mandibular vascular malformations present clinically as pulsatile, discolored swellings. On radiographic examination, the lesion is an irregular radiolucency. Smaller mandibular vascular malformations can be treated with sclerosing agents, radiotherapy, or cryotherapy. Larger lesions require embolization with subsequent surgical resection.

VASCULAR TUMORS. Other, much rarer mandibular vascular tumors include angiosarcoma, hemangioendothelioma, malignant hemangioendothelioma, epithelioid hemangioendothelioma, and histiocytoid hemangioma.[95]

Neurogenic Tumors

Benign neurogenic tumors of the mandible include schwannoma, neurofibroma, and traumatic neuroma. These are typically a group of slow-growing neural tissue tumors that cause pain or paresthesia. Schwannoma is encapsulated and has two distinct histologic components, Antoni type A and type B tissue. A neurofibroma arises from the connective tissue sheath of nerve fibers and is unencapsulated with axons traversing its length. Neurofibroma is typically solitary; multiple neurofibromas should raise the suspicion of neurofibromatosis. On radiographic examination, these lesions are radiolucencies associated with the inferior alveolar canal. All have the potential to enlarge, causing bone expansion, cortical perforation, and extension into the soft tissue. Treatment is surgical; smaller lesions can be removed with minimal nerve damage or hard tissue defect. Larger lesions may require en bloc resection coupled with reconstruction and microsurgical nerve repair.[96]

Primary Malignant Nonodontogenic Tumors

Primary malignant nonodontogenic tumors of the mandible are rare, aggressive neoplasms with an extremely poor prognosis. Included in this group are osteosarcoma, chondrosarcoma, fibrosarcoma of bone, Ewing sarcoma, Burkitt lymphoma, plasma cell neoplasms, and malignant lymphoma.

OSTEOSARCOMA. Osteosarcoma (osteogenic sarcoma) is the most common primary bone tumor. It is composed of malignant connective tissue cells producing osteoid and bone; 2.5% occur in the mandible (1 case per 3 million people per year). Whereas mandibular osteosarcoma can occur at any age, it typically presents during the third to fourth decade of life. There is a male predilection (2 : 1). The majority (60%) occur in the mandibular body. Mandibular osteosarcoma presents clinically as swelling and pain in the affected area. Associated symptoms include tooth mobility and paresthesia. The average duration of symptoms before diagnosis is 3 to 4 months.[97]

Radiographic findings vary on the basis of the amount of calcification within the lesion; mandibular osteosarcoma therefore can appear completely radiolucent, mixed radiopaque and lucent, or entirely radiopaque. Universally, however, its borders are ill-defined. A key radiographic finding in early-stage osteosarcoma is widening of the periodontal ligament around involved teeth due to tumor infiltration along the roots of teeth. A "sunburst" radiographic pattern is classically described for osteosarcoma, resulting from bone spicules perpendicular to its surface. On histopathologic study, all osteosarcomas contain a stroma rich in osteoid produced by malignant osteoblastic cells. In addition, chondroid and fibrous connective tissue are also produced. Osteosarcoma ranges from well defined to pleomorphic. On the basis of the amount of osteoid, chondroid, and connective tissue produced, osteosarcomas are divided into three histologic subtypes: osteoblastic, chondroblastic, and fibroblastic. Mandibular osteosarcoma is primarily chondroblastic. Differential diagnosis includes scleroderma, chronic osteomyelitis, chondrosarcoma, and fibrosarcoma. The 5-year survival rate of osteosarcoma treated with surgery alone ranges from 25% to 45%. Combination surgery and multiagent chemotherapy has survival rates of 60% to 70% (radiotherapy has no benefit). Osteosarcoma has a metastatic risk of 25% (metastasis is through the hematogenous route). The lung and brain are the typical sites of metastases; if metastatic disease occurs, the mean survival is about 6 months.

Juxtacortical Osteosarcoma.[98] Unlike standard osteosarcoma, juxtacortical osteosarcoma arises in the periphery of bone in the periosteum. This type of osteosarcoma represents 5% of all osteosarcomas and very rarely occurs in the mandible. There are two subgroups, parosteal and periosteal.

Parosteal osteosarcoma has a peak incidence at 39 years of age with a female predilection (3:2 female-to-male ratio). This type of osteosarcoma is found in the distal femur most often. Mandibular symptoms include a slowly progressive swelling associated with dull pain in the affected area. On radiographic examination, a radiodense mass is observed attached to the surface of bone by a broad base. A radiolucent space, representing periosteum, can be identified between tumor and bone cortex. On histologic evaluation, parosteal osteosarcoma is well differentiated with a spindle cell stroma. About 20% invade underlying bone.[99]

Periosteal osteosarcoma is even rarer than its parosteal counterpart. It has a peak incidence at 20 years of age and a 2:1 male-to-female ratio. This type of osteosarcoma is seen typically in the tibia and rarely the mandible. On radiographic examination, it is radiolucent because of its high cartilaginous composition. On histologic evaluation, periosteal osteosarcoma reveals malignant cartilage with minimal osteoid. In addition, there is no invasion into adjacent bone. There is rare metastasis to the lungs noted in the literature.

Treatment of both types of juxtacortical osteosarcoma includes either en bloc resection or radical excision. The 5-year survival rate after surgery is 80%.[100]

CHONDROSARCOMA. Chondrosarcoma is a rare malignant bone tumor characterized by cartilage formation by tumor cells. It makes up about 10% of all primary skeletal tumors, but less than 1% of chondrosarcomas involve the mandible. Mandibular chondrosarcoma occurs most frequently in the premolar-molar region, followed by the symphysis and coronoid process. The mean age at occurrence is 60 years. The typical presenting complaints include a painless swelling and expansion of the mandible causing tooth mobility. On radiographic examination, chondrosarcoma consists of a radiolucency with poorly defined borders. Widening of the periodontal ligament may also be noted. On histologic evaluation, chondrosarcoma demonstrates varying degrees of mature cartilage. Most mandibular chondrosarcomas are well differentiated. Chondrosarcomas are divided into three histopathologic grades of malignancy that correlate with rate of tumor growth and prognosis. Grade 1 is a well-differentiated chondrosarcoma, closely resembling a chondroma, composed of chondroid matrix and chondroblasts. Calcification or ossification of the cartilaginous matrix is often prominent, and metastasis does not occur. Grade 2 chondrosarcoma contains moderately sized nuclei and increased cellularity. The cartilaginous matrix is more myxoid with less hyaline compared with grade 1. There is minimal metastatic disease. Grade 3 chondrosarcoma is highly cellular and has a prominent spindle cell proliferation. Metastatic disease to the lungs usually develops. Mandibular chondrosarcoma is usually grade 1.[101]

Differential diagnosis includes chondroma and chondroblastic osteosarcoma. Chondrosarcoma is a radioresistant neoplasm. As a result, surgical excision is the treatment of choice. Death from this mandibular malignant neoplasm is usually due to uncontrolled local recurrence with extension to vital structures. The 5-year survival rate of mandibular chondrosarcoma is extremely poor, about 17%.[102]

Mesenchymal Chondrosarcoma. Mesenchymal chondrosarcoma is an extremely rare variant of chondrosarcoma. It occurs in the soft tissues as well as in bone. The most common skeletal sites of occurrence are the maxilla, mandible, and rib. Most mesenchymal chondrosarcomas occur between the ages of 10 and 30 years (unlike chondrosarcoma, with a mean age at occurrence of 60 years). The presenting complaint is a painful mandibular swelling. On radiographic examination, mesenchymal chondrosarcoma is a well-circumscribed radiolucency with poorly differentiated borders. The characteristic histologic appearance of this malignant neoplasm is that of anaplastic small cell sarcoma with well-formed malignant cartilage.[103]

Because of its aggressive malignant potential, treatment of mesenchymal chondrosarcoma is radical surgical resection. Like chondrosarcoma, it is radioresistant. Its highly malignant course is verified by an

80% mortality rate. Mesenchymal chondrosarcoma can both recur locally and metastasize to the lung.

EWING SARCOMA. Ewing sarcoma is a primary malignant sarcoma of bone first described by James Ewing in 1921. The etiology is unknown and the cell of origin unclear. It is thought that Ewing sarcoma derives from neuroectoderm because it shares a common karyotype translocation [t(11;12) (11;22) (q24;q12)] with the peripheral primitive neuroectoderm tumor. Clinically, 90% of Ewing sarcoma occurs between the ages of 5 and 30 years, with a 2 : 1 male-to-female ratio. It is also a disease unique to whites; this neoplasm is rarely encountered among blacks and Asians. The presenting symptoms of mandibular Ewing sarcoma include pain and swelling (a common theme among most malignant tumors of the mandible). In addition, there may be resulting facial asymmetry, alveolar bone loss with subsequent mobility of teeth, paresthesia, and mucosal ulceration; fever is also often noted. Laboratory studies reveal an increased erythrocyte sedimentation rate and an increased white blood cell count.[104]

Radiographic findings are nonspecific—irregular lytic cone destruction with ill-defined margins. Ewing sarcoma appears histologically as a proliferation of small round cells compartmentalized by fibrous bands, forming a lobular pattern. Large amounts of necrosis and hemorrhage are seen as well. Differential diagnosis includes lymphoma, leukemia, neuroblastoma, and mesenchymal chondrosarcoma. Ewing sarcoma is a highly malignant tumor. It often metastasizes to the lungs, long bones, and lymph nodes. Comprehensive treatment requires surgery of mandibular lesions, chemotherapy, and radiation. With proper combined treatment, the 5-year survival rate has improved from 10% to 60%. Metastasis, systemic symptoms, increasing lactate dehydrogenase, and thrombocytosis are indicators of a poor prognosis.[105]

BURKITT LYMPHOMA. Burkitt lymphoma is a high-grade non-Hodgkin lymphoma endemic to the African continent. Denis Burkitt in Uganda first diagnosed this neoplasm in 1958. There is also a rare North American form that is histologically identical to its African counterpart but has a different clinical course. Both forms of Burkitt lymphoma are characterized by a translocation of the distal part of chromosome 8 to chromosome 14. This tumor has the highest rate of cellular proliferation known of any human neoplasm, with a doubling time of 24 hours. Clinically, African Burkitt lymphoma has a peak incidence between 3 and 8 years of age with a 2 : 1 male-to-female predilection. The American form has a higher mean age (11 years). African Burkitt lymphoma occurs in the mandible, maxilla, abdomen, kidney, liver, ovaries, and endocrine glands. American Burkitt lymphoma occurs primarily in the abdomen and rarely in the mandible.[106]

The majority of African cases (90%) are associated with Epstein-Barr virus, whereas only 10% of the American type are. When it occurs in the mandible, symptoms include an expanding intraoral mass and mobility of teeth. Pain and paresthesia often occur as well. On radiographic examination, a moth-eaten poorly circumscribed mandibular radiolucency is noted. On histopathologic study, Burkitt lymphoma is a neoplastic B-cell proliferation. In addition, there are macrophages containing pyknotic debris, giving Burkitt lymphoma a "starry sky" histologic appearance. Differential diagnosis includes non-Hodgkin lymphoma, metastatic neuroblastoma, and acute leukemia. Burkitt lymphoma is an aggressive malignant neoplasm, and if it is left untreated, death occurs 4 to 6 months after diagnosis. Fortunately, this neoplasm is extremely sensitive to combination chemotherapy, improving the 2-year survival rate to 54%.[107,108]

PLASMA CELL NEOPLASMS. Plasma cell neoplasms are derived from bone marrow stem cells originating from B-cell lymphocytes and, as a result, secrete immunoglobulin. There are three distinct types: in the soft tissue, extramedullary plasmacytoma; in the bone, solitary plasmacytoma of bone; and systemically, multiple myeloma.

Multiple Myeloma. Multiple myeloma, a rare malignant neoplasm of plasma cell origin, is a disease of the hematopoietic marrow-bearing bone of the skeleton; 70% to 80% of cases have mandibular involvement. Multiple myeloma is usually diagnosed clinically after the fifth decade of life, with a mean age at occurrence of 63 years; there is a male predilection. Mandibular symptoms range from asymptomatic to include pain, swelling, bone expansion, tooth mobility, or pathogenic fracture. Generalized symptoms include fatigue, anemia, and weight loss. Multiple myeloma of the mandible appears radiographically as multiple, sharply punched out radiolucent areas of bone destruction. On histopathologic evaluation, multiple myeloma appears as diffuse monotonous sheets of plasmacytoid cells that invade and replace normal bone. The plasma cells may have a wide range of differentiation and are associated with small vessels and fibroblasts. Differential diagnosis includes metastatic carcinoma, lymphoma, and idiopathic histiocytosis. Treatment of multiple myeloma includes chemotherapy coupled with steroids; local irradiation is directed at painful bone lesions. Survival ranges from 2 to 5 years. Most often, patients with multiple myeloma die of renal failure, myeloma, cardiac failure, hemorrhage, or thrombosis.[109-112]

Solitary Plasmacytoma of Bone. Solitary plasmacytoma of bone is a solitary bone tumor of plasma cell origin. Similar to multiple myeloma, it occurs later in life at a mean age of 50 years. It has a male predominance. Solitary plasmacytoma of bone rarely occurs in the mandible; however, when it does, this tumor is located in the posterior body-ramus region. Mandibular symptoms include expansion of bone and pain. On radiographic examination, solitary plasmacytoma of bone is a well-circumscribed unilocular lucency. It is histologically identical to multiple myeloma. Diagnosis is based on histologic features and also a full-body skeletal survey revealing only an isolated bone lesion. Treatment involves local radiotherapy with or without surgical excision. Unfortunately, up to 75% of individuals with solitary plasmacytoma of bone develop multiple myeloma.

Fibrosarcoma of Bone. Fibrosarcoma of bone is a malignant tumor of fibroblasts that arise from the periosteum, endosteum, or periodontal ligament. It may occur as a primary lesion or secondary to irradiation of bone; varying amounts of collagen are produced. Fibrosarcoma of bone can occur at any age (mean age, 40 years). It primarily occurs in the long bones; 15% occur in the craniofacial skeleton, including the mandible. Symptoms include pain, swelling, paresthesia, and loosening of teeth. On radiographic examination, fibrosarcoma of bone is a radiolucent lytic lesion. Treatment involves wide surgical excision. Recurrence and metastases are rare.

Malignant Lymphoma. Primary malignant lymphoma of the mandible is an extremely rare neoplasm and is part of a group of lymphoid tumors that collectively make up non-Hodgkin lymphoma. The typical presenting complaint is localized bone pain. Systemic symptoms are rare. Paresthesia, bone expansion, or perforation may occur. On radiographic examination, primary malignant lymphoma of the mandible is a poorly defined radiolucency. On histologic evaluation, there are dense sheets of lymphoid cells. The treatment of choice is combination radiation therapy and chemotherapy. The 10-year survival is about 50%.

METASTATIC CARCINOMA OF THE MANDIBLE

Metastatic carcinoma of the mandible is rare—only 1% of malignant neoplasms metastasize to the jaws. In adults, mandibular metastases usually originate from primary malignant neoplasms of the breast and lung. Other less common primary sites include adrenal, bone, kidney, colon, prostate, and thyroid gland. In children younger than 10 years, neuroblastoma of the adrenal gland is the most common primary tumor of origin. For children in the second decade of life, long bone malignant neoplasms are the most common site of primary carcinoma. Adults who develop metastatic mandibular carcinoma are typically in the fifth to seventh decade of life; the mean age is 45 years.[113] The

mechanism of spread is hematogenous. The premolar-molar region of the mandible is most commonly affected. Pain, tooth mobility, paresthesia, gingival mass, swelling, or pathologic fracture may occur. Not uncommonly, the oral lesion is the first sign of malignant disease. Interestingly, the literature notes cases of metastasis occurring in postextraction sites in the mandible. It is postulated that local factors associated with wound healing of the dental extraction site attract metastatic tumor cells and further entrap them in the rich capillary network of healing granulation tissue.

On radiographic examination, metastatic carcinoma of the mandible is a poorly circumscribed, irregular moth-eaten radiolucency. The histopathologic appearance of metastatic disease is extremely variable, depending on the primary malignant neoplasm. A desmoplastic stroma is often seen. When diagnosis is difficult, immunoperoxidase staining is performed for cytokeratin, found in all types of tumor cells. Differential diagnosis includes other poorly differentiated carcinomas; anaplastic sarcoma, lymphoma, and amelanotic melanoma. Treatment of mandibular metastatic disease is twofold. First, the primary carcinoma must be identified with subsequent appropriate therapy. In addition, it is important to determine, by full skeletal bone scans, whether the metastatic lesion in the mandible is a solitary metastasis or whether the primary neoplasm has disseminated throughout the skeletal system. Prognosis for patients with mandibular metastases is extremely poor. The 5-year survival rate is 10%, and the majority are dead within a year of diagnosis.[114-116]

REFERENCES

1. Daley T, Wysocki GP: New developments in selected cysts of the jaws. J Can Dent Assoc 1997;63:526-532.
2. DelBalso A: Lesions of the jaws. Semin Ultrasound CT MR 1995;16:487-512.
3. Bell RC, Chauvin PJ, Tyler MT: Gingival cyst of the adult. J Can Dent Assoc 1997;63:533-555.
4. Cataldo E, Berkman MD: Cysts of the oral mucosa in newborns. Am J Dis Child 1968;116:44-48.
5. Suljak JP: Lateral periodontal cyst: a case report and review of the literature. J Can Dent Assoc 1998;64:48-50.
6. Angelopoulou E, Angelopoulos AP: Lateral periodontal cyst: review of the literature and report of a case. J Periodontol 1990;61:126-131.
7. Kusukawa J, Irie K, Morimatsu M, et al: Dentigerous cyst associated with a deciduous tooth. Oral Surg Oral Med Oral Pathol 1992;73:415-418.
8. Shear M: Cysts of the jaws: recent advances. J Oral Pathol 1985;14:43-59.
9. Main DM: Follicular cysts of mandibular third molar teeth. Dentomaxillofac Radiol 1989;18:156-159.
10. Bataineh AB, al Qudah M: Treatment of mandibular odontogenic keratocysts. Oral Surg Oral Med Oral Pathol Oral Radiol Endod 1998;86:42-47.
11. Crowley T, Kaugars GE, Gunsolley JC: Odontogenic keratocysts: a clinical and histologic comparison of the parakeratin and orthokeratin variants. J Oral Maxillofac Surg 1992;50:22-26.

12. Marker P, Brondum N, Clausen PP, Bastian HL: Treatment of large odontogenic keratocysts by decompression and later cystectomy: a long-term follow-up and histologic study of 23 cases. Oral Surg Oral Med Oral Pathol Oral Radiol Endod 1996; 82:122-131.

13. Ramer M, Montazem A, Lane SL, Lumerman H: Glandular odontogenic cyst. Oral Surg Oral Med Oral Pathol Oral Radiol Endod 1997;84:54-57.

14. Koppang HS, Johannessen S, Haugen LK, et al: Glandular odontogenic cyst. J Oral Pathol Med 1990;27:455-462.

15. Ficarra G, Chou L, Panzoni E: Glandular odontogenic cyst. Int J Oral Maxillofac Surg 1990;19:331-333.

16. el-Beialy RR, el-Mofty S, Refai H: Calcifying odontogenic cyst. J Oral Maxillofac Surg 1990;48:637-640.

17. Erasmus JH, Thompson IO, van Rensburg LJ, van der Westhuijzen AJ: Central calcifying odontogenic cyst. Dentomaxillofac Radiol 1998;27:30-35.

18. Lu Y, Mock D, Takata T, Jordan RC: Odontogenic ghost cell carcinoma. J Oral Pathol Med 1999;28:323-329.

19. Dahl EC: Diagnosing inflammatory and noninflammatory periapical disease. J Indiana Dent Assoc 1991;70:22-26.

20. High AS, Hirschmann PN: Age changes in residual radicular cysts. J Oral Pathol 1986;15:524-528.

21. Wolf J, Hietanen J: The mandibular infected buccal cyst (paradental cyst). Br J Oral Maxillofac Surg 1990;28:322-325.

22. Thompson IO, de Waal J, Nortje CJ: Mandibular infected buccal cyst and paradental cyst. J Dent Assoc S Afr 1997;52:503-506.

23. Gardner DG: An evaluation of reported cases of median mandibular cyst. Oral Surg Oral Med Oral Pathol 1987;63:545-550.

24. Padwa B, Denhart BC, Kaban LB: Aneurysmal bone cyst "plus"—a report of three cases. J Oral Maxillofac Surg 1997; 55:1144-1152.

25. Revel MP, Vanel D, Sigal R, et al: Aneurysmal bone cysts of the jaws. J Comput Assist Tomogr 1992;16:84-86.

26. Motamedi MH, Yazdi E: Aneurysmal bone cyst of the jaws: analysis of 11 cases. J Oral Maxillofac Surg 1994;52:471-475.

27. Saito Y, Hoshina Y, Nagamine T, et al: Simple bone cyst. Oral Surg Oral Med Oral Pathol 1992;74:487-491.

28. Sapp JP, Stark ML: Self-healing traumatic bone cysts. Oral Surg Oral Med Oral Pathol 1990;69:597-602.

29. Barker B, Jensen JL, Howell FV: Focal osteoporotic defects of the jaws. Oral Surg Oral Med Oral Pathol 1974;38:404-413.

30. Batsakis J, Hicks MJ, Flaitz CM: Peripheral epithelial odontogenic tumors. Ann Otol Rhinol Laryngol 1993;102:322-324.

31. Tomich CE: Benign mixed odontogenic tumors. Semin Diagn Pathol 1999;16:308-316.

32. Eversole L: Malignant odontogenic tumors. Semin Diagn Pathol 1999;16:317-324.

33. Philipsen HP, Reichart PA, Praetorius F: Mixed odontogenic tumours and odontomas. Oral Oncol 1997;33:86-99.

34. Melrose RJ: Benign epithelial odontogenic tumors. Semin Diagn Pathol 1999;16:271-287.

35. Philipsen HP, Reichart PA: Unicystic ameloblastoma: a review of 193 cases from the literature. Oral Oncol 1998;34:317-325.

36. Ferretti C, Polakow R, Coleman H: Recurrent ameloblastoma: report of two cases. J Oral Maxillofac Surg 2000;58:800-804.

37. Reichart PA, Philipsen HP, Sonner S: Ameloblastoma: biological profile of 3677 cases. Eur J Cancer B Oral Oncol 1995; 31B:86-99.

38. Lo Muzio L, Mignogna MD, Staibano S, De Rosa G: Granular cell ameloblastoma: a case report. Eur J Cancer B Oral Oncol 1996;32B:210-212.

39. Nagai N, Takeshita N, Nagatsuka H, et al: Ameloblastic carcinoma: a case report and review. J Oral Pathol Med 1991;20:460-463.

40. Bruce RA, Jackson IT: Ameloblastic carcinoma. J Craniomaxillofac Surg 1991;19:267-271.

41. Pindborg JJ, Vedtofte P, Reibel J, Praetorius F: The calcifying epithelial odontogenic tumor. A review of recent literature and report of a case. APMIS Suppl 1991;23:152-157.

42. Philipsen HP, Reichart PA: Calcifying epithelial odontogenic tumour: biological profile based on 181 cases from the literature. Oral Oncol 2000;36:17-26.

43. Hicks MJ, Flaitz CM, Wong ME, et al: Clear cell variant of calcifying epithelial odontogenic tumor. Head Neck 1994;16:272-277.

44. Schwartz-Arad D, Lustmann J, Ulmansky M: Squamous odontogenic tumor. Int J Oral Maxillofac Surg 1990;19:327-330.

45. Favia GF, Di Alberti L, Scarano A, Piattelli A: Squamous odontogenic tumor: report of two cases. Oral Oncol 1997;33:451-453.

46. Yamamoto H, Inui M, Mori A, Tagawa T: Clear cell odontogenic carcinoma. Oral Surg Oral Med Oral Pathol Oral Radiol Endod 1998;86:86-89.

47. Sadeghi EM, Levin S: Clear cell odontogenic carcinoma of the mandible. J Oral Maxillofac Surg 1995;53:613-616.

48. Kumamoto H, Yamazaki S, Sato A, et al: Clear cell odontogenic tumor of the mandible. J Oral Pathol Med 2000;29:43-47.

49. Favia G, Di Alberti L, Scarano A, Piattelli A: Ameloblastic fibro-odontoma. Oral Oncol 1997;33:444-446.

50. Haring JI: Ameloblastic fibro-odontoma. RDH 1999;19:12.

51. Awange DO: Adenomatoid odontogenic tumor—a review. East Afr Med J 1991;68:155-163.

52. Philipsen HP, Reichart PA, Zhang KH, et al: Adenomatoid odontogenic tumor. J Oral Pathol Med 1991;20:149-158.

53. Philipsen HP, Reichart PA: Adenomatoid odontogenic tumour. Oral Oncol 1999;35:125-131.

54. Philipsen HP, Reichart PA, Praetorius F: Mixed odontogenic tumors and odontomas. Oral Oncol 1997;33:86-99.

55. Miki Y, Oda Y, Iwaya N, et al: Clinicopathological studies of odontomas in 47 patients. J Oral Sci 1999;41:173-176.

56. Dunlap C: Odontogenic fibroma. Semin Diagn Pathol 1999; 16:293-296.

57. Handlers JP: Central odontogenic fibroma. J Oral Maxillofac Surg 1991;49:46-54.

58. Kaffe I: Clinical and radiological features of odontogenic myxomas of the jaws. Dentomaxillofac Radiol 1997;26:299-303.

59. Piattelli A, Scarano A, Antinori A, Trisi P: Odontogenic myxoma of the mandible. Acta Stomatol Belg 1994;91:101-109.

60. Barker BF: Odontogenic myxoma. Semin Diagn Pathol 1999; 16:297-301.

61. Piattelli A, D'Addona A, Piattelli M: Benign cementoblastoma. Acta Stomatol Belg 1990;87:209-215.

62. Berwick J, Maymi GF, Berkland ME: Benign cementoblastoma. J Oral Maxillofac Surg 1990;48:208-211.

63. El-Mofty S: Cemento-ossifying fibroma and benign cementoma. Semin Diagn Pathol 1999;16:302-307.

64. Mogi K, Belal E, Kano A, Otake K: Benign cementoblastoma. Aust Dent J 1996;41:9-11.

65. Ulmansky M, Hjorting-Hansen E, Praetorius F, Haque MF: Benign cementoblastoma. Oral Surg Oral Med Oral Pathol 1994;77:48-55.

66. Waldron CA: Fibro-osseous lesions of the jaws. J Oral Maxillofac Surg 1993;51:828-835.

67. Ferretti C, Coleman H, Dent M, Altini M: Cystic degeneration in fibrous dysplasia of the jaws: a case report. Oral Surg Oral Med Oral Pathol Oral Radiol Endod 1999;88:337-342.

68. MacDonald-Jankowski D: Fibrous dysplasia in the jaws of a Hong-Kong population: radiographic presentation and systematic review. Dentomaxillofac Radiol 1999;28:195-202.

69. Sozeri B, Ataman M, Ruacan S, Gedikoglu G: Ameloblastic fibrosarcoma. Int J Pediatr Otorhinolaryngol 1993;25:255-259.

70. Muller S, Parker DC, Kapadia SB, et al: Ameloblastic fibrosarcoma of the jaws. Oral Surg Oral Med Oral Pathol Oral Radiol Endod 1995;79:469-477.

71. Park HR, Shin KB, Sol MY, et al: A highly malignant ameloblastic fibrosarcoma. Oral Surg Oral Med Oral Pathol Oral Radiol Endod 1995;79:478-481.

72. Kaplan I, Calderon S, Buchner A: Peripheral osteoma of the mandible. J Oral Maxillofac Surg 1994;52:467-470.

73. Kondoh T, Seto K, Kobayashi K: Osteoma of the mandibular condyle. J Oral Maxillofac Surg 1998;56:972-979.

74. Chen Y, Lin LM, Lin CC: Osteoma of the mandibular coronoid process. Int J Oral Maxillofac Surg 1998;27:222-233.

75. Piattelli A, Scarano A, Di Alberti L, Piattelli M: Osteoma of the mandible. Acta Stomatol Belg 1993;92:13-15.

76. Peters T, Oliver DR, McDonald JS: Benign osteoblastoma of the mandible: report of a case. J Oral Maxillofac Surg 1995;53:1347-1349.

77. Ataoglu O, Oygur T, Yamalik K, Yucel E: Recurrent osteoblastoma of the mandible: a case report. J Oral Maxillofac Surg 1994;52:86-90.

78. Jainkittivong A, Langlais RP: Buccal and palatal exostoses: prevalence and concurrence with tori. Oral Surg Oral Med Oral Pathol 2000;90:48-53.

79. Shah DS, Sanghavi SJ, Chawda JD, Shah RM: Prevalence of torus palatinus and torus mandibularis in 1000 patients. Indian J Dent Res 1992;3:107-110.

80. Eversole LR, Leider AS, Nelson K: Ossifying fibroma: a clinicopathologic study of 64 cases. Oral Surg Oral Med Oral Pathol 1985;60:505-511.

81. Sciubba JJ, Younai F: Ossifying fibroma of the mandible and maxilla: review of 18 cases. J Oral Pathol Med 1989;18:315-321.

82. Hopkins K, Huttula CS, Kahn MA, Albright JE: Desmoplastic fibroma of the mandible: review and report of two cases. J Oral Maxillofac Surg 1996;54:1249-1254.

83. De Vito MA, Tom LW, Boran TV, Quinn PD: Desmoplastic fibroma of the mandible. Ear Nose Throat J 1989;68:553-556.

84. Karras S, Wolford LM, Cottrell DA: Concurrent osteochondroma of the mandibular condyle and ipsilateral cranial bone resulting in temporomandibular joint ankylosis. J Oral Maxillofac Surg 1996;54:640-646.

85. Kerscher A, Piette E, Tideman H, Wu PC: Osteochondroma of the coronoid process. Oral Surg Oral Med Oral Pathol 1993;75:539-564.

86. Whitaker SB, Waldron CA: Central giant cell lesions of the jaws. Oral Surg Oral Med Oral Pathol 1993;75:199-208.

87. Auclair PL, Cuenin P, Kratochvil FJ, et al: Giant cell lesions of the jaws. Oral Maxillofac Surg Clin North Am 1997,9.655-680.

88. Chuong R, Kaban LB, Kozakewich H, Perez-Atayde A: Central giant cell lesions of the jaws: a clinicopathologic study. J Oral Maxillofac Surg 1986;44:708-713.

89. Yamaguchi T, Dorfman HD, Eisig S: Cherubism—clinicopathological features. Skeletal Radiol 1999;28:350-353.

90. Yucel OT, Genc E, Kaya S: Cherubism—a radiologic and clinical presentation. Turk J Pediatr 1998;40:453-459.

91. Sellari-Franceschini S, Forli F, Pierini S, et al: Langerhans cell histiocytosis: a case report. Int J Pediatr Otorhinolaryngol 1999;48:85-87.

92. Martinez-Perez D, Mulliken JB, Arceci RJ: Langerhans cell histiocytosis: an uncommon disease commonly manifesting in the craniofacial skeleton. Plast Reconstr Surg 1996;98:211-216.

93. Mody R, Sathawane RS, Rai S: Central hemangioma. Ann Dent 1995;54:22-24.

94. Bunel K, Sindet-Pedersen S: Central hemangioma of the mandible. Oral Surg Oral Med Oral Pathol 1993;75:565-570.

95. Kaban L, Mulliken JB: Vascular anomalies of the maxillofacial region. J Oral Maxillofac Surg 1986;44:203-213.

96. Weber AL, Scrivani SJ, Aziz SR: Cysts, tumors, and nontumorous lesions of the jaw. In Som PM, Curtin HD, eds: Head and Neck Imaging, 4th ed, vol 1. St. Louis, Mosby, 2003:930-994.

97. Patterson A, Greer RO Jr, Howard D: Periosteal osteosarcoma of the mandible. J Oral Maxillofac Surg 1990;48:522-526.

98. Piattelli A, Favia GF: Periosteal osteosarcoma of the jaws. J Periodontol 2000;71:325-329.

99. August M, Magennis P, Dewitt D: Osteogenic sarcoma of the jaws: factors influencing prognosis. Int J Oral Maxillofac Surg 1997;26:198-204.

100. Kawasaki T, Ono N, Watanabe K, Hoshi K: Chondroblastic osteosarcoma of the mandible. J Oral Maxillofac Surg 1996; 54:1123-1127.

101. Zakkak T, Flynn TR, Boguslaw B, Adamo AK: Mesenchymal chondrosarcoma of the mandible. J Oral Maxillofac Surg 1998;56:84-91.

102. Gorsky M, Epstein JB: Craniofacial osseous and chondromatous sarcomas in British Columbia. Oral Oncol 2000;36:27-31.

103. Takahashi K, Sato K, Kanazawa H, et al: Mesenchymal chondrosarcoma of the jaw. Head Neck 1993;15:459-464.

104. Wood RE, Nortje CJ, Hesseling P, Grotepass F: Ewing's tumor of the jaws. Oral Surg Oral Med Oral Pathol 1990;69:120-127.

105. Vaccani JP, Forte V, de Jong AL, Taylor G: Ewing's sarcoma of the head and neck in children. Int J Pediatr Otorhinolaryngol 1999;48:209-216.

106. Shapira J, Peylan-Ramu N: Burkitt's lymphoma. Oral Oncol 1997;34:15-23.

107. Hanazawa T, Kimura Y, Sakamaki H, et al: Burkitt's lymphoma involving the mandible. Oral Surg Oral Med Oral Pathol Oral Radiol Endod 1998,85.216-220.

108. Shapira J, Peylan-Ramu N, Lustmann J: Retrospective study of Burkitt's lymphoma in Israel and diagnosis by conservative incisional biopsy. Eur J Cancer B Oral Oncol 1995;31B:319-322.

109. Kanazawa H, Shoji A, Yokoe H, et al: Solitary plasmacytoma of the mandible. J Craniomaxillofac Surg 1993;21:202-206.

110. Gonzalez J, Elizondo J, Trull JM, De Torres I: Plasma cell tumours of the condyle. Br J Oral Maxillofac Surg 1991;29:274-276.

111. Nofsinger YC, Mirza N, Rowan PT, et al: Head and neck manifestations of plasma cell neoplasms. Laryngoscope 1997;107:741-746.

112. Witt C, Borges AC, Klein K, Neumann HJ: Radiographic manifestations of multiple myeloma in the mandible: a retrospective study of 77 patients. J Oral Maxillofac Surg 1997;55:450-453.

113. Sanchez Aniceto G, Garcia Penin A, de la Mata Pages R, Montalvo Moreno JJ: Tumors metastatic to the mandible. J Oral Maxillofac Surg 1990;48:246-251.

114. Pruckmayer M, Glaser C, Marosi C, Leitha T: Mandibular pain as the leading symptom of metastatic disease. Ann Oncol 1998;9:559-564.

115. Hirshberg A, Leibovich P, Buchner A: Metastatic tumors of the jaw bones: analysis of 390 cases. J Oral Pathol Med 1994;23:337-341.

116. Hirshberg A, Leibovich P, Horowitz I, Buchner A: Metastatic tumors to postextraction sites. J Oral Maxillofac Surg 1993; 51:1334-1337.

Carcinoma of the Upper Aerodigestive Tract

STEVEN A. GOLDMAN, MD ✦ EDWARD A. LUCE, MD

The upper aerodigestive tract comprises the mouth, nose, paranasal sinuses, pharynx, larynx, trachea, and esophageal inlet. Carcinoma of the upper aerodigestive tract is a devastating disease, and its treatment may leave patients with difficulty in talking and swallowing or the inability to talk and swallow, obvious cosmetic defects, and sometimes a permanent tracheostome, all of which can have a profound impact on a patient's quality of life and psychological state. Treatment of head and neck carcinomas must address the functional importance of the affected structures. In general, patients are treated through the combined effort of a multidisciplinary team involving surgeons, radiation oncologists, medical oncologists, speech pathologists, nutritionists, and others. Medical consultation is often necessary because patients with head and neck cancer often have associated medical comorbidities, such as coronary atherosclerosis or chronic obstructive pulmonary disease, due to risk factors of smoking, alcohol abuse, and older age.

The predominant histopathologic change is squamous cell carcinoma arising from the stratified squamous epithelium that lines most of the upper aerodigestive tract. Tobacco abuse is the primary risk factor for development of a squamous cell tumor, and alcohol is a secondary synergistic carcinogen. The majority of patients are older men. Tumors can be characterized by site of origin and stage; the stage refers to the American Joint Committee on Cancer staging system based on the size and location of a tumor, the number and size of regional (lymphatic) metastases, and the presence of distant metastases. Survival is influenced by the size and location of the primary tumor and the presence or absence of lymph node metastases. Lymphatic metastases reduce survival rates by about half.[1]

Treatment options involve surgical extirpation or radiotherapy for small lesions and excision with adjuvant radiation for large lesions. Chemotherapy and immunotherapy are usually given as part of experimental protocols. Organ preservation protocols combining induction chemotherapy with radiation have produced encouraging results and are being used increasingly for advanced tumors.[1] Contemporary reconstructive techniques not only have improved the quality of life for patients with head and neck cancer, they have permitted more aggressive extirpation because complex wounds can now be closed. Effective reconstruction in these patients has great potential to improve quality of life by shortening recovery time, maximizing the potential for useful speaking and swallowing, minimizing cosmetic deformity, and limiting complications from surgery and adjuvant therapy. Thus, the plastic surgeon has a crucial role in contemporary treatment of the patient with head and neck cancer.

This chapter covers a broad subject, head and neck cancer. Textbooks have been dedicated to the topics of head and neck oncology, surgical treatment of tumors of the head and neck (i.e., extirpation), and reconstruction of head and neck defects.[2-4] The authors have attempted to distill the salient features of these subtopics in the following sections; however, this discussion is not intended to be comprehensive.

ANATOMY

The upper aerodigestive tract consists of the passages for food and air to the gastrointestinal tract and lower airway. The structures that serve this purpose are the oral and nasal cavities, paranasal sinuses, nasopharynx, oropharynx, hypopharynx, and larynx (Fig. 111-1). The larynx is further divided into the supraglottis, glottis, and subglottis. These structures have well-defined anatomic boundaries. Tumors arising from different sites within the upper aerodigestive tract have different rates of local, regional, and distant metastasis and mortality, so correct anatomic classification is crucial for accurate prognostic information to be provided to patients and for sound surgical planning. The anatomic boundaries of each region are described in detail in this section.[5]

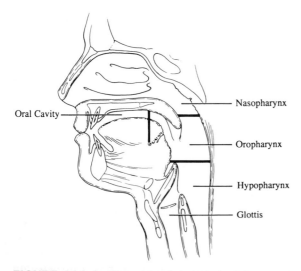

FIGURE 111-1. The anatomic subsites of the upper aerodigestive tract. (From Ariyan S, Chicarilli ZN: Cancer of the upper aerodigestive system. In McCarthy JG, ed: Plastic Surgery. Philadelphia, WB Saunders, 1990:3412.)

Oral Cavity and Oropharynx

The anterior border of the oral cavity is the vermilion border of the upper and lower lips. The posterior border is defined by the circumvallate papillae of the tongue inferiorly and the junction between the hard and soft palates superiorly. Structures of the oral cavity include the lips, gingivobuccal sulci, gingiva and teeth, buccal mucosa, floor of the mouth, ventral and dorsal oral tongue, retromolar trigone on each side, and hard palate (Fig. 111-2). The oropharynx begins at the posterior limit of the oral cavity and extends to the posterior and lateral walls of the pharynx. The oropharynx extends superiorly to the level of the soft palate and inferiorly to the level of the hyoid bone. Structures within the oropharynx include the posterior tongue and circumvallate papillae, base of tongue, valleculae, soft palate, uvula, tonsils, anterior and posterior tonsillar pillars, and lateral and posterior walls of the oropharynx.

Nasal Cavity and Nasopharynx

The nasal cavity begins anteriorly at the nostrils and ends posteriorly at the paired nasal choanae, which open into the nasopharynx. The paired nasal cavities contain the nasal vestibules, turbinates or conchae (inferior, middle, superior, and sometimes supreme), septum, and choanae. The septum is a midline structure composed of the quadrangular cartilage anteriorly, the perpendicular plate of the ethmoid bone posterosuperiorly, and the vomer posteroinferiorly. The nasopharynx is the superior aspect of the pharynx. Above the nasopharynx is the skull base. The inferior border is the level of the soft palate. The nasopharynx includes the nasal aspect of the soft palate, the adenoids, and the superior aspect of the posterior and lateral pharyngeal walls. The eustachian tube orifices are located in the lateral walls of the nasopharynx. The muscular ridge that forms their superior border is the torus tubarius. The retropharyngeal lymph nodes, also known as the nodes of Rouvière, are in the fossae of Rosenmüller, the sulci just superior to the torus tubarius. The presence of these nodes either clinically or radiographically is considered pathologic.

Hypopharynx and Larynx

The hypopharynx is the most inferior part of the pharynx. The hypopharynx forms a chute around the glottis through which food passes into the esophagus and is composed of the piriform sinuses, the postcricoid area, and the pharyngeal walls below the level of the tip of the epiglottis. The hypopharynx wraps around the anteriorly situated larynx. The supraglottic larynx extends from the tip of the epiglottis to the plane of the vocal cords and includes the epiglottis,

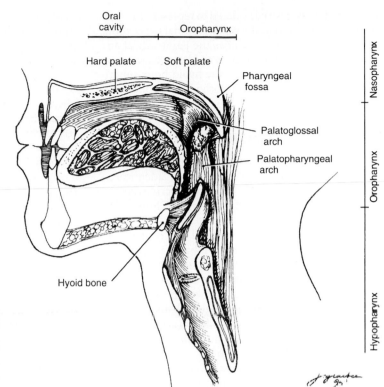

FIGURE 111-2. Sagittal view of the upper aerodigestive tract and some of the surface landmarks of the oropharynx. (From Civantos FJ, Goodwin WJ: Cancer of the oropharynx. In Myers EN, Suen JY, eds: Cancer of the Head and Neck. Philadelphia, WB Saunders, 1996:361.)

the arytenoepiglottic folds, the false vocal cords, and the ventricles. The floors of the ventricles are the true vocal cords. The glottis consists of the true vocal cords and the area extending below the plane of the true cords for 1 cm. It therefore includes the true cords, arytenoid cartilages, and anterior commissure. The subglottic larynx extends from 1 cm below the true cords to the trachea.

Cervical Lymphatics

The cervical lymphatics have been divided into six zones (Fig. 111-3). Zone I includes the submandibular and submental nodes, bounded superiorly by the inferior border of the mandibular body, inferiorly by the posterior belly of the digastric muscle, and anteriorly by the midline. Zones II, III, and IV comprise the cervical chain; they extend anteriorly to the strap musculature and posteriorly to the posterior border of the sternocleidomastoid muscle. Zone II is superior and extends from posterior to the mandibular angle to the level of the hyoid bone clinically or to the carotid bifurcation surgically; zone II contains the jugulodigastric nodes. Zone III extends down to the level of the cricoid cartilage clinically and to the omohyoid muscle surgically. Zone IV extends to the clavicle. Zone V nodes are in the posterior cervical triangle, between the sternocleidomastoid and trapezius

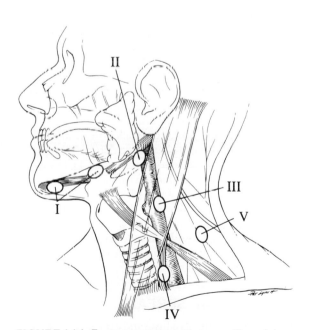

FIGURE 111-3. Cervical lymphatic zones. (From Ariyan S, Chicarilli ZN: Cancer of the upper aerodigestive system. In McCarthy JG, ed: Plastic Surgery. Philadelphia, WB Saunders, 1990:3412.)

muscles; they are also considered to represent the lymphatics that lie deep to the cervical spinal nerve roots. Zone VI (not labeled) includes the paratracheal and pretracheal nodes, lying deep to and between the strap musculature extending from the hyoid bone superiorly to the sternal notch inferiorly; it is the only non-paired lymph node group.

ONCOLOGIC CONSIDERATIONS

The majority of head and neck cancers are squamous cell carcinomas. Mucosal melanoma, adenocarcinoma, salivary gland tumors, neuroendocrine tumors, and other malignant neoplasms are also found. The primary risk factors are smoking and alcohol consumption. Most patients with head and neck cancer are older men with a history of tobacco and alcohol consumption. Alcohol by itself is a weak carcinogen, but it is synergistic with tobacco. Other carcinogens that have been weakly associated with head and neck cancers include industrial chemicals like arsenic, chromium, and radium. Wood dust has been associated with paranasal sinus lesions. Malnutrition and vitamin deficiencies have been associated with hypopharyngeal lesions. Ebstein-Barr virus has been linked to nasopharyngeal carcinoma. Prior irradiation has been associated with thyroid and skin cancers more than with aerodigestive tract lesions.

The concept of field cancerization is central to the pathogenesis of mucosal squamous cell carcinomas. This theory suggests that carcinogens like alcohol and tobacco affect all the mucosal surfaces of the aerodigestive tract with which they come in contact. Thus, when a carcinoma develops, it does so not as an isolated, coincidental event but as the end result of a multistep process that is occurring, to some degree, over all of the mucosal surfaces exposed to the carcinogens. The primary tumor thus arises in a field of abnormal mucosa. Mutations such as those in the *TP53* tumor suppressor gene have been detected at mucosal sites distant from primary carcinomas. Field cancerization may play the greatest role in the oral cavity, where gross evidence of this process is manifested by widespread leukoplakia and diffuse erythema often seen in conjunction with tumors. The concept of field cancerization has also been used to explain the incidence of second primaries in the head and neck, which is discussed in the next section.[6]

PATTERNS OF SPREAD

Changes in treatment of head and neck carcinoma have not appreciably affected survival rates since the advent of contemporary therapies but rather have resulted in a shift in recurrence patterns. Local and regional tumor control has greatly improved. Patients are now more likely to succumb to distant disease, such as lung or liver metastases. Local control refers to the primary tumor; regional control refers to the cervical lymphatics. Upper aerodigestive tract squamous cell carcinomas spread first to the cervical lymphatics and then to distant sites in a fairly predictable pattern based on the location and size of the primary tumor. This observation has a number of implications. When a patient presents with a primary tumor, one can focus treatment of the cervical lymphatics on those groups most at risk for metastasis based on the site of the primary. On the other hand, if a patient presents with a neck mass, the location of the mass suggests where the primary tumor may be found. The concept of elective or prophylactic neck dissection pertains to patients with no clinically palpable or radiographically suspicious lymph node enlargement. The nodal basins most at risk for subclinical metastasis, based on the known patterns of spread, are removed even though no clinically positive nodes are present. Pathologic examination of these nodes can guide further therapy and provide prognostic information for the patient according to the status of the lymph nodes. Elective radiotherapy can also be used to treat the nodal basins most at risk for metastasis.[1] The debate concerning when elective treatment of the neck is warranted and with what modality is discussed in the following section.

In general, oral cavity lesions spread to zones I, II, and III as the first echelon. Laryngeal and pharyngeal lesions spread to zones II, III, and IV. Skin lesions of the face and scalp spread to periparotid and zone I nodes when they are preauricular and to upper cervical and zone V nodes when they are postauricular. Nasopharyngeal and soft palate lesions spread to the retropharyngeal nodes and may also present in zone V. Aerodigestive tract squamous cell carcinomas rarely metastasize to distant sites without first presenting with regional lymph node metastases. The lungs, liver, and bones are the most common distant sites involved. Up to a third of head and neck tumors may ultimately develop clinically apparent distant metastases.[6]

GENERAL THERAPEUTIC GUIDELINES

In general, treatment must address the primary site and the regional lymphatics. For small lesions, radiation and surgery have similar efficacy but different morbidity, and the treatment of a given lesion often reflects local bias; some institutions use radiation more liberally, and some favor surgery. Larger tumors benefit from combined modality treatment with surgery and adjuvant radiotherapy. The most commonly used chemotherapeutic regimen is 5-fluorouracil and cisplatin; in general, chemotherapy is administered on protocol. Organ-sparing protocols using radiation and chemotherapy with surgical salvage are being more commonly used, especially for advanced laryngeal and tongue base tumors because of the severe adverse effects of surgical extirpation. Brachytherapy has been most commonly used in nasopharyngeal tumors (with molds) and tongue base tumors (with percutaneous catheters and radioisotope seeds). Immunotherapy, angiogenesis inhibitors, and tumor vaccines are currently being used experimentally.

The guiding principle of surgical extirpation is complete excision of the primary tumor with negative pathologic margins. Effective pathologic examination of a complex head and neck specimen in three dimensions requires good communication between the surgeon and pathologist and usually entails review of the specimen together. Frozen section margins are used, and the surgeon must identify questionable margins intraoperatively for frozen section. If the permanent section margins are positive, further resection should be considered because radiation will not necessarily eliminate residual tumor. The resection itself involves close visual inspection and palpation of the tumor to maintain adequate gross margins; a cuff of 1 cm of normal mucosa or muscle should be taken when possible to help ensure complete extirpation. This may be inappropriate in areas like the vocal folds or impossible in areas like the orbit or skull base. When tumors involve bone, most commonly the mandible, extirpation must include an adequate bone margin. Because the marrow space can be a route of local tumor spread, a wide bone margin is usually indicated. Frozen section cannot be used to assess bone because it must be decalcified for pathologic examination. The surgeon must also account for direct tumor extension along nerves. In the case of the mandible, frozen section examination of the inferior alveolar nerve is often warranted. In planning extirpation, wide exposure is essential to allow the best chance for complete excision with negative margins; the concept of tumor debulking has no role in the treatment of head and neck carcinoma.

Treatment of the cervical lymphatics depends on the nodal stage of the tumor at presentation. The N0 neck is clinically free of disease on both physical and radiographic examination (no palpable lymphadenopathy or evidence of enlargement, central necrosis, or distortion of the normal oval shape of the lymph nodes on scans). Treatment of the N0 neck has been a subject of ongoing debate. The argument for treatment of the cervical lymphatics electively, before there is clinical evidence of metastasis, is that observation of the N0 neck until nodal disease becomes apparent too often results in unresectable disease in the neck, with a consequentially dismal prognosis for the patient. Elective or prophylactic neck treatment by definition entails treatment of the neck before lymphatic disease is apparent and can be accomplished with either radiation or lymph node dissection. Elective neck dissection alone may be adequate treatment of the neck in the absence of extracapsular extension of lymph node disease and when fewer than four pathologically positive nodes are present. If either condition is evident on pathologic examination, postoperative radiotherapy is indicated.[7,8] Therapeutic neck dissections are, by definition, performed to remove clinically apparent disease. In general, a modified radical neck dissection is indicated. A radical neck dissection includes removal of the spinal accessory nerve, internal jugular vein, and sternocleidomastoid muscle. Modified radical neck dissections preserve one or more of these structures. As with elective neck dissection, if pathologic examination reveals extracapsular extension or more than four positive nodes, postoperative radiotherapy is indicated. Neck dissection is discussed in detail in Chapter 117.

RECONSTRUCTION

Reconstruction of extirpative defects of the head and neck poses some of the most difficult problems facing the plastic surgeon. Without reconstruction, extirpation would often be not only unreasonable but impossible. Reconstruction of the aerodigestive tract may affect speech and swallowing and may restore the integrity of the pharynx, isolating vital structures such as the carotid artery from saliva and food. Skull base defects often require isolation of neurovascular structures, including the central nervous system, from the nasopharynx or external environment by use of vascularized soft tissue. External defects may involve challenging aesthetic and functional problems, such as restoring an oral cavity defect that involves the full thickness of the lip and the underlying mandible. Modern reconstructive techniques rely heavily on free tissue transfer and pedicled muscle flaps.

Pectoralis Flap

The workhorse pedicled flap of head and neck reconstruction is the pectoralis muscle or musculocutaneous flap (Fig. 111-4). The dominant blood supply comes from the pectoral branch of the thoracoacromial artery, a branch of the subclavian artery. Secondary blood supply comes from segmental perforators of the internal mammary artery and from minor branches off the axillary artery. The secondary blood supply is ligated. The muscle is then transposed on the thoracoacromial artery, which is located near the junction of the middle and lateral thirds of the clavicle. The muscle is rotated above the clavicle. If a muscle-only flap is used, the muscle may be turned over on itself, folding it superiorly on the clavicle. If a musculocutaneous flap is used, the arc of rotation is approximately 180 degrees. The musculocutaneous flap is significantly more bulky than the muscle-only flap. The muscle flap may be skin grafted whether it is placed externally or

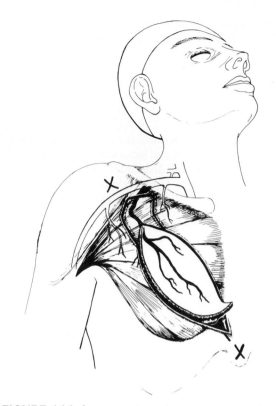

FIGURE 111-4. Pectoralis major myocutaneous flap. The pectoral branch of the thoracoacromial artery travels along a line drawn from the acromion to the xiphoid, as noted by the two X marks. The origin of the vascular pedicle starts roughly at the junction between the middle and lateral thirds of the clavicle. (From Ariyan S, Chicarilli ZN: Cancer of the upper aerodigestive system. In McCarthy JG, ed: Plastic Surgery. Philadelphia, WB Saunders, 1990:3412.)

intraorally, but in the oral cavity or pharynx, the muscle is rapidly covered with mucosa and does not often require grafting. The pectoralis flap will easily resurface defects of the neck or oral cavity, including glossectomy defects, but various authors state different superior limits of the flap. Most authors agree that the flap is unreliable superior to the zygoma and is probably not reliable above the external auditory meatus. Further superior reach may be obtained by delaying a randomly based skin paddle inferiorly on the upper abdomen. Further reach may also be obtained by removing a portion of the clavicle or by removing the superior attachments of the muscle to the clavicle and debulking the superficial muscle in this area.

Flap harvest is technically straightforward. The pedicle originates approximately between the lateral and central thirds of the clavicle and can be located on a line drawn between the acromion and the nipple. For the muscle-only flap, an incision is taken from the central clavicle inferiorly over the anterior surface of

the pectoralis muscle. The skin is raised off the muscle, leaving the fascia intact. The muscle's origin is divided from the sternum medially and rib cage inferiorly. Large medial perforators from the internal mammary artery (secondary pedicles) must be controlled near the sternum. Laterally, the insertion of the pectoralis onto the pectoral groove of the humerus is cut at the anterior axillary line, which is formed by the muscle. The subpectoral plane is readily entered by blunt dissection, which avoids trauma to the vascular pedicle that lies on the deep surface and allows dissection of the muscle from the pectoralis minor. The muscle fibers of origin from the clavicle are divided partially from the bone while the pedicle is protected. It may finally be rotated or flipped into the defect. If a skin paddle is used, this is designed on the chest wall, avoiding the nipple-areola complex. As mentioned, this skin island can extend past the muscle as a randomly based extension.

Other Pedicled Flaps

Multiple other muscle flaps are used in reconstruction of head and neck cancer defects, none of which is as versatile and reliable as the pectoralis. The arc of rotation of the latissimus muscle or musculocutaneous flap is the axilla (Fig. 111-5). The flap is based on the thoracodorsal artery of the subscapular system. Although its use has been described for defects as far superior as the vertex of the skull, the distal edge is unreliable once it is raised. The latissimus can be used reliably for coverage of the neck anteriorly or posteriorly and can provide intraoral lining. A skin island can be included, oriented obliquely or transversely. Harvest begins with an incision made from the axilla to a point a few centimeters above the iliac crest; this incision is made 2 or 3 cm posterior to the anterior border of the muscle. The skin is raised off the superficial aspect of the muscle. The muscle is then elevated from the chest wall, and the origin from the iliac crest and paraspinal area is transected. Large posterior paraspinous perforators must be ligated to minimize the risk of postoperative hematoma. The pedicle is identified on the deep surface of the muscle along the anterosuperior border. The branch of the thoracodorsal artery to the serratus anterior muscle is ligated to free the vascular pedicle with the muscle. The point of rotation is located where the subscapular vascular system originates from the axillary artery. Disinsertion of the muscle from the humerus can also increase rotation.

The trapezius muscle may be used to cover intraoral or external defects, in particular occipital or posterior scalp defects, but it may be less reliable than pectoralis and latissimus muscle or musculocutaneous flaps (see Fig. 111-5). The dominant vascular supply comes from the descending branches of the transverse

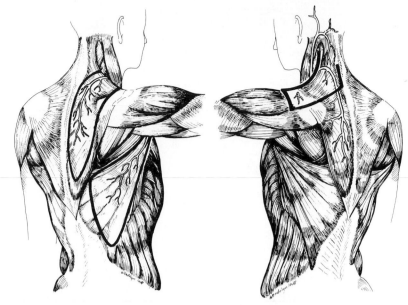

FIGURE 111-5. Outlines of the latissimus and trapezius muscles with their vascular supply from the lateral thoracic and transverse cervical arteries, respectively. (From Ariyan S, Chicarilli ZN: Cancer of the upper aerodigestive system. In McCarthy JG, ed: Plastic Surgery. Philadelphia, WB Saunders, 1990: 3412.)

cervical artery. Vascular supply also comes from the occipital artery, dorsal scapular artery, and posterior intercostal perforators. The standard flap incorporates transverse cervical branches by use of a vertically oriented strip of muscle, with or without overlying skin. The muscle is taken between the posterior trunk midline and the scapula. The arc of rotation is the posterior base of the neck. Preservation of the superior aspect of the trapezius muscle preserves shoulder function. If a neck dissection has been performed, the transverse cervical artery may have been ligated, preventing reliable use of the flap. The sternocleidomastoid muscle has triplicate blood supply from the transverse cervical, superior thyroid, and occipital arteries. With no dominant pedicle, it is unreliable when pedicled superiorly or inferiorly. It is also frequently sacrificed with a neck dissection. Nonetheless, it has been used for intraoral defects with a small skin paddle.

Nasolabial flaps can be turned intraorally to resurface the floor of mouth and cover the anterior mandible. One has to be careful not to sacrifice tongue mobility if these flaps are used because of the obvious adverse implications for articulation if the mobile tongue is tethered. Bilateral flaps can be used to provide adequate coverage. The flaps are usually based inferiorly with inflow from facial artery branches. They are turned in through a defect placed in the cheek. They can be placed in one stage with a de-epithelialized segment turned into the cheek defect, or the pedicle can be divided at approximately 14 days as a planned two-stage procedure (Fig. 111-6). The cheek defect is noticeable. The deltopectoral flap is a large fasciocutaneous advancement flap with random blood supply

(Fig. 111-7). It can be used to resurface the lower neck or to provide oral lining. It is unreliable distally, limiting its utility. A laterally based forehead flap (scalping flap) has also been used to line intraoral defects (Fig. 111-8). The skin of the forehead is elevated above the periosteum, based laterally on the superficial temporal artery. The flap is then tunneled into the oral cavity deep to the zygoma, and the defect is skin grafted. The donor defect is significant.

The temporoparietal fascia flap, based on the superficial temporal artery, can be used for small defects of the oral cavity, oropharynx, nasopharynx, and sometimes facial skin. The flap dissection begins with an incision from just above the tragus into the temporal hairline. Subcutaneous dissection lifts the scalp off the thin temporoparietal fascia, which is in turn elevated off the deep temporal fascia, identified by its dense, white appearance. The pedicle from the superficial temporal artery is preserved inferiorly. The flap is quite thin and is usually combined with a skin graft to replace facial skin defects and to cover exposed auricular cartilage. Alopecia is not uncommon at the donor site. If it is transposed to the oral cavity, the arc of rotation is the superficial temporal artery, the terminal branch of the external carotid artery, at the level of the superior aspect of the tragus. The flap is used when skin grafts alone will not suffice, such as with complex maxillary and orbital defects. As such, it is generally tunneled deep to the zygomatic arch by temporarily removing the arch and brought into the oral cavity or facial defect. The temporalis muscle flap can also be used for intraoral lining posteriorly and laterally, including around the posterior mandible, and for nasopharyngeal defects. It is based on the

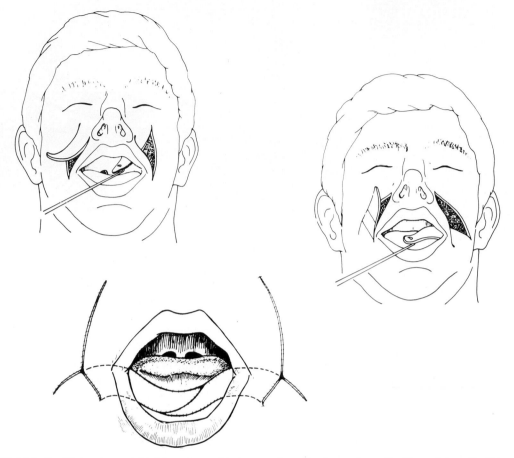

FIGURE 111-6. Bilateral nasolabial flaps turned in to resurface the floor of mouth. (From Ariyan S, Chicarilli ZN: Cancer of the upper aerodigestive system. In McCarthy JG, ed: Plastic Surgery. Philadelphia, WB Saunders, 1990:3412.)

anterior and posterior deep temporal branches of the internal maxillary artery. The temporalis flap is exposed by extending a linear or curvilinear skin incision from the preauricular area to the temporal scalp. Dissection through skin and the loose pretemporal fascia allows identification of the dense, white deep temporal fascia overlying the muscle. The muscle is divided from its origin along the temporal line of the skull. The arc of rotation can be increased by temporarily removing the zygomatic arch, which is then reattached with plate fixation. The frontal branch of the facial nerve is protected as it crosses over the arch

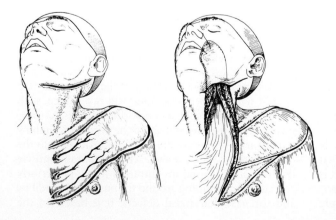

FIGURE 111-7. The deltopectoral flap, shown here as used for intraoral lining. (From Ariyan S, Chicarilli ZN: Cancer of the upper aerodigestive system. In McCarthy JG, ed: Plastic Surgery. Philadelphia, WB Saunders, 1990:3412.)

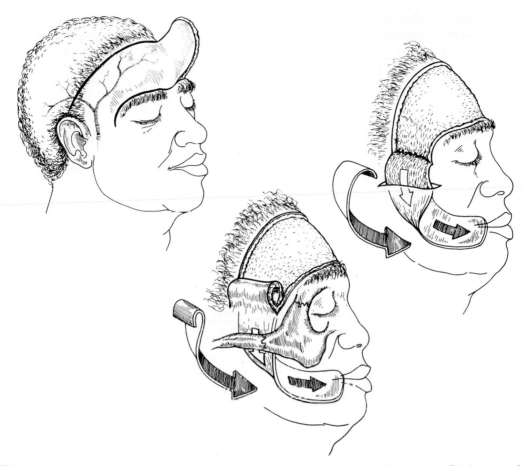

FIGURE 111-8. The laterally based forehead flap shown with its vascular supply, the superficial temporal artery, and used here for intraoral lining. (From Ariyan S, Chicarilli ZN: Cancer of the upper aerodigestive system. In McCarthy JG, ed: Plastic Surgery. Philadelphia, WB Saunders, 1990:3412.)

in the superficial layer of the deep temporal fascia by elevating the fascia with subperiosteal dissection off of the arch. The deep temporal arteries can be identified on the deep surface of the muscle inferior to the arch. The muscle can then be reflected inferiorly into the nasopharynx or oropharynx. The arc of rotation can be increased by transecting the insertion of the muscle from the coronoid process of the mandible. Note that if the external carotid artery has been transected from a neck dissection, this flap cannot be used because the deep temporal arteries are branches of the external carotid artery.

Free Tissue Transfer

Modern extirpative techniques, especially of large cancers of the head and neck, rely heavily on free tissue transfer for reconstruction. Free tissue transfer is indicated when local or regional flaps cannot provide adequate coverage or when free tissue allows improved quality of the reconstructive site.[9] The use of free flaps does require familiarity with microvascular techniques and instrumentation, but it avoids the morbidity of the use of local tissue from the head and neck and often provides more reliable vascularized tissue than the distal portion of a pedicled flap. For example, the donor morbidity of tongue flaps often results in difficulty with articulation and the oral phase of swallowing. The defect left by harvesting of a temporalis muscle flap is obvious temporal hollowing. Free flap donor sites are often more tolerable: a skin graft on the volar wrist for the radial forearm fasciocutaneous free flap, a lateral trunk scar for the latissimus muscle or musculocutaneous free flap. Also, free flaps in the head and neck especially have excellent vascularity. Although there is a risk of microvascular thrombosis, the failure rate is often lower than with pedicled flaps, for which distal flap necrosis may require salvage with another flap.[10,11] In the setting of salvage extirpative surgery after radiotherapy, free tissue transfer provides the additional benefit of delivering nonirradiated tissues into the irradiated field.

Although many different free flaps have been described, most of the reconstructive needs of the head and neck can be provided with a few specific flaps. The radial forearm fasciocutaneous flap can provide intraoral, pharyngeal, or external coverage and can be tubed to repair a pharyngectomy defect. A segment of free jejunum can also be used to fill a pharyngectomy defect. The rectus muscle or musculocutaneous flap can provide bulky coverage of skull base defects or glossectomy defects. The fibular osseous or osteoseptocutaneous flap can provide bone stock to reconstruct the mandible and lining for the oral cavity, although the reliability of the skin portion of the flap is variable, with a failure rate of approximately 10% to 30% for the cutaneous paddle.[12]

Immediate reconstruction with free tissue transfer allows definitive address of defects in a single stage to minimize the morbidity of extirpation. Free flaps also allow residual function to be maximized to facilitate rehabilitation. For instance, the continuity of the pharynx or mandible can be maintained, or the mobility of the tongue can be preserved (Table 111-1).

EVALUATION OF THE PATIENT WITH HEAD AND NECK CANCER

History and Symptoms

The initial evaluation of the patient with head and neck cancer requires knowledge of the risk factors, signs, symptoms, and physical findings associated with tumors of the various subsites within the head and neck. Familiarity with a complete head and neck physical examination, including indirect laryngoscopy, is a prerequisite. Diagnosis may not be difficult when a patient is referred for a suspected tumor, but when

patients present with symptoms like otalgia or persistent sore throat, the practitioner must maintain a high index of suspicion to detect an early cancer.

In addition to risk factors, the history of a patient with a potential head and neck cancer must focus on symptoms suggestive of that diagnosis. All patients should be asked about dysphagia (difficulty swallowing), odynophagia (pain on swallowing), weight loss, hoarseness, throat pain (especially if it is focal to a specific site or side), otalgia (ear pain), new cough, hemoptysis, and globus sensation (the sensation of something stuck in the throat). An early laryngeal cancer can present with hoarseness. Advanced laryngeal tumors may also cause dysphagia, odynophagia, or hemoptysis. Pharyngeal tumors may present with the same symptoms but more commonly present only with pain, persistent unilateral sore throat, or referred otalgia. Otalgia can be caused by base of tongue, pharyngeal wall, and supraglottic tumors. The mechanism of this referred pain involves the vagus and glossopharyngeal nerves. The internal branch of the superior laryngeal nerve provides sensation to the supraglottic larynx and adjacent pharyngeal wall and base of tongue. The afferent fibers travel as part of the vagus nerve. Pain from these areas is referred to the ear through Arnold nerve, a branch of the vagus that innervates the external auditory canal. Tumors of the base of tongue and oropharyngeal wall may produce pain that travels in the glossopharyngeal nerve, which sends branches to the tympanic membrane and middle ear through Jacobson nerve, also allowing pain to be referred to the ear. Thus, infectious, neoplastic, and other causes of mucosal inflammation in the throat may be associated with otalgia even when patients have little or no sore throat.

Patients may also present with symptoms of aural fullness, hearing loss, epistaxis, and unilateral or

TABLE 111-1 ◆ COMMONLY USED FLAPS IN UPPER AERODIGESTIVE TRACT RECONSTRUCTION, FLAP TYPE, AND PRIMARY APPLICATION BY SITE

Flap	Type	Sites
Pectoralis major	Muscle, musculocutaneous	Oral cavity, oropharynx, tongue base, neck (including pharyngocutaneous fistula), face
Latissimus dorsi	Muscle, musculocutaneous (pedicled or free)	Neck, face, oral cavity, cranial (free flap)
Trapezius	Muscle, musculocutaneous	Neck, occiput
Deltopectoral	Fasciocutaneous	Neck, oral cavity
Nasolabial	Fasciocutaneous	Oral cavity, face
Tongue	Muscle	Oral cavity
Temporalis	Muscle	Oral cavity, oropharynx, nasopharynx
Temporoparietal	Fascial	Face (especially ear), oral cavity
Radial forearm	Free fasciocutaneous	Oral cavity, pharynx (including total pharyngectomy), face
Fibula	Free osseous, osteoseptocutaneous	Mandible, oral cavity
Jejunum	Free visceral	Total pharyngectomy
Rectus abdominis	Free muscle, musculocutaneous	Oral cavity, oropharynx (especially tongue), craniofacial

bilateral nasal obstruction, all of which can be attributed to a nasal cavity or nasopharyngeal tumor. If adults complain of unilateral hearing loss, otologic examination is mandatory to assess for a middle ear effusion; if fluid is present, flexible nasopharyngoscopy is warranted to rule out a mass obstructing the eustachian tube orifice in the nasopharynx. Patients may present with the sole complaint of a neck mass. A neck mass in an adult should be treated as carcinoma until proven otherwise, although young adults can present with congenital masses, such as branchial cleft and thyroglossal duct cysts, as well as with inflammatory or infectious masses, such as actinomycosis or scrofula.

The patient should also be questioned about symptoms of gastroesophageal reflux, including heartburn, water brash (a bitter taste), and regurgitation. Reflux has been linked to head and neck cancer as a minor risk factor, and it may cause some of the same symptoms as a tumor, including chronic hoarseness, sore throat, and globus sensation.

Physical Examination

As with physical examination of the abdomen or other sites of the body, the head and neck examination should be performed in a consistent, systematic, and sequential fashion. General evaluation includes an assessment of overall health. The head and neck examination is commonly sequenced as follows. Otoscopic examination is performed to look for middle ear effusion or skin lesions of the external ear. Nasal examination is performed with a speculum and headlight or head mirror. Oral examination is performed with a tongue blade in each hand to encompass all mucosal surfaces including buccal, gingival, lip, floor of mouth, retromolar trigone, hard and soft palate, ventral and dorsal tongue, and posterior and lateral walls of the oropharynx. The neck is palpated for masses bilaterally; the examiner consciously rolls the sternocleidomastoid muscles between fingers and thumb to probe the cervical lymphatics. All zones must be assessed, including the submandibular, jugulodigastric, lower jugular, posterior, supraclavicular, and peritracheal nodes. The thyroid gland should also be palpated. Indirect nasopharyngoscopy and laryngoscopy with mirrors are also part of the routine head and neck examination. These techniques can easily be mastered with practice but do require the patient's cooperation. A headlight or head mirror with backlighting is used to illuminate the mirrors, which are warmed to prevent fogging. The smaller nasopharyngeal mirror is passed posterior to the free edge of the soft palate and rotated upward to visualize the eustachian tube orifices, the nasal choanae, and the adenoids, if present, while a tongue blade is used to depress the tongue. For examination of the hypopharynx, base of tongue, and larynx, a larger mirror is used, which can

be magnified. The patient is asked to lean forward and tilt the head forward and chin up. The tongue is gently grasped with a gauze pad while the patient pants to minimize the tendency to gag. The mirror is passed posterior to the tongue and tilted downward to visualize the base of tongue, valleculae, epiglottis, and larynx. The piriform sinuses, postcricoid area, subglottis, and posterior commissure are usually visualized but can be difficult to assess in some patients. All mucosal surfaces can be checked for lesions, and the vocal cords should be assessed carefully for mobility. The larynx can be brought anteriorly, making it easier to view, by having the patient say "eeeeee." This maneuver also helps with assessment of vocal cord mobility.

Office endoscopy is an indispensable tool in evaluation of the head and neck. Rigid rod lens telescopes include 0- and 30-degree nasal endoscopes and Hopkins rod lenses. Endoscopes provide a clear, magnified view of the nasal cavity and can be used to visualize the nasopharynx. Hopkins rod lenses are angled at 90 degrees and are used to evaluate the larynx and hypopharynx much the same way as with mirrors but with better optics. Flexible fiberoptic nasopharyngoscopes, however, are the workhorse scope for office evaluation of the patient who presents with a complaint in the head and neck, such as chronic sore throat or hoarseness. Although fiberoptics cannot provide the resolution of the rigid lens systems, fiberoptic examination is well tolerated by patients and can be used to visualize all the mucosa from the nares to the vocal folds. Because flexible endoscopy is well tolerated, accurate dynamic assessment of the airway, in particular vocal cord mobility, is obtained. The main limitation compared with rigid operative endoscopy is the inability to visualize the apices of the piriform sinuses or proximal esophagus. The flexible scope can provide a view that is more comprehensive than in mirror examination. The most sophisticated of the office endoscopy tools is the video stroboscope. This couples a 90-degree Hopkins rod lens with a xenon strobe paced by the fundamental frequency of the patient's own voice, as sensed by a microphone worn on the neck during the examination. For cancer diagnosis, this tool finds its greatest utility in diagnosis of early glottic primaries that can affect the mucosal wave propagation across the vocal fold, which can be seen only with stroboscopy. Nonetheless, video stroboscopy is not used routinely to examine the patient with head and neck cancer.

Studies

After the initial office evaluation is complete, radiographic and other studies may be warranted. It may be appropriate to perform biopsies in the office. If a mucosal mass is easily accessible, cup forceps biopsy under local anesthesia is safe and can provide pathologic diagnosis, without which definitive resection cannot be performed. If a neck mass is present, fine-needle aspiration biopsy is sensitive and specific for squamous cell carcinoma. Biopsy can also be performed at the time of operative rigid endoscopy.

Laboratory evaluation for a patient with a known or suspected head and neck carcinoma before definitive resection should include any tests necessary for preoperative medical risk evaluation as well as those that may find metastatic lesions or synchronous primaries. In general, this includes chest radiography, complete blood count, basic chemistry panel, coagulation panel, and electrocardiography. Liver function tests are warranted if the patient has a history of alcohol abuse to evaluate liver function; they are not as useful as a screening tool to detect metastases. Computed tomographic (CT) scan of the chest has proved more efficacious than chest radiography in detection of synchronous chest neoplasms and metastatic lesions; it should be used in patients with advanced and perhaps even early head and neck cancer.[13] The lungs are the most common site for a synchronous primary when patients have laryngeal primaries; this association has been attributed to the carcinogenic effects of tobacco. A resectable lung primary does not in general preclude resection of the head and neck tumor.

CT scan with contrast enhancement of the head and neck is obtained in almost every patient with head and neck cancer to characterize (or to search for) the primary tumor, to evaluate the cervical lymphatics for metastasis, and potentially to find second primaries. The CT scan has become an indispensable tool for staging and surgical planning. The determination as to whether a tumor is truly resectable is often based on the findings from scans. A specific, sequential surgical plan can be generated that includes both extirpation and reconstruction. Magnetic resonance imaging has been used more commonly because of superior soft tissue resolution and more options for planes in which to visualize the lesion; it has improved sensitivity for detection of bone marrow invasion, perineural spread, and intracranial involvement. One notable weakness of conventional scanning techniques is the inability to differentiate lymph node metastases from benign, reactive nodes. Cervical nodes are considered suspicious for metastasis if they are greater than 1 cm in size, have a hypodense (implying necrotic) center, or have an eccentric shape; the jugulodigastric nodes are an exception in that a diameter up to 1.5 cm is generally considered normal. Positron emission tomography may ultimately be more sensitive and specific for lymph node metastases but is not yet used routinely in most centers.

Clinically suspicious lymph nodes, or any neck mass, can be further evaluated with fine-needle aspiration biopsy under local anesthesia in the office. This is generally performed after scanning because edema, hematoma, or other minor trauma associated with the biopsy may compromise interpretation of the radiographs. An aspirate can yield important information in the work-up of the patient before any operative intervention. For instance, if squamous cells consistent with carcinoma are found in a neck mass, the subsequent work-up can be directed at identifying the mucosal primary. The aspiration is performed by first cleaning the skin and applying local anesthetic over the neck mass. A needle, commonly 20-gauge, is then passed percutaneously into the mass. Suction is applied with an attached syringe, 20 mL or larger. A "gun" device may be used to hold the syringe and more easily apply suction. The needle is maintained on suction while it is passed within the mass 10 to 15 times, without letting the needle come out of the dermis to avoid breaking the suction. The suction is let down; the needle is removed. The contents of the needle are sprayed onto a microscope slide and then sprayed with fixative. The needle and syringe are then flushed with a cytologic suspension solution. The microscope slides and suspension are then evaluated by the cytopathologist. Lymph node metastasis from a squamous cell carcinoma of the head and neck can readily be identified by this technique.

The final step in preparing the patient with head and neck cancer for definitive extirpation is operative endoscopy. Direct visualization of the aerodigestive tract is obtained under general anesthesia with rigid endoscopes. The goals of this procedure are to stage the primary tumor, to perform biopsy, and to look for synchronous primary tumors of the head and neck. Direct visualization of the primary allows the surgeon to accurately delineate the size and anatomic site of the primary tumor for staging purposes, evaluation of resectability, and surgical planning. A biopsy is performed, if a specimen was not obtained in the office, for tissue diagnosis. Extirpation should not be performed without first confirming the diagnosis of carcinoma. Endoscopy involves direct laryngoscopy, esophagoscopy, and sometimes bronchoscopy. Bronchoscopy may be performed with a flexible bronchoscope and may use bronchial washings. Bronchoscopy is not done routinely in most centers because it has not been shown to be more sensitive than chest radiography in identifying pulmonary metastasis. Esophagoscopy is deferred by some surgeons in lieu of a preoperative barium esophagogram to rule out mucosal lesions; performing both is generally not necessary. Endoscopy can be performed just before surgical extirpation; frozen section diagnosis is used if a biopsy specimen has not previously been obtained. Modern scanning and in-office flexible nasopharyngoscopy often allow accurate surgical planning before endoscopy.

SITE-SPECIFIC DISCUSSION

Oropharynx

ANATOMY

The oropharynx includes the base of tongue, faucial arches, tonsillar fossae, and posterior and lateral pharyngeal walls. The faucial arches include the anterior tonsillar pillars, soft palate, and uvula. The oropharynx extends superiorly to the plane of the soft palate and inferiorly to the plane of the hyoid bone. The anterior border is a ring formed by the circumvallate papillae of the tongue, the anterior tonsillar pillars laterally, and the border of the hard and soft palates superiorly.

GENERAL CONSIDERATIONS

The biology of squamous cell carcinoma of the oropharynx is aggressive.[14] Tumors tend to present at an advanced stage; they are undetected when small and are not detected until they enlarge enough to cause pain and dysfunction or to be visible in the back of the mouth. Local pain is the most common presenting symptom. Patients may also present with sore throat, otalgia, odynophagia, dysphagia, trismus, or neck mass. Physical examination should include visual inspection and careful palpation of the base of tongue and pharyngeal walls because submucosal extension of these tumors is common; a large lesion may have only a small visible mucosal component. Access is critical for adequate resection and may involve transhyoid pharyngotomy, lateral pharyngotomy, mandible-splitting approaches, and, in select patients, transoral excision. Resections that involve the base of tongue can have a deleterious effect on swallowing. Reconstruction commonly involves skin grafts, the pectoralis muscle or musculocutaneous flap, or free flaps. Organ preservation therapy is primarily used for advanced lesions.

STAGING

The American Joint Committee on Cancer staging system for primary tumors of the oropharynx is as follows:

Tis   Carcinoma in situ
T1   Tumor 2 cm or less in greatest dimension
T2   More than 2 cm but less than 4 cm
T3   Greater than 4 cm
T4   Invasion of bone, deep tongue muscles, skin

Nodal staging is the same regardless of the primary tumor site and is as follows:

N0   No clinically detectable nodes
N1   Single ipsilateral node, less than or equal to 3 cm in diameter
N2a   Single ipsilateral node, greater than 3 cm but less than 6 cm
N2b   Multiple ipsilateral nodes, none greater than 6 cm
N2c   Bilateral or contralateral nodes, none greater than 6 cm
N3   One or more nodes greater than 6 cm present

Clinical evaluation of lymph nodes includes palpation as well as radiographic evaluation, as discussed before. Finally, distant metastases are classified as M0, no known metastases, or M1, metastases present.

The American Joint Committee on Cancer staging schema (TNM staging) is as follows and applies to all head and neck primaries:

Stage I   T1 N0 M0
Stage II   T2 N0 M0
Stage III   T3 N0 M0 or T1, T2, or T3 N1 M0
Stage IV   Any T4, N2 or N3, or M1 lesions

The staging system, like any oncologic staging system, allows more accurate recording and analysis of outcome data to assist in counseling patients about prognosis, to communicate with other physicians and services, and to evaluate treatment efficacy.

TREATMENT

Surgery and radiation are the two principal treatment options for oropharyngeal primaries or, for that matter, any squamous cell carcinoma of the head and neck. The choice of surgical treatment or radiotherapy is a complex and controversial topic, a detailed discussion of which is beyond the scope of this chapter. Different institutions rely more or less heavily on one modality. Surgeons tend to favor surgery. Radiation oncologists tend to favor radiation. The use of a multidisciplinary tumor board can allow enlightened discussion of treatment options by medical oncologists, surgical oncologists, and radiation oncologists. However, it is generally agreed that smaller head and neck lesions can be treated with equivalent efficacy by radiation or surgery, whereas tumors of advanced stage are best controlled with a combination of surgery, radiation, and sometimes chemotherapy.[5,6] The debate over whether to use surgery or radiation therefore traditionally focuses on patients with early-stage lesions. It is the authors' preference to use surgery alone when possible for early lesions to avoid the sequelae of radiotherapy and to preserve this powerful modality for salvage therapy in the case of recurrence. Treatment of small head and neck carcinomas with surgery has disadvantages: general anesthesia, discomfort, hospitalization, possible temporary tracheostomy, often a period of dysfunction characterized by aspiration and decreased ability to talk or swallow, and cost. Radiation, on the other hand, tends to have less short-term morbidity but significantly worse long-term morbidity, especially progressive radiation-induced fibrosis, which can cause wound healing problems, long-term dysphagia, hoarseness, pain, or xerostomia. From a plastic surgery perspective, the soft tissue fibrosis that characterizes an irradiated wound is often more of a problem than the scarring that characterizes a surgical wound. Furthermore, once used, radiation cannot subsequently be used at appropriate doses if local or regional recurrence develops. Finally, without surgical extirpation, the tumor cannot be pathologically staged, which can result in undertreatment of lesions that are not properly staged clinically. Thus, from a plastic surgery perspective, single-modality treatment with surgery is generally preferable to radiotherapy.

On the other hand, stage III and stage IV tumors are most effectively treated with multimodality therapy, and some stage IV tumors are best treated with organ preservation protocols of chemotherapy and radiation.[1,15,16] Specifically, patients with large tumors of the tongue base that would require total glossectomy and laryngectomy should be considered for such protocols. Survival with any treatment modality is poor for stage IV tumors, and the inability to speak and eat is a devastating and profound psychosocial insult, so if locoregional control can be attained without complete loss of speech and deglutition, this is generally a better option. Surgery is reserved for salvage, although recurrent lesions may be nonresectable. Patients treated with organ preservation protocols usually must undergo tracheostomy and gastrostomy tube placement, but compromised speech is usually possible. Other advanced lesions aside from those of the tongue may be suitable for organ preservation protocols. Of note, immunotherapeutic agents are being used in experimental protocols, including cytokines (i.e., interferon gamma), tumor vaccines, and cellular agents like activated killer cells and dendritic cells.

The guiding principle for surgical resection is en bloc excision with adequate margins. As with most other head and neck sites, a mucosal and deep muscle margin of 1 cm is acceptable for the oropharynx; however, this may not be feasible when tumor is adjacent to structures like the mandible, prevertebral fascia, skull base, or larynx. Margins must be verified on pathologic section. This requires a pathologist experienced

in evaluating head and neck tumors and good communication between the surgeon and pathologist to orient the specimen in three dimensions and direct closer examination of questionable margins. In the end, only the surgeon can determine the true adequacy of margins. It is often essential to send additional margins at the time of definitive resection.

Small lesions of the tonsil, soft palate, or tongue may be amenable to transoral excision, but larger and more posterior lesions require better access. Options for this access include lateral pharyngotomy, transhyoid (or suprahyoid) pharyngotomy, and mandible-splitting procedures with or without a median glossotomy. Mandibulectomy may also be used, but it causes functional and aesthetic morbidity unwarranted if the mandible does not require excision for oncologic reasons. All of these procedures require a temporary tracheotomy because of the potential for postoperative airway obstruction secondary to edema as well as to provide pulmonary toilet and to maintain control of the airway if postoperative bleeding occurs. Patients are decannulated once they can maintain their airway and pulmonary toilet.

Transhyoid or suprahyoid pharyngotomy may be used to approach small lesions of the base of tongue or posterior wall of the oropharynx. Extension of tongue base lesions anterior to the circumvallate papillae is a relative contraindication to this approach because it is difficult to reach this far anteriorly. Extension of posterior wall lesions onto the lateral wall or tonsil may require an extended approach, like a lateral pharyngotomy. In general, large lesions require mandible-splitting procedures. Oropharyngeal lesions are aggressive and generally require selective or modified radical neck dissection, which is performed before the extirpation of the primary lesion. After neck dissection, the hyoid bone is identified. The central portion of the bone can be resected, or the suprahyoid musculature can be transected, leaving a few millimeters of muscle cuff on the superior aspect of the bone to facilitate subsequent closure (Fig. 111-9). As dissection proceeds laterally, the hypoglossal nerve is protected by anteriorly retracting the lateral cornu

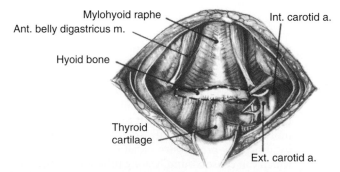

Mylohyoid raphe
Ant. belly digastricus m.
Hyoid bone
Int. carotid a.
Thyroid cartilage
Ext. carotid a.

FIGURE 111-9. Exposure of the hyoid bone as the suprahyoid musculature is transected for the suprahyoid pharyngotomy approach. (From Loré JM, ed: An Atlas of Head and Neck Surgery. Philadelphia, WB Saunders, 1988.)

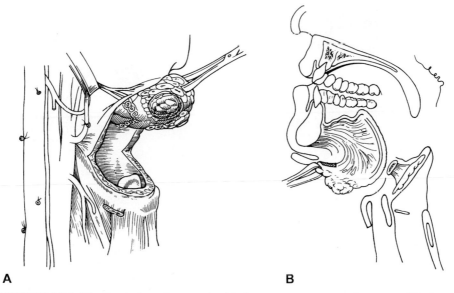

A   **B**

FIGURE 111-10. Depiction of a suprahyoid pharyngotomy approach to a small lesion of the base of tongue. *A*, The tongue base as retracted with an Allis clamp after separation of the suprahyoid musculature from the hyoid bone and pharyngotomy at the junction of the tongue base and vallecula. *B*, A lateral schematic view of the approach. (From Myers EN: Suprahyoid pharyngotomy. In Myers EN, ed: Operative Otolaryngology: Head and Neck Surgery. Philadelphia, WB Saunders, 1997:241.)

of the hyoid. The nerve can be identified deep to the digastric muscle. Transection of the hypoglossal nerve produces ipsilateral tongue paralysis, which can contribute to aspiration and problems with articulation. Ideally, the superior laryngeal nerve is identified and preserved to maintain ipsilateral supraglottic sensation, loss of which can contribute to postoperative aspiration. The superior laryngeal nerve branches off the vagus nerve near the level of the carotid bifurcation and travels medially in the vicinity of the superior thyroid artery, deep to the carotid arteries. The internal branch pierces the thyrohyoid membrane. Once the hypoglossal and superior laryngeal nerves are identified, the suprahyoid musculature is transected with impunity; this basically separates the tongue base off the hyoid until the pharynx is entered at the level of the vallecula (Fig. 111-10). Once the oropharyngeal or hypopharyngeal lesion is resected, the mucosa can be closed primarily (small defects), left to granulate, or reconstructed with a split-thickness skin graft. If one of the last two options is chosen, the cut mucosal edges are tacked to the pharyngeal wall to prevent the risk of dissection and contamination of the deep neck planes (Table 111-2).

Lateral pharyngotomy is used primarily to approach the lateral and posterior walls of the oropharynx and hypopharynx but can also be used for access to the base of tongue or supraglottic larynx. Extensive lesions or those with laryngeal involvement generally require laryngopharyngectomy. Even if part of

the larynx can be preserved, the entire larynx will need to be removed if aspiration is inevitable. For lateral pharyngotomy, skin incisions are placed in a horizontal neck skin crease and altered to accommodate neck dissection if necessary. Skin flaps are elevated in the usual subplatysmal plane. Because these are aggressive lesions, neck dissection is generally performed: modified radical dissection if clinically positive nodes are present, selective neck dissection for the N0 neck. The carotid sheath is retracted posteriorly after neck dissection (or identified deep to the sternocleidomastoid muscle if neck dissection is not performed). The strap muscles are retracted anteriorly (Fig. 111-11). The thyroid cartilage is identified and retracted anteriorly with wide double skin hooks on its lateral

TABLE 111-2 ✦ KEY STEPS IN SUPRAHYOID PHARYNGECTOMY

Tracheostomy
Subplatysmal skin flaps
Neck dissection
Release of suprahyoid musculature
Identification and protection of superior laryngeal and
 hypoglossal nerves
Pharyngotomy through the vallecula
Direct visualization of tumor and resection with
 adequate margins
Closure in layers (mucosa, muscle, skin)—primarily or
 with skin graft or flap

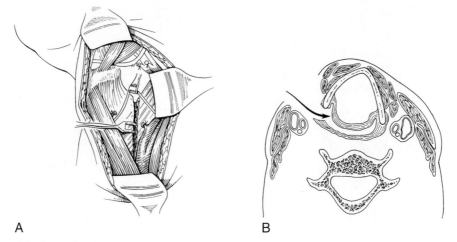

FIGURE 111-11. The lateral pharyngotomy approach is shown. *A,* The thyroid ala is retracted with a double hook, the carotid bifurcation is retracted posteriorly, the superior laryngeal nerve is retracted superiorly, and a myotomy of the inferior constrictor muscle is shown. *B,* The approach is depicted in an axial view, showing the inferior constrictor myotomy. (From Carrau RL: Lateral pharyngotomy. In Myers EN, ed: Operative Otolaryngology: Head and Neck Surgery. Philadelphia, WB Saunders, 1997:247.)

edge. The superior laryngeal and hypoglossal nerves are identified and preserved. The inferior pharyngeal constrictor inserts along the thyroid ala. It is cut by placing a Yankauer suction tube through the mouth and along the lateral pharyngeal wall to tent-up the muscle and underlying mucosa. An incision is made just posterior to the thyroid ala; this site corresponds to the lateral wall of the piriform sinus. The tumor is palpated and visualized as the pharynx is opened to ensure an adequate margin of resection (Fig. 111-12).

For lesions of the hypopharynx, the pharynx is entered through the inferior pharyngeal constrictor at the piriform sinus. The tumor is visualized, and a margin of 1 cm of mucosa is obtained. This is usually feasible along the posterior and lateral pharyngeal walls and tongue base, but if the tumor lies too close to the larynx, a laryngopharyngectomy may be indicated. Similarly, if the tumor enters the esophageal introitus, an esophagectomy may be indicated. These determinations are ideally made before surgery

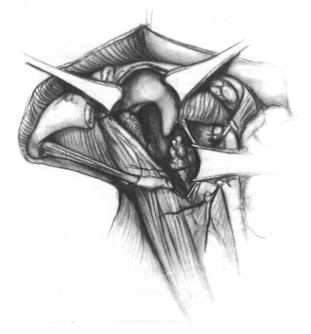

FIGURE 111-12. A pharyngotomy is made through the lateral wall of the piriform sinus to visualize a posterior pharyngeal wall tumor by the lateral pharyngotomy approach. (From Loré JM, ed: An Atlas of Head and Neck Surgery. Philadelphia, WB Saunders, 1988.)

on the basis of the findings of scans and direct laryngoscopy.

The pharyngotomy is closed in layers. The mucosa is closed with a Connell stitch. The muscle is closed as a separate layer. If the pharyngotomy defect cannot be closed without excess tension, which will lead to stenosis, reconstruction is necessary with skin grafts, pedicled flaps, or free flaps. Advocates of skin graft favor its relative simplicity, minimal donor site morbidity, and lack of bulk (Fig. 111-13). The pectoralis muscle flap can be used without a skin paddle to decrease bulk; the raw muscle surface is covered secondarily by mucosa. The muscle is generally used to restore bulk if a large base of tongue defect exists. The muscle's bulk can interfere with swallowing and direct food boluses toward the larynx, contributing to aspiration. The most useful free flap for reconstruction of the oropharynx, especially pharyngeal wall defects, is the radial forearm fasciocutaneous flap because of its relative thinness and pliability (Table 111-3).

Mandible-splitting procedures have a variety of indications and provide good visualization of even large tumors. The procedure can be used to approach oropharyngeal lesions, oral cavity lesions, and the skull base. If the mandible is not involved by tumor, it may be split to gain access posteriorly. The osteotomy is

TABLE 111-3 ✦ KEY STEPS IN LATERAL PHARYNGOTOMY

Tracheostomy
Subplatysmal skin flaps
Neck dissection
Identification and retraction of carotid sheath posteriorly and strap musculature anteriorly
Anterior rotation of thyroid cartilage
Identification and protection of superior laryngeal nerve and hypoglossal nerve
Detachment of inferior constrictor muscle from posterior edge of thyroid cartilage
Pharyngotomy at lateral wall of piriform sinus, carried into vallecula superiorly
Visualization of tumor and resection with adequate margins
Layered closure of mucosa, muscle, and skin with skin graft or flap if needed

then reconstituted with plate fixation. Rigid fixation minimizes problems with bone healing or occlusion; intermaxillary fixation is unnecessary. The preferred approach is a midline or paramedian mandibulotomy, which can be combined with a median glossotomy if necessary. Access to the mandible can be obtained through either a lip-splitting incision or a visor flap. The visor flap is performed through a transverse skin crease incision in the neck. The skin flap, raised in the subplatysmal plane, is lifted superiorly to expose the mandible. The mental nerves are usually transected for adequate exposure. The primary disadvantage of the lip-splitting incision is an often conspicuous scar, but this approach preserves the mental nerves. This incision is performed as follows. The vermilion border is marked. The lip is incised full thickness in the midline. A step-cut can be performed at the vermilion border to diminish the chance of a vertical scar contracture. The skin incision is taken across the chin either vertically or curved around the mental crease and inferiorly onto the neck, then transversely in an existing horizontal skin crease. A mucosal cut is then made in the lower gingivobuccal sulcus, leaving an adequate cuff of mucosa next to the gingiva to facilitate subsequent closure. The mucosal cut is taken to the mandible. Before the mandibulotomy is performed, a mandibular plate is bent to conform to the site of the mandibulotomy, and the screw holes are drilled. The plate should be marked to identify left-right orientation so that it is placed properly at closure. The osteotomy is easily made in a straight, vertical line; some authors prefer a step-cut, but rigid fixation has obviated the need for this (Fig. 111-14). Once the osteotomy has been performed, the mandible is retracted laterally, like opening a book. The mucosa is cut along the floor of the mouth, leaving a cuff of mucosa on the lingual aspect of the gingiva for subsequent closure. The mylohyoid muscle lies deep to the mucosa and is cut with it. Dissection

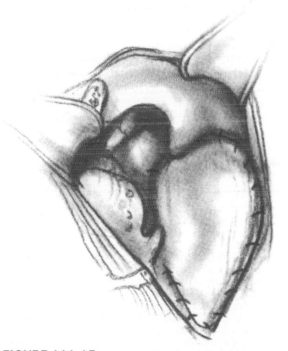

FIGURE 111-13. A skin graft is used to reconstruct a posterior and lateral pharyngeal wall defect exposed with a lateral pharyngotomy. A tie-over bolster is placed on the graft. This is removed in the operating room if necessary. (From Loré JM, ed: An Atlas of Head and Neck Surgery. Philadelphia, WB Saunders, 1988.)

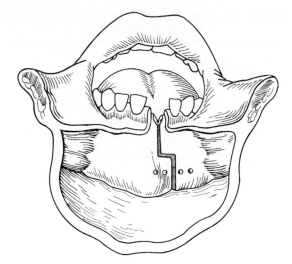

FIGURE 111-14. A vertical paramedian osteotomy is performed for the mandibular swing approach. A fixation plate was adapted to the mandible and predrilled before osteotomy for use at closure. (From Johnson JT: Mandible-splitting approaches. In Myers EN, ed: Operative Otolaryngology: Head and Neck Surgery. Philadelphia, WB Saunders, 1997:294.)

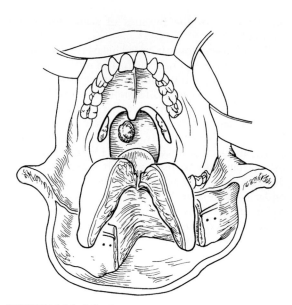

FIGURE 111-16. Exposure of an oropharyngeal tumor by the median glossotomy and mandible-splitting approach. (From Johnson JT: Mandible-splitting approaches. In Myers EN, ed: Operative Otolaryngology: Head and Neck Surgery. Philadelphia, WB Saunders, 1997:294.)

proceeds from anterior to posterior, and the mandible is swung further laterally (Fig. 111-15). This is done until the appropriate point is reached to enter the tongue, tongue base, or pharynx for tumor resection (Table 111-4).

Alternatively, a midline glossotomy can be used (Fig. 111-16). This approach may be used for the skull base (in particular the clivus), anterior cervical spine, oropharynx, hypopharynx, and nasopharynx; the latter requires the addition of a palatal split or Le Fort I osteotomies. The median glossotomy is preferred to the more lateral approach when the tumor is toward the midline. The disadvantages of splitting the tongue are the consequent edema, discomfort, and interference with swallowing and articulation during early postoperative healing. When it is used, the mandibulotomy is performed as described before, the floor of mouth mucosa is incised in the midline, and the tongue is cut in the midline until tumor is reached or until the entire tongue is bisected, exposing the pharynx.

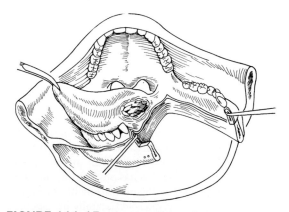

FIGURE 111-15. The mandible-splitting approach to a posterior tongue lesion is shown. (From Johnson JT: Mandible-splitting approaches. In Myers EN, ed: Operative Otolaryngology: Head and Neck Surgery. Philadelphia, WB Saunders, 1997:294.)

TABLE 111-4 ✦ KEY STEPS IN MANDIBULAR SWING APPROACH

Tracheostomy
Lip-splitting incision or elevation of visor flap and subplatysmal neck flaps
Neck dissection
Incision of gingiva to expose mandible and subperiosteal elevation of gingival mucosal cuffs
Adaptation and predrilling of mandibular miniplate at anticipated osteotomy site
Median or paramedian mandibulotomy
Incision of mucosa and mylohyoid muscle along floor of mouth
(Median glossotomy uses incision in midline tongue, as opposed to floor of mouth incision)
Lateral retraction of mandible (opens like a book)
Exposure of tumor and resection with adequate margins in three dimensions
Closure in layers with skin graft or flap if needed

The lingual arteries and lingual and hypoglossal nerves are avoided by maintaining the midline plane.

MANDIBULECTOMY

Fixation of a mucosal tumor to bone on palpation, not associated with visible changes to the bone cortex on CT scan, implies periosteal involvement without gross bone invasion; this warrants marginal mandibulectomy. Evidence of bone invasion, detected through CT or magnetic resonance imaging, necessitates a composite or segmental mandibulectomy. Radiation alone is a poor choice for treatment of tumors with bone involvement because the relative hypoxia of bone and its high density interfere with the ionizing radiation, resulting in poor control rates. The approach to segmental resection of the mandible is either a lip-splitting or visor incision as with mandibulotomy approaches. The mucosal incisions are placed on the gingival mucosa (keeping adequate margins around the tumor) and taken down to bone. Subperiosteal elevation exposes the bone; elevation is minimized over any area that is not to be resected to preserve periosteal blood supply. The mucosal cuts are designed so that a cuff of mucosa covers the osteotomy sites. The osteotomies are placed at least 2 cm away from tumor. The posterior osteotomy is often performed at the sigmoid notch (Fig. 111-17). Frozen section margins should include the inferior alveolar nerve to rule out perineural invasion within the remaining mandible. Bone margins cannot be obtained on frozen section. Touch preparation from the cut ends of the bone can be used, but false-negative results

TABLE 111-5 ◆ KEY STEPS FOR SEGMENTAL MANDIBULECTOMY

Tracheostomy
Lip-splitting incision or visor flap and subplatysmal neck skin flaps
Elevation of cheek flap off of involved mandible
Gingival incisions down to bone with adequate margin around tumor
Floor of mouth incisions, into tongue if needed, maintaining margins
Osteotomies 2 cm or more from tumor, anteriorly and posteriorly
En bloc delivery of specimen
Closure primarily or with skin graft or flap

can occur. The optimal method to obtain negative bone margins is to plan an adequate resection (Table 111-5).

Reconstruction may involve primary closure, skin grafting, and pedicled or free flaps. Skin grafts cannot be placed directly on bone, although there is often enough soft tissue to cover exposed bone. The most commonly used pedicled flap is the pectoralis muscle or musculocutaneous flap. Latissimus or temporalis flaps may occasionally be used but present significant technical difficulties. Others, such as the forehead, deltopectoral, and tongue flaps, are for the most part of historical significance. Free flap reconstruction often uses the radial forearm free fasciocutaneous flap, which provides thin, supple lining. This flap is asensate, although end-to-end or end-to-side coaptation of the

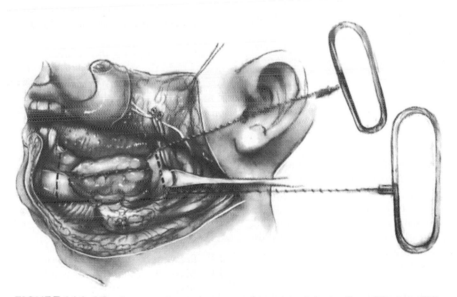

FIGURE 111-17. Osteotomies and exposure for segmental resection of the mandible are shown, although the authors generally use power saws. (From Loré JM, ed: An Atlas of Head and Neck Surgery. Philadelphia, WB Saunders, 1988.)

medial or lateral antebrachial cutaneous nerves to a sensory nerve in the neck, commonly the lingual nerve, can ultimately produce limited sensation. When resection involves the anterior mandible, a free fibular osseous or osteoseptocutaneous flap is the flap of choice to reconstitute the mandibular ring. The fibular flap may need to be combined with a radial forearm free flap to adequately reconstruct bone and mucosa defects. Lateral mandibular defects may not require bone reconstruction but will result in aesthetic deformity as well as significant mandibular deviation, much like a subcondylar fracture, because the medial pterygoid muscle is separated from the anterior mandible. Deviation of the mandible toward the resected side will result in malocclusion with a crossbite if the patient has intact dentition. Temporary intermaxillary fixation or a glide plane (a device attached to the maxillary and mandibular dentition on the intact side that prevents medial or lateral deviation) can be used to maintain occlusion, but reconstruction is preferred for larger lateral bone defects, particularly involving the angle.

The free fibular osseous flap is the most commonly used method of bone reconstruction. A reconstruction plate can be molded to fit the intact mandible before resection, and the screws can be predrilled to the uninvolved bone to ensure an exact fit after resection. The reconstruction plate is removed for the resection, then replaced to serve as a template to which the fibula can be molded. The fibula receives segmental periosteal blood supply, so it can tolerate multiple closing wedge osteotomies, allowing it to conform to the plate. Miniplates can be placed across each osteotomy, instead of a large reconstruction plate, but predrilling is not possible. Other methods of bone reconstruction include free cortical bone grafts and cancellous bone grafts placed in carrier trays; unacceptably high resorption rates, especially when radiation was used, have rendered these methods largely obsolete.

GLOSSECTOMY

This topic is discussed further in Chapter 109 but deserves mention here because total glossectomy may be required in extensive tumors of the tongue base. Such tumors can be approached by the techniques described for access to the oropharynx. These tumors may extend to involve the larynx, preepiglottic space, or mandible. Even with no laryngeal involvement, laryngectomy was traditionally performed with any total glossectomy to prevent intractable aspiration postoperatively. Nonetheless, total glossectomy without laryngectomy has been effective in properly selected patients. In such patients, reconstruction with a bulky (although asensate and immobile) flap is required to protect the larynx and to afford placement of a tongue

replacement prosthesis. The pectoralis musculocutaneous pedicled flap and free transverse rectus abdominis musculocutaneous flaps are the most commonly used. After acute healing is over, an acrylic tongue replacement prosthesis is fashioned. The prosthesis provides further bulk to the floor of the mouth so that some articulation is possible with appropriate speech therapy. Recurrent aspiration, the loss of the ability to articulate and taste food, and in some cases the additional morbidity of a laryngectomy cause a significant diminution in quality of life in patients with total glossectomy. Serious consideration on the part of the surgeon, patient, and multidisciplinary head and neck cancer team must be given to organ preservation protocols in these patients, with resection reserved for salvage.

Hypopharynx

Hypopharyngeal tumors present late with odynophagia, dysphagia, referred otalgia, hoarseness, globus sensation, or a neck mass. The majority of hypopharyngeal tumors involve the piriform sinus. Of note, the apex of the piriform sinus cannot be well visualized with flexible nasopharyngoscopy; rigid endoscopy is required to evaluate this site. Because these tumors are aggressive and advanced at presentation, treatment most often consists of combined surgery and radiotherapy.

ANATOMY

The hypopharynx comprises the piriform sinuses, postcricoid area, and posterior and lateral hypopharyngeal walls. The larynx lies anterior to the hypopharynx; the hypopharynx wraps around and behind the larynx. The postcricoid mucosa forms the upper part of the esophageal introitus; the underlying cricopharyngeus muscle constitutes the upper esophageal sphincter and inserts onto the posterior aspect of the cricoid cartilage. The piriform sinuses are the chutes through which a food bolus passes after hitting the epiglottis and proceeding around the larynx. The first echelon of lymphatic drainage is zone II and zone III, with common extension to zone IV.

STAGING

Primaries of this site are staged as follows:

T1 Confined to the site of origin
T2 Spread to an adjacent subsite or region without vocal cord fixation
T3 Fixation of the ipsilateral vocal cord
T4 Massive tumor with invasion of bone or the soft tissues of the neck

Nodal staging remains the same as for any tumor of the head and neck.

TREATMENT

Because of the aggressive nature of hypopharyngeal lesions, a combination of surgery and radiation therapy is often used to treat these lesions. Whether combination therapy is to be used for early lesions is often a determination made by a multidisciplinary team including a head and neck surgeon, radiation oncologist, and medical oncologist. The surgical options for treatment vary according to the size of the lesion. Small lesions can be treated with limited resection. Large lesions may require laryngectomy or laryngopharyngectomy. For such lesions, organ preservation protocols using combination chemotherapy-radiation therapy with surgical salvage may be appropriate in an attempt to preserve the larynx and avoid a permanent laryngostome. Of course, the chance of cure should not be compromised in attempting to avoid a stoma. Extirpation of piriform sinus lesions often entails laryngectomy; the principal, and uncommon, exception is a small (T1) lateral wall lesion. This can be removed with a partial pharyngectomy or even by endoscopic carbon dioxide laser excision. Extirpation of postcricoid lesions requires a laryngectomy because this area composes the posterior aspect of the larynx. If the lesion extends onto the lateral and posterior wall, a partial or total pharyngectomy will also be required. The total laryngopharyngectomy can be reconstructed with a free jejunal transfer or tubed radial forearm free flap.[17] Pedicled flaps like the tubed pectoralis or latissimus muscle flaps are mainly of historical significance. If a postcricoid lesion extends into the cervical esophagus, esophagectomy is required. The pharyngoesophagectomy defect is generally reconstructed with a gastric pull-up. Free flaps are not possible because the distal mucosal anastomosis cannot be performed below the level of the esophageal inlet; this would place this repair in the mediastinum. The gastric pull-up alone has a mortality rate, so patients must be counseled accordingly.

Lesions of the posterior or lateral wall of the hypopharynx can be resected with partial pharyngectomy through a lateral pharyngotomy or mandible-splitting approach. Closure may be obtained primarily in some cases, but if there is significant tension, pharyngeal stricture will be likely, especially if adjuvant radiotherapy is planned. Pedicled flaps may suffice for small defects. More often, a radial forearm free flap or free jejunal segment is needed. For the latter, the remaining pharyngeal mucosa is sacrificed at that level to establish a circumferential defect.

Larynx

Glottic tumors have a better prognosis than do those of most other head and neck sites, perhaps because these tumors tend to present early with hoarseness and because the vocal fold lymphatics are sparse, which may delay metastatic spread.

ANATOMY

The larynx is divided into the glottis, supraglottis, and subglottis (Fig. 111-18). The anterior limit of the larynx includes the suprahyoid epiglottis, thyrohyoid membrane, inner perichondrium of the thyroid cartilage, cricothyroid membrane, and anterior aspect of the cricoid cartilage. The preepiglottic space is important for staging supraglottic tumors; it extends from the thyrohyoid membrane anteriorly to the epiglottis posteriorly with the hyoepiglottic ligament superiorly. The glottis comprises the true vocal cords,

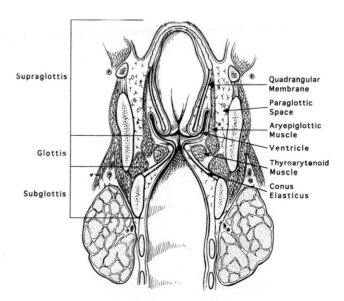

FIGURE 111-18. Coronal view of the larynx and its subsites. (From Sinard JR, Netterville JL, Garrett CG, Ossoff RH: Cancer of the larynx. In Myers EN, ed: Operative Otolaryngology: Head and Neck Surgery. Philadelphia, WB Saunders, 1997:381.)

anterior commissure, and posterior commissure. The superior limit of the glottis is the plane of the superior surface of the true vocal folds, which constitutes the floor of the laryngeal ventricles. The inferior limit is arbitrarily set as a plane 1 cm inferior to the first plane. The supraglottis extends from the tip of the epiglottis to the floor of the ventricles and includes the epiglottis, arytenoepiglottic folds, cuneiform and corniculate cartilages, arytenoids, false vocal cords, and preepiglottic space. The subglottis extends from the plane 1 cm below the vocal folds to the inferior edge of the cricoid cartilage. Below this is trachea, which is rarely the source of a primary tumor but is not uncommonly involved by inferior spread of large laryngeal tumors.

The lymphatic drainage of the larynx separates into an inferior and superior grouping. The supraglottis and glottis drain into the jugulodigastric (zone II) and paratracheal (zone VI) nodes as the first echelon and then into the entire cervical chain (zones II, III, and IV). The subglottis drains into the pretracheal (Delphian) and paratracheal nodes as the first echelon and then to the cervical chain.

STAGING

Staging of laryngeal cancers varies by subsite. For supraglottic cancers, tumor staging is as follows:

T1   Confined to site of origin with normal vocal cord mobility
T2   Involving adjacent sites without cord fixation
T3   Limited to the larynx with spread to the hypopharynx (medial wall of the piriform sinus or postcricoid area) or preepiglottic space and/or vocal cord fixation
T4   Massive tumor extending beyond the larynx to involve the thyroid cartilage, soft tissues of the neck, or oropharynx (e.g., tongue base)

For glottic carcinomas, tumor staging is as follows:

T1   Confined to one or both vocal cords with normal mobility
T2   Supraglottic or subglottic extension with normal or impaired vocal cord mobility
T3   Fixation of one or both vocal cords but confined to the larynx
T4   Massive tumor with thyroid cartilage invasion or extension beyond the larynx

For subglottic carcinoma, tumor staging is as follows:

T1   Confined to the subglottis
T2   Extending to the vocal cords, with normal or impaired mobility
T3   Confined to the larynx with cord fixation
T4   Massive tumor with cartilage invasion or extension beyond the larynx

Assessment of vocal cord mobility requires that the patient actively move the cords and therefore cannot be done under general anesthesia; but it can be accomplished easily in the office by indirect laryngoscopy with a mirror or flexible nasopharyngoscope, or a flexible or rigid scope can be used in the operating room to examine the cords for spontaneous movement as the patient is induced or awakens from general anesthesia during panendoscopy. Clear definition of the limits of the tumor is critical to staging and surgical planning. Physical examination, laryngoscopy, CT scanning, and rigid endoscopy all serve to characterize the tumor. Endoscopy also affords the opportunity for biopsy because a pathologic diagnosis must be established before all or part of the larynx can be removed. Several lesions, including sarcoidosis, tuberculosis, blastomycosis, and rare neoplasms like clear cell carcinoma, can mimic squamous cell carcinoma. The neck must also be evaluated for nodal metastasis by physical examination and scanning. Contrast-enhanced CT scans are most commonly used to evaluate the neck and primary lesion, but magnetic resonance imaging and positron emission tomography are potentially more sensitive in evaluating soft tissue changes, especially in the lymph nodes.

TREATMENT

Small, superficial laryngeal lesions are treated with equal efficacy by radiation or surgery. Surgery has short-term morbidity including perioperative pain, inpatient hospitalization, and anesthetic risk. Radiation has more long-term morbidity, including chondroradionecrosis, hypothyroidism, xerostomia, and progressive neck fibrosis. Advanced tumors are usually best treated with surgery or combined modality therapy with surgery and radiation. Chemotherapy may be used as adjuvant therapy for advanced tumors or with radiation in organ conservation protocols. Immunotherapy is still experimental. A multidisciplinary approach, with evaluation by a surgeon, medical oncologist, and radiotherapist with input from pathology, radiology, speech pathology, and dental prosthetics, is the standard of care for the complex patient with head and neck cancer. The choice of surgery versus radiation is controversial, and preferences vary by institution and surgeon. The details of this debate are beyond the scope of this chapter, but from the perspective of the plastic surgeon, the sequelae of radiotherapy are not insignificant. The progressive fibrosis impairs wound healing and can result in varying degrees of chondroradionecrosis, although it is uncommon. Conservation laryngeal procedures such as hemilaryngectomy and supraglottic laryngectomy, when they are feasible, will preserve speech and swallowing and avoid a permanent tracheostomy. Radiation sequelae are less severe if the primary site alone, not the cervical lymphatics, requires irradiation.

Organ preservation therapy is relatively new. Especially with tumors for which survival is poor regardless of the therapeutic modality chosen, quality of life concerns must be factored in to treatment decisions. In advanced tumors that would require laryngectomy or total glossectomy, organ preservation can allow enough speech and swallowing function to permit a better quality of life than with radical resection, especially if a permanent tracheostome can be avoided. Temporary tracheotomy and feeding tube placement are generally needed during treatment and sometimes permanently. If there is local recurrence after a conservation protocol, surgical salvage can be difficult and has a significant rate of wound healing complications.

Surgical Treatment of Laryngeal Subsites

SUPRAGLOTTIS

As with any head and neck tumor, the size and subsite of the tumor determine which procedure is appropriate for resection. Small tumors of the suprahyoid epiglottis are amenable to endoscopic laser epiglottectomy. Lesions that involve the supraglottis anterior to the arytenoids may be treated with supraglottic laryngectomy. Involvement of both arytenoids necessitates total laryngectomy because resection of both arytenoids would result in intractable aspiration. If the supraglottis including a single arytenoid is involved, an extended supraglottic laryngectomy may be appropriate in patients whose pulmonary status will tolerate significant chronic aspiration postoperatively. Tumors that involve the arytenoepiglottic fold often extend onto the adjacent medial wall of the piriform sinus and can be treated by supraglottic laryngectomy as well if the apex is not involved. If extension onto the lateral wall of the piriform sinus is present, a partial pharyngectomy can be included with the supraglottic laryngectomy. However, if the tumor extends inferiorly to the apex of the piriform sinus, the tumor is actually below the plane of the floor of the laryngeal ventricles (the inferior limit of the supraglottic laryngectomy), and a total laryngectomy is indicated. If there is extensive involvement of the pharyngeal wall, laryngopharyngectomy may be necessary. If a supraglottic tumor extends in the other direction, anteriorly and superiorly into the preepiglottic space, vallecula, or tongue base, resection of these sites will be necessary. Of note, all patients who undergo supraglottic laryngectomy will aspirate postoperatively, although this improves with time. If resection extends into the tongue base, aspiration will be worse. Furthermore, the extent of resection at the tongue base can be difficult to predict preoperatively because submucosal spread of tumor is common and difficult to assess clinically. The surgeon and patient must be prepared preoperatively for a total laryngectomy if an extensive tongue base resection is needed. With good preoperative clinical and radiographic assessment, this eventuality should rarely be unanticipated.

Last, the clinician must specifically assess for paraglottic spread of tumor. The paraglottic space is the space bounded by the true and false vocal cords medially and the thyroid cartilage laterally. The thyroarytenoid muscles are within this space deep to the vocal ligament of the true cords. Deep to the ventricular folds, or false vocal cords, is paraglottic fat. Tumor involvement of the paraglottic space can impair vocal cord mobility through invasion of the thyroarytenoid muscle, vocal cord mucosa, or arytenoids. Vocal cord mobility can be difficult to assess. Some authors advocate the use of video stroboscopy to assess symmetry and propagation of the mucosal wave produced by the true cord on phonation. CT and magnetic resonance scanning can visualize the paraglottic space with precision. The paraglottic fat, especially, can be assessed because tumor is more radiodense on CT scanning and because fat, but not tumor, enhances on T1 images with magnetic resonance imaging not using fat suppression. Paraglottic spread should not be missed because the inferior limit of a supraglottic laryngectomy is through the most inferior aspect of the laryngeal ventricles, just above the true cords. The paraglottic space extends farther inferior, to the level of the superior aspect of the cricoid cartilage, where the cricothyroid membrane and conus elasticus insert. If paraglottic involvement with tumor exists, microscopic or macroscopic disease will remain at the inferior resection margin at the level of the vocal cords or below, and an incomplete resection will result.

Preoperative assessment of patients who are to undergo laryngeal conservation surgery or partial glossectomy must include an evaluation of the patient's overall medical and functional status as well as pulmonary status. Laryngeal conservation procedures will result in postoperative aspiration. In the early postoperative period, aspiration is copious and obvious and is one of the indications for perioperative tracheostomy. After postoperative healing is complete, patients must have adequate pulmonary reserve to tolerate chronic low-level aspiration. Most patients with head and neck cancer have some chronic obstructive pulmonary disease secondary to smoking. Pulmonary reserve must be evaluated preoperatively, and poor function may contraindicate conservation laryngeal procedures, in particular supraglottic laryngectomy. Medical consultation, pulmonary function tests, and baseline arterial blood gas analysis are commonly used. Cardiopulmonary screening also includes an assessment of exercise tolerance by history, a chest radiograph, and an electrocardiogram. Cardiac evaluation with stress testing or coronary angiography may be indicated. Interpretation of these test results is somewhat controversial. Probably the best predictor of whether a patient will tolerate chronic aspiration is overall functional status.

Surgical Technique

Supraglottic laryngectomy is an effective, straightforward procedure (Table 111-6). A tracheostomy can be placed at the beginning or end of the procedure; the beginning is preferable to visualize the tumor more adequately without interference from an endotracheal tube. A superiorly based apron flap is constructed and is designed to give access for neck dissection. Supraglottic tumors have a high propensity for cervical metastasis, including contralateral metastases. Thus, bilateral selective neck dissections should be performed for the N0 neck. Neck irradiation can be avoided if elective neck dissection reveals three or fewer metastatic nodes without extracapsular extension. Modified radical neck dissection and postoperative neck irradiation are indicated for clinically positive nodes. The apron flap is incised, and the subplatysmal skin flap is elevated superiorly and inferiorly. The inferior subplatysmal elevation is stopped above the level of the tracheostomy to prevent contamination of the neck wounds with tracheal secretions postoperatively.

TABLE 111-6 ✦ KEY STEPS IN SUPRAGLOTTIC LARYNGECTOMY

Tracheostomy
Repeated endoscopy to re-examine tumor
Subplatysmal neck flaps
Neck dissection
Release of suprahyoid musculature and delivery of hyoid bone
Incision of thyroid perichondrium and elevation of perichondrial flap
Transverse incision of thyroid cartilage at midportion; curve superiorly to preserve posterior edge on noninvolved side
Pharyngotomy at vallecula through suprahyoid dissection or piriform sinus through inferior constrictor
Retraction of epiglottis with Allis clamp
Direct visualization of tumor
Resection of epiglottis and preepiglottic space into tongue base if necessary
Incision down through arytenoepiglottic fold, with resection of arytenoid mucosa if necessary (extended supraglottic laryngectomy)
Cut across floor of ventricle, above anterior commissure, and across contralateral floor of ventricle, in front of contralateral arytenoid, across contralateral arytenoepiglottic fold, and into vallecula to deliver specimen en bloc, maintaining adequate margins
Closure by suturing perichondrial flap to base of tongue

The hyoid bone is identified. The infrahyoid and suprahyoid strap muscles are transected. The superior laryngeal nerve on the less involved side is identified and preserved to maintain ipsilateral supraglottic sensation. The greater cornu of the hyoid is retracted anteriorly to protect the hypoglossal nerve. The thyroid cartilage is identified, and the perichondrium on the anterior face of its superior edge is incised (Fig. 111-19). Subperichondral dissection is performed. The cartilage is cut transversely with a No. 10 blade or oscillating saw at the level of the vertical midpoint of the thyroid cartilage in men or the junction of the upper and middle thirds in women. The transverse cut is taken across the lateral edge of the thyroid cartilage on the involved side; the cut is carried superiorly to preserve the superior horn on the contralateral side (Fig. 111-20).

The pharynx is then entered through the valleculae or the piriform sinus, depending on the tumor and the surgeon's preference. For the valleculae to be used, there must be no preepiglottic space involvement. The suprahyoid musculature is separated from the hyoid bone, which is resected en bloc with the rest of the larynx. The contralateral greater cornu can be preserved. If the piriform sinus is entered first, the surgeon must be careful to maintain an adequate mucosal margin around the primary. Note that the lateral wall of the piriform sinus is the medial surface of the ala of the thyroid cartilage. The epiglottis is retracted anteriorly with an Allis clamp. If the lingual surface of the epiglottis is uninvolved, the resection cut is carried across the valleculae. If there is tongue

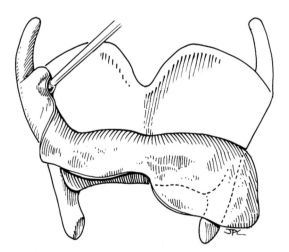

FIGURE 111-19. The thyroid cartilage anterior perichondrium is incised to begin elevation of the perichondrial flap that will be used to close the supraglottic laryngectomy. (From Johnson JT: Surgery for supraglottic cancer. In Myers EN, ed: Operative Otolaryngology: Head and Neck Surgery. Philadelphia, WB Saunders, 1997:403.)

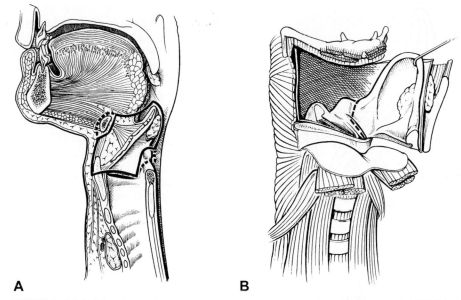

FIGURE 111-20. Outline of the resection performed in a supraglottic laryngectomy. *A*, Sagittal view. *B*, Anterior oblique view. The resection is as marked by the black line in *A* and dotted line in *B*. The dotted lines in *A* show possible inclusion of the hyoid bone or part of one arytenoid cartilage. (From Sinard JR, Netterville JL, Garrett CG, Ossoff RH: Cancer of the larynx. In Myers EN, ed: Operative Otolaryngology: Head and Neck Surgery. Philadelphia, WB Saunders, 1997:381.)

base involvement or spread onto the lingual surface of the epiglottis, the necessary margin is obtained across the tongue base under direct visualization. The cut is continued across the arytenoepiglottic fold, just anterior to the arytenoid if it is not involved.

If the arytenoid mucosa is involved, an extended supraglottic partial laryngectomy is performed by carrying the mucosal cut posterior to the arytenoid before continuing it along the floor of the laryngeal ventricle, resecting the false vocal cord. The posterior cut edge of the true vocal cord is fixed to the cricoid cartilage with a fine Vicryl or PDS suture to prevent it from bowstringing postoperatively. For a conventional supraglottic laryngectomy, the arytenoid is preserved, and the mucosal cut that was taken across the arytenoepiglottic fold is carried inferiorly, in front of the arytenoid, across the laryngeal ventricle just above the floor or true vocal fold. This mucosal cut corresponds to the transverse cut through the thyroid cartilage; it can be made with scalpel or scissors. The cut is carried across the midline, just superior to the anterior commissure, and across the floor of the contralateral ventricle, arytenoepiglottic fold, and piriform sinus mucosa into the vallecular incision (Fig. 111-21). Dissection often proceeds bilaterally from the valleculae and piriform sinuses, across the larynx to be completed in the midline, delivering the specimen. Margins of 2 or 3 mm are ideally maintained. Frozen section control is essential.

Closure is attained by suturing the superior cut edge of the thyroid perichondrium to dense fibrofatty tissue at the tongue base. The skin is closed in layers. A cricopharyngeal myotomy can be performed before closure. The operator's finger is placed in the esophageal introitus, and the inferior constrictor muscle fibers are then cut until the submucosal plane is reached. The surgeon's glove can usually be visualized through the translucent mucosa. This maneuver facilitates postoperative swallowing, although it can contribute to aspiration in patients with severe gastroesophageal reflux. A nasogastric feeding tube is also inserted before closure. Insertion later can cause disruption of the suture line by a misdirected tube. Because closure is not airtight, the tracheostomy must be maintained with the cuff inflated for at least 5 days. Attempts at initiating decannulation early may result in aspiration, coughing, and disruption of the suture line.

Some patients are also candidates for endoscopic laser-assisted supraglottic laryngectomies. This is truly a minimally invasive approach and avoids the open access incisions. Early series suggest that this is an oncologically sound procedure with less morbidity and faster recovery than with open approaches.

GLOTTIC TUMORS

Glottic tumors present with hoarseness. Any patient with prolonged hoarseness deserves indirect

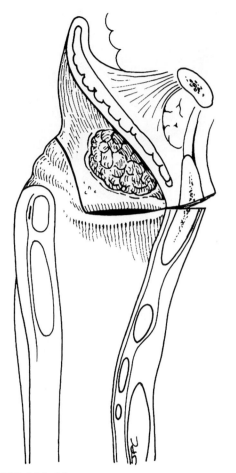

FIGURE 111-21. Excision of the supraglottic larynx proceeds with an incision through the laryngeal ventricles. (From Johnson JT: Surgery for supraglottic cancer. In Myers EN, ed: Operative Otolaryngology: Head and Neck Surgery. Philadelphia, WB Saunders, 1997:403.)

laryngoscopy with mirror or flexible scope. These tumors tend to be well differentiated, grow slowly, and metastasize late. The sparse lymphatics of the true cords probably explain the late metastasis. Late symptoms include sore throat, dysphagia, hemoptysis, and odynophagia. Early lesions can be treated with radiation or surgery. Even relatively advanced lesions may be treated with surgery alone, depending on deep invasion and the status of the cervical lymphatics. Tumor persistence after radiation has been attributed to understaging, especially failure to recognize involvement of the paraglottic space.

The principal surgical treatment options include total laryngectomy, vertical partial or "hemi-" laryngectomy, supracricoid laryngectomy, laryngofissure and cordotomy, and microlaryngoscopy with endoscopic vocal cord stripping by laser or steel. Patients who undergo surgery or radiation will be left with hoarseness to varying degrees. Those who undergo

laryngectomy will be unable to phonate without some sort of speech rehabilitation, such as by learning esophageal speech (which is essentially talking by eructating), with use of an electrolarynx, or through placement of a tracheoesophageal puncture—a one-way valve that allows the patient to force air from the trachea into the esophagus, through the neopharynx, and out of the mouth, causing vibrations in the neopharynx modulated by the tongue and mouth to produce speech similar to esophageal speech. Development of speech techniques postoperatively is critical to maintaining effective interpersonal communication, without which patients are more likely to become isolated and depressed. Because rehabilitation is intense, not all patients develop useful speech. However, the tracheostome has the most negative impact on quality of life after laryngectomy. Tracheopulmonary secretions are not simply swallowed unnoticed as with an intact upper aerodigestive tract. Coughing and wheezing are common, and secretions must be managed by the patient. The stoma tends to isolate patients from society. This observation has been the motivating factor in the search for laryngeal preservation techniques. The most significant advance in this realm is probably development of the supracricoid laryngectomy, in which the vocal cords themselves can be resected, leaving either one or two arytenoids behind to serve as the neoglottis.

Surgical Technique

As opposed to supraglottic carcinoma, which has a propensity toward early metastasis, glottic carcinoma does not metastasize until late, so elective neck dissection is unnecessary for T1, T2, and perhaps T3 lesions. For T1 lesions, radiotherapy or surgery is appropriate. One advantage of surgical resection is that tissue is obtained for pathologic assessment of margins. For T1 lesions that involve just the membranous true vocal cord, not the arytenoid, anterior commissure, ventricle, or subglottis, transoral excision with suspension microlaryngoscopy is appropriate. The carbon dioxide laser is a useful adjunct to this procedure, although sharp excision by use of microlaryngoscopy instruments is also feasible and permits more accurate examination of margins. Suspension laryngoscopy is used in which a rigid laryngoscope is suspended from the Mayo stand or a framework attached to the bed. An operating microscope allows magnified, binocular visualization of the vocal cords while permitting the surgeon to use both hands. The lesion or adjacent mucosa is grasped with a microlaryngoscopy cup forceps, normal mucosa is incised sharply or with the laser, and a plane is developed between the mucosa and the thyroarytenoid muscle in Reinke space. A 1- or 2-mm margin is adequate grossly, and negative pathologic margins must be obtained. If the lesion invades muscle, an adequate deep margin must also be maintained. If negative margins cannot be obtained because of extension of tumor beyond the membranous cord, a larger resection will be necessary, and the patient must be counseled appropriately. Pathologic examination will reveal whether the tumor was initially understaged, an opportunity not afforded if the tumor is treated with radiotherapy. After adequate resection, patients must be observed with monthly office examination for at least 1 year, with less frequent examinations ideally for the remainder of the patient's life. Any suspicious changes warrant return to the operating room.

Tumors that involve one true vocal cord with extension onto the anterior commissure, vocal process of the arytenoid cartilage, or floor of the laryngeal ventricle may be resected with a hemilaryngectomy. The procedure can be extended to include up to one third of the anterior aspect of the contralateral true cord. The tumor cannot extend more than 5 mm below the plane of the true vocal fold or extend onto the false vocal fold and be safely resected with this technique. Slight impairment of vocal cord mobility is not an absolute contraindication to this procedure because direct involvement of the thyroarytenoid muscle, which is resected, can result in impaired cord mobility, but patients must be carefully evaluated for preepiglottic space extension or paraglottic space involvement as discussed previously. In select patients, more than one third of the contralateral vocal cord may be resected, although postoperative aspiration is worse.

Hemilaryngectomy begins with a tracheostomy placed through a separate incision so that it does not soil the laryngeal wound with secretions. If the patient was intubated before tracheostomy, the endotracheal tube is now removed to allow appropriate visualization of the endolarynx, which can be re-examined with direct laryngoscopy at this time. A transverse incision is made in a preexisting skin crease over the thyroid ala. Subplatysmal flaps are elevated superiorly and inferiorly. The strap muscles are separated in the midline, revealing the thyroid cartilage. The perichondrium is incised vertically in the midline and along the superior and inferior rim of the thyroid ala. The perichondrium is elevated posteriorly to 3 or 4 mm from the posterior edge of the cartilage on the involved side and for a few millimeters from midline on the contralateral side. The cartilage is divided vertically in the midline with a No. 10 blade or oscillating saw and vertically approximately 4 mm from its posterior border on the affected side (Fig. 111-22). The larynx is entered through the cricothyroid membrane. A transverse cut is made here below the inferior aspect of the tumor. The midline cartilage cut is carried through the mucosa from inferior to superior, allowing the thyroid cartilage to be retracted laterally (Fig. 111-23), permitting visualization of the endolarynx with a headlight. The anterior cut is made in the midline, across the anterior aspect of the contralateral true vocal fold, or between the ipsilateral true fold and the anterior commissure, depending on the anterior extent of the tumor. If the anterior aspect of the contralateral cord is taken, this constitutes an extended or frontolateral vertical partial laryngectomy. The anterior cut edge of the true cord is then suture fixated to the thyroid cartilage to prevent retraction and bowstringing. In this instance, the anterior cartilage cut is not made in the midline but instead 2 or 3 mm lateral to midline on the less involved side. The superior and posterior mucosal cuts are then made. The superficial aspect of the superior cut travels along the superior border of the thyroid cartilage. The deep aspect of this incision extends through the mucosa of the false vocal cord. This must be resected for an adequate oncologic margin and because this mucosa can become markedly edematous postoperatively and contribute to airway obstruction, delaying decannulation, if it is left

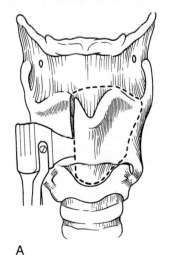
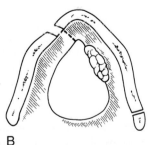

FIGURE 111-22. The incisions for a hemilaryngectomy are shown with dotted lines. *A,* An anterior view of the thyroid cartilage and associated structures. *B,* An axial schematic of the cut through the thyroid cartilage and underlying vocal cord just lateral to the anterior commissure on the uninvolved side. (From Eibling DE: Surgery for glottic carcinoma. In Myers EN, ed: Operative Otolaryngology: Head and Neck Surgery. Philadelphia, WB Saunders, 1997:416.)

A   B

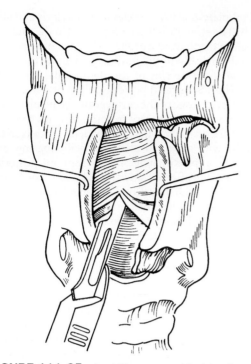

FIGURE 111-23. A midline mucosal incision is made from inferior to superior as the previously cut thyroid cartilage is retracted laterally to expose the endolarynx. (From Eibling DE: Surgery for glottic carcinoma. In Myers EN, ed: Operative Otolaryngology: Head and Neck Surgery. Philadelphia, WB Saunders, 1997:416.)

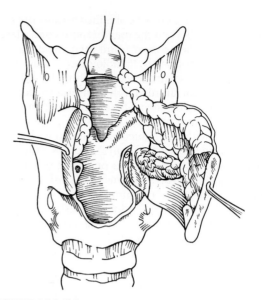

FIGURE 111-24. Mucosal incisions are carried through the false vocal cord and across the vocal process of the arytenoid. (From Eibling DE: Surgery for glottic carcinoma. In Myers EN, ed: Operative Otolaryngology: Head and Neck Surgery. Philadelphia, WB Saunders, 1997:416.)

redundant. Posteriorly, the cartilage incision 4 mm anterior to the posterior aspect of the thyroid cartilage is connected to a mucosal cut now made across the vocal process (Fig. 111-24), the insertion of the true vocal cord on the arytenoid cartilage, unless the arytenoid is involved, in which case the arytenoid is taken en bloc by disarticulating the cricoarytenoid joint with a No. 15 blade. Closure is accomplished by suturing the flap of anterior thyroid perichondrium to the contralateral perichondrium. The strap muscles can be closed as a second layer. Skin is closed in layers. A nasogastric feeding tube is inserted before mucosal closure. As with the supraglottic laryngectomy, a tracheostomy tube is left in with cuff inflated for at least 5 days postoperatively because this is not an airtight closure (Table 111-7).

Total laryngectomy is the "gold standard" in the treatment of glottic tumors to which all other treatments are compared (Table 111-8). Total laryngectomy is an elegant procedure from which recovery is rapid. Aspiration does not occur postoperatively because the airway and the pharynx have no connection. All tracheopulmonary secretions are eliminated externally, through the stoma. Rehabilitation of speech can be accomplished as discussed previously. When this and

other head and neck tumor procedures are performed, the airway must be considered. If the patient has an obstructive lesion, it is safest to perform an awake tracheostomy with local anesthesia before induction of general anesthesia. If the patient can be safely intubated, the tracheostomy may be deferred until a point in the procedure when the trachea is well exposed. The skin incision used for laryngectomy depends, as usual, on the surgeon's preference, but a

TABLE 111-7 ✦ KEY STEPS IN HEMILARYNGECTOMY

Tracheostomy
Endoscopy repeated if necessary
Subplatysmal flaps
Neck dissection if indicated
Straps separated in midline
Thyroid perichondrium incised and perichondrial flap elevated, with incisions made along superior margin of ala, midline, and 3 to 4 mm anterior to posterior border (midline incision placed 3 to 4 mm onto contralateral side for extended hemilaryngectomy)
Cricothyroid membrane cut transversely
Tumor visualized from cricothyrotomy as mucosal incision is made in midline and carried inferior to superior, opening the larynx progressively like a book
Posterior mucosal cut from inferior to superior across vocal process of arytenoid or posterior to (including) arytenoid, delivering specimen en bloc
Closure by suturing perichondrial flap to contralateral perichondrium

superiorly based apron flap works well. Neck dissection can be performed through this incision, and vertical extensions can be placed laterally to improve exposure. The transverse component of the apron flap can be placed at the level of the anticipated tracheostome. Subplatysmal flaps are elevated. Neck dissections are performed if indicated. Modified radical neck dissection is used if three clinically pathologic nodes are present. Selective neck dissection of zones II, III, and IV is performed for T4 and some T3 glottic lesions. There is potential therapeutic benefit; if fewer than three nodes without extracapsular extension are present, postoperative radiotherapy is not generally necessary.

With or without neck dissection, the laryngectomy begins by skeletonization of the larynx. The strap muscles are transected a couple fingerbreadths above the clavicles. The thyroid gland is identified and split at the isthmus. The ipsilateral gland is generally resected with the larynx on the involved side. The underlying thyroid cartilage is rotated anteriorly, exposing the attachment of the inferior constrictor to its posterior border. The muscle is incised (Fig. 111-25), initially with preservation of the underlying mucosa of the lateral wall of the piriform sinus. If this mucosa is uninvolved, it can be bluntly dissected free of the cartilage and preserved to construct a larger neopharynx on closure. Dissection proceeds superiorly. The superior laryngeal neurovascular bundle is ligated. The hyoid bone is identified, grasped, and

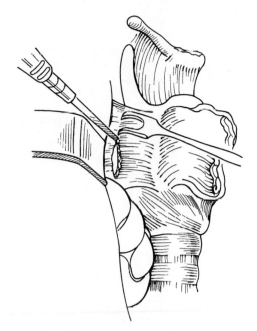

FIGURE 111-25. Separation of the inferior pharyngeal constrictor muscle off of the lateral aspect of the thyroid cartilage. (From Eibling DE: Surgery for glottic carcinoma. In Myers EN, ed: Operative Otolaryngology: Head and Neck Surgery. Philadelphia, WB Saunders, 1997-416.)

TABLE 111-8 ✦ KEY STEPS IN TOTAL LARYNGECTOMY

Awake tracheostomy or intubation
Subplatysmal flaps
Neck dissection if needed
Straps transected inferiorly
Thyroid isthmus transected and gland on involved side removed with specimen
Thyroid cartilage rotated anteriorly and inferior constrictor cut
Piriform sinus mucosa incised on uninvolved side
Suprahyoid musculature released and hyoid bone delivered
Vallecular mucosa entered
Tumor visualized to maintain margins
Piriform sinus and vallecular incisions joined
Piriform incisions carried inferiorly to postcricoid area
Trachea transected in beveled fashion with endotracheal tube now replaced through tracheotomy unless patient already has tracheostomy
Common wall between trachea and esophagus separated
Specimen delivered with transverse cut across postcricoid mucosa
Tracheoesophageal puncture
Neopharynx closed with inverted running suture
Skin flaps closed, incorporating tracheostoma

retracted anteriorly to facilitate transection of the suprahyoid musculature. Once accomplished, this leaves the vallecular mucosa exposed. The pharynx can then be entered through either the vallecula or piriform sinus, whichever is not involved with tumor. Once the pharynx is opened, the tumor is visualized and a margin of a few millimeters is maintained. Cuts connect the vallecula to the piriforms and then inferiorly along the medial wall of the piriforms to the level of the cricoid cartilage and hypopharyngeal mucosa. The trachea can then be transected, beveling superiorly as the cut proceeds posteriorly, so that the trachea is actually transected obliquely to provide a wide stoma. The common wall between the trachea and esophagus and pharynx is bluntly dissected superiorly until the mucosal cuts from the piriforms are reached, and the larynx is delivered by transection of the postcricoid mucosa transversely (Fig. 111-26). Frozen section margins are sent. A nasogastric feeding tube is placed before closure.

At this point, a tracheoesophageal puncture is generally performed. A stab incision is made on the posterior wall of the trachea into the esophagus. This incision should be placed several millimeters away from the cut edge of the trachea. Placement of the incision is facilitated by a right-angled clamp in the proximal esophagus, pushed anteriorly to tent the posterior wall of the trachea outward at the anticipated location. The

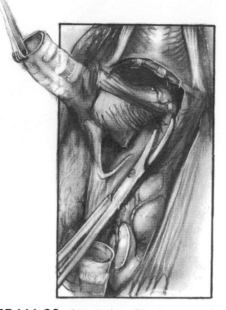

FIGURE 111-26. Completion of laryngectomy by incision of the postcricoid mucosa. (From Loré JM, ed: An Atlas of Head and Neck Surgery. Philadelphia, WB Saunders, 1988.)

common tracheoesophageal wall in this area must not have been separated during the laryngectomy, or secretions from the puncture site will be able to leak into the neck wound. A 14 French red rubber catheter is secured through the puncture site and into the esophagus. The catheter is changed to a Blom-Singer or similar valve approximately 2 weeks postoperatively in the office. Some authors routinely perform a cricopharyngeal myotomy before closure, as described previously. The pharyngeal mucosa is then closed with a running inverted suture (Connell stitch) of 3-0 Vicryl on a tapered needle. The mucosa can be closed vertically, horizontally, or in a T shape, depending on the defect and the surgeon's preference. The constrictor muscle should not be closed because closure interferes with swallowing and speech rehabilitation. The tracheostome is then created by suturing the cut edge of the trachea to the skin flaps. The inferior skin flap forms the inferior and lateral sides of the stoma. Half-vertical mattress or "pie crust" sutures are used through the skin into the deep aspect of the tracheal wall and out tracheal mucosa as a simple stitch, then back in the deep aspect of the skin and out.

The supracricoid laryngectomy is indicated for lesions that involve the supraglottis and glottis but spare at least one arytenoid. The entire thyroid cartilage and the membranous vocal cords, including the anterior commissure, are resected. The classic indication is a tumor that involves the anterior commissure with inferior extension. The primary difference between the supracricoid laryngectomy and the other conservation laryngeal procedures is that the entire thyroid cartilage and the underlying true vocal cords are resected, but as opposed to the total laryngectomy, the cricoid cartilage, hyoid bone, and one or both arytenoids are preserved (Fig. 111-27). The access incisions are essentially the same as for a laryngectomy, as are the initial mucosal incisions. The cricothyroid joints are then separated, with care taken not to damage the recurrent laryngeal nerves. The mucosal cuts are taken through the vocal processes of the arytenoids; one arytenoid can be resected if needed. They are continued to the level of the cricoid cartilage, resecting the true cords. The cricoid cartilage is wider posteriorly than anteriorly; it is shaped like a signet ring. Thus, significant inferior extension of a posteriorly located tumor is a contraindication to this procedure because an adequate margin cannot be obtained while preserving the cricoid. Closure, as with the other conservation laryngeal procedures, is not watertight. A cricohyoidopexy or cricohyoidoepiglottopexy is employed; the cricoid is suspended to the hyoid bone. If there is minimal supraglottic involvement and the epiglottis is preserved, the cricoid is then suspended to the petiole of the epiglottis. Phonation and airway protection are surprisingly efficacious once healing is complete, and failure to decannulate is rare.

Nasopharynx

Nasopharyngeal tumors seem to be qualitatively different from other aerodigestive tract tumors. Smoking and industrial exposure to wood dust and various chemicals are risk factors, similar to other head and neck tumors, as are a diet high in salted fish, Asian ancestry, and exposure to the Epstein-Barr virus, antibodies to which were detected in some studies in almost all patients with nasopharyngeal tumors. The histopathology is also different; typical keratinizing squamous cell carcinoma accounts for about 50% of these tumors. Approximately 30% are nonkeratinizing or poorly differentiated squamous cell carcinomas.[6] The remainder are mostly lymphomas and occasionally adenoid cystic carcinomas, melanomas, and other tumors. These tumors are thought to originate not just from the mucosa but from the lymphoid tissue prevalent in the nasopharynx. Presentation may be with a unilateral serous middle ear effusion and the resultant unilateral conductive hearing loss, aural fullness, otalgia, or dysequilibrium. Any patient, especially an adult, who presents with a chronic unilateral middle ear effusion should undergo nasopharyngoscopy for evaluation of a nasopharyngeal mass. A neck mass, especially in the suboccipital nodes or posterior triangle (zone V), may be the first sign of a nasopharyngeal mass. Lymph node involvement has

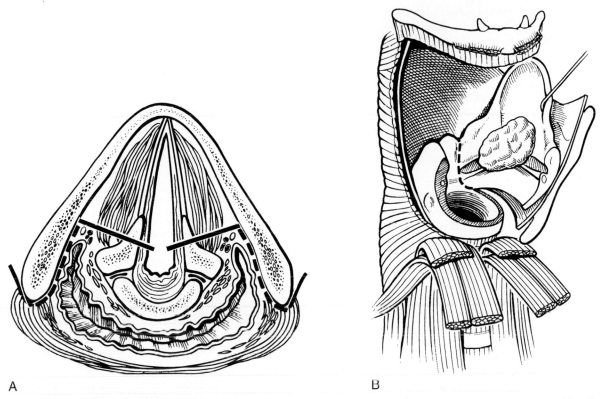

A   B

FIGURE 111-27. Supracricoid laryngectomy is shown from anterior oblique *(A)* and axial *(B)* views. (From Sinard JR, Netterville JL, Garrett CG, Ossoff RH: Cancer of the larynx. In Myers EN, ed: Operative Otolaryngology: Head and Neck Surgery. Philadelphia, WB Saunders, 1997:381.)

been estimated to occur in 80% of these patients.[6] Of note, the retropharyngeal lymph nodes (nodes of Rouvière), which are not included in a standard neck dissection, are the first echelon for lymphatic metastasis. Nasal obstruction, epistaxis, and cranial nerve deficits from skull base or cavernous sinus involvement are late findings of nasopharyngeal carcinoma.

ANATOMY

The nasopharynx is cuboidal. The anterior limit is the paired nasal choanae, which form the posterior limit of the nasal cavities. The roof is the skull base. The posterior limit is the posterior pharyngeal wall, over the vertebral atlas, where the adenoid pad is found in children and young adults. The roof and posterior wall constitute the vault. The lateral walls compose the remainder of the nasopharynx. The medial ends of the eustachian tubes open in the lateral walls. The superior lip of the eustachian tube orifice is the torus tubarius. Superior to this, marked topographically by a sulcus, is the fossa of Rosenmüller, where the retropharyngeal nodes are found. These nodes are the first echelon for lymphatic drainage of the nasopharynx, although the jugulodigastric nodes can also drain the nasopharynx directly.

STAGING

The staging system is as follows:

T1   Confined to one site
T2   Two sites (vault and lateral wall) involved
T3   Skull base extension (bone or cranial nerve involvement)

TREATMENT

Because of the relative inaccessibility of the nasopharynx, the difficulty in treating the retropharyngeal nodes surgically, and the radiosensitivity of nasopharyngeal tumors, radiotherapy is usually the first line of treatment. Surgery can be reserved for salvage in the neck or nasopharynx. Skull base techniques are needed for access to the nasopharynx and include Le Fort I osteotomies and transfacial approaches.

Paranasal Sinuses

The majority of paranasal sinus tumors are squamous cell carcinomas. Sinonasal undifferentiated carcinoma, adenocarcinoma, minor salivary gland tumors including adenoid cystic carcinoma, mucosal melanoma, and sarcomas are much less common.

Approximately 80% of paranasal sinus carcinomas arise in the maxillary antrum. In addition to smoking, industrial exposure to heavy metals (especially nickel and chromium), wood processing dust, and radium have been linked to sinus tumors. Treatment of these tumors is problematic because of the proximity of the sinuses to the skull base, orbits, and cranial nerves, and survival rates are poor. Preoperative imaging with CT or magnetic resonance scanning is crucial to staging and treatment planning.

ANATOMY

The paranasal sinuses include the maxillary, ethmoid, frontal, and sphenoid sinuses. Approximately 4% of adults have no frontal sinus.[18] The maxillary sinuses are pyramidal with the apex laterally and base medially. The roof of the maxillary sinus is the floor of the orbit, and the floor is the palate. The ethmoid sinus forms the medial wall of the orbit and part of the medial wall of the maxillary sinus. The sphenoid sinus is posterior to the ethmoid sinuses and nasal cavity. The roof of the sphenoid sinus abuts the sella turcica and optic chiasm. The lateral walls are adjacent to the cavernous sinuses and sphenoid portion of the carotid arteries. The frontal sinus is between the anterior cranial fossa and the frontal bone of the forehead and may extend posteriorly to form part of the orbital roofs.

STAGING

There is no generally accepted staging system for ethmoid, sphenoid, and frontal sinus tumors. Staging for maxillary sinus tumors is as follows:

T1 Tumor confined to the antral mucosa
T2 Tumor confined to the superior wall without bone involvement or lateral and inferior walls with bone invasion but no further extension
T3 Invasion of the cheek, orbit, anterior ethmoid sinuses, or pterygoid muscles
T4 Invasion of the skull base, posterior ethmoid or sphenoid sinuses, or pterygoid plates

Nodal staging is the same as for other head and neck sites.

TREATMENT

Combined therapy with surgery and radiation is used for most paranasal sinus carcinomas because of the difficulty in obtaining wide surgical margins. Radiation alone is generally used for palliation. Surgery alone is used only for small T1 lesions. The advent of craniofacial approaches with modern reconstructive techniques, including free flaps, has broadened the indications for extirpation. Maxillary antrum lesions can be excised with a lateral rhinotomy and medial maxillectomy. Transoral or transpalatal approaches can

remove lesions that involve the floor of the maxillary sinus alone. Midfacial degloving affords access to the inferior and medial maxillary walls. The Weber-Fergusson approach involves a standard lateral rhinotomy incision combined with a lip-splitting incision through the philtral column or a lower eyelid incision (Fig. 111-28). This can extend exposure to include the lower orbit and anterior zygoma. Craniofacial approaches combine facial incisions with a bicoronal incision. Pericranial flaps are often used for closure. Through these approaches, total or partial maxillectomy, orbital exenteration, and en bloc resection of the anterior cranial base can be performed. The last is most commonly indicated for olfactory neuroblastoma (esthesioneuroblastoma).

Perineural invasion along cranial nerves can lead to intracranial involvement. Direct extension into the orbit is also common with advanced sinus tumors. Preoperative CT or magnetic resonance scans should allow identification of such deep extension preoperatively, with special attention paid to the courses of the cranial nerves. The goal of reconstruction is watertight separation of the central nervous system from the sinus cavities and their colonizing flora. The pericranial flap, temporalis muscle flap, dural repair with fascia lata free grafts, and vascularized free tissue transfer may all be used toward the goal of cranionasal separation. Postoperative lumbar puncture may also

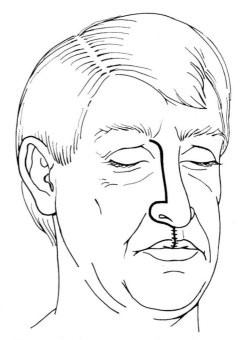

FIGURE 111-28. The Weber-Fergusson incision. (From Myers EN: Medial maxillectomy. In Myers EN, ed: Operative Otolaryngology: Head and Neck Surgery. Philadelphia, WB Saunders, 1997:100.)

decrease the incidence of postoperative cerebrospinal fluid leak.

SPECIAL TOPICS
Complications of Head and Neck Cancer Treatment

Complications of head and neck cancer treatment include the medical complications of surgery in general, such as myocardial infarction, pulmonary embolus, and drug reactions. Common complications also include wound infection, seroma, and hematoma. Complications unique to surgery in this area must also be considered. Airway obstruction may occur from large lesions, especially during induction of general anesthesia. Awake tracheostomy is often necessary. Postoperative airway complications, including decannulation and obstruction, can be devastating. Healing problems may also occur with laryngopharyngeal closures, resulting in pharyngocutaneous fistulas, which may resolve with expectant care or require closure, most commonly with a pectoralis flap. The incidence of fistula is higher in irradiated fields. Chyle leak is a potentially life-threatening complication of neck dissection that often requires re-exploration and ligation of the thoracic duct or its tributaries. Cranial nerve injury can occur from extirpation of the primary tumor or neck dissection. Cerebrovascular accident may occur, especially with neck dissection, secondary to intimal dissection of the carotid artery, embolism of an atherosclerotic plaque, or hypotension. Air embolism can occur if the internal jugular vein is lacerated intraoperatively and can be life-threatening. Cerebrospinal fluid leak, meningitis, and subarachnoid hemorrhage can result from skull base procedures. One must consider the potential complications and their treatment when caring for the patient with head and neck cancer.

Second Primaries and the Unknown Primary

The concept of field cancerization suggests that patients with head and neck cancer have premalignant changes throughout the mucosal surfaces of the upper aerodigestive tract because of exposure to smoking, alcohol, or other carcinogens, as discussed previously. Dysplastic changes can be detected by conventional pathology stains and immunohistochemistry. Second primary tumors may arise within the field of abnormal mucosa. By definition, a second primary is geographically separate from the first primary. If the lesions are present at they same time, they are referred to as synchronous primaries. If they present more than 6 months apart, they are considered metachronous primaries. The initial evaluation of a patient with head and neck cancer therefore includes endoscopy and chest radiography or CT scan to look for synchronous primaries. The chest work-up can also identify lung metastases. The risk for development of a second primary is estimated at 10% to 40% during the lifetime of the patient with head and neck cancer and is approximately 5% to 6% per year, although up to half of second primaries may occur within the first 2 years after initial treatment.[6] Oral cavity tumors have the highest rate of second primaries, most of which occur in the head and neck. Laryngeal cancers also have a high rate of second primaries, with the lung being the most common site of the second lesion, presumably because of the carcinogenic effects of tobacco on the lung. Of note, chemoprevention of second primaries with vitamins C and E, retinoids, and beta-carotene has been studied with mixed results, but patients with head and neck cancer should be monitored for good nutritional intake during short- and long-term follow-up. In addition, patients are more at risk for development of a second primary if they continue to smoke and consume alcohol.

The unknown primary in the head and neck refers to a tumor that presents with metastatic tumor in the cervical lymphatics (i.e., a neck mass) but no identifiable primary. Meticulous physical examination and endoscopy will often reveal gross evidence of a small primary, but several strategies are employed to help make a diagnosis. First, the pathologic process must be verified, which is readily achieved by fine-needle aspiration biopsy; this technique is sensitive and specific for squamous cell carcinoma, although patients are often referred after excision elsewhere of a neck mass revealing squamous cell carcinoma. If the pathologic examination shows lymphoma, this usually represents a primary tumor. If the pathologic examination shows melanoma, closer examination of the skin is warranted. The surgeon must remember also that cutaneous squamous cell carcinoma can metastasize to regional lymphatics, although this generally occurs with advanced, readily apparent lesions. The location of the involved cervical lymph node will give some indication of the site of the primary. Upper cervical nodes come from oral cavity, oropharynx, supraglottic, or laryngeal lesions. Midjugular nodes commonly originate from laryngeal lesions. Central, or zone VI, nodes come from laryngeal and thyroid lesions. Zone V nodes generally metastasize from nasopharyngeal tumors. The majority of supraclavicular metastases result from primaries below the clavicles, specifically breast, lung, or gastrointestinal lesions. Another consideration is that certain primary sites are more likely than others to present as an unknown primary with a neck mass, specifically the tonsil, tongue base, and nasopharynx. Tonsillectomy and random biopsies of the tongue base and nasopharynx may therefore be warranted in the search for the unknown primary.

SUMMARY

Carcinoma of the upper aerodigestive tract is a complex problem that is usually treated through a multidisciplinary approach. Evaluation of the patient with head and neck cancer requires knowledge of the risk factors for these tumors and their symptoms and signs as well as familiarity with the head and neck physical examination, including indirect laryngoscopy and office endoscopy. Work-up often includes radiographic scanning, biopsy, and rigid endoscopy. Treatment may involve surgery, radiation, chemotherapy, or a combination of multiple modalities. Surgical extirpation requires a familiarity with the complex anatomy of this region as well as an understanding of the appropriate indications for the multiple procedures available. Contemporary reconstructive techniques have expanded the indications for surgical extirpation and improved the quality of life of these patients, a crucial concern when survival remains poor for advanced lesions and given the potentially devastating nature of this disease and its treatment, especially with respect to speech, swallowing, and airway concerns.

REFERENCES

1. Adelstein DJ, Lavertu P, Saxton JP, et al: Mature results of a phase II randomized trial comparing concurrent chemoradiotherapy with radiation therapy alone in patients with stage III and IV squamous cell carcinoma of the head and neck. Cancer 2000;88:876-883.
2. Myers EN, ed: Operative Otolaryngology: Head and Neck Surgery. Philadelphia, WB Saunders, 1997.
3. Loré JM, ed: An Atlas of Head and Neck Surgery, 3rd ed. Philadelphia, WB Saunders, 1988.
4. Bailey BJ, ed: Atlas of Head and Neck Surgery—Otolaryngology. Philadelphia, Lippincott-Raven, 1996.
5. Cummings CW, Fredrickson JM, Harker LA, et al, eds: Otolaryngology—Head and Neck Surgery. St. Louis, Mosby, 1998.
6. Myers EN, Suen JY, eds: Cancer of the Head and Neck, 3rd ed. Philadelphia, WB Saunders, 1996.
7. Pitman KT, Johnson JT, Myers EN: Effectiveness of selective neck dissection for management of the clinically negative neck. Arch Otolaryngol Head Neck Surg 1997;123:917-922.
8. Hostal AS, Carrau RL, Johnson JT, Myers EN: Selective neck dissection in the management of the clinically node-negative neck. Laryngoscope 2000;110:2037-2040.
9. Schusterman MA, ed: Microsurgical reconstruction of the cancer patient. Philadelphia, Lippincott-Raven, 1997.
10. Schusterman MA, Kroll SS, Weber RS, et al: Intraoral soft tissue reconstruction after cancer ablation: a comparison of the pectoralis major flap and the free radial forearm flap. Am J Surg 1991;162:397-399.
11. Kroll SS, Reece GP, Miller MJ, Schusterman MA: Comparison of the rectus abdominis free flap with the pectoralis major myocutaneous flap for reconstruction in the head and neck. Am J Surg 1992;164:615-618.
12. Schusterman MA, Reece GP, Miller MJ, Harris S: The osteocutaneous free fibula flap: is the skin paddle reliable? Plast Reconstr Surg 1992;90:787-793.
13. Johnson JT: Proposal of standardization of screening tests for detection of distant metastases from head and neck cancer. ORL J Otorhinolaryngol Relat Spec 2001;63:256-258.
14. Perlmutter MA, Johnson JT, Snyderman CH, et al: Functional outcomes after treatment of squamous cell carcinoma of the base of tongue. Arch Otolaryngol Head Neck Surg 2002;128:887-891.
15. Adelstein DJ, Saxton JP, Lavertu P, et al: Maximizing local control and organ preservation in stage IV squamous cell head and neck cancer with hyperfractionated radiation and concurrent chemotherapy. J Clin Oncol 2002;20:1405-1410.
16. Gokhale AS, Lavertu P: Surgical salvage after chemoradiation of head and neck cancer: complications and outcomes. Curr Oncol Rep 2001;3:72-76.
17. Reece GP, Schusterman MA, Miller MJ, Kroll SS: Morbidity and functional outcome of free jejunal transfer reconstruction for circumferential defects of the pharynx and cervical esophagus. Plast Reconstr Surg 1995;96:1307-1316.
18. Schaeffer JP: The Embryology, Development and Anatomy of the Nose, Paranasal Sinuses, Nasolacrimal Passageways and Olfactory Organs in Man. Philadelphia, P. Blakiston's, 1920.

Benign Tumors of the Skin

Pablo León, MD

A plastic surgeon needs essential diagnostic elements for the accurate diagnosis and treatment of the patient with skin lesions, and an overview of these elements is provided. Knowledge of the structure and function of normal skin is crucial to the understanding of cutaneous disease.

As in other specialties, medical history is important; however, the ability to interpret what is observed is even more important. The diagnosis of skin disease must be approached in an orderly and logical manner. A brief history noting duration, onset location, symptoms, family history, allergies, occupation, and previous treatment is obtained. The skin should be examined methodically. An eye scan over wide areas is inefficient. It is most productive to mentally divide the skin surface into several sections and carefully study each section. For example, in studying the face, the area around each eye, the nose, the mouth, the cheeks, and the temples should be examined. A complete skin examination is performed for all patients who present with a skin lesion. The examination starts with the hair and scalp and then moves to the face. The back, chest, abdomen, and extremities, including palms, soles, and nails, are examined. Skin generally covered by undergarments must also be examined because serious lesions, such as melanoma, can arise in these areas.

In each region of the body, the physical examination includes three maneuvers:

1. observation for color or surface changes;
2. touching or light stroking to detect texture changes, warmth, and moisture, with an understanding that the smoothness or roughness of the skin depends on factors such as normal keratinization, proper hydration of the stratum corneum, and normal cutaneous blood flow; and
3. palpation and stretching of the skin to determine its consistency and pliability, with the appreciation that elasticity depends on the normal structure and function of dermal connective tissue and ground substance and that certain infiltrates can be detected by palpation.

PRIMARY LESIONS AND SURFACE CHARACTERISTICS

Lesions should be examined carefully. Valuable information about the distribution is provided by standing back and viewing a disease process. Close examination with a magnifying device provides much more information. The plastic surgeon should learn the surface characteristics of all the common entities and gain experience by examining known entities. A flesh-colored papule might be a wart, sebaceous hyperplasia, or basal cell carcinoma. Because there are many hundreds of dermatoses, a logical process of elimination is required to narrow the possibilities, first to specific categories of lesions and then, it is hoped, to one final diagnosis. Identify the patient's specific lesion by looking for distinctive features, such as the distribution, any unusual shape, the arrangement of several lesions (annular, serpiginous, dermatomal), the dominant hue and color, and the surface characteristics (particularly the appearance of scales or verrucous or vegetative changes).

Clinical indications for biopsy include lesions that fail to heal, increase in size, bleed easily, or ulcerate spontaneously and tumors or growths of uncertain nature. Three types of biopsies can be performed. The choice of technique determines the size and shape of the specimen obtained. The procedure selected should secure the tissue most likely to contain the pathologic alterations and leave the smallest cosmetic defect. For the most complete histopathologic assessment, an elliptical, full-thickness excision is best because, in one procedure, the entire lesion is removed and secured for diagnosis and the remaining defect is easily sutured. The excisional biopsy technique is indicated when malignant melanoma is suggested or when a lesion is deep in skin or subcutaneous tissue and its orientation in surrounding tissue is relevant for diagnosis. Another biopsy method is the shave or parallel incision, in which lidocaine is injected locally under the lesion to lift it above the skin surface and a scalpel (the knife horizontal to the skin surface) is used to "shave" off the protruding part of the skin and lesion. This technique is useful for diagnosis of malignant and benign tumors when subsequent treatment by curettage and electrodesiccation is anticipated. It should never be used when melanoma is suspected because the specimen obtained is too superficial for adequate histologic grading. Shave biopsy is convenient for removal of superficial benign tumors such as seborrheic keratoses and skin tags. In the third technique, punch biopsy, the clinician uses a tubular blade to cut out a circular plug of skin by slightly rotating and pushing the cutting edge deep into the dermis. The specimen is clipped off at its base with scissors, and the defect can readily be closed with sutures. Punch biopsies are used to diagnose inflammatory diseases and tumors. If a first skin biopsy does not provide an answer, it is often necessary and appropriate to resample the area.

VIRAL TUMORS
Verruca Vulgaris

Verruca vulgaris or the common wart is a benign epidermal neoplasm. Warts are caused by the human papillomavirus. Many different types of human papillomavirus have been identified by their DNA composition, and each is associated with a particular set of clinical and pathologic entities. Viral warts are tumors initiated by a viral infection of keratinocytes. The cells proliferate to form a mass, but the mass remains confined to the epidermis. Thrombosed vessels are seen as black dots on the surface of some warts. Although warts remain confined to the epidermis, the growing mass can protrude and displace the dermis. The undersurface of a wart is a smooth round mass.

INCIDENCE AND EPIDEMIOLOGY

Warts commonly occur during childhood and early adulthood but may occur at any age. Warts are transmitted by touch and commonly occur at sites of trauma. Warts may be found at sites of nail biting, picking of the skin, or plantar pressure caused by poorly fitting shoes or faulty weight bearing.

CLINICAL DESCRIPTION

There are several clinical types of warts. Verruca vulgaris is the most commonly seen. Common warts begin as smooth, flesh-colored papules and evolve into dome-shaped, gray-brown, hyperkeratotic growths with black dots on the surface. The black dots, which are thrombosed capillaries, are a useful diagnostic sign. The hands are the most commonly involved areas, but warts may be found on any skin surface (Fig. 112-1; see also Color Plate 112-1). In general, warts are few in number, but it is not unusual for common warts to become so numerous that they become confluent and obscure large areas of normal skin.

TREATMENT

Because warts are benign lesions, one should strive for minimal destruction of normal tissue. Topical salicylic acid preparations, liquid nitrogen, and light electrocautery are the best methods for initial therapy. Treatment with tretinoin cream has met with limited success. Treatment with 5-fluorouracil cream may produce dramatic clearing of flat warts,[1] although hyperpigmentation may persist. Direct excision is used for resistant or large lesions.

Molluscum Contagiosum
CLINICAL DESCRIPTION

Molluscum contagiosum is a virus infection of the skin characterized by discrete, 2- to 5-mm, slightly

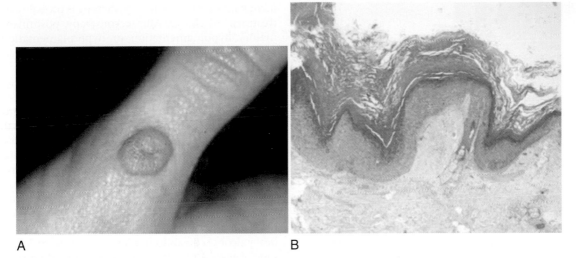

A   B

FIGURE 112-1. *A* and *B,* Verruca vulgaris. (See also Color Plate 112-1.)

umbilicated, flesh-colored, dome-shaped papules (Fig. 112-2). It spreads by autoinoculation, by scratching, or by touching a lesion. The areas most commonly involved are the face, trunk, axillae, extremities in children, and pubic and genital areas in adults. Lesions are frequently grouped. Unlike warts, it does not involve the palms and soles. The individual lesion begins as a smooth, dome-shaped, white to flesh-colored papule. An important clinical characteristic is that with time, the center becomes soft and umbilicated. Most lesions are self-limited and clear spontaneously in 6 to 9 months, but they may last much longer.

DIAGNOSIS

If necessary, the diagnosis can be established easily by laboratory methods. The virus infects epithelial cells, forming large intracytoplasmic inclusion bodies and disrupting cell bonds by which epithelial cells are

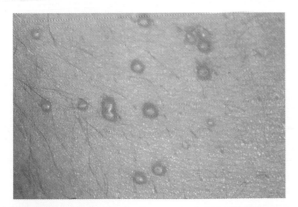

FIGURE 112-2. Molluscum contagiosum.

generally held together. This lack of adhesion causes the central core of the lesion to be soft. The infected cells are dark and round and disperse easily with slight pressure, whereas normal epithelial cells are flat and rectangular and tend to remain stuck together in sheets.

TREATMENT

Spontaneous resolution is known to occur. Small papules can be removed with a curet in adults. Children can be treated after application of a lidocaine-prilocaine cream (EMLA) for analgesia.[2] Curettage is useful when there are a few lesions because it provides the quickest, most reliable treatment. A small scar may form; therefore, this technique should be avoided in cosmetically important areas. Liquid nitrogen is also effective as in treatment of the common wart. Carbon dioxide laser therapy has been used to treat genital lesions.[3] Another method of treatment is the trichloroacetic acid peel, which has been used in patients with human immunodeficiency virus infection with extensive facial molluscum contagiosum.[4]

SEBORRHEIC KERATOSIS

Clinical Description

Seborrheic keratosis, also known as senile wart, senile keratosis, or basal cell papilloma, is the most common benign cutaneous neoplasm. In general, the lesions appear after the fourth decade. Most people will develop at least one such tumor in their lifetime. These lesions can appear on any part of the body except the mucous membranes. Seborrheic keratosis consists of a sharply circumscribed, rough or smooth papule or plaque that is 1 mm to several centimeters in size

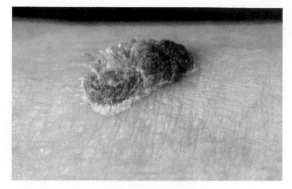

FIGURE 112-3. Seborrheic keratosis.

and dirty yellow to dark brown (Fig. 112-3). The lesions often have the appearance of being stuck on and are characterized by prominent follicular plugging. They are most common in light-skinned races and are not thought to be photoinduced. A biopsy may be required to rule out a pigmented basal cell carcinoma or an inflamed seborrheic keratosis, malignant melanoma, or squamous cell carcinoma. Patients who present with dark, irregular, sometimes irritated seborrheic keratosis may worry that it is melanoma. Seborrheic keratosis can show many of the features of a malignant melanoma, including an irregular border and variable pigmentation. The key differential diagnostic features are the surface characteristics. Melanomas have a smooth surface that varies in elevation and in color density and shade. Seborrheic keratoses preserve a uniform appearance over their entire surface.

Epidemiology

The etiology of seborrheic keratosis is not known. In patients with a great number of lesions, it is sometimes noted that there is a positive family history. This may well reflect a genetic propensity. There does not seem to be a relationship with skin type or with areas of exposure. Basal cell carcinoma and other common skin cancers have been reported, rarely, in association with seborrheic keratoses.[5-7] Multiple eruptive seborrheic keratoses, also known as the sign of Leser-Trélat, have been mentioned in association with multiple internal malignant neoplasms.[8] The most frequent associations are adenocarcinomas of the stomach, colon, and breast.

Treatment

Lesions are removed for cosmetic purposes or to eliminate a source of irritation. Adequate treatment of seborrheic keratosis consists of shave excision, curettage, superficial electrodesiccation, or freezing with liquid nitrogen because this lesion does not undergo malignant degeneration. Cryotherapy is probably the treatment of choice. After cryotherapy, postinflammatory hypopigmentation or hyperpigmentation, which is usually temporary, may develop.

RHINOPHYMA

The word *rhinophyma* is derived from the Greek words *rhis,* meaning nose, and *phyma,* meaning growth. Rhinophyma is a glandular form of acne rosacea affecting the nose, in which the sebaceous glands hypertrophy to such an extent that the nose becomes bulbous and lobulated. It is characterized by sebaceous hyperplasia, fibrosis, follicular plugging, and telangiectasias of the skin of the nose (Fig. 112-4). This was once thought to be an unfounded association with heavy alcohol consumption. There is a male-to-female ratio of about 12:1, although acne rosacea is three times more common in women than in men. The reported incidence of occult cancer in the setting of rhinophyma varies from 15% to 30%.[9-12] Basal carcinoma is the most common malignant neoplasm.

Many different techniques have been used to treat this condition, including dermabrasion,[13] excision and reconstruction with full-thickness skin grafts, carbon dioxide and argon laser excision,[14-16] electrocautery, and paring with the scalpel.[17] In many patients, a good cosmetic result is achieved by paring off the excess tissue and leaving the area to re-epithelialize. This occurs within 2 to 3 weeks; the remnants of the hypertrophied sebaceous glands act as multiple foci for epithelialization. Excessive resection of underlying sebaceous tissue can lead to considerable pain and disfigurement due to scarring. The risk of scarring and hypopigmentation appears to be least with use of the scalpel because there is no chance of thermal injury to surrounding tissue.[18] A dermabrader is useful in feathering the edges. Local infiltration of epinephrine is used for hemostasis. A postoperative wound dressing such as bacitracin ointment with Xeroform should be applied to keep the wound bed moist and clean.

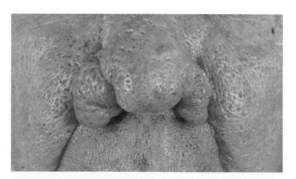

FIGURE 112-4. Rhinophyma.

CYSTS

Epidermal Cysts

CLINICAL DESCRIPTION AND EPIDEMIOLOGY

The epidermal or sebaceous cyst is the most common form of cyst and occurs primarily on the face, back or base of the ears, chest, and back where the sebaceous glands are most numerous and active (Fig. 112-5). Epidermal cysts are the result of the proliferation of surface epidermal cells within the dermis. Production of keratin within a circumscribed space results in a cyst. The cyst wall is lined with stratified squamous epithelium, which produces keratin. Epidermal cysts may arise from occlusion of pilosebaceous follicles, from implantation of epidermal cells into the dermis after penetration injury, and from trapping of epidermal cells along embryonal fusion planes. The first mechanism is the most common. Epidermal cysts are rare in children but common in adults. Both sexes are affected equally. Children who are brought to the physician with epidermal cysts or patients with epidermal cysts in unusual areas, such as the legs, should be suspected of having Gardner syndrome. Epidermal cysts may be intradermal or subcutaneous tumors. The round, protruding, smooth-surfaced mass is movable and varies in size from a few millimeters to several centimeters. The cyst communicates with the surface through a narrow channel, and the surface opening appears as a small, round, sometimes imperceptible keratin-filled orifice (i.e., a blackhead). Epidermal cysts may originate from comedones; such lesions are superficial, with a large, black, keratinous plug on the surface. They are referred to as giant comedones and are commonly found on the back.

Epidermal cysts are slow growing and usually not symptomatic. Some cysts may become inflamed and secondarily infected. This occurs most frequently on the face and neck in association with acne vulgaris. These cysts may rupture and induce an inflammatory response. Spontaneous rupture of the wall results in discharge of the soft, yellow keratin into the dermis.

TREATMENT

Fluctuant, inflamed cysts should be incised, drained, and cultured. The initial antibiotic treatment should be directed against *Staphylococcus aureus* because this is the most common pathogen. Removal of the cyst is usually best deferred until the inflammation and infection have subsided. Excision is the procedure of choice for noninflamed cysts. The entire epidermal lining should be removed to prevent recurrence.

Pilar Cysts

CLINICAL DESCRIPTION AND EPIDEMIOLOGY

Pilar cysts occur in the scalp and, like epidermal cysts, are freely movable. They are frequently multiple and may become large masses. The epithelium-lined wall resembles the outer root sheath of the hair and produces keratin of a quality different from that of the epidermal cyst. The cyst contains concentric layers of dry keratin, which over time may become macerated and soft. They are reportedly more common in women and usually present in middle age. Pilar cysts may become inflamed and may suppurate, but this is uncommon. Proliferating pilar cyst may develop from an ordinary pilar cyst.[19,20] This condition is usually seen in the elderly and is clinically recognized as a progressively enlarging lobulated mass that may ulcerate and resemble a squamous cell carcinoma. Although considered biologically benign, it may be locally aggressive. Very rarely, malignant transformation may occur, and this is heralded by rapid enlargement of the nodule.[21]

TREATMENT

Treatment is the same as for an epidermal cyst. A proliferating epidermal cyst must be excised with a narrow margin to ensure complete removal.

MILIA

Milia are small superficial keratin cysts. The etiology is unknown, but these lesions are believed to arise from the pilosebaceous follicle. Secondary milia may represent retention cysts that follow injury to the skin and are believed to be derived from a hair follicle, sweat gland, sebaceous duct, or epidermis. Secondary milia may be seen after dermabrasion and in areas of chronic glucocorticoid-induced atrophy.[22]

Milia are commonly found on the skin and mucosa of infants. They also commonly occur in adults and show no sexual predisposition.

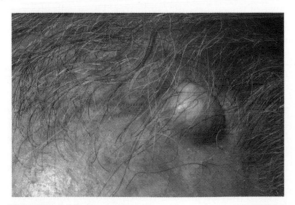

FIGURE 112-5. Epidermal cyst.

Clinically, they are superficial white papules, generally only 1 to 2 mm in diameter. They are most common on the eyelids and cheeks. Milia in the newborn are commonly seen on the nose. They may also appear on other parts of the body, including palatal and gingival mucosa.

On histologic evaluation, milia resemble epidermal cysts, varying only in size. These lesions are lined with mature epithelium with few cell layers and central keratin material.

Treatment usually consists of incision with a No. 11 blade or needle. Multiple lesions may be treated with light electrodesiccation.

EPIDERMAL APPENDAGE TUMORS

Sebaceous Hyperplasia

Senile sebaceous hyperplasia consists of small tumors composed of enlarged sebaceous glands. They begin as pale yellow, slightly elevated papules; with time, they become yellow, dome shaped, and umbilicated. Senile sebaceous hyperplasia with telangiectasia may be mistaken for a basal cell carcinoma. The lesions occur after the age of 30 years in 25% of the population and gradually become more numerous. There is no relationship between the skin type and the occurrence of these lesions. They are commonly found on the forehead, cheeks, lower lid, and nose. The etiology remains unclear; chronic solar exposure is not a likely cause.[23] The lesions consist of lobules of mature sebaceous glands situated around a sebaceous duct that opens to the surface epidermis or the mucous epithelium.

Treatment consists of eradication by electrodesiccation and curettage, cryosurgery, or simple excision.

Epidermal Nevus

EPIDEMIOLOGY

Epidermal nevus is a developmental (hamartomatous) disorder characterized by hyperplasia of epidermal structures (surface epidermis and adnexal structures) in a circumscribed area of the skin. The term nevus is used here to denote a congenital defect of the skin characterized by the localized excess of one or more types of cells; there is no proliferation of nevocellular nevus cells (melanocytes) in the lesion.

The term epidermal nevus is commonly used to describe a group of cutaneous hamartomas linked by common clinical and histologic features. Linear epidermal nevus or nevus unius lateris (a linear, unilateral, wart-like nevus) and nevus verrucosus (a localized, wart-like nevus) are some of the names given to variants of epidermal nevus.

The cause of epidermal nevus syndrome is unknown. Possible explanations are the faulty migration and development of embryonic tissue and a developmental error in separation of the ectoderm from the neural tube.

The incidence of epidermal nevi is estimated to be 1 per 1000 live births.[24] The majority of epidermal nevi occur sporadically; familial occurrences of the disease have been described.[24] Epidermal nevi affect both sexes equally. Most epidermal nevi are present at birth or infancy, but the lesions rarely appear as late as puberty.[24,25]

CLINICAL DESCRIPTION

These well-circumscribed growths are present at birth or appear in infancy or childhood. They are round, oval, or oblong and elevated, flat-topped, and yellow-tan to dark brown; they have a uniformly warty or velvety surface with sharp borders. They appear more commonly on the head and neck; 13% of patients have widespread lesions. These lines represent a developmental growth pattern of the skin. Epidermal nevi may spread beyond their original distribution; further progression is unlikely after late adolescence. Nevi present at birth and those on the head are less likely to spread. In spite of their unusual appearance and occasional itching, they are generally inconsequential. On occasion, the growths are large and disfiguring. Patients with epidermal nevi are at significant risk of having other anomalies in other organ systems.[26] Abnormalities are more likely in patients with widespread nevi. The most common systems involved are skeletal, neurologic, and ocular.

PATHOLOGY

The cells are histologically identical to or closely resemble normal cells. Epidermal nevus should be used as a general term to designate an excess of one type of epidermally derived cells. However, the term is commonly reserved for congenital growths in which the predominant cell is the keratinocyte. These nevi arise from the pluripotential germinative cells in the basal layer of the embryonic epidermis. These cells give rise to keratinocytes and skin appendages (hair follicles, sweat glands).

GENETIC COUNSELING

The rare epidermal nevus syndrome consists of extensive epidermal nevi associated with skeletal, ocular, and central nervous system disorders.[24,27,28] Small lesions are sporadic. Patients do not have a family history of epidermal nevi. Most instances of epidermal nevus syndrome occur sporadically, but there is some suspicion that an autosomal dominant transmission may be present. Inform patients that genetic transmission is possible with large epidermal nevi but that the data are inadequate for an accurate determination to be made.

TREATMENT

Reported therapeutic approaches include dermabrasion, cryotherapy, laser therapy, and partial-thickness excision. Full-thickness surgical excision is effective definitive treatment.[29,30]

Verrucous Nevus

The lesion consists of closely set verrucous papules that may coalesce to form well-demarcated plaques. They may be skin colored, brown, or gray-brown (Fig. 112-6). A linear configuration is common, especially for lesions on the limb. Such lesions may appear to follow skin tension lines. Verrucous epidermal nevi may be localized or diffuse. When the lesions are distributed on half of the body, it is termed nevus unius lateris. A verrucous epidermal nevus may enlarge slowly during childhood. By adolescence, the lesion usually reaches a stable size, and further extension is unlikely.[24] Rarely, basal cell and squamous cell carcinomas have been reported to develop in a verrucous epidermal nevus; this malignant transformation should be suspected when sudden localized growth, nodules, or ulcers appear.[24] On histologic evaluation, there is hyperkeratosis, acanthosis, and papillomatosis. The rete edges are elongated. The histologic appearance is essentially that of a benign papilloma.

Excision is the most reliable treatment. This may not be practical or advisable if the lesion is extensive or at sites not amenable to simple surgery. The excision should extend to the deep dermis; otherwise, the lesion may recur. Alternative treatments have included laser,[31] cryotherapy, and electrodesiccation dermabrasion. These treatments usually remove only the superficial portion of the nevus, and recurrence is common. Because epidermal nevus is associated with

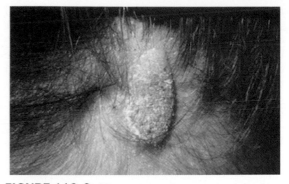

FIGURE 112-6. Verrucous nevus.

a small risk of malignant change, biopsy should be performed of suspect areas of any lesion.

Nevus Sebaceus

Nevus sebaceus is a distinctive growth most commonly found on the scalp, followed by the forehead and retroauricular region[32] (Fig. 112-7; see also Color Plate 112-2). Involvement of the neck and trunk is exceptional. A nevus of epithelial and nonepithelial skin components, nevus sebaceus sustains age-related modifications in morphologic appearance. The nevus occurs singly and is asymptomatic. Two thirds are present at birth; the remaining third develop in infancy or early childhood. Males and females are equally affected. The rare nevus sebaceus of Jadassohn syndrome consists of the triad of a linear sebaceous nevus, convulsions, and mental retardation. A variety of congenital malformations of the ocular, skeletal, vascular, and urogenital systems have been described in association with nevus sebaceus.[33,34]

Lesions are oval to linear, varying from 0.5 × 1 cm to 7 × 9 cm. The three-stage evolution of the nevoid condition (newborn, puberty, and adult) parallels

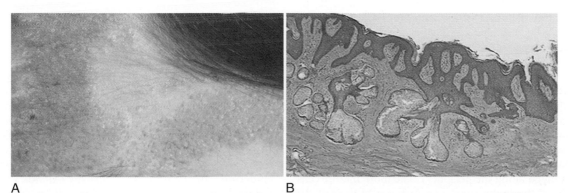

A   B

FIGURE 112-7. *A* and *B,* Nevus sebaceus. (See also Color Plate 112-2.)

the natural histologic differentiation of normal sebaceous glands. The lesions in infants and younger children are smooth to gently papillated, waxy, hairless thickenings. During puberty, there is a massive development of sebaceous glands with epidermal hyperplasia within the lesions. At this stage, they change clinically by developing a verrucous mulberry irregularity of the surface covered with numerous, closely aggregated, yellow to dark brown papules. When this transformation becomes noticeable, parents become worried and seek medical attention. In approximately 20% of patients, a third phase of evolution involves the development of secondary neoplasia in the mass of the nevus. A number of benign and malignant "nevoid tumors" may occur, the most common of which is the basal cell epithelioma. The malignant degenerations are relatively low grade; only a few instances of metastasis have been reported.[35] Most lesions are sporadic, but instances of inherited nevus sebaceus have been reported.[36]

On histologic evaluation, the epidermis shows papillomatous hyperplasia. In the dermis, there are increased numbers of mature sebaceous glands. In childhood, the sebaceous glands are underdeveloped, and the histologic finding may consist of only immature hair structures.

Surgical excision of a nevus sebaceus is recommended because of the high potential for development of basal cell carcinoma and other tumors. The lesion should preferably be excised before puberty because it may enlarge, and the risk of malignant transformation increases after puberty.[37]

Pilomatricoma

Pilomatricoma, or benign calcifying epithelioma of Malherbe, is a firm, deep-seated nodule covered with normal skin.[38] It can occur anywhere but is found most commonly on the face and upper extremities (Fig. 112-8). In general, the lesions are 0.5 to 5 cm in diameter. When the nodule is more superficial, it may appear dark blue. The tumor may arise at any age, but the onset is frequently found during childhood.[39] There have been a few instances of familial occurrence, some of which were associated with myotonic dystrophy.[38]

On the basis of histologic features, pilomatricoma has become accepted as a tumor differentiating toward hair structure.[40] The tumor is found in the dermis and may extend into the subcutaneous fat. The tumor is sharply demarcated and sometimes even encapsulated. Two types of epithelial cells are present, basophilic and shadow. The basophilic cells stain intensely and are arranged along the periphery. The more mature cells toward the center show a gradual loss of their nuclei and appear as shadow cells. They possess an unstained

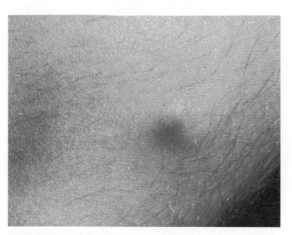

FIGURE 112-8. Pilomatricoma.

central area as a shadow of the lost nucleus. Calcification is found mainly in older tumors.

Treatment is by surgical excision.

SWEAT GLAND TUMORS

Syringoma

Syringomas are sweat duct tumors composed of small, firm, flesh-colored or yellow dermal papules that occur on the lower lids and less commonly over the face and trunk. They occur more frequently in women than in men. Lesions may develop at any age, but they initially appear most frequently during adolescence or early adult life, then slowly become more numerous. The tumors have no malignant potential. On histologic evaluation, there is benign proliferation of the eccrine ducts. The lesions are small ducts embedded in a fibrous stroma. The walls of the ducts are lined by rows of epithelial cells. The lesions may be removed for cosmetic purposes by electrodesiccation and curettage[41] or excised by gently elevating the small mass with the curved bevel of a 25-gauge needle. The oval wound is left to heal by secondary intention.[42,43]

Eccrine Poroma

Eccrine poroma occurs as a solitary lesion usually on the sole of the foot or the palm of the hand in persons older than 40 years. It may also occur on the chest, the neck, or other locations.[44] Eccrine poromas are seen as firm papules less then 2 cm in size. Lesions may occasionally be pedunculated and have a normal or erythematous color and a firm consistency (Fig. 112-9). Ulceration may occur at points of pressure.

Eccrine poroma may be located entirely within the epidermis[45] or the dermis.[46] It usually extends from the epidermis deeply into the dermis. It consists of broad bands of uniformly small cuboidal cells

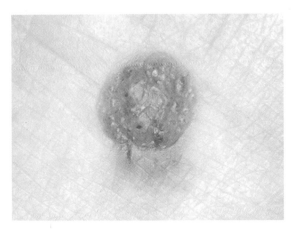

FIGURE 112-9. Eccrine poroma.

Nodules may also present on the face and rarely on the extremities.[48] In the solitary lesion type, there is no familial history. The lesion appears in adult life. The surface is smooth and may be telangiectatic. Cylindromas are usually benign, but malignant changes have been reported.[49]

The tumors are composed of islands of epithelial cells, which are surrounded by a thick hyaline sheath. The tumor cells are of two types. Small basal cells are found in the periphery, and cells with large nuclei lie

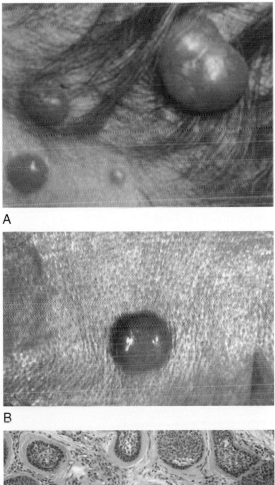

connected by intracellular bridges. The tumor cells have a cuboidal appearance, are strongly basophilic, and are smaller than the epidermal squamous cells. A characteristic feature is the significant amount of glycogen[47] and the eccrine-type enzymes contained within the tumor cell. In rare instances, malignant eccrine poroma or porocarcinoma develops either spontaneously or from long-standing benign eccrine poroma.

Eccrine poromas are treated by surgical excision.

Clear Cell Hidradenoma

Clear cell hidradenoma is an eccrine sweat gland tumor. It occurs as a slow-growing, usually solitary nodule. The tumors measure 0.5 to 2 cm or more in diameter and are firm to touch. Some tumors discharge serous material, whereas others tend to ulcerate. Lesions may occur anywhere.

The term *clear cell* indicates that cells appear empty under the light microscope. They contain large amounts of glycogen and all the eccrine-type enzymes. The tumor is well circumscribed and often encapsulated. It consists of lobulated masses in the dermis within which are tubular lumens of various sizes. The lumens often show branching or cystic spaces. One type of cell at the periphery has an elongated nucleus and basophilic cytoplasm. The other type of cell has a round nucleus and clear cytoplasm.

The treatment of choice is surgical excision.

Cylindroma

Cylindroma presents as either solitary or multiple lesions (Fig. 112-10; see also Color Plate 112-3). The multiple-lesion type has a genetic component. They are classically found on the scalp as numerous small papules or large nodules and may cover the entire scalp like a turban (turban tumor).

FIGURE 112-10. *A to C,* Cylindroma. (See also Color Plate 112-3.)

in the center. The tumor is consistent with an immature sweat gland epithelioma with eccrine and apocrine features.

For solitary lesions, treatment is by excision or electrosurgery. For small cylindromas, the carbon dioxide laser may be used. Multiple cylindromas usually require extensive plastic surgery that may be obviated by progressively excising a group of nodules in multiple procedures.

Trichoepithelioma

Trichoepithelioma usually presents as multiple, yellowish pink, translucent papules distributed symmetrically on the cheeks, eyelids, and nasolabial areas (Fig. 112-11). It is often inherited as an autosomal dominant trait. The lesions first appear at puberty and are more frequently seen in women. Lesions are benign but can be confused with basal cell carcinomas clinically and histologically.

The lesions are well circumscribed. A characteristic histologic feature is horn cysts, which consist of a fully keratinized inner shell surrounded by an outer shell of flattened basophilic cells. The keratinization in the horn cysts is abrupt and complete.

A single or localized lesion may be removed by electrodesiccation and curettage, but multiple lesions may be difficult to treat.

DERMATOFIBROMA

Dermatofibroma, also called histiocytoma, is a firm, skin-colored or reddish brown sessile papule or nodule that arises spontaneously or after minor trauma, such

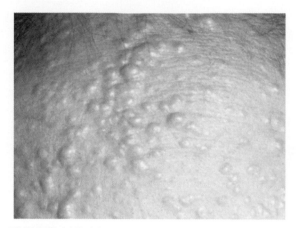

FIGURE 112-11. Trichoepithelioma.

as after an insect bite (Fig. 112-12; see also Color Plate 112-4). They are benign, asymptomatic lesions occurring more frequently in women. They vary in number from 1 to 10 and can be found anywhere on the extremities and trunk, but they are most likely to occur on the anterior surface of the lower legs. They appear as 3- to 10-mm slightly raised, pink-brown, sometimes scaly, hard growths that retract beneath the skin surface during attempts to compress and elevate them. They tend to remain stable for years as discrete solitary lesions.

Dermatofibromas demonstrate mixtures of fibroblasts, collagen, capillaries, and histiocytes under light microscopy. The overlying epidermis often contains significant hyperplasia.

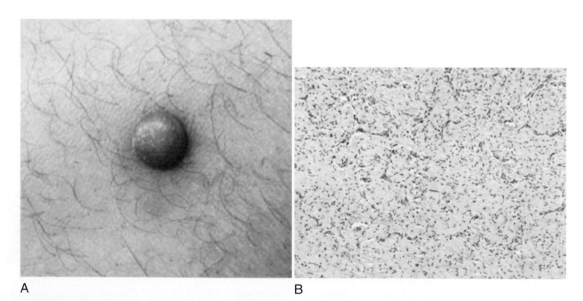

A   B

FIGURE 112-12. *A* and *B,* Dermatofibroma. (See also Color Plate 112-4.)

Lesions are usually treated for cosmetic reasons by surgical excision.

SKIN TAGS (ACROCHORDON)

Skin tags, also called acrochordon, commonly occur as multiple skin-colored or tan, filiform or smooth-surfaced papules that are 2 to 3 mm in diameter. They are found in approximately 25% of men and women. They can begin in the second decade, with a steady increase in frequency up to the fifth decade.[50] Lesions are often located on the neck or axillae but may also appear on the groin or in the extremities, often as isolated larger polypoid growths. The fibrous stalk consists of loose connective tissue with dilated capillaries. Lesions may become irritated or are traumatized from twisting of the stalk. Biopsy is performed if the clinical diagnosis is uncertain. Skin tags may be removed for cosmetic reasons by use of electrocautery or the scalpel.

NEVOCELLULAR NEVI AND SELECTED PIGMENTED LESIONS

Freckles (Ephelides)

Freckles, or ephelides, are small, red or light brown macules that are promoted by sun exposure and fade during the winter months. They are usually confined to the face, arms, and back. The number varies from a few spots on the face to hundreds of confluent macules on the face and arms (Fig. 112-13). They occur as an autosomal dominant trait and are most often found in individuals with fair complexions. The use of sunscreens prevents the appearance of new freckles and helps prevent the darkening of existing freckles that typically accompanies sun exposure.

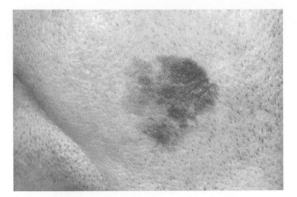

FIGURE 112-14. Lentigo.

Lentigo

Lentigo, or liver spot, occurs in sun-exposed areas of the face, arms, and hands. The lesions vary in size from 0.2 to 2 cm and become more numerous with advancing age (Fig. 112-14). Lentigo simplex is an acquired or congenital brown macule consisting of intraepidermal melanocytic hyperplasia, increased melanin production, and epidermal hyperplasia. There is no need to treat benign-appearing lentigo. A biopsy specimen should be taken from any lentigo that develops a highly irregular border, localized increase in pigmentation, or localized thickening to rule out lentigo maligna melanoma.

Melanocytic Nevi or Nevomelanocytic Nevus

Nevi, or moles, are benign tumors composed of nevus cells that are derived from melanocytes. The nevus cell differs from melanocytes in a number of ways. The nevus cell is larger, lacks dendrites, has more abundant cytoplasm, and contains coarse granules. Nevus cells aggregate in groups (nests) or proliferate in a nonnested pattern in the basal region at the dermal-epidermal junction.

INCIDENCE

Moles are so common that they appear on virtually every person (Fig. 112-15). They are present in 1% of newborns and increase in incidence throughout infancy and childhood, reaching a peak at puberty. Size and pigmentation may increase at puberty and during pregnancy. A few may continue to appear throughout life. Nevi may occur anywhere on the cutaneous surface. There is a strong correlation between sun exposure and the number of nevi. Acquired nevi on the buttock or female breast are unusual. A difference in frequency distribution of nevi according to sex is not clear, although most series show an equal

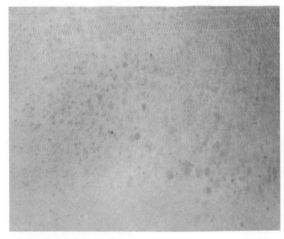

FIGURE 112-13. Freckles.

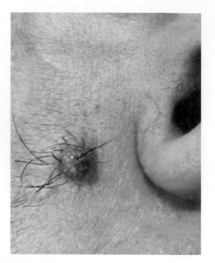

FIGURE 112-15. Melanocytic nevus (nevus cell nevus).

incidence in males and females. The prevalence of nevi varies according to race. There is evidence that the size and frequency distribution patterns of acquired nevi tend to aggregate in families.

ETIOLOGY AND PATHOGENESIS

There has been a continual debate as to whether nevomelanocytes in the dermis are derived from epidermal melanocytes and drop down from the epidermis to dermis or whether epidermal melanocytes and dermal nevomelanocytes have a dual origin. Demonstration of basement membrane around nevomelanocytes in the dermis based on routine and electron microscopy[51] provides evidence that nevomelanocytic nevi consist of a benign neoplastic proliferation of nevomelanocytes that may occupy epidermis, dermis, or both sites.

Overlying epidermal melanocytes usually produce visible pigmentation of nevomelanocytic nevi. In contrast to congenital nevi, pigmentation of acquired nevi occurs later. Epidermal melanocytes in acquired nevi may be stimulated to produce melanin and thus appear suddenly or become more prominent in response to sun exposure,[52] steroids, and other factors that are not well defined.[53]

Common acquired nevi may be papillomatous, dome shaped, pedunculated, or flat topped and are usually flesh colored, pink, or pigmented. Dark brown and black are unusual colors for common acquired nevi in lightly pigmented people. In contrast, dark pigmentation is usual for common acquired nevi in people who have darkly pigmented skin. Blue-gray, red, and white areas in a nevus are not typical features and ought to be viewed with suspicion. More elevated acquired nevi tend to be more lightly pigmented, and flatter acquired nevi tend to be more darkly pigmented. More elevated and less pigmented lesions tend to have a prominent intradermal nevus component, whereas flatter and darker lesions have a more prominent junctional melanocytic or nevomelanocytic component and a less prominent dermal component.

Multiple studies demonstrate that prominent numbers of nevi indicate increased melanoma risk. The risk is increased 10- to 60-fold with the differences related to both size and number of lesions.[54] Absence of direct site specificity of nevi and melanoma suggests that nevus proneness indicates a general melanoma risk[55] largely independent of hair and eye color and overall sun exposure.[56]

There may be relatively sudden changes in nevi that are unrelated to malignant transformation. These changes may be physiologic in nature, such as pregnancy, puberty, or systemic glucocorticoid administration. In these patients, all of the nevi in a given location should change together. Any single nevus that is noted to change independently should be cause for concern.

PATHOLOGY

Nevomelanocytes in the epidermis have nuclei similar in size to or larger than nuclei of melanocytes. They have abundant eosinophilic cytoplasm with dendritic extensions; the nuclei are pale staining.

Although the epidermis overlying nevomelanocytic nevi may be associated with a lentiginous pattern, a more common pattern is a normal or thickened epidermis.

The dermal component has an orderly progression from top to bottom; larger epithelioid cells above blend into a pattern of smaller cells in the deeper dermis. Features that suggest atypicality of nevomelanocytes in the dermis are nests or fascicles pushing and compressing collagen in the reticular dermis, lack of maturation with descent into the deep dermis, persistence of pigment production in the deep dermis, irregularity of size and shape of cells, and desmoplasia or fibrosis in the dermis. Nevomelanocytes in the dermis of typical acquired nevi have a monotonous similarity one to another within the same anatomic level and an overall symmetry of architecture from top to bottom and side to side.

It may be difficult to differentiate relatively flat nevomelanocytic nevi that are pale brown from solar lentigo, lentigo simplex, or café au lait macule. Oblique lighting will usually reveal some skin surface distortion in nevomelanocytic nevi. In addition, high magnification of nevi usually consists of speckles of darker pigment on a lighter background, whereas the patterns of café au lait macule and lentigo are uniform tan background.

TREATMENT

Most acquired nevi may be left alone. Biopsy should be performed of any pigmented lesion suspected of being malignant, or referral should be made for a second opinion. Suspicious lesions should be completely removed by excisional biopsy down to and including subcutaneous tissue. Leaving a partially excised nevus can lead to repigmentation or regrowth simulating neoplasia (pseudomelanoma).[57] Indications for excision of nevi include cosmetic removal, continual irritation, atypical appearance, atypical evolution, lesions at high risk for development of melanoma, large number of prominent nevi, and anatomic site.

Patients frequently request removal of nevi for cosmetic purposes. It is good practice to perform biopsy of all pigmented lesions; therefore, total removal by electrocautery should be avoided. Nevi exposed to continual physical irritation and that demonstrate periodic enlargement or discoloration are best excised to avoid confusion with neoplasia. Atypical appearance is reason enough to recommend excision. The most important gross features in a given lesion that may suggest an increased likelihood of atypical histologic features are dark pigmentation and haphazard distribution of pigmentation. Other atypical features, in combination with pigment pattern, include irregular borders and poor demarcation from surrounding skin, heterogeneous and symmetric topography, and large size (>5 mm). Absolute size and presence or absence of hair are usually less specific indicators of dysplasia or malignancy than are pigment pattern and overall architecture.

Nevi usually grow in proportion to growth of a given anatomic location. Any nevus undergoing independent growth may require excisional biopsy for definition. In general, a sudden and rapid change in color, size, or topography should be suggestive of atypical evolution if it occurs in an individual lesion.

There are well-defined and clinically recognizable melanocytic and nevomelanocytic lesions that appear to have a high risk for development of melanoma. Such lesions require either prophylactic excision or careful photographic follow-up indefinitely. High-risk lesions include lentigo maligna, congenital nevomelanocytic nevus, cellular blue nevus, nevus of Ota, nevus of Ito, spindle cell nevus, and dysplastic nevus. Increased melanoma risk is also indicated by a large number of prominent nevi, family history of melanoma, prior melanoma, and sun-induced freckles.

With regard to anatomic site, darkly pigmented nevi on acral or mucosal surfaces should be viewed with suspicion and evaluated.

Congenital Nevomelanocytic Nevus

Congenital nevomelanocytic nevi are nevomelanocytic nevi present at birth. They vary in size from a few millimeters to several centimeters, covering wide areas of the trunk, extremity, or face. Synonyms for congenital nevomelanocytic nevi include garment nevus, verrucous nevus, and giant hairy nevus. Not all pigmented lesions present at birth are congenital nevi; café au lait spots may also be present at birth.

HISTORICAL ASPECTS

In 1832, Aibert described a giant nevus. In 1861, Rokitansky described a patient with a giant congenital nevomelanocytic nevus and leptomeningeal hyperpigmentation. The malignant potential of giant congenital nevomelanocytic nevi was documented as early as 1879 by Jablokoff and Klein, and there were at least 53 instances of the disease reported by 1959.[58]

Baker reported staged excision of large congenital nevomelanocytic nevi in 1878. Tissue expansion techniques have revolutionized the management of extensive skin defects after surgical excision of giant congenital nevomelanocytic nevi.

EPIDEMIOLOGY

Most congenital nevomelanocytic nevi are small and singular; 2.5% of newborns have pigmented lesions,[59] but only 1% have a biopsy-confirmed nevomelanocytic nevus.[60,61]

CLINICAL DESCRIPTION

Congenital nevomelanocytic nevi are on average larger than acquired nevi. Nevi attaining a diameter of more than 1.5 cm are likely to be dysplastic, congenital, or malignant.

Except for size, overall appearance of congenital nevomelanocytic and acquired nevi is similar. Congenital nevomelanocytic nevi are usually round or oval; outlines are usually smooth, regular, and sharply demarcated. Some have coarse long hairs, whereas others are relatively hairless. Congenital nevomelanocytic nevi usually have a uniform pigmented pattern consisting of medium or dark brown speckles similar to acquired nevi.

There is a significant association between neurofibromatosis and giant congenital nevomelanocytic nevi. Large congenital nevomelanocytic nevi of the head may be associated with underlying cranial or spinal leptomeningeal melanocytosis. This phenomenon may be asymptomatic or give rise to communicating hydrocephalus, seizures, focal neurologic deficits, mental retardation, or even melanoma.[62-66] Symptomatic leptomeningeal melanocytosis carries a poor prognosis even in the absence of melanoma.

PATHOLOGY

Congenital nevomelanocytic nevi are characterized by the presence of nevomelanocytes in the epidermis as well as ordered theques of nevomelanocytes in the dermis as sheets, nests, cords, or single cells. Although histologic features are cited as being useful in distinguishing nevi as congenital or acquired, there are no known features that have demonstrated 100% specificity and 100% sensitivity for diagnosis.

TREATMENT

The treatment of large and small congenital nevomelanocytic nevi depends on the perceived risk of melanoma plus cosmetic and functional considerations. The most important consideration for treatment of congenital nevomelanocytic nevi relates to the perceived malignant potential. Melanoma may arise in large congenital nevomelanocytic nevi even in the first several years of life. Therefore, surgical excision should be considered as early as possible. Management of large congenital nevomelanocytic nevi must be individualized on a patient by patient basis. Tissue expansion is invaluable in repair of large wound defects. The treatment goal is to remove as much of the nevus as possible while preserving function and improving cosmetic appearance. Indications for surgical excision of large congenital nevomelanocytic nevi other than to prevent melanoma include chronic pruritus, ulceration, and infection.

All congenital nevomelanocytic nevi should be documented at birth. Suspicious changes in color, surface, or size require urgent evaluation. Atypical-appearing congenital nevomelanocytic nevi should be considered for immediate prophylactic excision because even small congenital nevomelanocytic nevi may give rise to melanoma during early childhood. All small congenital nevomelanocytic nevi should be evaluated for prophylactic excision before the age of 12 years, after which time the risk for melanoma rises sharply.

ASSOCIATION BETWEEN CONGENITAL NEVI AND MELANOMA

The risk for melanoma development is proportional to the size of the congenital nevus,[67] with evidence of increased risk in patients with congenital nevi that involve more than 5% of the body surface.[68] The lifetime risk for melanoma of patients with large congenital nevomelanocytic nevi has been estimated to be at least 6.3%. Melanoma may develop in large congenital nevomelanocytic nevi at any time, but the diagnosis of melanoma was made in the first 3 to 5 years of life in half of affected patients who ultimately developed melanoma in association with giant congenital nevomelanocytic nevi.[69-71] The prognosis for patients who develop melanoma in association with giant congenital nevomelanocytic nevi is poor.[62]

Malignant degeneration of large congenital nevomelanocytic nevi may be associated with the relatively sudden appearance of a dermal or subcutaneous nodule, dark pigmentation, itching, pain, bleeding, or ulceration. Detection of melanoma in association with giant congenital nevomelanocytic nevi may be impossible until a dermal nodule or metastatic disease appears. A causal relationship between established small congenital nevomelanocytic nevi and melanoma is more difficult to establish than for large congenital nevomelanocytic nevi.

Blue Nevus

CLINICAL DESCRIPTION

The common blue nevus occurs as a solitary, sharply circumscribed, blue-black papule (Fig. 112-16). This malformation consists of a group of melanocytes with long, thin surface projections in the middle and lower thirds of the dermis and in the subcutaneous fat. The brown pigment absorbs longer wavelengths of light and scatters blue light (Tyndall effect). The blue nevus appears in childhood and is most common on the extremities and dorsum of the hands. No tendency toward malignant transformation exists. A rare variant, the cellular blue nevus, is larger (usually more than 1 cm), nodular, and frequently located on the buttock. There are reported instances of malignant degeneration of these larger blue nevi into melanomas.[72]

EPIDEMIOLOGY

Blue nevi are present in fewer than 1 in 3000 newborns, 1% to 2% of white schoolchildren, and 0.5% to 4% of white adults. Most blue nevi are single, small, deep blue macules or papules and 1 to 2 mm in diameter.

Blue nevus is believed to represent an ectopic accumulation of melanin-producing melanocytes in the dermis during their migration from the neural crest to sites in the skin.

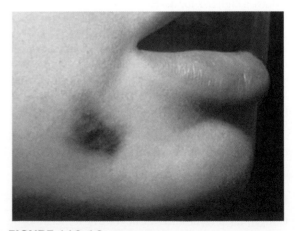

FIGURE 112-16. Blue nevus.

PATHOLOGY

In common blue nevus, dermal melanocytes appear as melanin-containing fibroblast-like cells grouped in irregular bundles admixed with melanin-containing macrophages associated with fibrous tissue in the reticular dermis. The epidermis in the common blue nevus appears normal.

TREATMENT

A common blue nevus that is stable for many years in an adult requires no therapy. The sudden appearance of a blue nodule, the expansion of a pre-existing blue nodule, a congenital blue nodule, or a relatively large blue nodule should be examined by biopsy.

Halo Nevus

CLINICAL DESCRIPTION AND PATHOLOGY

A halo nevus consists of an acquired zone of hypopigmentation surrounding a pigmented tumor. This phenomenon often indicates the onset of involution and subsequent regression of the central nevus. The depigmented halo is symmetric and round or oval with a sharply demarcated border. The halo of depigmentation is variable in size, usually a radial zone 0.5 to 5 cm from the central lesion (Fig. 112-17). Most halo nevi are located on the trunk; they never occur on palms or soles. Halos develop spontaneously, most commonly during adolescence. The number of halo nevi per person may be one or many; the frequency of multiple lesions is 25% to 50% of patients.[73] The halo lesion typically involutes during a period of months in the absence of clinical signs of inflam-

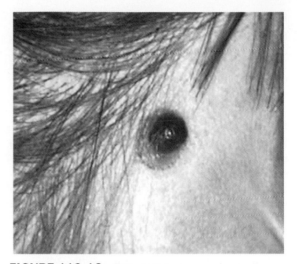

FIGURE 112-18. Spitz nevus.

mation. On histologic evaluation, a chronic lymphocytic infiltrate surrounds the nevus, which may represent an autoimmune phenomenon. There are no melanocytes in the halo area.

EPIDEMIOLOGY

The overall prevalence rate is 0.9%.[74] The disease develops in most patients before the age of 20 years. The most common condition associated with halo nevus is vitiligo, occurring in 18% to 26% of patients.[73] In a halo nevus, the central tumor may persist unchanged, become less pigmented with time, or flatten and totally disappear. Areas of depigmentation may persist unchanged for months or years or become repigmented totally.

TREATMENT

Benign-appearing nevi associated with halo depigmentation need not be removed. It is reasonable to recommend periodic examination of affected individuals for dysplastic nevus, vitiligo, and melanoma. Atypical-appearing lesions in halo nevi should be considered for biopsy.

Spindle Cell Nevus (Spitz Nevus)

CLINICAL DESCRIPTION

Spindle cell nevus usually arises in childhood as a pink or reddish brown, smooth or slightly scaly, firm papule with a predilection for the face, especially the cheeks (Fig. 112-18). Other terms for spindle cell nevus are Spitz nevus and benign juvenile melanoma. The term *melanoma* is used because of the similar appearance to melanoma clinically and histologically, although it usually follows a benign course.

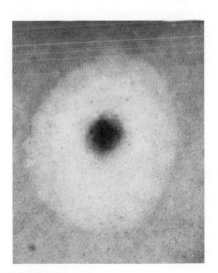

FIGURE 112-17. Halo nevus.

EPIDEMIOLOGY

Spindle cell nevi are not restricted to children, and there appears to be no sexual predilection. The frequency in the general population is unknown. Among nevi excised in children, 1% to 8% are interpreted as spindle cell nevi.[75]

PATHOLOGY

Histologic features and the frequent occurrence of dermal inflammation in spindle nevi may cause diagnostic confusion, but they can usually be differentiated from melanoma. Spindle cell nevi contain well-circumscribed nested melanocytic elements in the epidermis and dermis. The epidermis is usually hyperplastic. Edema in the epidermis and dermis is marked in most patients. Unlike in ordinary nevus and melanoma, nevomelanocytes in spindle cell nevus are large, often twice the size of epidermal basal keratinocytes.[76]

Features believed to distinguish spindle cell nevus from melanoma include presence of bizarre mononuclear and multinucleated giant cells, maturation of tumor cells with increasing depth, and absence of atypical mitoses. Favoring the diagnosis of melanoma are deep dermal invasion, intense melanin production in the dermis, atypical mitoses, and lack of maturation of nevomelanocytes with increasing tumor depth.

TREATMENT

Total excision is the treatment of choice for a spindle cell nevus because it is often indistinguishable from melanoma. Incompletely excised lesions may recur up to 15% of the time.[75]

Dysplastic Nevus (Atypical Mole)

Dysplastic nevi are acquired and have clinical features that are indistinguishable from those of malignant melanoma (Fig. 112-19). Dysplastic nevi are found on the skin of 90% of patients with hereditary melanomas. The lifetime risk for development of cutaneous melanoma among the white population in the United States is approximately 0.8% or 1 in 125. Dysplastic nevi in patients with no family history have a 6% risk for development of melanoma.[77] Those with a family history have a 15% risk. Dysplastic nevi are larger than common nevi. They have a mixture of colors, including tan, brown, pink, and black. The border is indistinct and often fades into the surrounding skin. The surface is complex and variable, with both macular and papular components. Dysplastic nevi are not present at birth but begin to appear in the mid-childhood years as typical common moles. The appearance changes at puberty, and newer lesions continue to appear well after the age of 40 years.[77]

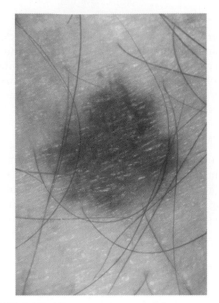

FIGURE 112-19. Dysplastic nevus.

The histologic features include architectural disorder with asymmetry, subepidermal fibroplasia, and lentiginous melanocytic hyperplasia. Melanocytic atypia may be present to a variable degree.

Because atypical moles are common and patients may have several, it is impractical and unnecessary to remove all atypical moles. Patients should have yearly total body photographs and examinations. Any lesion that changes should undergo excisional biopsy.

BOWEN DISEASE

Bowen disease, also known as squamous cell carcinoma in situ, is found most often on the lower limbs of women and on the scalp and ears of men.[78] Typical lesions are slightly elevated, red, scaly plaques with surface fissures and foci of pigmentation. The borders are well defined, and lesions closely resemble psoriasis, chronic eczema, carcinoma, seborrheic keratosis, and malignant melanoma (Fig. 112-20). The lesion grows slowly by lateral extension and may eventually invade the dermis, producing induration and ulceration.

Lesions are treated by excision.

ACTINIC KERATOSIS
Clinical Description and Epidemiology

Actinic keratoses are sun-induced premalignant lesions that increase with age. Years of sun exposure are required to induce sufficient damage to cause lesions. Actinic keratoses may undergo spontaneous remission

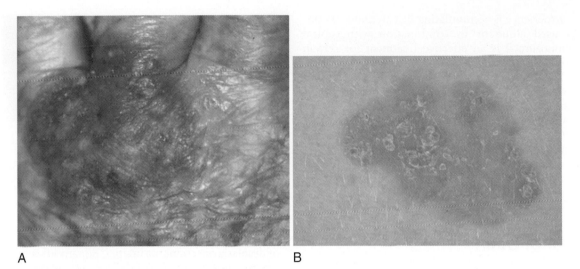

A   B

FIGURE 112-20. *A* and *B,* Bowenoid papulosis.

if sunlight exposure is reduced. Actinic keratoses begin as an area of increased vascularity with the skin surface becoming slightly rough. An adherent yellow crust forms that may cause bleeding on removal. Lesions vary in size from 3 to 6 mm. Induration and inflammation suggest degeneration into malignancy (Fig. 112-21).

After several years, a small percentage of lesions may degenerate into squamous cell carcinomas. A low yearly transformation rate for single lesions can translate into a substantial lifetime risk of transformation for patients with several actinic keratoses. Up to 60% of squamous cell carcinomas develop from actinic keratosis.[79] Squamous cell carcinomas that evolve from actinic keratosis are not aggressive but may eventually metastasize.[80] All patients with actinic keratosis should be examined carefully for basal cell carcinomas.

Pathology

On histologic evaluation, actinic keratoses consist of atypical squamous cells confined to the epidermis. Penetration through the dermal-epidermal junction and into the dermis indicates the development of a squamous cell carcinoma.

Treatment

Because actinic keratoses sometimes undergo spontaneous remission, definitive treatment may be delayed for patients with a few superficial lesions. Small lesions should be re-examined at a later date for spontaneous remission. Patients should make every effort to prevent further sun damage. Cryotherapy is the treatment of choice for most isolated, superficial actinic keratoses. Actinic keratosis resides in the epithelium. Cryotherapy with liquid nitrogen causes the separation of the epidermis and dermis, resulting in a highly specific, nonscarring method of therapy for superficial lesions. Patients with darker complexions may have hypopigmented areas after freezing, and treatment of multiple lesions on the faces of such patients may result in white-spotted faces.

Individual indurated lesions or those with thick crusts should be removed with minor surgical procedures. It is unnecessary to perform biopsy of lesions less than 0.5 cm. Larger lesions or those occurring about or on the vermilion border of the lips should be examined.

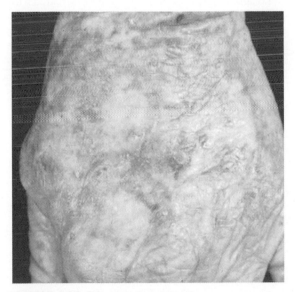

FIGURE 112-21. Actinic keratosis.

Experience is accumulating that tretinoin (Retin-A) used alone or in combination with topical 5-fluorouracil is an effective treatment for certain actinic keratoses.

Regular use of sunscreens prevents the development of solar keratoses.[81] Sunscreens that contain a combination of ingredients to block both the A and B spectra of ultraviolet light are most effective.

Glycolic acid is an alpha-hydroxy acid that is useful as a chemical peeling agent. Actinic keratoses involve epidermal hyperplasia and retention of stratum corneum. Alpha-hydroxy acids applied topically in high concentrations (30% to 70% glycolic acid) cause epidermolysis and elimination of keratosis.[82]

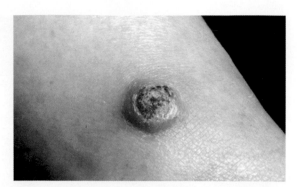

FIGURE 112-23. Keratoacanthoma.

LEUKOPLAKIA

Leukoplakia is a clinical term used to describe a range of nonspecific white lesions, from slightly raised, white, translucent areas to dense, white, opaque lesions, with or without ulceration on the vermilion border of the lips, oral mucosa, or vulva. It can be simply defined as a white patch on the mucosa that cannot be rubbed off. The most common sites of oral leukoplakia are the commissures and the buccal mucosa (Fig. 112-22). Smoking is the most common cause of oral lesions, but chronic irritation from carious teeth or misaligned dentures is also a cause. Leukoplakia is seen most commonly in people 50 to 70 years of age. Histologic changes range from mild scaling and epidermal thickening with minimal inflammation to varying degrees of dysplasia or carcinoma in situ.[83] Squamous cell carcinoma develops in 17% of all patients with leukoplakia.[84,85] Leukoplakia on the floor of the mouth and the ventral surface of the tongue is associated with the highest risk of cancer.[86] Degeneration to carcinoma takes 1 to 20 years. Clinically, the patches are white, slightly elevated, usually well-defined plaques that show little tendency to extend peripherally. The white color is due to increased epithelial water uptake. The differential diagnosis includes candidiasis, lichen planus, habitual cheek biting, white sponge nevus, and secondary syphilis. The clinical appearance of leukoplakia does not generally correlate well with the histopathologic change; therefore, biopsy should be performed for all patients to determine which lesions are precancerous.[87] Small lesions may be examined by biopsy and simply observed if the histologic appearance is benign. Plaques that exhibit atypical histologic features should be excised, destroyed with the laser,[88] or frozen with liquid nitrogen.[89]

Localized dysplastic oral leukoplakia is treated with surgical excision. Leukoplakia of the lip can be successfully treated with 5-fluorouracil. Many lesions clear spontaneously when cigarette or pipe smoking is stopped.[90] Long-term follow-up is desirable to check for recurrences.

KERATOACANTHOMA

Keratoacanthoma is a relatively common, benign epithelial tumor, possibly of viral origin,[91] that was previously considered to be a variant of squamous cell carcinoma.[92] It is a disease of the elderly (mean age, 64 years) with an annual incidence rate of 104 per 100,000. It is not associated with internal malignant disease.

Keratoacanthoma begins as a smooth, dome-shaped, red papule that resembles molluscum contagiosum. In a few weeks, the tumor may rapidly expand to 1 or 2 cm and develop a central keratin-filled crater that is frequently filled with crust (Fig. 112-23). The

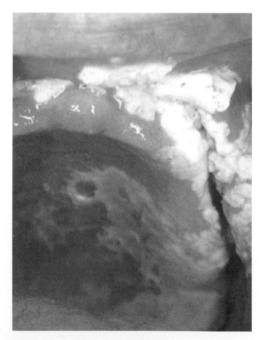

FIGURE 112-22. Leukoplakia.

growth retains its smooth surface, unlike a squamous cell carcinoma. Untreated, growth stops in approximately 6 weeks, and the tumor remains unchanged for an indefinite period. In the majority of patients, it then regresses slowly during 2 to 12 months and frequently heals with scarring. The limbs, particularly the hands and arms, are the most common site; the trunk is the second most common site, but keratoacanthoma may occur on any skin surface. On occasion, multiple keratoacanthomas appear, or a single lesion extends over several centimeters. These rare variants resist treatment and are unlikely to undergo spontaneous remission.

Keratoacanthomas can be difficult to distinguish histologically from squamous cell carcinoma. A keratoacanthoma is typically composed of well-differentiated squamous epithelium showing little pleomorphism and excessive keratin formation. Keratoacanthomas generally have a smooth, well-demarcated infiltration of tumor into the dermis with limited depth that does not extend beyond the level of the hair follicles. Adequate biopsy is essential to provide sufficient tissue for proper clinical and histopathologic confirmation.

Although keratoacanthomas may regress spontaneously, the tumor should be excised for histopathologic confirmation. Excision of the lesion can limit the resultant scar of spontaneous regression. Keratoacanthomas can recur.

SUMMARY

An overview of the essential elements a plastic surgeon needs for the accurate diagnosis and treatment of the patient with skin lesions has been provided. The key to successful management of benign skin tumors is a thorough understanding of their biologic behavior and natural history. This knowledge is based on accurate physical diagnosis and histologic evaluation.

REFERENCES

1. Lockshin NA: Flat facial warts treated with fluorouracil. Arch Dermatol 1979;115:929-930.
2. de Waard-van der Spek FB, Oranje AP, Lillieborg S, et al: Treatment of molluscum contagiosum using a lidocaine/prilocaine cream (EMLA) for analgesia. J Am Acad Dermatol 1990;23(pt 1):685-688.
3. Amstey MS, Trombetta GC: Laser therapy for vulvar molluscum contagiosum infection. Am J Obstet Gynecol 1985;153:800-801.
4. Garrett SJ, Robinson JK, Roenigk HH Jr: Trichloroacetic acid peel of molluscum contagiosum in immunocompromised patients. J Dermatol Surg Oncol 1992;18:855-858.
5. Rao BK, Freeman RG, Poulos EG, et al: The relationship between basal cell epithelioma and seborrheic keratosis. A study of 60 cases. J Dermatol Surg Oncol 1994;20:761-764.
6. Sloan JB, Jaworsky C: Clinical misdiagnosis of squamous cell carcinoma in situ as seborrheic keratosis. A prospective study. J Dermatol Surg Oncol 1993;19:413-416.
7. Maize JC, Snider RL: Nonmelanoma skin cancers in association with seborrheic keratoses. Clinicopathologic correlations. Dermatol Surg 1995;21:960-962.
8. Schwartz RA: Sign of Leser-Trélat. J Am Acad Dermatol 1996;35:88-95.
9. Acker DW, Helwig EB: Rhinophyma with carcinoma. Arch Dermatol 1967;95:250-254.
10. Plenk HP: Rhinophyma, associated with carcinoma, treated successfully with radiation. Plast Reconstr Surg 1995;95:559-562.
11. Broadbent NR, Cort DF: Squamous carcinoma in longstanding rhinophyma. Br J Plast Surg 1977;30:308-309.
12. Rees TD: Basal cell carcinoma in association with rhinophyma. Plast Reconstr Surg 1955;16:283-287.
13. Dolezal R, Schultz RC: Early treatment of rhinophyma—a neglected entity? Ann Plast Surg 1983;11:393-396.
14. Lloyd KM: Surgical correction of rhinophyma. Arch Dermatol 1990;126:721-723.
15. Har-El G, Shapshay SM, Bohigian RK, et al: The treatment of rhinophyma. "Cold" vs laser techniques. Arch Otolaryngol Head Neck Surg 1993;119:628-631.
16. Amedee RG, Routman MH: Methods and complications of rhinophyma excision. Laryngoscope 1987;97:1316-1318.
17. Odou BL, Odou ER: Rhinophyma. Am J Surg 1961;102:3-16.
18. Redett RJ, Manson PN, Goldberg N, et al: Methods and results of rhinophyma treatment. Plast Reconstr Surg 2001;107:1115-1123.
19. Brownstein MH, Arluk DJ: Proliferating trichilemmal cyst: a simulant of squamous cell carcinoma. Cancer 1981;48:1207-1214.
20. Leppard BJ, Sanderson KV: The natural history of trichilemmal cysts. Br J Dermatol 1976;94:379-390.
21. Weiss J, Heine M, Grimmel M, Jung EG: Malignant proliferating trichilemmal cyst. J Am Acad Dermatol 1995;32(pt 2):870-873.
22. Tsuji T, Kadoya A, Tanaka R, et al: Milia induced by corticosteroids. Arch Dermatol 1986;122:139-140.
23. Burton CS, Sawchuk WS: Premature sebaceous gland hyperplasia: successful treatment with isotretinoin. J Am Acad Dermatol 1985;12(pt 2):182-184.
24. Solomon LM, Esterly NB: Epidermal and other congenital organoid nevi. Curr Probl Pediatr 1975;6:1-56.
25. Submoke S, Piamphongsant T: Clinico-histopathological study of epidermal naevi. Australas J Dermatol 1983;24:130-136.
26. Rogers M, McCrossin I, Commens C: Epidermal nevi and the epidermal nevus syndrome. A review of 131 cases. J Am Acad Dermatol 1989;20:476-488.
27. Goldberg LH, Collins SA, Siegel DM: The epidermal nevus syndrome: case report and review. Pediatr Dermatol 1987;4:27-33.
28. Happle R: How many epidermal nevus syndromes exist? A clinicogenetic classification. J Am Acad Dermatol 1991;25:550-556.
29. Fox BJ, Lapins NA: Comparison of treatment modalities for epidermal nevus: a case report and review. J Dermatol Surg Oncol 1983;9:879-885.
30. Lee BJ, Mancini AJ, Renucci J, et al: Full-thickness surgical excision for the treatment of inflammatory linear verrucous epidermal nevus. Ann Plast Surg 2001;47:285-292.
31. Hohenleutner U, Landthaler M: Laser therapy of verrucous epidermal naevi. Clin Exp Dermatol 1993;18:124-127.
32. Alessi E, Sala F: Nevus sebaceus. A clinicopathologic study of its evolution. Am J Dermatopathol 1986;8:27-31.
33. Kang WH, Koh YJ, Chun SI: Nevus sebaceus syndrome associated with intracranial arteriovenous malformation. Int J Dermatol 1987;26:382-384.
34. Diven DG, Solomon AR, McNeely MC, Font RL: Nevus sebaceus associated with major ophthalmologic abnormalities. Arch Dermatol 1987;123:383-386.
35. Tarkhan II, Domingo J: Metastasizing eccrine porocarcinoma developing in a sebaceous nevus of Jadassohn. Report of a case. Arch Dermatol 1985;121:413-415.

36. Sahl WJ Jr: Familial nevus sebaceus of Jadassohn: occurrence in three generations. J Am Acad Dermatol 1990;22(pt 1):853-854.

37. Thomson HG: Common benign pediatric cutaneous tumors: timing and treatment. Clin Plast Surg 1990;17:49-64.

38. Chiaramonti A, Gilgor RS: Pilomatricomas associated with myotonic dystrophy. Arch Dermatol 1978;114:1363-1365.

39. Moehlenbeck FW: Pilomatrixoma (calcifying epithelioma). A statistical study. Arch Dermatol 1973;108:532-534.

40. Forbis R Jr, Helwig EB: Pilomatrixoma (calcifying epithelioma). Arch Dermatol 1961;83:606-618.

41. Stevenson TR, Swanson NA: Syringoma: removal by electrodesiccation and curettage. Ann Plast Surg 1985;15:151-154.

42. Moreno-Gonzalez J, Rios-Arizpe S: A modified technique for excision of syringomas. J Dermatol Surg Oncol 1989;15:796-798.

43. Maloney ME: An easy method for removal of syringoma. J Dermatol Surg Oncol 1982;8:973-975.

44. Okun MR, Ansell HB: Eccrine poroma. Report of three cases, two with an unusual location. Arch Dermatol 1963;88:561-566.

45. Coburn JG, Smith JL: Hidroacanthoma simplex; an assessment of a selected group of intraepidermal basal cell epitheliomata and of their malignant homologues. Br J Dermatol 1956;68:400-418.

46. Winkelmann RK, McLeod WA: The dermal duct tumor. Arch Dermatol 1966;94:50-55.

47. Freeman RG, Knox JM, Spiller WF: Eccrine poroma. Am J Clin Pathol 1961;36:444-450.

48. Baden HP: Cylindromatosis simulating neurofibromatosis. Nord Hyg Tidskr 1962;267:296-297.

49. Galadari E, Mehregan AH, Lee KC: Malignant transformation of eccrine tumors. J Cutan Pathol 1987;14:15-22.

50. Banik R, Lubach D: Skin tags: localization and frequencies according to sex and age. Dermatologica 1987;174:180-183.

51. Lea PJ, Pawlowski A: Human melanocytic naevi. I. Electron microscopy and 3-dimensional computer reconstruction of naevi and basement membrane zone from ultrathin serial sections. Acta Derm Venereol Suppl (Stockh) 1986;127:5-15.

52. Kopf AW, Lazar M, Bart RS, et al: Prevalence of nevocytic nevi on lateral and medial aspects of arms. J Dermatol Surg Oncol 1978;4:153-158.

53. Coskey RJ: Eruptive nevi [letter]. Arch Dermatol 1975;111:1658.

54. Grulich AE, Bataille V, Swerdlow AJ, et al: Naevi and pigmentary characteristics as risk factors for melanoma in a high-risk population: a case-control study in New South Wales, Australia. Int J Cancer 1996;67:485-491.

55. Weinstock MA, Colditz GA, Willett WC, et al: Moles and site-specific risk of nonfamilial cutaneous malignant melanoma in women. J Natl Cancer Inst 1989;81:948-952.

56. Swerdlow AJ, English J, MacKie RM, et al: Benign melanocytic naevi as a risk factor for malignant melanoma. Br Med J (Clin Res Ed) 1986;292:1555-1559.

57. Kornberg R, Ackerman AB: Pseudomelanoma: recurrent melanocytic nevus following partial surgical removal. Arch Dermatol 1975;111:1588-1590.

58. Russell JL, Reyes RG: Giant pigmented nevi. JAMA 1959;171:2083-2086.

59. Walton RG, Jacobs AH, Cox AJ: Pigmented lesions in newborn infants. Br J Dermatol 1976;95:389-396.

60. Clemmensen OJ, Kroon S: The histology of "congenital features" in early acquired melanocytic nevi. J Am Acad Dermatol 1988;19:742-746.

61. Alper J, Holmes LB, Mihm MC Jr: Birthmarks with serious medical significance: nevocellular nevi, sebaceous nevi, and multiple cafe au lait spots. J Pediatr 1979;95(pt 1):696-700.

62. Reed WB, Becker SW Sr, Becker SW Jr, Nickel WR: Giant pigmented nevi, melanoma, and leptomeningeal melanocytosis: a clinical and histopathological study. Arch Dermatol 1965;91:100-119.

63. DeDavid M, Orlow SJ, Provost N, et al: Neurocutaneous melanosis: clinical features of large congenital melanocytic nevi in patients with manifest central nervous system melanosis. J Am Acad Dermatol 1996;35:529-538.

64. Kudel TA, Bingham WT, Tubman DE: Computed tomographic findings of primary malignant leptomeningeal melanoma in neurocutaneous melanosis. AJR Am J Roentgenol 1979;133:950-951.

65. Hoffman HJ, Freeman A: Primary malignant leptomeningeal melanoma in association with giant hairy nevi. J Neurosurg 1967;26:62-71.

66. Kadonaga JN, Frieden IJ: Neurocutaneous melanosis: definition and review of the literature. J Am Acad Dermatol 1991;24(pt 1):747-755.

67. Marghoob AA, Schoenbach SP, Kopf AW, et al: Large congenital melanocytic nevi and the risk for the development of malignant melanoma. A prospective study. Arch Dermatol 1996;132:170-175.

68. Swerdlow AJ, English JS, Qiao Z: The risk of melanoma in patients with congenital nevi: a cohort study. J Am Acad Dermatol 1995;32:595-599.

69. Lanier VC Jr, Pickrell KL, Georgiade NG: Congenital giant nevi: clinical and pathological considerations. Plast Reconstr Surg 1976;58:48-54.

70. Hori Y, Nakayama J, Okamoto M, et al: Giant congenital nevus and malignant melanoma. J Invest Dermatol 1989;92(suppl):310S-314S.

71. Quaba AA, Wallace AF: The incidence of malignant melanoma (0 to 15 years of age) arising in "large" congenital nevocellular nevi. Plast Reconstr Surg 1986;78:174-181.

72. Rapini RP: Spitz nevus or melanoma? Semin Cutan Med Surg 1999;18:56-63.

73. Kopf AW, Morrill SD, Silberberg I: Broad spectrum of leukoderma acquisitum centrifugum. Arch Dermatol 1965;92:14-33, discussion 33-35.

74. Larsson PA, Liden S: Prevalence of skin diseases among adolescents 12-16 years of age. Acta Derm Venereol 1980;60:415-423.

75. Sagebiel RW, Chinn EK, Egbert BM: Pigmented spindle cell nevus. Clinical and histologic review of 90 cases. Am J Surg Pathol 1984;8:645-653.

76. Spitz S: Melanomas of childhood. 1948. CA Cancer J Clin 1991;41:40-51.

77. Halpern AC, Guerry D 4th, Elder DE, et al: Natural history of dysplastic nevi. J Am Acad Dermatol 1993;29:51-57.

78. Kossard S, Rosen R: Cutaneous Bowen's disease. An analysis of 1001 cases according to age, sex, and site. J Am Acad Dermatol 1992;27:406-410.

79. Marks R, Rennie G, Selwood TS: Malignant transformation of solar keratoses to squamous cell carcinoma. Lancet 1988;1:795-797.

80. Moller R, Reymann F, Hou-Jensen K: Metastases in dermatological patients with squamous cell carcinoma. Arch Dermatol 1979;115:703-705.

81. Thompson SC, Jolley D, Marks R: Reduction of solar keratoses by regular sunscreen use. N Engl J Med 1993;329:1147-1151.

82. Moy LS, Murad H, Moy RL: Glycolic acid peels for the treatment of wrinkles and photoaging. J Dermatol Surg Oncol 1993;19:243-246.

83. Zakrzewska JM, Lopes V, Speight P, Hopper C: Proliferative verrucous leukoplakia: a report of ten cases. Oral Surg Oral Med Oral Pathol Oral Radiol Endod 1996;82:396-401.

84. Silverman S Jr, Gorsky M, Lozada F: Oral leukoplakia and malignant transformation. A follow-up study of 257 patients. Cancer 1984;53:563-568.

85. Dorey JL, Blasberg B, Conklin RJ, Carmichael RP: Oral leuko-plakia. Current concepts in diagnosis, management, and malignant potential. Int J Dermatol 1984;23:638-642.
86. Schepman KP, van der Meij EH, Smeele LE, van der Waal I: Malignant transformation of oral leukoplakia: a follow-up study of a hospital-based population of 166 patients with oral leukoplakia from the Netherlands. Oral Oncol 1998;34:270-275.
87. Shklar GS: Oral leukoplakia. N Engl J Med 1986;315:1544-1546.
88. Horch HH, Gerlach KL: CO_2 laser treatment of oral dysplastic precancerous lesions: a preliminary report. Lasers Surg Med 1982;2:179-185.
89. Al-Drouby HA: Oral leukoplakia and cryotherapy. Br Dent J 1983;155:124-125.
90. Martin GC, Brown JP, Eifler CW, Houston GD: Oral leukoplakia status six weeks after cessation of smokeless tobacco use. J Am Dent Assoc 1999;130:945-954.
91. Magee KL, Rapini RP, Duvic M, Adler-Storthz K: Human papillomavirus associated with keratoacanthoma. Arch Dermatol 1989;125:1587-1589.
92. Schwartz RA: Keratoacanthoma. J Am Acad Dermatol 1994;30:1-19, quiz 20-22.

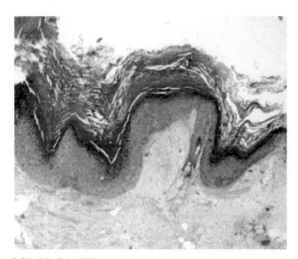

COLOR PLATE 112-1. Verruca vulgaris.

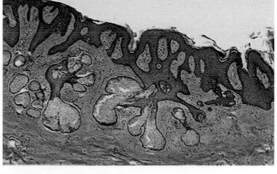

COLOR PLATE 112-2. Nevus sebaceus.

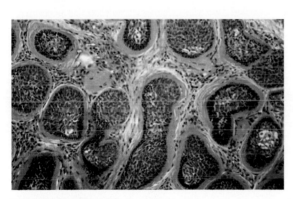

COLOR PLATE 112-3. Cylindroma.

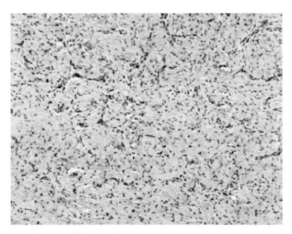

COLOR PLATE 112-4. Dermatofibroma.

CHAPTER 113

Malignant Tumors of the Skin

RONALD M. BARTON, MD

In the United States, there has been an overall decrease in the incidence of cancer and mortality rate since the early 1990s.[1] However, the incidence of malignant tumors of the skin has been steadily increasing. An estimate for the year 2003 reveals that 1,334,100 new instances of invasive cancer will be diagnosed in the United States.[2] The estimate also predicts that the lifetime probability of developing cancer is higher in men (43.5%) than in women (38.5%). New instances of skin cancer, excluding basal and squamous cell skin carcinoma, total 58,800 (32,300 in men, 26,500 in women). Of these newly diagnosed patients, 54,200 will have melanoma. In addition, more than 1 million patients will be diagnosed with basal cell carcinoma (BCC) or squamous cell carcinoma (SCC) in the United States. The exact number of people who develop BCCs and SCCs is not known because these cancers are not reported to registries. Therefore, all statistics related to BCCs and SCCs are estimates.

The American Cancer Society (*http://www.cancer.org*) and the Skin Cancer Foundation (*http://www.skincancer.org*) provide a great deal of statistical information about skin cancer. BCC and SCC primarily arise in white populations. When they are seen in pigmented persons, they are usually associated with unusual causes and anatomic sites. Men are about twice as likely to develop BCCs or SCCs as are women. The number of BCCs and SCCs is believed to be rising at a rate of 5% per year. Cancer of the skin (including melanoma and nonmelanoma skin cancer) is the most common, probably accounting for more than 50% of all cancers. Death is uncommon in patients with BCCs or SCCs (approximately 1000 to 2000 patients per year); however, it may occur among the elderly or in patients with compromised immune systems (e.g., transplant recipients).

The statistics for global cancer rates are similar. There are an estimated 8,000,000 new patients with cancer evenly divided between developing and developed countries.[3] The estimated rate of growth of patients newly diagnosed with skin cancer is 2.1% per year, which outstrips the growth rate of the world population at 1.7% per year. Worldwide rates of melanoma are highest in Australia and New Zealand with an age-standardized incidence rate of 27.9 per 100,000 men and 25 per 100,000 women; in North America, it is 10.9 per 100,000 men and 7.7 per 100,000 women. Australia and New Zealand also have the best survival rates (85%), which has been attributed to the educational campaigns resulting in early diagnosis.

Developing countries have a lower survival rate of approximately 40% thought to be due to lack of early diagnosis and access to therapy and the incidence of acral melanoma with a worse prognosis. Globally, in the year 2000, it was expected that approximately 100,000 new patients would be diagnosed with melanoma, resulting in approximately 33,000 deaths. The overall incidence of BCC to SCC is approximately three to one.[3]

The following discussion primarily focuses on the most common malignant skin cancers, BCC and SCC and their premalignant precursors. The final section provides an overview of the less common malignant skin tumors that tend to lack specific etiologic factors, are not easily diagnosed on clinical grounds, and often have an unpredictable prognosis. A thorough discussion of the diagnosis and treatment of malignant melanoma is contained elsewhere in this volume (see Chapter 114).

ETIOLOGIC FACTORS

Ultraviolet Radiation

The carcinogenic effect of sunlight is well known. An interval of several years to decades between the exposure and the tumor expression is noted. The effects of radiation appear to be on cellular DNA. This damage is potentiated by other factors that block the normal DNA repair mechanisms. Authors have found that more than 90% of SCCs and more than 50% of BCCs have mutations in the *p53* tumor suppressor gene. Brash et al[4] propose that sunlight acts as both a tumor initiator and a promoter. Because of a *p53* mutation, cells can no longer correct DNA damage, which would ordinarily lead to apoptosis of precancerous cells.

Ultraviolet (UV) radiation has long been known to have a causative effect related to melanoma as well as to squamous cell and basal cell skin cancers. The sun emits two types of UV light that can reach the earth's surface, UVA (320 to 400 nm) and UVB (290 to 320 nm). UVB radiation is thought to be the primary although not the only etiologic agent in the development of nonmelanoma skin cancer.[5] There is evidence, however, that UVA light also contributes to the carcinogenic potential of UV radiation.[6,7] Most UVB light is absorbed by the stratospheric ozone layer, although some does reach the surface of the earth. UVA radiation is not absorbed by the stratospheric ozone layer; however, some of the more energetic wavelengths of UVA light (UVA II, 320 to 340 nm) are partly absorbed by ozone. The quantity of UV light striking the earth's surface depends on several factors including atmospheric and environmental conditions, time of day, season, latitude, and continued ozone layer depletion.[8] It has been estimated that the ozone layer over the United States decreased by 4.8% and 7.4% during the period 1979 to 1992.[9]

Basal cell and squamous cell skin cancers are primarily diseases of white populations. In 1971, Urbach[10] reported that the susceptibility of skin cancer varied with the melanocyte content of the skin. Epstein[11] subsequently reported that the amount of melanin the skin contains is an important determinant of susceptibility to UV radiation. Those persons with more melanin have more protection.

Pathak and Fitzpatrick[12] classified skin into multiple types according to the sensitivity to UV light and melanin content. This classification ranges from type I, in which the skin is white and reactions to the first sun exposure are always burning without tanning, to type VI, in which the skin is black and does not burn but tans easily. Asian, Indian, and Hispanic persons or light-skinned persons of African descent are classified as type V, in which the skin is dark brown and very rarely burns but tans easily. The types were further modified by Cesarini in 1977 (Table 113-1).[13,14]

Exposure to Radiation

It has been known for nearly a century that skin cancer could be induced by radiation. The first such episode

TABLE 113-1 ✦ CLASSIFICATION OF PHOTOTYPES

Hair Color	Complexion	Freckles	Sunburn	Tan	Phototype
White	Albino	No	Constant	No	0
Red	"Creamy"	Numerous	Constant	No	I
Blond	Light	Numerous	Constant	Slight tan	II
Blond	Light	Some	Frequent	Light/dark	IIIa
Chestnut	Medium	Some	Frequent	Light/dark	IIIb
Brown	Medium	No	Rare	Dark	IV
Brown	Medium	No	Exceptional	Very dark	V
Black	Black	No	No	Black	VI

From Malvy J, Guinot C, Preziosis P, et al.: Epidemiologic determinants of skin photoaging: baseline data of the SU.VI.MAX. cohort. J Am Acad Dermatol 2000;42:47. Copyright 2000, with permission from The American Academy of Dermatology, Inc.

was reported in a radiology technician.[15] Persons exposed to radiation in the workplace (e.g., radiologists and pilots) and those treated in the past with radiation for benign conditions were predisposed to later development of both BCCs and SCCs.[16] Workplace monitoring of radiation levels and recognition of the potentially dangerous practice of using radiation for benign conditions have had a limited effect on this co-carcinogen.

Immune Response

The immune system has a great effect on the development and progression of skin cancer. It has been reported that UV radiation-induced skin cancers in mice incite a response from the immune system to these highly antigenic tumors and that the immune response is capable of controlling the growth of these malignant neoplasms.[17,18] However, there has yet to be a direct extrapolation from the murine model to humans.

It has been demonstrated that Langerhans cells are able to recognize and present antigens to T lymphocytes. Chronic UV exposure reduces the number and the function of Langerhans cells during the initial exposure.[19] Soluble mediators liberated into the circulation by keratinocytes after UV irradiation have the potential to increase and decrease immune functions. The most important host defense mechanism against skin cancer is cell-mediated immunity. Tumor growth is reduced or prevented by natural killer cells and T cells. The infiltrate surrounding skin tumors contains large numbers of T cells that can produce interferon and interleukin-2.[18]

Cytokines are soluble factors that act in multiple ways, including up-regulation and down-regulation of other immune functions. They also influence Langerhans cells by promoting their translocation from skin to lymph nodes after contact with an allergen. These cytokines are principally interleukin-12 and interleukin-15. Cytokines may have a direct effect on immune cells or an indirect effect by increasing other factors that suppress immunity.[18] If anti-inflammatory agents are used or the release of prostaglandin E_2 is prevented, the UV-induced immune suppression is blocked.[20,21]

UV radiation has at least two effects in skin tumor generation—it causes genetic alterations within cells, and it inhibits the immune response. UV radiation has immunosuppressive effects caused by cross-links between adjacent pyrimidines and DNA molecules. Persons with xeroderma pigmentosum have a genetic inability to repair the damaged DNA (see section entitled "Xeroderma Pigmentosum"). DNA may be damaged in other ways, such as breaks in the double strand, psoralen adducts, and cross-links.[18]

The use of immunosuppressive drugs, such as those used in solid organ transplantation, has been shown to increase the appearance and growth of BCC and SCC. Patients who have received an organ transplantation have a 50- to 100-fold increase in the incidence of skin cancer.[22] The biologic behavior of tumors in these patients appears to be more aggressive.[23]

Human immunodeficiency virus (HIV) has been associated with increased incidence of skin cancers, Kaposi sarcoma being the most notable. However, both SCC and BCC have a higher occurrence in patients with HIV infection along with increased morbidity and mortality.[24] Franceschi et al[25] reported that although the incidence of nonmelanoma skin cancer is significantly increased in patients with HIV infection, it is lower than the rate in transplant recipients.

Chronic Wounds and Scars

The development of carcinoma in chronic wounds most commonly occurs after burns, but it may occur after any open wound has failed to heal for many years. In 1828, Jean-Nicolas Marjolin characterized the malignant degeneration of chronic ulcers.[26] SCCs are the most common forms of cancer found in scars (Fig. 113-1).[27] SCCs found in scars have a greater tendency to metastasize than do SCCs resulting from sun exposure. Although most scar malignant neoplasms are SCCs, a BCC will occasionally form in scars. Malignant transformation of scars into BCC is rare compared with the more common transformation to SCC.[28]

The latent period between the occurrence of the wound and development of cancer ranges from 20 to 40 years.[27] One series reported the mean development time between initial wound formation and development of carcinoma to be 26 years in a series of 10 patients.[29] Another series of 19 patients with Marjolin ulcers reported that burn scars accounted for 52% of the carcinomas; chronic fistula and osteomyelitis accounted for 32%.[30] The mean latent period was 31.5 years. At the time of diagnosis, 32% had metastasized. A local recurrence that averaged 8.8 months from the time of initial surgery developed in 25% of the patients treated with surgical procedures.

Chronic sinus tracks also have the potential for development of SCC. When sinus tracks are associated with osteomyelitis, the rate of metastasis has been noted to be 20%.[30]

Chemicals

Polycyclic aromatic hydrocarbons are organic compounds consisting of three or more aromatic rings that contain only carbon and hydrogen and share a pair of carbon atoms.[31] One such compound is creosote, which is used extensively as a wood preservative, usually by high-pressure impregnation of lumber, and as a constituent of fuel oil, lubricant for die molds, and pitch for roofing. Creosote contains more than 300

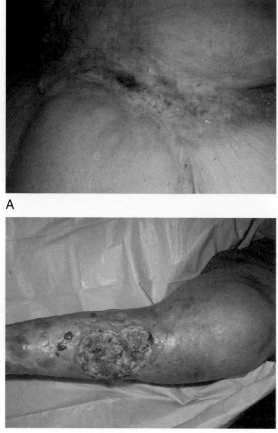

FIGURE 113-1. *A,* Marjolin ulcer in a burn scar. *B,* Marjolin ulcer (invasive SCC) of the left lower leg in 40-year-old burn scar.

different compounds, the major components of which are polycyclic aromatic hydrocarbons, phenols, cresols, xylenols, and pyridines. Occupational creosote exposure is a risk for squamous papilloma and carcinoma of the skin.[31] As early as 1775, Sir Percival Pott found a high incidence of scrotal cancer in chimney sweeps.[32] Polycyclic aromatic hydrocarbons were found to be some of the active ingredients in, among other things, the soot in the environment of the chimney sweeps. Polycyclic aromatic hydrocarbons are also present in a variety of other tars, oils, and waxes.

Dermal photocarcinogenicity (the process by which skin tumors are induced by exposure to UV radiation) is believed to be enhanced by certain substances. Such substances are considered to act as photocarcinogens.[33] The compound 8-methoxypsoralen, used in psoralen-ultraviolet A (PUVA) therapy, has been shown to be a photocarcinogen in animal models and is classified as a known human carcinogen.[34,35] PUVA is often used in the treatment of psoriasis. An increase in the incidence of SCC in patients treated with PUVA

has been reported.[34] Patients undergoing PUVA treatment should be monitored carefully for potential adverse effects.

Animal and human evidence during the past 15 to 20 years suggests that formaldehyde may be carcinogenic.[36] SCCs of the nasal epithelium were induced in rats and mice exposed for prolonged periods (up to 2 years).[36] Malignant melanoma of the nasal mucosa has also been reported in three persons occupationally exposed to formaldehyde; however, the International Agency for Research on Cancer found sufficient evidence in animals, but not in humans, for the carcinogenicity of formaldehyde.[37]

PREVENTION

The primary prevention strategy against skin cancer consists of reducing one's exposure to the sun. Protective clothing and the use of sunscreen are important factors in the prevention of skin cancer (Table 113-2). The American Academy of Dermatology and Centers for Disease Control and Prevention Conference[38] recommends the following:

- Limit exposure to UV radiation, especially between 10 AM and 4 PM.
- Wear protective clothing and sunglasses.
- Use sunscreens (SPF 15 or higher) including SPF lip balms.
- Avoid artificial tanning devices.
- For children younger than 6 months, use hats, clothing, and shading rather than sunscreen.
- Encourage children to practice the shadow rule: seek shade when your shadow is shorter than you are tall. Provision of shady areas and preservation of the ozone layer should contribute to primary prevention of skin cancer.

Other types of prevention include chemoprevention and diet. Secondary prevention consists of early detection of skin cancer through self-examination and public education.

Sunscreen

UV radiation is by far the leading cause of skin cancer. Sunscreens may be applied topically and offer some measure of protection by a variety of methods, such as absorption, reflection, and scattering. Sunscreens are given a numerical rating known as a sun protection factor (SPF), which measures the amount of UVB radiation causing minimal erythema. The SPF number is a ratio of the minimal erythema dose of radiation for sunscreen-protected skin to that for unprotected skin. There is some question as to whether there is a strictly mathematical relationship between the SPF number assigned to any compound and the actual protection that it affords. When sunscreen is used, it

TABLE 113-2 ✦ ACTIVE INGREDIENTS IN SIX COMMON SUNSCREENS

Sunscreen	Chemical Agent	Physical Agent
A	Mexoryl SX 3.3% 4-Methylbenzylidene camphor 5.0% Parsol 1789 (butylmethoxy-dibenzoylmethane) 3.5%	Titanium dioxide 4.1%
B	Octyl methoxycinnamate 7.5% Octyl salicylate 5.0%	Titanium dioxide
C	Homosalate 8.0% Ethythexyl p-methoxycinnamate 7.5% Oxybenzone 6.0% Octyl salicylate 5.0%	
D	Parsol 1789 (butylmethoxy-dibenzoylmethane) 3.0% Octyl methoxycinnamate 7.5% Octyl salicylate 5.0% Oxybenzone 3.0%	
E	—	Titanium dioxide 9.6% Zinc oxide 1.5%
F	—	Titanium dioxide 12.0%

From Bissonnette R, Allas S, Moyal D, Provost N: Comparison of UVA protection afforded by high sun protection factor sunscreens. J Am Acad Dermatol 2000;43:1036-1038. Copyright 2000, with permission from The American Academy of Dermatology, Inc.

is important to apply 2 mg/cm^2.[39] In addition to application of the correct amount, it should be replenished if the skin is cleaned or washed.

Mutations in the *p53* tumor suppressor gene may contribute to the development of human skin cancer. These mutations have been found in actinic keratoses, leading some authors to conclude that the mutations arise early in the progression from sun-damaged skin to cancer. A study by Ananthaswamy et al[40] showed that these *p53* mutations could be detected months before the appearance of skin tumors. The application of sunscreens with SPF 15 before the UV radiation treatment resulted in an 88% to 92% reduction in the number of *p53* mutations.

Sunscreens may be effective in skin cancer reduction. However, in the murine model, sunscreens have been shown to reduce the erythema of sunburn. They are less effective in reducing the decrease in immune function due to UV irradiation.[41] This observation may result in a false sense of security among some sunscreen users. Because sunscreens reduce the erythema of sunburn, people may tend to believe they are also being protected from the carcinogenic potential of UV irradiation.

Chemoprevention

Green tea contains polyphenolic antioxidants that may reduce the carcinogenesis of UV irradiation and prevent UV-induced immune suppression.[42,43] Extracts of the aloe plant appear to prevent immunosuppressive cytokine release from skin after UV irradiation in a murine model.[44]

Retinoids can modulate differentiation and carcinogenesis in vitro and in vivo and may be considered useful as chemopreventive agents in skin cancer. The mechanisms by which these effects occur are incompletely understood but probably involve retinoid binding to nuclear receptors, leading to gene expression for cytodifferentiation and growth regulation. Vitamin A has been evaluated in patients with a history of multiple actinic keratoses that have not advanced to skin cancers. Pharmacologic doses of vitamin A were found to protect these patients from subsequent SCCs but did not prevent BCCs. Vitamin A and isotretinoin have been evaluated as preventive agents in patients with a history of multiple skin cancers. Unfortunately, neither vitamin A nor isotretinoin prevented the development of new skin cancers. Therefore, it appears that retinoids can alter skin cancer progression, but only in the relatively early stages.[45]

Another promising use of retinoids as a chemopreventive agent is in patients with diseases associated with multiple cutaneous malignant neoplasms. High-dose isotretinoin is effective in the prevention of additional primary tumors in patients with SCC of the aerodigestive tract and in patients with xeroderma pigmentosum or nevoid BCC syndrome. Relapses are common after therapy is discontinued. Systemically administered retinoids have produced some remissions in SCC and BCC, but the results are incomplete and of short duration. In general, the response of established tumors to retinoids has been disappointing. Future directions for retinoid therapy include trials with new synthetic retinoids with receptor specificity to enhance efficacy against cutaneous tumors.[45]

Diet

The question of whether dietary fat intake can influence the development of skin cancer has been investigated. In a 2-year clinical trial, those who adopted a diet consisting of 20% total calorie intake as fat had a significantly lower number of new actinic keratoses as well as a lower incidence of nonmelanotic skin cancer.[46]

PREMALIGNANT LESIONS

Actinic Keratoses

Actinic keratoses are precancerous lesions developing on sun-exposed skin areas as a result of excessive exposure to sunlight. Approximately 16% of actinic keratoses will become invasive SCC, but no reliable method exists to determine which actinic keratosis will progress to invasive SCC.[47] Actinic keratosis is a collection of neoplastic keratinocytes confined to the epidermis. When these cells extend to involve the papillary or reticular dermis, they are classified as SCC.[48] The transformation into neoplasia occurs as a mutation in the *p53* gene. Thus, actinic keratoses and SCC are different points along the continuum of cell morphology.

In a review of 1011 SCCs, Guenthner et al[49] found that nearly 100% of lesions on sun-damaged skin contained SCC in situ at the periphery or within the confines of the SCC. The authors reported that the malignant changes began in single layers of the lower epidermis and then evolved into the dermis. Further evidence that actinic keratosis and SCC are close in the continuum was shown by histologic studies in which 165 instances of cutaneous SCC were reviewed for concomitant actinic keratosis. Actinic keratosis was found in 82.4% of the specimens. Of this group, 26.7% had superficial SCC arising within an actinic keratosis. The authors concluded that there is a strong correlation between these two lesions and that early aggressive treatment for actinic keratosis is warranted because of the substantial number of these lesions that will progress to SCC.[50]

Actinic keratoses present as a slightly reddened, scaly, rough lesion that can vary in size from a few millimeters to a centimeter or more. Some lesions may produce so much keratin that a cutaneous "horn" develops (Color Plate 113-1A). They are often indistinguishable from SCC without performance of a biopsy (Fig. 113-2). There is often a gradual transition from the lesion into normal surrounding skin without sharp delineation between the lesion and surrounding skin.

The measurement of matrix metalloproteinase (MMP-1) expression may help differentiate actinic keratosis and SCC. Tsukifuji et al[51] have speculated that MMP-1 expression could be an early event in the

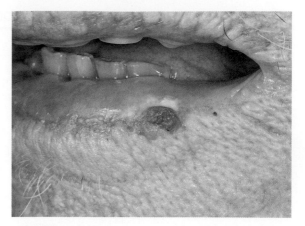

FIGURE 113-2. Actinic keratosis. The type and depth of this lesion are difficult to judge by physical examination alone. (From Habif TP: Clinical Dermatology, 4th ed. Philadelphia, Mosby, 2004.)

development of SCC and that actinic keratoses demonstrating MMP-1 messenger RNA may have an increased chance of progression to SCC. The presence of actinic keratosis at the margin of SCC does not predict the risk of metastasis. Dinehart et al[52] reviewed lesions in 22 patients with metastatic SCC and found actinic keratosis in 44% of the specimens. They concluded that actinic keratosis is not useful in predicting the metastatic behavior of these lesions and that tumor thickness and depth of invasion are more prognostic of the behavior of SCC.

There are several histologic variances of actinic keratosis, including hypertrophic, atrophic, bowenoid, and lichenoid (Color Plate 113-1B and C).[53] Actinic keratoses may also be pigmented (Fig. 113-3) and potentially lead to confusion in diagnosis between pigmented BCCs and melanoma. Histopathologic criteria have been used to distinguish actinic keratosis from BCC; however, both lesions have downwardly budding dysplastic keratinocytes.[54]

Actinic keratoses should be treated. A common treatment for single or multiple actinic keratoses is the topical application of 5-fluorouracil (5-FU), which is available in either 2% or 5% solution. This has proved to be an effective treatment for actinic keratoses, and it may also be useful for superficial early BCCs. Careful follow-up is mandatory, and any lesion that is not effectively treated with 5-FU should be surgically excised or irradiated.[55]

Although actinic keratoses are generally characterized as premalignant lesions, there is considerable evidence that this lesion is the earliest clinically recognizable manifestation of SCC.[56,57] In addition, there is some evidence that actinic keratosis can progress to other tumor types, such as sebaceous carcinoma.[58]

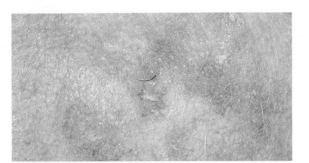

FIGURE 113-3. Pigmented actinic keratosis. (From Habif TP: Clinical Dermatology, 4th ed. Philadelphia, Mosby, 2004.)

Leukoplakia

The word *leukoplakia* is derived from the Greek meaning "white patch." These lesions may occur on either the oral or vulvar mucosa. Leukoplakia is a clinical description, but it carries the implication that persistent lesions should be examined histologically. They often occur in the setting of chronic irritation from use of tobacco or mechanical irritation by dentures (Color Plate 113-2). Analysis of these lesions shows that some react to papillomavirus antibodies.[59] On examination, approximately 80% of the oral leukoplakia lesions are benign; 17% show in situ anaplasia, and 3% show infiltrating SCC.[60] Leukoplakia should be differentiated from erythroplakia of the oral mucosa, which demonstrates in situ anaplasia in approximately half of the patients observed and invasive carcinoma in the other half.[60]

When leukoplakia develops into SCC of the oral mucosa, it has a greater tendency to metastasize than does SCC that develops from a solar keratosis of the skin.[61] The effect of cessation of smoking and chewing betel nuts was examined by Shiu et al.[62] The study examined 435 patients in a leukoplakia cohort. They found 60 oral carcinomas. Using a survival model, they determined the relevant risk factors and stated that cessation of smoking could reduce the incidence of leukoplakias by 36%, whereas the cessation of chewing betel nuts could prevent 62% of leukoplakias and 26% of malignant transformations.

Treatment of oral leukoplakia has been examined by Saito et al,[63] who studied 142 patients with oral leukoplakia; some did not receive any treatment, whereas others received surgical excision, cryosurgery, or cryosurgery and surgical excision. The authors concluded that surgical excision of oral leukoplakia may reduce the risk of subsequent development of carcinoma. Lenz et al[64] studied 11 malignant tumors and 16 premalignant lesions (leukoplakias) by fluorescence in situ hybridization to look for alterations in certain chromosomes. They found an increasing number of chromosome aberrations as they progressed from simple leukoplakias to dysplastic leukoplakias and finally to malignant tumors. They postulated that fluorescence in situ hybridization analysis would be a useful adjunct in the characterization of the malignant potential of leukoplakias.

Xeroderma Pigmentosum

Xeroderma pigmentosum is a genetic disorder in which individuals are unable to repair the DNA damage done by UV irradiation.[65,66] The hallmark of xeroderma pigmentosum, which is autosomal recessive, is extreme photosensitivity of the skin and eyes with premature cutaneous aging and a 1000-fold increased frequency of cutaneous BCCs, SCCs, and melanomas, especially in sun-exposed areas (Color Plate 113-3). In the United States, 1 in 250,000 live births are affected by xeroderma pigmentosum.[67]

The diagnosis of xeroderma pigmentosum is often based on clinical findings, but other tests are warranted in patients who have mild symptoms of xeroderma pigmentosum or who have chronic sun exposure without the disease. Photo testing is one modality that can be used. Traditionally, UVB is the waveband thought to cause most of the damage in xeroderma pigmentosum. However, one report indicates that in some patients, despite the diagnosis of xeroderma pigmentosum, no abnormal erythema responses are present.[68] One patient showed severe photosensitivity from 330 to 400 nm but normal UVB response. The conclusion was that erythemal responses in xeroderma pigmentosum are highly variable and therefore not always a reliable screening test.

Cell fusion analysis has identified seven xeroderma pigmentosum complementation groups (A through G) among patients with nucleotide excision repair-deficient xeroderma pigmentosum. In addition, there is a nucleotide excision repair-proficient form of xeroderma pigmentosum, the XP variant (XP-V).[69] Xeroderma pigmentosum is one of a family of diseases collectively termed the chromosome breakage syndromes or the DNA repair disorders. This group includes such diseases as Fanconi anemia, ataxia-telangiectasia, Bloom syndrome, Cockayne syndrome, and trichothiodystrophy. The common feature is the inability to repair certain types of DNA.[70] Patients affected with xeroderma pigmentosum may produce a wide variety of tumors including melanoma and sarcomas in the subcutaneous tissue. Internal malignant neoplasms are reported to have an incidence 10 to 20 times greater than in nonaffected individuals.[71]

The prevention of initial lesions in patients with xeroderma pigmentosum involves avoidance of UV light; however, by the time many children are diagnosed, they have already received significant sun exposure. Medical treatments for lesions include 5-

FU and retinoic acid.[72] Enzymes such as T4 endonuclease V have shown some promise. Because affected individuals have a genetic defect in DNA repair, an attempt has been made to lower the development rate of cancer by the topical application of T4 endonuclease V in liposomes.[73] This enzyme increases the rate of repair of sunlight-induced DNA damage in human cells. The results revealed that the treated group had an annualized rate of new actinic keratosis of 8.2%, whereas those in the placebo group had a rate of 25.9%. In addition, BCC had an annualized rate of new lesions of 3.8% in the treatment group and 5.4% in the placebo group.

The mainstay of treatment remains surgical excision of lesions, and an attempt should be made to excise as many of the lesions as possible at an early stage. Unfortunately, in spite of treatment, the longevity of these patients is not great, and many succumb to their disease by the age of 20 years.

Keratoacanthoma

Keratoacanthoma was originally described by Hutchinson[74] in 1889. It is a rapidly growing tumor with a predilection for sun-exposed areas of light-skinned individuals. The period of rapid growth usually lasts 4 to 8 weeks. Historically, keratoacanthoma has been considered a benign neoplasm (a pseudomalignancy) with the potential for spontaneous involution, usually within 4 to 6 months.[75] However, because of the recognized malignant potential of keratoacanthoma, it is often termed pseudobenignity or keratocarcinoma.[76,77]

Clinically, keratoacanthoma is usually a solitary tumor but may be multifocal, including a generalized eruptive form. It is a raised lesion often described as bud or dome shaped (Fig. 113-4). Keratoacanthoma is histologically similar to SCC, and Schwartz[75] stated that there is no sufficiently sensitive and specific criterion to distinguish keratoacanthoma from

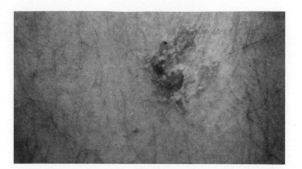

FIGURE 113-5. Bowen disease (carcinoma in situ), an asymptomatic lesion on thigh. No history of injury existed. Biopsy confirmed diagnosis. (From Davis JH, ed: Clinical Surgery. St. Louis, CV Mosby, 1987.)

SCC. Strieth et al[78] stated further that there is no immunohistochemical means of differentiating keratoacanthoma and SCC. Classically, keratoacanthomas are symmetric with a keratin plug, but this is not a universal finding and cannot be completely relied on for a definitive diagnosis.

Keratoacanthomas are thought to be derived from hair follicles, which helps explain the keratin plug found in many lesions. The pathogenesis has been linked to UV irradiation, trauma, chemicals, viral infections, and immunosuppression.[79] There is also a genetic predisposition in the Ferguson Smith type of multiple eruptive keratoacanthomas.[80] Persons with multiple keratoacanthomas or those with sebaceous differentiation should be evaluated for Muir-Torre syndrome because there is an association with visceral malignant neoplasms.[75]

Treatment of keratoacanthoma is largely surgical, but whether traditional excision or Mohs fresh tissue technique, laser ablation, or desiccation-curettage is used, the best approach is to consider keratoacanthoma a type of SCC and achieve total removal with careful follow-up. If an incisional biopsy is performed, it is best to include a margin of normal skin at the periphery as well as the central portion of the tumor. Total excision is preferred for cosmetic reasons because spontaneous regression will often leave a depressed scar.[61] Keratoacanthomas rarely metastasize. In a study of 40 patients with keratoacanthoma with perineural invasion, Godbolt et al[81] found no metastatic disease.

Bowen Disease

Bowen disease is considered SCC in situ. It presents as an erythematous patch with an irregular border that can become scaly, crusted, and elevated, usually on sun-exposed areas (Fig. 113-5). The junction between the epidermis and dermis is histologically sharp and well demarcated in spite of acanthosis (Fig. 113-6). Bowen disease that occurs on the glans penis, vulva,

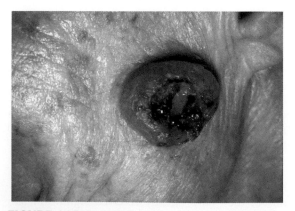

FIGURE 113-4. Keratoacanthoma.

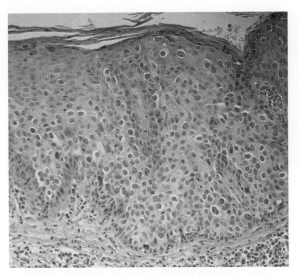

FIGURE 113-6. Bowen disease. Atypical cells are present throughout the entire thickness of the epidermis. The dermal-epidermal junction remains distinct and intact. (From Habif TP: Clinical Dermatology, 4th ed. Philadelphia, Mosby, 2004.)

or oral mucosa may also be referred to as erythroplasia of Queyrat and is histologically identical. The term has survived because it was described 1 year before Bowen disease (Color Plate 113-4).[61]

Another common site of occurrence is the nail folds or nail beds of the digits.[82] Only about 3% to 11% of lesions become invasive SCC, and this occurs only after many years. There are scattered reports in the literature suggesting that there is an increased incidence of internal malignant neoplasms associated with Bowen disease,[83,84] but most authors have not found a high correlation. The preferred treatments are 5-FU and surgical excision.

Epidermodysplasia Verruciformis

Epidermodysplasia verruciformis is a rare disease in which patients have a decreased ability to resist infections caused by the human papillomavirus. Skin eruptions resembling plain warts with minimal hyperkeratosis develop in a generalized pattern. Human papillomavirus lesions consist of more than seven different types, some of which can evolve into malignant tumors including SCC. In epidermodysplasia verruciformis, the function of T cells is impaired. This disease is inherited as an autosomal recessive trait in 25% of patients and X-linked recessive in others.[85] Diagnosis is usually made by histologic examination as well as by testing for viral DNA.[86]

Medical treatments have included etretinate in the early stages and interferon. However, surgical excision still remains the mainstay of therapy. SCCs that evolve from this disorder may metastasize, leading to mortality.

Nevus Sebaceus of Jadassohn

Nevus sebaceus of Jadassohn is a congenital lesion that most often occurs on the scalp or face. It is usually a well-circumscribed lesion that is waxy with a yellowish plaque appearance (Fig. 113-7). It may become verrucous or nodular. Approximately 10% to 15% will undergo malignant degeneration.[61] These malignant neoplasms often occur in adolescents (Fig. 113-8). Most often, the transformation is into a BCC. However, a study by Jaqueti et al[87] revealed trichoblastoma to be the most common neoplasm in a series of 155 patients with nevus sebaceus of Jadassohn. They could not identify any patients with BCC. However, in addition to trichoblastomas, cutaneous hamartomas, hyperplasias, and lesions of adnexal structures without any malignant neoplasm were also found. Because of these findings, they question the traditional wisdom of early excision to prevent malignant transformation. An additional series,[88] in which 596 patients were studied from 1932 to 1998, cited evidence that conversion of nevus sebaceus to BCC may not be as common as was once believed. Of the lesions studied, 49.8% were on the scalp. Basal cell cancers were found in only five patients, representing 0.8%, with the mean age at occurrence of 39.3 years. There were 81 benign tumors representing 13.6%. The most common benign tumors were syringocystadenoma papilliferum (30 were found) and trichoblastoma (28 were found). They concluded that the rate of malignant transformation in nevus sebaceus is low, and they questioned the benefit of prophylactic surgery in young children.

Other authors analyzed 62 patients with nevus sebaceus with contrasting results.[89] The study showed

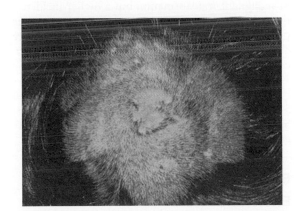

FIGURE 113-7. Nevus sebaceus (of Jadassohn) of the scalp. It is yellowish, not hair bearing, and elevated above the surrounding skin. (From Casson PR, Robins P: Malignant tumors of the skin. In McCarthy JG, ed: Plastic Surgery. Philadelphia, WB Saunders, 1990:3614.)

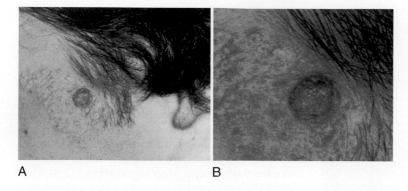

A   B

FIGURE 113-8. *A* and *B,* Nevus sebaceus (of Jadassohn) of the temporal skin in a 17-year-old male patient. A nodule that had appeared 4 months before presentation was determined to be BCC. (From Casson PR, Robins P: Malignant tumors of the skin. In McCarthy JG, ed: Plastic Surgery. Philadelphia, WB Saunders, 1990: 3614.)

that the risk of degeneration into BCC justified surgical treatment. Further argument for early excision comes from Beer et al,[90] who encountered 4 malignant tumors occurring from 18 sebaceous nevi during a period of 9 years. None of them was suggestive of cancer macroscopically.

Porokeratosis

Porokeratosis is a premalignant lesion that forms annular plaques with distinct keratitic ridges. There are five variances, all of which may lead to malignant neoplasia, including porokeratosis of Mibelli, disseminated superficial actinic porokeratosis, porokeratosis palmaris et plantaris disseminata, porokeratosis punctata palmaris et plantaris, and linear porokeratosis.[53] In one study of the literature concerning patients with porokeratosis, linear porokeratosis was found to have a high rate of malignant degeneration. This helps support the argument that the genetic mechanism of allelic loss giving rise to linear porokeratosis may represent an initial step in the development of cancer.[91] Disseminated superficial actinic porokeratosis, described by Chernosky,[92] has a lower frequency of malignant transformation but a higher incidence than of the other types. Disseminated superficial actinic porokeratosis has been associated with sun exposure and tanning bed use; it is an autosomal dominant disorder whose locus has been identified at chromosome 12q23.2-24.[93]

Medical treatment for porokeratosis includes topical 5-FU, topical vitamin D analogues, and oral retinoids. Surgical excision is essential for lesions that have undergone malignant degeneration.

BASAL CELL CARCINOMA

Etiologic Factors

BCC is the most prevalent malignant neoplasm, including all other skin cancers.[2] The primary cause of BCC is exposure to UV radiation from sunlight. BCC occurs almost exclusively on the hair-bearing skin,

most frequently in sun-exposed areas. There is a direct correlation between a person's residence relative to the equator and the development of BCC. Other predisposing factors are light skin that has a tendency to burn rather than to tan, fair hair, and blue eyes. BCCs may also result from specific syndromes and diseases, including xeroderma pigmentosum and basal cell nevus syndrome.

Pinkus,[94] in 1953, proposed that basal cell (and squamous cell) carcinomas arise from pluripotential cells in the epithelium and hair follicles. Their growth is dependent on the surrounding connective tissue stroma because isolated BCCs will not survive if transplanted alone.[95]

The majority of BCCs occur in men, but the incidence in women is increasing because of changing fashions in clothing and time spent out of doors in recreation or specific occupations.[2]

Histopathology

BCC, also referred to as basal cell epithelioma or basaloma, is characterized by large nuclei that are oval and compose most of the cellular matrix, with little cytoplasm. There is a higher nucleus-to-cytoplasm ratio in malignant cells compared with normal cells. Masses of tumor are surrounded by a peripheral cell layer in which the nuclei form a palisade or picket fence-type arrangement.

Tumors can be categorized into differentiated and undifferentiated, although there is not a clear division between the two. The differentiated tumors take on the characteristics of glandular appendages or hair follicles. Tumors classified as noduloulcerative, nevoid basal cell syndrome, and Bazex syndrome may be differentiated or undifferentiated. However, BCCs such as the pigmented, fibrosing, superficial, and fibroepitheliomas are usually undifferentiated.[61]

The basal cells are surrounded by connective tissue stroma containing fibroblasts arranged in parallel. Type IV collagen is present within the stroma. There is evidence of an inflammatory response in tumors that have ulcerated.

TABLE 113-3 ✦ BASAL CELL CARCINOMA: HISTOLOGIC SUBTYPES

Type*	Percentage of BCCs
Nodular	21
Superficial	17
Micronodular	15
Infiltrative	2
Morpheaform	1

*A mixed pattern (two or more major histologic patterns) is present in 38.5% of patients.

From Habif TP: Clinical Dermatology, 4th ed. Philadelphia, Mosby, 2004.

Basal cell cancers have been classified into five types according to their histologic characteristics and include nodular, superficial, micronodular, infiltrative, and morpheaform (Table 113-3 and Color Plate 113-5). Many patients (approximately 38%) have a mixed pattern consisting of two or more histologic patterns.[96]

Clinical Features

The head and neck account for nearly 85% of tumors. The nose is the area with the highest frequency (up to 25%) of primary tumors; the periorbital area and ear have the highest incidence of recurrent lesions.[97] Nearly all BCCs occur in white individuals, and those that occur in blacks are usually associated with burns, chronic wounds, or albinism. BCCs that do develop in blacks also occur preferentially on the head and neck.

Basal cell cancer usually occurs as an isolated lesion in a single area. The concept of superficial multicentric BCCs has been challenged. Kimura[98] has shown connections between nests of cells along the rete ridges. However, metachronous lesions are common, and it is estimated that about 40% of patients who have a BCC will develop another cutaneous tumor within 10 years.[2]

Growth of these tumors is characteristically slow, evolving for months to years. The actively growing tissue is at the periphery of the lesion, with cellular apoptosis and resultant ulceration in the central region. In treating these lesions, it is important to eradicate the farthest marginal areas because these tend to have the most aggressively behaving cells. Growth may continue for months or even years, gradually invading and destroying bone as well as soft tissue. There is a predilection for invasion along tissue planes, periosteum, and nerves. A common theory states that the embryonic fusion planes, such as the nasolabial fold, are more susceptible to tumor growth.

Basal cell cancers rarely metastasize. The incidence of metastases ranges from 0.0028% to 0.1%, depending on the series and group of patients studied, and is twice as common in men.[99] The low incidence of metastases is probably in part due to the requirement for a connective tissue stroma for the cells to survive and multiply. The average length of time from initial presentation of the cutaneous lesion to development of a metastasis is approximately 10 years. As opposed to SCCs, which usually spread initially to the regional nodal basin, about half of all metastatic BCCs spread by hematogenous means, usually to lung and bones. A typical scenario for metastases is that a slow-growing lesion ulcerates, is incompletely treated, and becomes locally invasive and recurs.

SPECIFIC TYPES

Clinical subtypes include nodular, cystic, pigmented, sclerosing or morpheaform, and superficial BCC. There is a great deal of overlap in the clinical categories; however, the clinical type will often indicate biologic behavior and preferred modes of treatment.[61]

Nodular BCC is by far the most common type, representing more than 50% of all BCCs (Fig. 113-9; see also Color Plate 113-6). This lesion usually starts as a small nodule, often pale with telangiectatic vessels on the surface. It gradually enlarges and may eventually ulcerate, giving rise to the descriptive term "rodent ulcer" (Fig. 113-10). The irregular borders of the ulcer may give the impression that the tissue was chewed on by a rat. The lesion customarily has elevated, white, rolled edges surrounding the central ulceration and may contain small areas of brown or bluish pigment.

Superficial BCCs, representing 10% of all BCCs, are flat, scaly, and erythematous and may be confused with eczematous dermatitis. They spread by irregular growth patterns, and as opposed to other types, they occur on the trunk more often than on the head and neck. The initial growth pattern is horizontal, but they may ulcerate. The lesions may have areas of spontaneous regression that appear like flat scars.

Pigmented BCCs, representing about 5% of all BCCs, are usually brown because of the melanin content but may range from blue to black and are occasionally confused with melanoma for that reason. The coloration is explained by the fact that melanocytes are present in the epidermis and in hair matrix in 75% of tumors. They vary from nodular BCC only in color (Color Plate 113-7 and Fig. 113-11).

Morpheaform or sclerosing BCCs, accounting for 2% of BCCs, present as a flat, whitish or yellow plaque with ill-defined borders. The surface is often shiny and scar-like. Ulceration, when it occurs, happens late in the course. Because of its more indolent appearance, it is often misdiagnosed, undertreated, and recurrent (Color Plate 113-8 and Fig. 113-12).

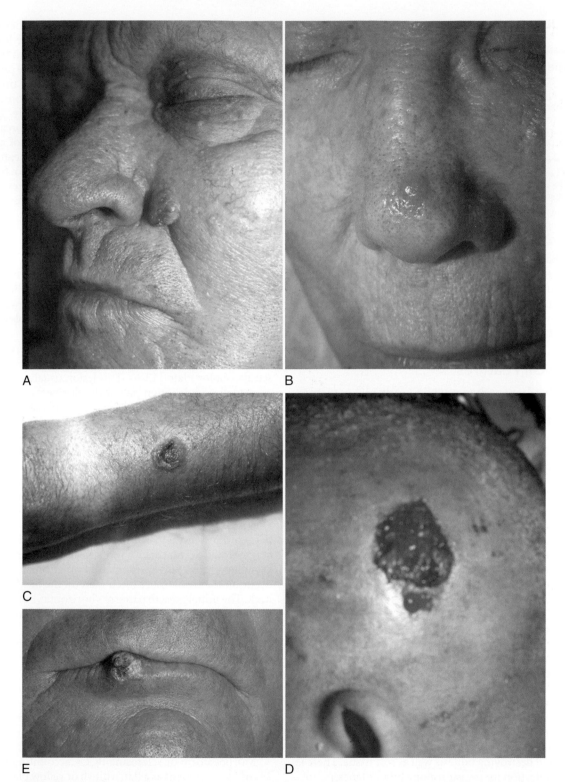

FIGURE 113-9. *A,* Nodular BCC of the cheek. (See also Color Plate 113-6*A.*) *B,* Nodular BCC of the nose. *C,* Nodular BCC of the forearm. *D,* Nodular BCC of the scalp. *E,* Nodular BCC of the lower lip. (See also Color Plate 113-6*B.*)

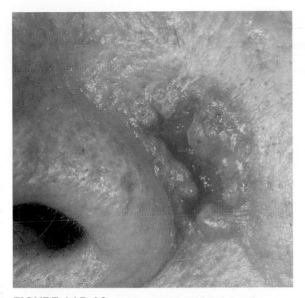

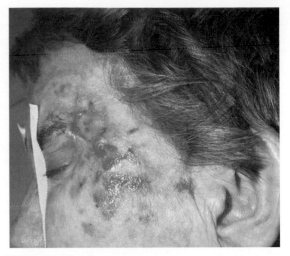

FIGURE 113-12. Recurrent sclerosing BCC of forehead, temple, and cheek.

FIGURE 113-10. BCC consisting of a deep ulcer surrounded by a nodular tumor. In the past, this type of lesion was referred to as a rodent ulcer. (From Habif TP: Clinical Dermatology, 4th ed. Philadelphia, Mosby, 2004.)

Treatment

Because of the rarity of metastases in patients with BCC, control of the local disease will often cure the patient. The treatments of choice for BCC include curettage and electrodesiccation, conventional surgical techniques, micrographic surgery, 5-FU, radiation therapy, and cryosurgery (Table 113-4).

CURETTAGE AND ELECTRODESICCATION

The technique of curettage and electrodesiccation is most commonly employed among dermatologists. The

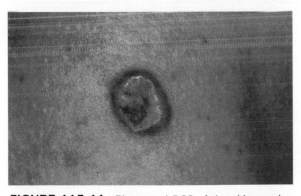

FIGURE 113-11. Pigmented BCC of the skin overlying the trapezius muscle in a 26-year-old woman of European parentage. This was diagnosed clinically as a nodular melanoma. (From Casson PR, Robins P: Malignant tumors of the skin. In McCarthy JG, ed. Plastic Surgery. Philadelphia, WB Saunders, 1990:3614.)

gross tumor is removed with a curet, and the base is desiccated with a cautery. Tumor may or may not be sent for histologic examination. Some practitioners prefer to perform a shave biopsy before curettage to allow better diagnosis. Others send specimens from the margins of the defect after curettage as a check on the effectiveness of removal, the so-called Mohs micrographic technique, in which the fresh tissue technique is then employed to ensure completeness of excision. The wound is left to heal secondarily.

The advantages of this technique are that it is quick and easy to learn. The disadvantages are that without biopsy and orientation of the specimen, histologic control is poor or absent, and hypertrophic scars and hypopigmentation may occur.[100] Wounds left to heal secondarily that are near normal tissue margins (eyelids, nasal ala, lips, and ears) will often develop a notch deformity that results in a scar unacceptable to many patients.

The consensus is that this technique is most useful for primary tumors of small size. The exact measurement of "small size" has been debated; some propose that 1 cm be the limit.[101] Recurrent tumors with strands of cancer cells growing within dense scar tissue or along tissue planes are less suitable candidates for curettage.

SURGICAL EXCISION

Surgical excision is the treatment modality most favored by surgeons. It has the advantage of being a single-stage procedure, and the wound is usually closed primarily and can therefore produce a better cosmetic result. The key element in the success of this method is the ability of the surgeon to correctly identify the lesion and extent of tumor spread. In a 1998 study by Hallock and Lutz,[102] clinical diagnosis of all

TABLE 113-4 ✦ TREATMENT OF BASAL CELL CARCINOMA

Treatment	Indications	Advantages	Disadvantages	Cure Rate
Surgical excision	Most tumors	Wounds closed primarily; better cosmetic result; single stage	Higher recurrence rates in some types compared with Mohs surgery; removes some normal tissue; limited histologic control	Up to 98% for nodular, primary 80% for recurrences
Mohs surgery	Large, invasive (morpheaform), or recurrent; high-risk areas; when patient is not a candidate for surgery	Histologic control of tumor excision	May leave large defects requiring surgical repair; time-consuming; requires special techniques and training	Up to 99% for primary
Curettage and electrodesiccation	Small (2-4 mm), primary, localized tumors; superficial multicentric	Commonly available, widely used	Poor histologic control; hypertrophic scarring, hypopigmentation; delayed wound healing	100% (<2 mm) 50% (>3 cm)
5-FU	Superficial, multicentric (very limited)	Noninvasive	Long treatment; pigmentation changes; not for invasive or recurrent tumors	Low
Radiation therapy	Nonsurgical candidates; inoperable tumors; palliation	"Spares" normal tissue	Requires special expertise; ulceration; poor cosmesis	95% (<5 mm) 85% (15 mm) 75%-90% recurrent
Cryosurgery	Localized, primary tumors; patient is poor surgical risk	"Spares" normal tissue	"Blind" treatment; not effective for sclerosing tumors or recurrences	Up to 95% (<2 cm) in primary lesions
Chemotherapy	Uncontrolled local and metastatic disease	May prolong survival; palliation	Toxicity	N/A
Photodynamic therapy	Superficial lesions	Noninvasive	Limited penetration of light source; lack of histologic control; patient photosensitized	10%-40% in nodular, higher in superficial

lesions (benign, premalignant, and malignant) was accurate in only 65% of those studied (Table 113-5). Benign lesions were correctly identified in 73%, premalignant in 42%, and malignant in 54% of the lesions studied. Basal cell cancers were correctly diagnosed in 70% and, when excised, had positive margins in 18% of patients. However, only 3% of lesions called benign by the surgeon actually were malignant on histologic examination. This study also found that basal cell cancers were more accurately diagnosed preoperatively than were squamous cell cancers.

In a series of 1039 consecutive neoplasms studied by Sexton et al,[103] the adequacy of excision was a function of histologic type. Superficial BCCs had the lowest percentage of positive margins after excision (3.6%), whereas morpheaform had the highest (33.3%) (Table 113-6).

Silverman et al[104] analyzed 588 primary and 135 recurrent BCCs that were treated by surgical excision. Primary treated tumors had a cumulative 5-year

TABLE 113-5 ✦ ACCURACY OF CLINICAL DIAGNOSIS OF SKIN LESIONS

Actual Diagnosis	Total (%)	Clinical Correct (%)
Benign	1313 (64)	967 (74)
Nevus	353 (17)	317 (90)
Seborrheic keratosis	289 (14)	221 (76)
Other	671 (33)	429 (64)
Premalignant	312 (15)	103 (33)
Bowen	98 (5)	12 (12)
Solar keratosis	208 (10)	87 (42)
Other	6 (0)	4 (67)
Malignant	433 (21)	260 (60)
Basal cell	309 (15)	206 (67)
Melanoma	10 (0)	3 (30)
Squamous cell	106 (5)	44 (42)
Other	8 (0)	7 (88)
Total	2058 (100)	1330 (65)

From Hallock GG, Lutz DA: Prospective study of the accuracy of the surgeon's diagnosis in 2000 excised skin tumors. Plast Reconstr Surg 1998;101:1255.

TABLE 113-6 ✦ PERCENTAGE OF POSITIVE MARGINS OF EXCISED BASAL CELL CARCINOMAS BASED ON HISTOLOGIC SUBTYPE

Histologic Pattern	No. of Excisions	Positive Margins (%)
Nodular	94	6.4
Micronodular	59	18.6
Superficial	56	3.6
Infiltrative	34	26.5
Morpheic	6	33.3
Nodular-micronodular	115	16.5
Mixed with infiltrative	103	30.1
Total	467	17.1

From Sexton M, Jones DB, Maloney ME: Histologic pattern analysis of basal cell carcinoma: study of a series of 1039 consecutive neoplasms. J Am Acad Dermatol 1990;23:1118-1126.

recurrence rate of 4.8%, whereas recurrent tumors recurred at a rate of 11.6%, a statistically significant difference. Recurrences were higher for head and neck tumors, with ear (42.9%) and nasolabial groove (20.2%) being the highest (Table 113-7). There was no significant difference with regard to size of the primary lesion. This conflicts with results of a study by Dubin and Kopf,[105] which found increasing recur-

TABLE 113-7 ✦ RECURRENCE RATES FOR PRIMARILY EXCISED BASAL CELL CARCINOMAS

Anatomic Site	5-Year Recurrence Rate (%)	No. of Patients
Ear	42.9	10
Nasal-labial groove	20.2	11
Scalp	14.7	22
Forehead	8.4	68
Paranasal	5.8	52
Nose	5.5	44
Periocular	5.3	21
Malar	4.0	81
Neck	2.5	47
Pre-/postauricular	0	15
Perioral	0	24
Chin-mandible	0	31
Canthi	0	7
Trunk	0	93
Extremities	0	47
Genitalia	0	2
Not recorded	NA	13
Total	4.8	588

From Silverman MK, Kopf AW, Bart RS, et al: Recurrence rates of treated basal cell carcinomas. Part 3: Surgical excision. J Dermatol Surg Oncol 1992;18:471-476.

TABLE 113-8 ✦ RECURRENCE OF BASAL CELL CARCINOMA AFTER SURGICAL EXCISION

Lesion Diameter (mm)	No. Recur/Total Excised	Recurrence (%)
<2	0/1	0
2-5	3/47	6.4
6-10	9/102	8.8
11-15	4/51	7.8
16-30	4/33	12.1
>30	3/13	23.1

From Dubin N, Kopf AW: Multivariate risk score for recurrence of cutaneous basal cell carcinomas. Arch Dermatol 1983;119:373.

rence rates of BCCs with increasing lesion size. Lesions smaller than 2 mm did not recur, lesions 6 to 10 mm had a recurrence rate of 8.8%, and lesions larger than 30 mm recurred 23.1% of the time (Table 113-8).

The concept of an "adequate surgical margin" is one of probability. Margins will depend on size of the lesion, anatomic location, clinical features, ulceration, and apparent depth of penetration. Practically speaking, margins are usually 2 to 10 mm, with smaller lesions requiring smaller margins. For early, primary lesions, a margin of 3 to 4 mm seems reasonable and supportable by the literature. Small, primary lesions are usually confined to the dermis, so that excision of the entire thickness of skin with a narrow margin of subcutaneous tissue is adequate. More important, the question is what is done with the histologic information and when that information is gained by the surgeon. Many surgeons simply excise the lesion and close the wound primarily. The specimen is sent to the pathology laboratory with the results transmitted within a few days. Surgical decisions are then made on the basis of these results. This method is popular because it conserves the surgeon's time.

Another method is to excise the tumor and submit the tissue for a "frozen section," which takes a half-hour or more. It also requires more timely communication between surgeon and pathologist regarding the clinical appearance and orientation of the lesion. Positive margins require immediate re-excision, with further histologic examination. There are some inevitable inaccuracies in this method because the pathologist cannot examine the specimen in as great detail as can be accomplished with permanent sections. Frozen section monitoring of margins may lead to findings of negative margins that are subsequently revealed to be positive a few days later. If a flap has been used to close the wound, it is re-elevated, and further resection is performed. It is questionable whether some of the tissue of the flap must also be removed. For this reason, reconstruction is occasionally delayed or a skin graft placed on the wound, and a flap is used only after the final margins are negative.

Traditional wisdom has stated that of incompletely excised BCCs, only 30% to 50% recur (however, one large series by Shanoff et al[106] found a recurrence rate of 67%), and if further resection is performed after positive margins, tumor is found in only half of the specimens. The reasons for these findings are multiple: (1) although the tumor extended to the surgical margin, it was, in fact, completely excised; (2) the small amount of residual tumor was destroyed by the host's immunity (although possible, it is less likely, since the most actively dividing and aggressive portions of the tumor are at the periphery); and (3) the tissue submitted after re-excision did actually contain a small focus of tumor, but because not every cell can be examined, it was not seen by the pathologist.

Pascal et al,[107] in a study that is often quoted, found that the closeness of the tumor to the surgical margin made a difference in recurrence. Of the lesions within one high-power field (400×) of the margin, 12% recurred; 33% recurred when the tumor involved the margin, and only 1.2% recurred when they were adequately excised.

In an attempt to more precisely define which patients have the highest potential for recurrence, Dellon et al[108] evaluated excised BCCs by histologic criteria of irregularities in the peripheral palisade, lymphocytic infiltration, and clinical ulceration of the tumor. They found that recurrence developed in 93% of patients with greater than 75% irregularities in the peripheral palisade (Fig. 113-13). This was a 39-fold increase in recurrence. Tumors that had ulcerated had a 2.8-fold incidence of recurrence.

If the surgeon decides not to re-excise the tumor, diligent follow-up is mandatory. However, this system is not foolproof. The patient has to present for frequent examination, and when a recurrence is detected, it may be far advanced and more difficult to treat because it has been relatively hidden by normal tissue or a flap or graft. Therefore, complete re-excision of incompletely excised tumors is the safest course of action.

MICROGRAPHIC SURGERY

Micrographic surgery, as first described by Frederic Mohs,[109] involved excising tissue, fixing it with a paste containing zinc chloride, and examining it histologically. A detailed map of the tumor site was made to record the positive margins and to direct the next excision. The original technique could take several days because of the time required (up to 24 hours) for fixation before each new tumor margin excision, and the paste was painful. Tromovitch and Stegman[110] eliminated the chemical fixative, shortened the entire

process, and renamed the procedure micrographic surgery. Nonetheless, the basic principles have remained the same in that histologically examined tissue directs further resection until all margins are clear of tumor.

Micrographic surgery finds its greatest utility in the treatment of BCCs that are more aggressive (e.g., morpheaform), in areas where recurrences would be more difficult to eradicate, for preservation of skin in areas adjacent to specialized structures (e.g., medial canthal region of the eye), and for lesions that have recurred and growth of the tumor is surrounded by scar tissue. High cure rates for primary excisions, approaching 100%, have been claimed by its proponents. The technique has been proposed for resection of dermatofibrosarcoma protuberans, melanoma, and Merkel cell carcinoma. However, this technique may not be effective where tumors spread along lymphatic vessels or nerves.

5-FLUOROURACIL

5-FU has been advocated by some investigators as a useful agent in the treatment of BCC. Its use should be confined to superficial lesions because the penetration of the agent is limited. It has no place in the treatment of invasive or recurrent lesions. Epstein[111] has reported a 5-year recurrence rate of 21% for thin BCCs treated with 25% fluorouracil for 3 weeks. However, if curettage was used before 5-FU treatment, the recurrence rate was 6%. Perhaps the main value of 5-FU is to determine which suspicious lesions require surgical excision. After a course of treatment lasting 3 to 6 weeks, biopsy of any remaining lesion should be performed.

RADIATION THERAPY

Radiation therapy is used in the treatment of recurrent BCCs, as an adjunctive measure after surgical excision, in patients who are not surgical candidates, and in those patients whose main goal is palliation.[112] The overall 5-year recurrence rate for BCCs treated with radiation therapy has been reported as 7.4%. This rate was not significantly different from that of patients with recurrent BCCs (previously treated), who had a re-recurrence rate of 9.5%. For the patients with primary BCCs, multivariate analysis showed that increasing BCC diameter is the only independent risk factor for high recurrence rates.[113]

A noted advantage of radiation therapy is that it spares normal tissue. Although adjacent normal tissue is not removed, it is subjected to the adverse effects of radiation, which can lead to dermatitis, pain, and, in extreme instances, ulceration. The good initial cosmetic result can deteriorate with time, such that in 10 years, skin may show hypopigmentation, atrophy, and telangiectasia.

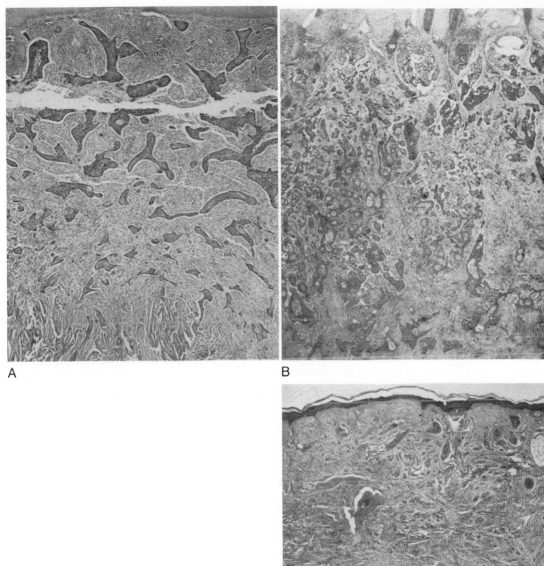

A

B

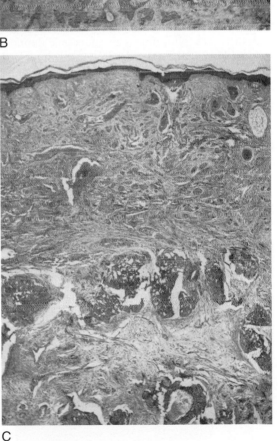

C

FIGURE 113-13. *A,* Positive-margin BCC graded as squamous differentiation 0% to 25%, irregularities in the peripheral palisade 75% to 100%, lymphocytic infiltration absent. It did recur (×30). *B,* Positive-margin BCC graded as squamous differentiation 75% to 100%, irregularities in the peripheral palisade 75% to 100%, lymphocytic infiltration absent. It did recur (×40). *C,* Positive-margin BCC graded as squamous differentiation 50% to 75%, irregularities in the peripheral palisade 50% to 75%, lymphocytic infiltration absent. It did recur (×30). (From Dellon AL, DeSilva S, Connolly M, Ross A: Prediction of recurrence in incompletely excised basal cell carcinoma. Plast Reconstr Surg 1985;75:860.)

As in other treatments, such as surgical excision, incomplete eradication of tumor can predispose the patient to a recurrence. Therefore, some have advocated pretreatment and post-treatment biopsies of the lesion.

CRYOSURGERY

Cryosurgery is a highly effective treatment for a broad range of benign skin problems. Although it is often used for premalignant lesions such as actinic keratoses, it is not the preferred method of treatment for BCCs because of the likelihood of recurrent or possibly invasive disease. One does not obtain a pathologic specimen when this method is used. In addition, pigment changes also introduce the possibility of less than desirable cosmetic outcome for many patients.[114]

Basal Cell Nevus Syndrome

Basal cell nevus syndrome, also known as nevoid BCC syndrome or Gorlin syndrome, is an inherited disorder complex that presents with multiple BCCs, pitting of the palmar and plantar surfaces, jaw cysts, and other musculoskeletal and neurologic abnormalities (Fig. 113-14).[85] This syndrome is an autosomal dominant disease. Loss of the normal PTC allele results in the development of multiple BCCs.[115]

Jaw cysts, odontogenic keratocysts, are part of the syndrome of nevoid BCC syndrome. Lo Muzio et al[116] described 14 patients in 5 families with the nevoid BCC syndrome. In 11 patients (78%), the first evidence of the syndrome was an odontogenic keratocyst. Only one of these patients had a BCC at the time of the study. They concluded that odontogenic keratocysts are often the first sign of BCC syndrome and their presence can be detected in the first decade of life.[116] In a series of 37 Italian patients, jaw cysts and calcification of the falx cerebri were the most frequently observed anomalies.[117] Next in order were BCCs and palmar or plantar pits. This study also speculates that the low frequency of BCCs in the Italian population is related to their darker skin pigmentation compared with northern Europeans.

Because BCCs of the palm are rare, there are a small number of reported instances. Thus, the finding of a BCC of the palm is strongly suggestive of basal cell nevus syndrome.

In patients with the nevoid BCC syndrome, BCCs most often occur on sun-exposed areas, but not exclusively so. Metastasis from these lesions is rare; however, these lesions can be locally invasive. There does not appear to be a relationship between sun exposure and the number of BCCs occurring in these patients.[118]

The treatment of choice for patients with BCCs arising from basal cell nevus syndrome is surgical excision and careful monitoring. Lesions of the face should be aggressively treated. The pits that occur on the palmar surface of the hand may contain BCC. These pits are on the order of 1 to 3 mm in depth.

Some patients with the nevoid BCC syndrome have hundreds of BCCs. For these patients, an alternative to surgery has been investigated. The application of imiquimod 5% cream has been used effectively in eradicating superficial, nonfacial BCCs.[119]

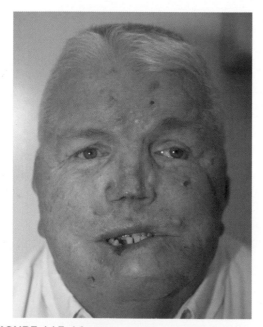

FIGURE 113-14. Basal cell nevus syndrome.

SQUAMOUS CELL CARCINOMA

Etiologic Factors

Squamous cell skin cancers are caused by both genetic and environmental factors. As with basal cell cancers, genetic defects in DNA repair, such as xeroderma pigmentosum, are associated with SCC. However, by far the most frequent causes are agents such as UVB radiation and x-irradiation.[120] These external causes of SCC may have increased propensity to cause malignant degeneration if there is an underlying immunosuppression, whether it is drug induced, through organ transplantation, or by lymphoproliferative disease.

Squamous cell cancers usually arise from damaged skin. That damage is most often caused by sunlight in the UVB (290 to 320 nm) range, but carcinogenesis may be stimulated by the UVA range (320 to 400 nm). Actinic keratoses often herald the development of SCC and are a marker for sun-damaged skin.[121] Other causes may be ionizing radiation, chemicals (particularly arsenicals), smoking, chronic irritation, and papillomavirus.

Direct correlation has been established between sun exposure and development of SCC. This may be further demonstrated by the incidence of SCC in individuals living closer to the equator (e.g., persons in Australia have a higher incidence than those living in northern United States).[8] Sun-exposed areas of the skin, such as the head and neck and hands, also have a higher incidence. SCCs also have a predilection for those persons with fair skin who do not tan readily.

Iatrogenic immunosuppression as given for organ transplantation and autoimmune diseases has long been associated with an increased risk of SCC.[122] Hartevelt et al[123] reported a 253-fold increase in SCC in those patients. In addition, cancers in the immunosuppressed patients tend to be more aggressive. The interplay between immunosuppression, infection with papillomavirus, development of keratoacanthomas, and lifelong sun exposure produces a more virulent clinical presentation.

Human papillomavirus (HPV) has been associated with nonmelanoma skin cancers. HPVs produce epithelial tumors of the skin and mucous membranes. More than 100 HPV types have been detected, and the genomes of almost 70 have been sequenced completely. The current classification system, which is based on similarities in the genomic sequences, generally correlates with the three categories used to describe HPV clinically: anogenital or mucosal, nongenital cutaneous, and epidermodysplasia verruciformis (EV) (Table 113-9).[124]

The earliest evidence for the involvement of specific HPV types in human skin cancer originates from observations for patients suffering from EV[125] (see previous section entitled "Epidermodysplasia Verruciformis"). About one third of patients with EV develop multifocal cutaneous SCCs mainly on sun-exposed parts of the body. These patients are commonly infected with a group of genotypically related HPV types (EV-associated HPVs) that induce characteristic macular skin lesions disseminated over the body.[125] EV HPV has been identified in cells of nonmelanoma skin cancer from immunocompetent patients as well as from more than 90% of organ transplant recipients.[126] The exact contribution to the formation of cancer from gene functions and UV radiation needs to be further investigated, but it does appear that prolonged UV irradiation is needed to activate the viral gene as well as to decrease cellular genes controlling cell growth.[127]

A study conducted by Feltkamp et al[128] examined the relationship between EV HPV infection and nonmelanoma skin cancer. They looked for HPV infection in 540 patients with a history of skin cancer and 333 control subjects. By measuring seroreactivity to L1 virus-like particles of EV HPV types 5, 8, 15, 20, 24, and 38 and the genital type HPV-16 and by estimating the skin cancer relative risk among HPV seropositives, they analyzed whether EV HPV serorecognition is associated with nonmelanoma skin cancer. Seroreactivity to five of the six EV HPV types tested (HPVs 5, 8, 15, 20, and 24) was significantly increased in the patients with SCC. After adjustment for age and sex, the estimated SCC relative risk was significantly increased in HPV-8 and HPV-38 seropositives (odds ratio = 14.7 [95% confidence interval, 1.6 to 135] and odds ratio = 3.0 [95% confidence interval, 1.1 to 8.4], respectively). The estimated relative risk for nodular and superficial multifocal BCC was also significantly increased in the HPV-8 seropositives (odds ratio = 9.2 [95% confidence interval, 1.1 to 78.2] and odds ratio = 17.3 [95% confidence interval, 2.1 to 143], respectively) and in the HPV-20 seropositives (odds ratio = 3.2 [95% confidence interval, 1.3 to 7.9] and odds ratio = 3.4 [95% confidence interval, 1.2 to 9.5], respectively). Their results indicate that EV HPV serorecognition is nonspecifically associated with nonmelanoma skin cancer and suggest that EV HPV-directed seroresponses are induced on skin cancer formation rather than on infection.

Histopathology

SCCs arise from the epidermis of skin and mucous membranes that have squamous epithelium. SCCs may also present as adenoid or mucin-producing cancers. Tumors are graded histologically by the degree of differentiation of individual cells (Color Plate 113-9). The more keratinization, the greater the degree of differentiation. In 1921, Broders[129] proposed a system of grading tumors from 1 to 4, depending on the percentage of cells that were differentiated (>75%, >50%, >25%, and <25% in grades 1 through 4, respectively). Other factors are also considered, such as the degree of atypicality of cells[61] and architecture of the tumor. The shape of cells as well as the number of mitotic figures and hyperchromasia are also important differentiating factors regarding degree of malignancy. Some undifferentiated tumors must be analyzed by immunohistochemical assays or antibodies to distinguish SCC from other tumors such as melanoma and spindle cell carcinomas.

Neural invasion is an important histologic criterion that has clinical relevance, with approximately an eightfold increase in metastases with invasion, and is reported in 2% to 10% of tumors.[130] Mendenhall et al[131] reported that patients with early perineural invasion are most often asymptomatic and that the diagnosis of perineural invasion is usually diagnosed on pathologic examination. Surgery and irradiation of asymptomatic patients result in a cure rate of 80%, whereas symptomatic patients had a cure rate of 45%.[131]

SCC and actinic keratosis are two points along a continuum of histologic morphology. They differ in the degree of atypicality of cells in that only SCC invades

TABLE 113-9 ✦ DISEASES AND ASSOCIATED HPV SUBTYPES

	HPV Type
Nongenital Cutaneous Disease	
Common warts (verruca vulgaris)	1, 2, 4, 26, 27, 29, 41, 57, 65
Plantar warts (myrmecia)	1, 2, 4, 63
Flat warts (verruca plana)	3, 10, 27, 28, 38, 41, 49
Butcher warts (common warts of people who handle meat, poultry, and fish)	1, 2, 3, 4, 7, 10, 28
Mosaic warts	2, 27, 57
Ungual squamous cell carcinoma	16
Epidermodysplasia verruciformis (benign)	2, 3, 10, 12, 15, 19, 36, 46, 47, 50
Epidermodysplasia verruciformis (malignant or benign)	5, 8, 9, 10, 14, 17, 20, 21, 22, 23, 24, 25, 37, 38
Nonwarty skin lesions	37, 38
Nongenital Mucosal Disease	
Respiratory papillomatosis	6, 11
Squamous cell carcinoma of the lung	6, 11, 16, 18
Laryngeal papilloma	6, 11, 30
Laryngeal carcinoma	16, 18
Maxillary sinus papilloma	57
Squamous cell carcinoma of the sinuses	16, 18
Conjunctival papillomas	6, 11
Conjunctival carcinoma	16
Oral focal epithelial hyperplasia (Heck disease)	13, 32
Oral carcinoma	16, 18
Oral leukoplakia	16, 18
Squamous cell carcinoma of the esophagus	16, 18
Anogenital Disease	
Condylomata acuminata	6, 11, 30, 42, 43, 44, 45, 51, 52, 54
Bowenoid papulosis	16, 18, 34, 39, 42, 45
Bowen disease	16, 18, 31, 34
Giant condylomata (Buschke-Löwenstein tumors)	6, 11
Unspecified intraepithelial neoplasia	30, 34, 39, 40, 53, 57, 59, 61, 62, 64, 66, 67, 68, 69
Low-grade intraepithelial neoplasia	6, 11, 43
Intermediate intraepithelial neoplasia	31, 33, 35, 42, 44, 45, 51, 52
High-grade intraepithelial neoplasia	16, 18, 56, 58
Carcinoma of vulva	6, 11, 16, 18
Carcinoma of vagina	16
Carcinoma of cervix	16, 18, 31
Carcinoma of anus	16, 31, 32, 33
Carcinoma in situ of penis (erythroplasia of Queyrat)	16
Carcinoma of penis	16, 18

From Orth G, Jablonska S, Jarzabek-Chorzelska M, et al: Characteristics of the lesions and risk of malignant conversion associated with the type of human papillomavirus involved in epidermodysplasia verruciformis. Cancer Res 1979;39:1074.

the reticular dermis. Tumor thickness correlates with both local recurrence and lymph node metastasis.

Clinical Features

The clinical appearance of squamous cell cancers is varied (Fig. 113-15; see also Color Plate 113-10). Early lesions may appear as erythematous plaques but may become raised papules or verrucous lesions. A useful clinical test that the author has used is to abrade the questionable area with a surgical sponge; if bleeding

occurs, it is often an indication of the extent of spread of the tumor. Eventually, most squamous cancers ulcerate, but they do not have the pearly white edge that is characteristic of BCCs (Fig. 113-16).

Treatment

Treatments for SCC are analogous to those for BCC. However, treatment plans must take into consideration the more aggressive nature of SCC, which may require wider skin margins at initial excision, more

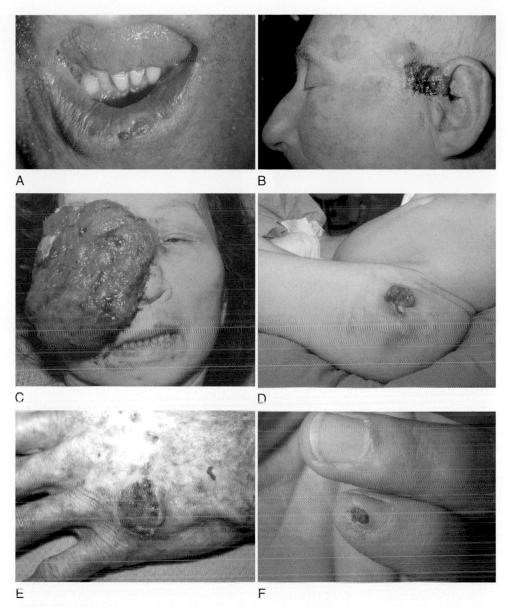

FIGURE 113-15. *A,* SCC of the lower lip. (See also Color Plate 113-10*A.*) *B,* SCC involving the ear and parotid. *C,* Extensive SCC of the face. *D,* SCC of the left hip. *E,* SCC of dorsum of the hand. (See also Color Plate 113-10*B.*) *F,* Localized SCC of the nail bed.

extensive removal of subcutaneous tissues, evaluation and treatment of regional lymph nodes, and more vigilant follow-up.

Surgical excision has been the traditional treatment of choice. Tumors that are less than 2 cm in diameter are usually successfully excised 95% of the time with a margin of 4 mm,[132] although the range may be 3 to 10 mm, depending on the original size of the tumor.[133] Luce[132] also cautions against the expectant treatment of positive margins after resection. The expectation of a majority of positive margins may be acceptable for

BCC, but in SCCs, this expectation may lead to increased morbidity and mortality.

Micrographic surgery has been used effectively with high cure rates. BCCs, recurrent SCCs, and tumors occurring on the face are most appropriate candidates for micrographic excision. Desiccation and curettage have been used successfully in lesions less than 2 cm in diameter. A cure rate of 97% was achieved by Freeman et al[134] and 98.8% by Chernosky.[135] Cryosurgery has been used in SCC. The same provisions and cautions exist as in treatment of BCC, in that

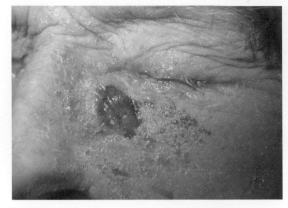

FIGURE 113-16. Recurrent SCC of the cheek.

the lesions must be well localized and do not invade deeper structures. It is not generally recommended for most SCCs.

Verrucous Carcinoma

Verrucous carcinoma is a well-differentiated SCC and was first described as an oral lesion of indolent nature that was less aggressive than invasive SCC.[136] It has since been shown to arise most commonly on the soles of the feet, the palms of the hands, and the urogenital-perineal region (Fig. 113-17). Early lesions appear wart-like and progress to polypoid masses that may be invasive. The oral form has been associated with the use of snuff and chewing tobacco; cutaneous lesions are often in areas of trauma. The human papillomavirus has been isolated in some types, but there is not a clear causative relationship. Distant metastases are uncommon and are associated with irradiation of oral lesions.[136]

Treatment of verrucous carcinoma is usually surgical, including micrographic surgery. Radiation therapy has been controversial, with some reports of anaplastic transformation.[137]

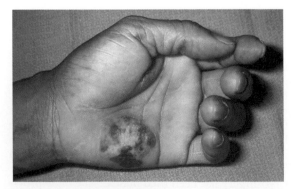

FIGURE 113-17. Verrucous carcinoma of the palm.

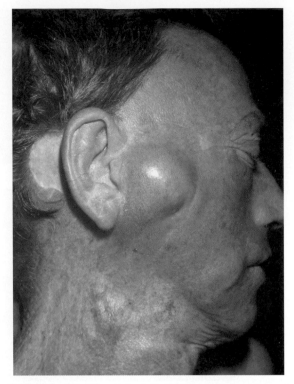

FIGURE 113-18. Metastatic SCC involving parotid and mandible. (Note previous excision and skin graft in post-auricular area.)

Metastatic Disease

The rate of metastases from SCC varies greatly with the cause of the lesion, the location, and whether the lesion is primary or secondary (Fig. 113-18). When SCC results from sun exposure, the metastatic rate is 0.1% to 3%; those arising in chronic ulcers, such as burn scars and osteomyelitis, have a much higher rate, approaching 20%.[61] The overwhelming majority of metastases are to lymph nodes (85%), with the remaining 15% to visceral organs.[138,139] The 5-year survival rate of patients with metastatic disease is approximately 25%.[140]

The decision to perform a regional lymphadenectomy should be based on the size, site, and biologic behavior of the primary tumor. Tumors of small caliber (<2 cm) can usually be treated by excision alone. However, larger lesions, or those with a higher metastatic potential, should be considered for prophylactic lymphadenectomy. Bessede et al[141] described 13 patients with SCC of the head and neck who presented with metastases or developed them later. All patients underwent tumor excision and radical neck dissection, and 92% had radiotherapy. The survival rate at 2 years was 62%.

Studies have indicated that sentinel lymph node biopsy is a useful tool in identifying occult regional lymph node disease in select patients with non-melanoma malignant skin cancer.[142-144] A report by Werner et al[145] noted that the majority of patients with head and neck SCC who have a clinical N0 neck undergo neck dissection even though no lymph node metastases may be detected. The investigators studied 90 patients with head and neck SCC, all staged with an N0 neck, who underwent intraoperative technetium Tc 99m-radiolabeled detection of up to three hot nodes (SN1-3) during elective neck dissection and primary site resection. The results were impressive. Sentinel lymphadenectomy (SN1-3) detected occult metastatic spread in 20 (22%) of 90 patients, whereas failure occurred in 3 of 90 patients. Metastatic spread was directed to level II in the majority (66.7%) of patients. If only the SN1 had been examined, the procedure would have failed in 9 (39%) of 23 patients. In this study, sentinel lymphadenectomy correctly identified the stage of metastatic disease in 97% of patients in those patients with up to three sentinel nodes identified. If only the lymph node with the highest tracer activity had been excised, 39% of cancer-positive necks would have been missed. Selective neck dissection identified metastatic disease in the additional 3% of patients.[145] In select patients with non-melanoma cutaneous malignant neoplasms, sentinel lymph node biopsy is a minimally invasive and highly sensitive staging tool.

OTHER MALIGNANT SKIN TUMORS

Paget Disease

Mammary Paget disease is a rare skin cancer that occurs unilaterally on the female breast. There have been only a few men who have developed the disease. It origi-nates on the nipple or areola but may spread to surrounding breast skin. It is clinically characterized by eczema-like skin changes (Fig. 113-19). It can be confused with erosive adenomatosis of the nipple, a benign condition. When the skin is involved, there is often underlying breast cancer. On histologic examination, Paget cells are located within the epidermis. These are large cells with large nuclei and abundant cytoplasm. Mastectomy is often necessary treatment for mammary Paget disease. Alternatively, it can be widely locally excised along with samples of axillary lymph nodes. Conservative treatment, such as partial nipple excision, wedge excision, cone excision, radiotherapy, or a combination of these, may be used in women with less advanced stages of the disease. However, recurrence is common in these patients.[146]

Extramammary Paget disease is also rare and displays Paget cells in the epidermis. It usually appears in the vulva and male genital area where apocrine glands are found and often has a more favorable prognosis than mammary Paget disease (Color Plate 113-11). Margin-controlled surgical excision of the affected area by Mohs surgery is the standard treatment for extramammary Paget disease. The margin is sometimes difficult to define, particularly when lesions are spread sporadically throughout the anogenital region. Recurrence is common, so patients should be re-examined every 3 months after surgery for the next 2 years, after which annual follow-ups are recommended. The immune response modifier imiquimod cream appears to be a promising additional therapy.[146]

Adnexal Carcinomas

MERKEL CELL CARCINOMA

Merkel cell carcinoma is a rare tumor, with only 600 instances of the disease reported between 1972 and 1995. It occurs more frequently in patients older than 65 years, with a range of 7 to 97 years, and equal male and female distribution.[147] Merkel cell carcinoma appears most often on sun-exposed sites on white skin; 50% occur on the head and neck (with 20% in the periocular region) and 40% on the trunk (Fig. 113-20).[147] Merkel cell carcinoma has been reported in sites previously treated with radiation, and UV exposure has been implicated as a contributing factor; however, the presence of this neoplasia in the larynx, esophagus, calvaria, and oral and genital mucosa implies that non-UV factors are also important in the development of this disease.[147,148]

Merkel cell carcinoma usually consists of painless, indurated, solitary dermal nodules approximately 2 to 4 mm in size. These nodules normally have a smooth surface, but cystic-appearing presentations have been reported.[149]

Merkel cell carcinoma is an aggressive tumor; metastases to regional lymph nodes are noted on initial

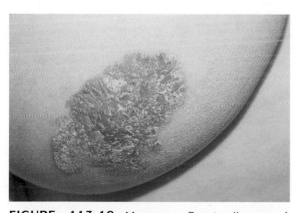

FIGURE 113-19. Mammary Paget disease. A red, scaling plaque drains serous fluid and forms a crust. The lesion appears eczematous but, unlike eczema, is unilateral. (From Habif TP: Clinical Dermatology, 4th ed. Philadelphia, Mosby, 2004.)

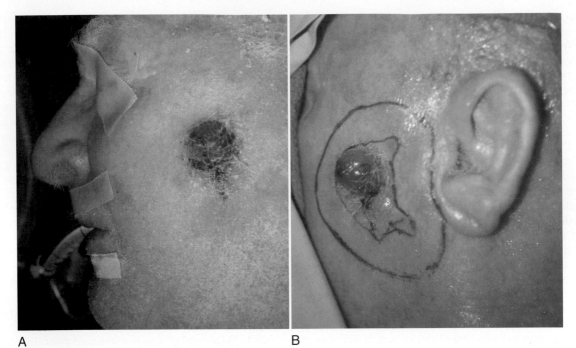

A   B

FIGURE 113-20. *A,* Merkel cell carcinoma. *B,* Extent of resection.

diagnosis in 12% to 15% of patients.[147] Regional metastasis eventually occurs in one half to two thirds of patients. Local recurrence after primary excision develops in 24% to 44% of patients. Time from diagnosis of the primary tumor to clinically apparent regional nodal metastases is approximately 7 to 8 months.[147,148] Distant metastases ultimately occur in one third of patients, in order of frequency, to lymph, liver, bone, brain, lung, and skin. The mean time from diagnosis to systemic involvement is 18 months, with death occurring 6 months later. Five-year survival has been reported as 30% to 64%. Two thirds or more of patients with local or regionally recurrent disease ultimately die.[147]

Surgical excision is the treatment of choice for primary tumors. The prevailing opinion regarding Merkel cell cancers is that they should be excised with margins similar to those for melanoma. Shaw,[150] in 1991, recommended surgical margins of 2.5 to 3 cm with irradiation if regional disease exists, coupled with prophylactic lymphadenectomy. Kahn et al[151] recommended a surgical margin of 3 cm, followed by local irradiation. Ott et al[152] recommended 2-cm margins combined with local or regional irradiation and sentinel lymph node biopsy with lymphadenectomy for patients with positive nodes. However, they could not demonstrate a survival advantage with node dissection. Boyer et al[153] advocated the use of Mohs technique and achieved a marginal recurrence of 4% and a local recurrence (marginal recurrence plus in-transit

metastases) of 16%. Their mean surgical margin of "clinically normal skin" was 16.7 mm.

Merkel cell carcinomas are radiosensitive, and radiation therapy should be considered for all patients. Chemotherapy has been effective for metastatic disease; however, its role in localized disease is undefined.[147]

SEBACEOUS CARCINOMAS

Sebaceous carcinoma, or meibomian gland carcinoma, is a malignant tumor derived from the adnexal epithelium of the sebaceous gland. Although sebaceous glands are found throughout the hair-bearing areas of the skin, 75% of all sebaceous carcinomas are on the eyelid.[154] The incidence of ocular sebaceous carcinoma ranks fourth, behind BCC, SCC, and malignant melanoma.[155] Ocular sebaceous carcinoma is generally seen in older patients (ranging from 60 to 80 years, with a mean age at occurrence of 63 years).[156] Other sites of sebaceous carcinoma include the head and neck, external genitalia, parotid and submandibular glands, external auditory canal, trunk, and upper extremity.[154]

Clinically, ocular sebaceous carcinoma presents as a small, firm, slowly enlarging deep-seated nodule of the eyelid (Fig. 113-21). It may also resemble many other types of tumors including keratoconjunctivitis, blepharoconjunctivitis, SCC, and BCC. Because this tumor has a presentation that is common to less aggres-

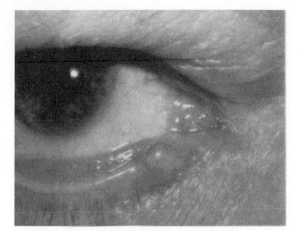

FIGURE 113-21. Sebaceous carcinoma of right medial lower lid. (From Nelson BR, Hamlet KR, Gillard M, et al: Sebaceous carcinoma. J Am Acad Dermatol 1995;33:1. Copyright 1995, with permission from The American Academy of Dermatology, Inc.)

sive carcinomas, the mean delay from onset of disease to diagnosis varies between 1.0 and 2.9 years.[157]

On histologic examination, sebaceous carcinoma is a dermal, nonencapsulated tumor with lobular, basaloid, and spindle cell patterns. Use of fresh tissue to prevent lipid dissolution and staining with special lipid stains, including oil red O and Sudan IV, aid in the diagnosis of sebaceous carcinoma (Fig. 113-22).[158]

Surgical excision is the preferred treatment, but there is controversy about the appropriate margins required for control of the disease. Although irradiation should not be considered for primary therapy, it may be useful for postoperative management and palliative care. Metastatic disease may be treated with a combination of excision, radiation therapy, and chemotherapy.[151]

Sebaceous carcinoma is considered an aggressive tumor, and local recurrences tend to occur within 5 years in 9% to 36% of patients. Metastasis occurs in

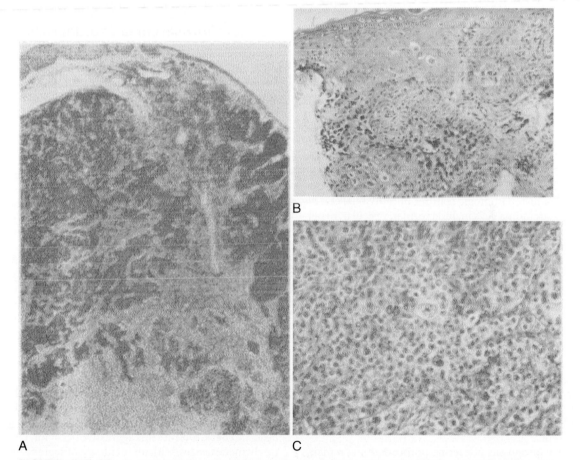

A   C

FIGURE 113-22. *A,* Basaloid type of sebaceous carcinoma. Note basaloid features and resemblance to BCC. (Hematoxylin and eosin stain; magnification ×150.) *B,* Sebaceous carcinoma of the eyelid demonstrates squamous features. (Hematoxylin and eosin stain; magnification ×250.) *C,* Well-differentiated sebaceous carcinoma. Note resemblance to mature sebocytes. (Hematoxylin and eosin stain; magnification ×250.) (From Nelson BR, Hamlet KR, Gillard M, et al: Sebaceous carcinoma. J Am Acad Dermatol 1995;33:1. Copyright 1995, with permission from The American Academy of Dermatology, Inc.)

14% to 25% of patients. Sites for metastases are the regional lymph nodes, liver, lung, brain, and bone. Metastasis may occur through lymphatic, hematogenous, lacrimal secretion, and excretory systems.[154]

ECCRINE CARCINOMAS

Eccrine carcinomas arise from the eccrine sweat glands. This is a rare tumor, representing approximately 0.005% of epithelial cutaneous neoplasms. Eccrine porocarcinoma is the most common variant. It originates from the intraepidermal ductal portion of the eccrine sweat gland (acrosyringium).[159]

The average age of a patient with eccrine porocarcinoma is 67.5 years.[160] In contrast to benign eccrine poroma, the location of malignant change is not correlated with the highest concentration of eccrine sweat glands (palmar and plantar areas). The main localizations are the lower limbs (55%, especially legs), followed by the head (nose, forehead, cheeks) and scalp (20%), then the upper limbs (12%) and the trunk and the abdomen (10%).[159]

Clinically, eccrine porocarcinoma may appear as a nodule or a verrucous, dome-shaped, cauliflower-like, infiltrated or erosive plaque or as a polypoid growth that is frequently ulcerated. Multinodularity, ulceration, and rapid growth may be associated with either locally recurrent or metastatic disease. Approximately 20% of eccrine porocarcinomas recur locally 4 months to 12 years after removal.[161] Another 20% metastasize to regional lymph nodes. In patients with lymph node involvement, there is a high mortality rate (approximately 67%).[160] Multiple cutaneous metastases can also develop.[162]

The histopathologic features of individual eccrine porocarcinoma cells include regular, vesicular, hyperchromatic, pleomorphic nucleus and abundant clear cytoplasm (Fig. 113-23). In some instances, variable amounts of glycogen contained in granules are seen in the cytoplasm of tumor cells. Another histologic feature of eccrine porocarcinoma is the presence in the tumor masses of many duct-like lumens.[163]

Because of the propensity for development of local recurrences, wide local excision of the primary tumor with histologic confirmation of tumor-free margins is the treatment of choice. Prophylactic lymphadenectomy should be done if regional nodes are enlarged or when a recurrent or poorly differentiated tumor with intralymphatic permeation is present.[164,165]

The prognosis of eccrine porocarcinoma remains difficult to assess. Tumors present for only a few weeks can be accompanied by both regional and visceral metastases, whereas others that may be present for many years have no evidence of metastatic spread. Once the tumor has metastasized, the outlook is poor.[163]

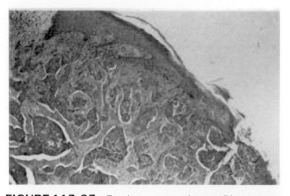

FIGURE 113-23. Eccrine porocarcinoma. Biopsy specimen showing well-demarcated nests of anaplastic tumor cells in dermis invading overlying epidermis and plugging some vessels. (Hematoxylin and eosin stain; original magnification ×10.) (From Huet P, Dandurand M, Pignodel C, Guillot B: Metastasizing eccrine porocarcinoma: report of a case and review of the literature. J Am Acad Dermatol 1996;35:860. Copyright 1996, with permission from The American Academy of Dermatology, Inc.)

Dermatofibrosarcoma Protuberans

Dermatofibrosarcoma protuberans (DFSP) is a locally aggressive fibroblastic tumor of the dermis. It is a rare tumor with an estimated incidence of 0.8 to 5 per 1 million persons per year.[166] There does not appear to be a hereditary or familial predisposition. It is predominantly a cancer of the young; most patients develop the disease between the ages of 20 and 50 years. Tumors in patients younger than 16 years are exceedingly rare, yet DFSP in newborns has been documented.[166] There appears to be a slight male predominance at 5:4.[167]

DFSP is found on the trunk (50% to 60%), the proximal extremities (20% to 30%), and the head and neck (10% to 15%).[166] Although up to 20% of patients provide a history that includes a trauma at the site of DFSP development, a definitive causal relationship has not been established.[166]

DFSP is a slowly enlarging malignant neoplasm. Growth can occur during months to decades. The tumor spreads with projections of neoplastic cells beneath clinically normal-appearing skin, making complete removal difficult. Recurrence rates of up to 60% are reported after standard surgical excision and 23% after wide excision with margins of more than 4 cm.[168,169] Uncontrolled local disease may result in death from spread into vital structures, especially the head and neck. Despite this aggressive behavior, DFSP rarely metastasizes, with an incidence of regional and distant metastases of 1% and 4%. Most patients who developed regional lymph node disease died within 2 years. For patients with distant metastases, survival ranged from 1 to 48 months with a mean of 14 months. The lung is the primary site of distant metastases, with

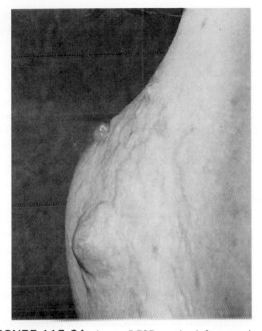

FIGURE 113-24. Large DFSP on the left upper back in a young woman—elevated firm papules and nodules that were initially misdiagnosed as cystic acne. (Courtesy of Kenneth E. Greer, MD. From Townsend CM: Sabiston Textbook of Surgery, 16th ed. Philadelphia, WB Saunders, 2001.)

reports of metastases to brain, bone, and peritracheal regions noted.[166]

DFSP presents clinically as an asymptomatic indurated red-brown or violaceous plaque (Fig. 113-24). It is usually a solitary lesion with a multicentric, firm nodule and soft plaque outgrowths. A high clinical suspicion is needed for early diagnosis because the indolent behavior and nonspecific features often cause DFSP to be dismissed by both the patient and the physician, leading to significant delay in diagnosis. DFSP has the histologic appearance of a well-differentiated fibrosarcoma (Fig. 113-25). The tumor arises from the dermis and is composed of a dense, uniform array of cells with spindle-shaped nuclei in a classic storiform pattern.[166]

Treatment for DFSP is surgical excision. Mohs micrographic surgery is the surgical method of choice for DFSP, with recurrence rates of 0.6% to 1.8%.[170] Prophylactic regional lymphadenectomy is not indicated. Adjuvant radiation therapy after excision is gaining acceptance, but it seems to be of limited benefit.

Kaposi Sarcoma

The definition of Kaposi sarcoma has undergone a dramatic revision during the past 20 years. Before the 1980s, it was a rare finding in the United States. However, with the AIDS epidemic, Kaposi sarcoma has become a frequent finding. Nonetheless, with sup-

pression of HIV replication, the incidence of Kaposi sarcoma is decreasing.[171]

This lesion was first described in 1872 by Moritz Kaposi. The so-called classic variety occurs in Jewish men of eastern European or Mediterranean descent. It develops in persons between the ages of 50 and 70 years and is most common on the lower extremities but can involve the gastrointestinal tract and lymph nodes.[172] The African variety of Kaposi sarcoma occurs in equatorial Africa, predominantly in men of younger age than with the classic variety. It has various manifestations ranging from localized skin tumors to a pediatric form that is more aggressive.[172]

AIDS-related Kaposi sarcoma has been termed an AIDS-defining condition by the Centers for Disease Control and Prevention; the presence of this lesion in persons who are HIV positive indicates that they have AIDS. These lesions most often involve skin and mucous membranes (oral and gastrointestinal) but can also involve solid organs, lymph nodes, and lung. The head and neck is a common site; the lesions are pigmented (purple to brownish black) and range in size from millimeters to a few centimeters. Lesions may be either flat (plaque-like) or raised as papules or nodules (Fig. 113-26).

On histologic evaluation, the tumor produces angiogenesis, inflammatory cells, and CD34 tumor spindle cells.[173] Human herpesvirus type 8 is an etio-

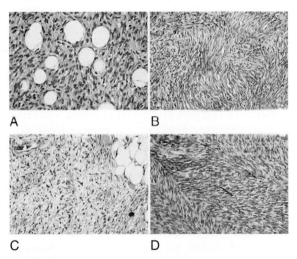

FIGURE 113-25. *A,* Bland spindle-shaped cells of DFSP intercalating between individual adipocytes in a honeycomb fashion. *B,* Classic storiform growth pattern of DFSP. *C,* Loose myxoid area within DFSP. Similar areas can be seen in spindle cell lipoma. *D,* Herringbone pattern of spindled cells with increased mitotic activity *(arrows)* characteristic of fibrosarcomatous transformation of DFSP. (From Harvell JD: Multiple spindle cell lipomas and dermatofibrosarcoma protuberans within a single patient: evidence for a common neoplastic process of interstitial dendritic cells. J Am Acad Dermatol 2003;48:82. Copyright 2003, with permission from The American Academy of Dermatology, Inc.)

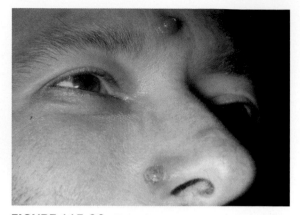

FIGURE 113-26. Kaposi sarcoma.

logic agent and is present within the tissues.[174] Kaposi sarcoma in this setting is not curable. However, local and systemic control can be achieved by a variety of therapies; the most important is antiretroviral therapy aimed at the underlying disease. Other therapies include alitretinoin topical gel (1%), which is applied to the lesion on a daily basis; radiation therapy may cause remission, but it can also cause toxicity and local fibrosis. Intralesional injection of vinblastine has produced some response; cryotherapy and liquid nitrogen have also been used with some success.[175] Surgical excision may result in local control, but it does nothing for the systemic disease, and recurrence is frequent.

Cutaneous T-Cell Lymphoma

Cutaneous T-cell lymphoma includes mycosis fungoides and Sézary syndrome, which are cancers of T4 helper cells. This type of skin cancer is rare, occurring in approximately 3.6 per 1 million people.[176] The incidence is higher in blacks than in whites, and it rarely occurs in Asians.[177]

The initial clinical appearance of cutaneous T-cell lymphoma is as a patch or plaque. The lesion may appear erythematous and eczematous or may be similar to a mild psoriatic lesion with elevation and scale. Additional clinical symptoms include persistent itching and a lesion that remains in the same location for an extended period. Diagnosis of cutaneous T-cell lymphoma is commonly delayed because it mimics other cutaneous disorders.[178] Whereas the initial course of this lesion may be slow, it can progress over time to frank lymphoma with bone marrow, blood lymphocyte, lymph node, and visceral involvement or Sézary syndrome, which is the corresponding progression to leukemia.

Patients with early disease, characterized by skin lesions with limited or generalized plaque, have 5-year survival rates ranging from 40% to 100%. However,

advanced disease carries a worse prognosis, especially in patients with lymph node involvement. The median survival in these patients is 3 years (Fig. 113-27).[179]

The several different treatment modalities for cutaneous T-cell lymphoma include topical nitrogen mustard, PUVA, PUVA plus interferon, total skin electron beam therapy, interferons and retinoids, and combined modality therapy.[180] Therapy is much more effective in patients with early disease as opposed to patients with advanced disease, in whom relapse-free survival is uncommon.[180]

SUMMARY

The successful plastic surgeon who cares for patients with cutaneous malignant neoplasms must become well versed in an increasing array of diagnostic and treatment modalities. The specialty must continue to be aware of progress in immunology and histochemistry as well as in allied fields of radiation therapy, chemotherapy, and dermatopathology.

Patients must be educated about the causes of skin cancers, and plastic surgeons must become advocates for prophylactic measures to reduce the incidence of skin malignant neoplasms. Greater numbers of persons are becoming immunosuppressed, either from iatrogenic causes such as treatment after transplantation or because of the AIDS epidemic. As a result, the susceptibility to the formation of skin cancers is also rising. Considering the increasing incidence of skin cancers in the United States alone, with an estimated 1 million new diagnoses per year, advances in technology and public health are required to reverse this course. Heightened public awareness will help, but it will also place increasing demands on the medical profession in general and on the plastic surgeon.

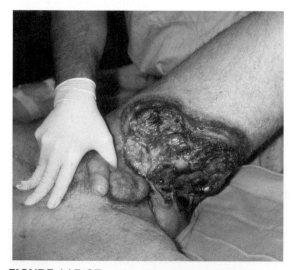

FIGURE 113-27. Cutaneous T-cell lymphoma.

REFERENCES

1. Cole P, Rodu B: Declining cancer mortality in the United States. Cancer 1996;78:2045.

2. Jemal A, Murray T, Samuels A, et al: Cancer statistics, 2003. CA Cancer J Clin 2003;53:5.

3. Parkin DM, Pisani P, Ferlay J: Global cancer statistics. CA Cancer J Clin 1999;49:33.

4. Brash DE, Ziegler A, Jonason AS, et al: Sunlight and sunburn in human skin cancer: p53, apoptosis, and tumor promotion. J Invest Dermatol Symp Proc 1996;1:136.

5. Kelner A, Taft EB: Influence of photoreactivating light on type and frequency of tumors induced by ultraviolet radiation. Cancer Res 1956;16:860.

6. Pathak MA, Fitzpatrick TB, Parrish JA: Topical and systemic approaches to protection of human skin against harmful effects of solar radiation. In Regan JD, Parrish JA, eds: The Science of Photomedicine. New York, Plenum, 1982:441.

7. Willis I, Menter JM, Whyte I IJ. The rapid induction of cancers in the hairless mouse utilizing the principle of photoaugmentation. J Invest Dermatol 1981;76:404.

8. Lim HW, Cooper K: The health impact of solar radiation and prevention strategies. J Am Acad Dermatol 1999;41:81.

9. Madronich S, de Gruijl FR: Stratospheric ozone depletion between 1979 and 1992: implications for biologically active ultraviolet B and non-melanoma skin cancer incidence. Photochem Photobiol 1994;59:541.

10. Urbach F: Geographic distribution of skin cancer. J Surg Oncol 1971;3:219.

11. Epstein JH: Photocarcinogenesis, skin cancer and aging. J Am Acad Dermatol 1983;9:487.

12. Pathak MA, Fitzpatrick TB: The role of natural photoprotective agents in human skin. In Pathak MA, et al, eds: Sunlight and Man: Normal and Abnormal Photobiologic Responses. Tokyo, University of Tokyo Press, 1976:725.

13. Cesarini JP: Soleil et peau. J Med Esthet 1977;14:5.

14. Malvy J, Guinot C, Preziosis P, et al: Epidemiologic determinants of skin photoaging: baseline data of the SU.VI.MAX. cohort. J Am Acad Dermatol 2000;42:47.

15. Conway H, Hugo NE: Radiation dermatitis and malignancy. Plast Reconstr Surg 1966;28:255.

16. Ron E, Modan B, Preston D, et al: Radiation-induced skin carcinomas of the head and neck. Radiat Res 1991;125:318.

17. Kripke ML: Immunology of murine skin cancers. In Conti C, Slaga T, Klein-Szanto AJ, eds: Skin Tumors: Experimental and Clinical Aspects. New York, Raven Press, 1989:273.

18. Strickland FM, Kripke ML: Immune response associated with nonmelanoma skin cancer. Clin Plast Surg 1997;24:637.

19. Alcalay J, Craig JN, Kripke ML: Alterations in Langerhans cells and thy-1+ dendritic epidermal cells in murine epidermis during the evolution of ultraviolet radiation-induced skin cancers. Cancer Res 1989;49:4591.

20. Mukhtar H, Agarwal R: Skin cancer chemoprevention. J Invest Dermatol Symp Proc 1996;1:209.

21. Nakamura T, Pinnell SR, Streilein JW: Antioxidants can reverse the deleterious effects of ultraviolet B (UVB) radiation on cutaneous immunity. J Invest Dermatol 1995;104:600.

22. Birkeland SA, Storm HH, Lamm LU, et al: Cancer risk after renal transplantation in the Nordic countries, 1964-1986. Int J Cancer 1995;60:183.

23. Marshall V: Pre-malignant and malignant skin tumors in immunosuppressed patients. Transplantation 1974;17:272.

24. Wang CY, Brodland DG, Su WP: Skin cancers associated with acquired immunodeficiency syndrome. Mayo Clin Proc 1995;70:766.

25. Franceschi S, Dal Maso L, Arniani S, et al: Risk of cancer other than Kaposi's sarcoma and non-Hodgkin's lymphoma in persons with AIDS in Italy. Cancer and AIDS registry linkage study. Br J Cancer 1998;78:966.

26. Marjolin JN: Ulcere. In Le Berne P, ed: Dictionnaire de medicine, vol 21. Paris, Bechet, 1828:46.

27. Konigova R, Rychterova V: Marjolin's ulcer. Acta Chir Plast 2000;42:91.

28. Ozyazgan I, Kontacs O: Basal cell carcinoma arising from surgical scars: a case and review of the literature. Dermatol Surg 1999;25:965.

29. Akguner M, Barutcu A, Yilmaz M, et al: Marjolin's ulcer in chronic burn scarring. J Wound Care 1998;7:121.

30. Hahn SB, Kim DJ, Jeon CH: Clinical study of Marjolin's ulcer. Yonsei Med J 1990;31:234.

31. Hall EJ: From chimney sweeps to astronauts: cancer risks in the work place: the 1998 Lauriston Taylor lecture. Health Phys 1998;75:357.

32. Mastrangelo G, Fadda E, Marzia V: Polycyclic aromatic hydrocarbons and cancer in man. Environ Health Perspect 1996;104:1166.

33. Epstein JH: Phototoxicity and photoallergy. Semin Cutan Med Surg 1999;18:274.

34. Peters BP, Weissman FG, Gill MA: Pathophysiology and treatment of psoriasis. Am J Health Syst Pharm 2000;57:645.

35. Chignell CF, Haseman JK, Sik RH, et al: Photocarcinogenesis in the Tg.AC mouse: lomefloxacin and 8-methoxypsoralen. Photochem Photobiol 2003;77:77.

36. McLaughlin JK: Formaldehyde and cancer: a critical review. Int Arch Occup Environ Health 1994;66:295.

37. IARC: Formaldehyde. IARC Monogr Eval Carcinog Risks Hum 1995;62:217.

38. Goldsmith L, Koh HK, Bewerse B, et al: Proceedings from the national conference to develop a national skin cancer agenda: American Academy of Dermatology and Centers for Disease Control and Prevention, April 8-10, 1995. J Am Acad Dermatol 1996;34:822.

39. Stenberg C, Larkö O: Sunscreen application and its importance for the sun protection factor. Arch Dermatol 1985;121:1400.

40. Ananthaswamy HN, Loughlin SM, Ullrich SE, Kripke ML: Inhibition of UV-induced p53 mutations by sun screens: implications for skin cancer prevention. J Invest Dermatol Symp Proc 1998;3:52.

41. Bestak R, Barnetson SR, Nearn MR, Halliday GM: Sunscreen protection of contact hypersensitivity responses from chronic solar-simulated ultraviolet irradiation correlates with the absorption spectrum of the sun screen. J Invest Dermatol 1995;105:345.

42. Mukhtar H, Agarwal R: Skin cancer chemoprevention. J Invest Dermatol Symp Proc 1996;1:209.

43. Ahmad N, Mukhtar H: Cutaneous photochemoprotection by green tea: a brief review. Skin Pharmacol Appl Skin Physiol 2001;14:69.

44. Strickland FM, Pelley RP, Kripke ML: Prevention of ultraviolet radiation-induced suppression of contact and delayed hypersensitivity by Aloe barbadensis gel extract. J Invest Dermatol 1994;102:197.

45. Levine M: The evolving role of retinoids in the management of cutaneous conditions. J Am Acad Dermatol 1998;39:s62.

46. Black HS: Influence of dietary factors on actinically-induced skin cancer. Mutat Res 1998;422:185.

47. Glogau RG: Actinic keratoses—scientific evaluation and public health implications: the risk of progression to invasive disease. J Am Acad Dermatol 2000;42:23.

48. Cockerell CJ: Histopathology of incipient intraepidermal squamous cell carcinoma (actinic keratosis). J Am Acad Dermatol 2000;42:11.

49. Guenthner ST, Hurwitz RM, Buckel LJ, Gray HR: Cutaneous squamous cell carcinomas consistently show histologic evidence of in situ changes: a clinicopathologic correlation. J Am Acad Dermatol 1999;41:443.

50. Mittelbronn MA, Mullins DL, Ramos-Caro FA, Flowers FP: Frequency of preexisting actinic keratosis in cutaneous squamous cell carcinoma. Int J Dermatol 1998;37:677.

51. Tsukifuji R, Tagawa K, Hatamochi A, Shinkai H: Expression of matrix metalloproteinase-1, -2 and -3 in squamous cell carcinoma and actinic keratosis. Br J Cancer 1999;80:1087.

52. Dinehart SM, Nelson-Adesokan P, Cockerell C, et al: Metastatic cutaneous squamous cell carcinoma derived from actinic keratosis. Cancer 1997;79:920.

53. Callen JP: Possible precursors to epidermal malignancies in cancer of the skin. In Friedman RJ, Rigel DS, Kopf AW, et al, eds: Cancer of the Skin. Philadelphia, WB Saunders, 1991:27.

54. Tope WD, Nowfar-Rad M, Kist DA: Ber-EP4-positive phenotype differentiates actinic keratosis from superficial basal cell carcinoma. Dermatol Surg 2000;26:415.

55. Barta U, Grafe T, Wollina U: Radiation therapy for extensive actinic keratosis. J Eur Acad Dermatol Venereol 2000;14:293.

56. Lober BA, Lober CW: Actinic keratosis is squamous cell carcinoma. South Med J 2000;93:650.

57. Hurwitz RM, Monger LE: Solar keratosis: an evolving squamous cell carcinoma: benign or malignant? Dermatol Surg 1995;21:183.

58. Ansai S, Mihara I: Sebaceous carcinoma arising on actinic keratosis. Eur J Dermatol 2000;10:385.

59. Löning T, Ikenberg H, Becker J, et al: Analysis of oral papillomas, leukoplakias, and invasive carcinomas for human papilloma virus type related DNA. J Invest Dermatol 1985;84:417.

60. Waldron CA, Shafer WG: Leukoplakia revisited. A clinicopathologic study of 3,256 leukoplakias. Cancer 1975;36:1386.

61. Lever WF: Tumors and cysts of the epidermis. In Lever WF, Schaumberg-Lever S, eds: Histopathology of the Skin, 7th ed. Philadelphia, JB Lippincott, 1990:546.

62. Shiu MN, Chen TH, Chang SH, Hahn LJ: Risk factors for leukoplakia and malignant transformation to oral carcinoma: a leukoplakia cohort in Taiwan. Br J Cancer 2000;82:1871.

63. Saito T, Sugiuria C, Hirai A, et al: Development of squamous cell carcinoma from preexistent oral leukoplakia: with respect to treatment modality. Int J Oral Maxillofac Surg 2001;30:49.

64. Lenz C, Dietz A, Pfuhl A, et al: Detection of numerical chromosome aberrations in leukoplakia and squamous epithelial carcinomas of the head-neck area using fluorescence in situ hybridization. HNO 2000;48:367.

65. Robbins JH, Kraemer KH, Lutzner MA, et al: Xeroderma pigmentosum. An inherited disease with sun sensitivity, multiple cutaneous neoplasms, and abnormal DNA repair. Ann Intern Med 1974;80:221.

66. Robbins JH: Xeroderma pigmentosum. Defective DNA repair causes skin cancer and neurodegeneration. JAMA 1988;260:384.

67. Cleaver JE, Volpe JP, Charles WC, Thomas GH: Prenatal diagnosis of xeroderma pigmentosum and Cockayne syndrome. Prenat Diagn 1994;14:921.

68. Stone N, Reed J, Mahood J, et al: Xeroderma pigmentosum, the role of photo testing. Br J Dermatol 2000;143:595.

69. Cleaver JE, Thompson LH, Richardson AS, States JC: A summary of mutations in the UV-sensitive disorders: xeroderma pigmentosum, Cockayne syndrome, and trichothiodystrophy. Hum Mutat 1999;14:9.

70. Mathur R, Chowdhury MR, Singh G: Recent advances in chromosome breakage syndrome and their diagnosis. Indian Pediatr 2000;37:615.

71. Kramer KH, Lee MM, Scotto J: DNA repair protects against cutaneous and internal neoplasia: evidence from xeroderma pigmentosum. Carcinogenesis 1984;5:511.

72. De Luca LM: Multiple mechanisms: the example of vitamin A. Basic Life Sci 1993;61:17.

73. Yarosh D, Klein J, O'Connor A, et al: Effect of topically applied T4 endonuclease V in liposomes on skin cancer in xeroderma pigmentosum: a randomized study. Xeroderma Pigmentosum Study Group. Lancet 2001;357:926.

74. Hutchinson J: Morbid growths and tumours: 1: the "crateriform" ulcer of the face, a form of acute epithelial cancer. Trans Pathol Soc London 1889;40:275.

75. Schwartz RA: Keratoacanthoma: a clinico-pathologic enigma. Dermatol Surg 2004;30:2.

76. Kwitten J: Dermatologic pseudobenignities. Mt Sinai J Med 1980;47:34.

77. Kwitten J: A histologic chronology of the clinical course of the keratocarcinoma (so-called keratoacanthoma). Mt Sinai J Med 1975;42:127.

78. Strieth S, Hartschuh W, Pilz L, Fusenig NE: Carcinoma-like vascular density in atypic keratoacanthoma suggests malignant progression. Br J Cancer 2002;87:1301.

79. Schwartz RA: Keratoacanthoma. J Am Acad Dermatol 1994;30:1.

80. Goudie DR, Yuille MAR, Leversha MA, et al: Multiple self-healing squamous epitheliomata (ESS1) mapped to chromosome 9q22-q31 in families with common ancestry. Nat Genet 1993;3:165.

81. Godbolt AM, Sullivan JJ, Weedon D: Keratoacanthoma with perineural invasion: a report of 40 cases. Australas J Dermatol 2002;43:155.

82. Sau P, McMarlin SL, Sperling LC, et al: Bowen's disease of the nail bed and periungual area: a clinicopathologic analysis of 7 cases. Arch Dermatol 1994;130:204.

83. Graham JH, Helwig EB: Bowen's disease and its relationship to systemic cancer. Arch Dermatol 1959;80:133.

84. Graham JH, Helwig EB: Precancerous skin lesions and systemic cancer. In M.D. Anderson Hospital and Tumor Institute: Tumors of the Skin; a Collection of Papers Presented at the Seventh Annual Clinical Conference on Cancer, 1962, at the University of Texas M.D. Anderson Hospital and Tumor Institute, Houston, Texas. Chicago, Year Book, 1964:209.

85. Gherardini G, Bhatia N, Stal S: Congenital syndromes associated with nonmelanoma skin cancer. Clin Plast Surg 1997;24:655.

86. Nuovo GJ, Ishag M: The histologic spectrum of epidermodysplasia verruciformis. Am J Surg Pathol 2000;24:1400.

87. Jaqueti G, Requena L, Sanchez Yus E: Trichoblastoma is the most common neoplasm developed in nevus sebaceus of Jadassohn: a clinicopathologic study of a series of 155 cases. Am J Dermatopathol 2000;22:108.

88. Cribier B, Scrivener Y, Grosshans E: Tumors arising in nevus sebaceus: a study of 596 cases. J Am Acad Dermatol 2000;42(pt 1):263.

89. Labbe D, Badie Modiri B, Betit F: Sebaceous nevus of Jadassohn apropos of 62 surgically treated cases and review of the literature. Rev Stomatol Chir Maxillofac 1999;100:175.

90. Beer GM, Widder W, Cierpka K, et al: Malignant tumors associated with nevus sebaceus: therapeutic consequences. Aesthetic Plast Surg 1999;23:224.

91. Happle R: Cancer proneness of linear porokeratosis may be explained by allelic loss. Dermatology 1997;195:20.

92. Chernosky ME: Porokeratosis. Arch Dermatol 1986; 122:869.

93. Xia JH, Yang YF, Deng H, et al: Identification of a locus for disseminated superficial actinic porokeratosis at chromosome 12q23.2-24.1. J Invest Dermatol 2000;114:1071.

94. Pinkus H: Premalignant fibroepithelial tumors of the skin. Arch Dermatol 1953;67:598.

95. Miller SJ: Biology of basal cell carcinoma (part I). J Am Acad Dermatol 1991;24:1.

96. Habif TP: Clinical Dermatology, 4th ed. Philadelphia, Mosby, 2004.

97. Shanoff LB, Spira M, Hardy SB: Basal cell carcinoma: a statistical approach to rational management. Plast Reconstr Surg 1976;39:619.

98. Kimura S: Three-dimensional architecture of epithelial skin tumors: an application of epidermal separation. J Dermatol 1981;8:13.

99. Roenigk RK, Ratz JL, Bailin PL, et al: Trends in the presentation and treatment of basal cell carcinoma. J Dermatol Surg Oncol 1986;12:860.

100. Lang PG Jr, Maize JC: Basal cell carcinoma. In Friedman RJ, Rigel DS, Kopf AW, et al, eds: Cancer of the Skin. Philadelphia, WB Saunders, 1991:61.

101. Salasche SJ: Status of curettage and desiccation in the treatment of primary basal cell carcinoma. J Am Acad Dermatol 1984;10:285.

102. Hallock GG, Lutz DA: Prospective study of the accuracy of the surgeon's diagnosis in 2000 excised skin tumors. Plast Reconstr Surg 1998;101:1255.

103. Sexton M, Jones DB, Maloney ME: Histologic pattern analysis of basal cell carcinoma: study of a series of 1039 consecutive neoplasms. J Am Acad Dermatol 1990;23:1118.

104. Silverman MK, Kopf AW, Bart RS, et al: Recurrence rates of treated basal cell carcinomas. Part 3: Surgical excision. J Dermatol Surg Oncol 1992;18:471.

105. Dubin N, Kopf AW: Multivariate risk score for recurrence of cutaneous basal cell carcinomas. Arch Dermatol 1983;119:373.

106. Shanoff LB, Spira M, Hardy SB: Basal cell carcinoma: a statistical approach to rational management. Plast Reconstr Surg 1967;39:619.

107. Pascal R, Hobby L, Lattes R, Crikelair G: Prognosis of incompletely excised versus completely excised basal cell carcinoma. Plast Reconstr Surg 1968;41:328.

108. Dellon AL, DeSilva S, Connolly M, Ross A: Prediction of recurrence in incompletely excised basal cell carcinoma. Plast Reconstr Surg 1985;75:860.

109. Mohs FE: Chemosurgery: a microscopically controlled method of cancer excision. Arch Surg 1941;42:279.

110. Tromovitch TA, Stegman SJ: Microscopic-controlled excision of cutaneous tumors: chemosurgery, fresh tissue technique. Cancer 1978;41:653.

111. Epstein E: Fluorouracil paste treatment of thin basal cell carcinomas. Arch Dermatol 1985;121:207.

112. Caccialanza M, Piccinno R, Grammatica A: Radiotherapy of recurrent basal and squamous cell skin carcinomas: a study of 249 re-treated carcinomas in 229 patients. Eur J Dermatol 2001;11:25.

113. Silverman MK, Kopf AW, Gladstein AH, et al: Recurrence rates of treated basal cell carcinomas. Part 4: X ray therapy. J Dermatol Surg Oncol 1992;18:549.

114. Andrews MD: Cryosurgery for common skin conditions. Am Fam Physician 2004;69:2365.

115. Takata M: Nevoid basal cell carcinoma syndrome. Nippon Rinsho 2000;58:1876.

116. Lo Muzio L, Nocini P, Bucci P, et al: Early diagnosis of nevoid basal cell carcinoma syndrome. J Am Dent Assoc 1999;130:669.

117. Lo Muzio L, Nocini PF, Savora A, et al: Nevoid basal cell carcinoma syndrome: clinical findings in 37 Italian affected individuals. Clin Genet 1999;55:34.

118. Goldstein AM, Bale SJ, Peck GL, et al: Sun exposure and basal cell carcinomas in the nevoid basal cell carcinoma syndrome. J Am Acad Dermatol 1993;29:34.

119. Kagy MK, Amonette R: The use of imiquimod 5% cream for the treatment of superficial basal cell carcinomas in a basal cell nevus syndrome patient. Dermatol Surg 2000;26:577.

120. Roth JJ, Granick MS: Squamous cell and adnexal carcinomas of the skin. Clin Plast Surg 1997;24:687.

121. Marks R, Ronnie G, Selwood T: The relationship of basal cell carcinomas and squamous cell carcinomas to solar keratoses. Arch Dermatol 1988;124:1039.

122. McGregor JM, Morris R, Smith CH, MacDonald DM: Skin cancer morbidity amongst renal allograft recipients—a 25-year retrospective follow-up study. Br J Dermatol 1995;133:40.

123. Hartevelt MM, Bavinck JN, Kootte AM, et al: Incidence of skin cancer after renal transplantation in the Netherlands. Transplantation 1990;49:506.

124. Gearhart PA, Randall TC: Human papillomavirus. Available at: http://www.emedicine.com. Accessed August 8, 2004.

125. Orth G, Jablonska S, Jarzabek-Chorzelska M, et al: Characteristics of the lesions and risk of malignant conversion associated with the type of human papillomavirus involved in epidermodysplasia verruciformis. Cancer Res 1979;39:1074.

126. Berkhout RJ, Bavinck JN, ter Schegget J: Persistence of human papillomavirus DNA in benign and (pre)malignant skin lesions from renal transplant recipients. J Clin Microbiol 2000;38:2087.

127. de Villiers EM: Human papillomavirus infections in skin cancers. Biomed Pharmacother 1998;52:26.

128. Feltkamp MC, Broer R, di Summa FM, et al: Seroreactivity to epidermodysplasia verruciformis-related human papillomavirus types is associated with nonmelanoma skin cancer. Cancer Res 2003;63:2695.

129. Broders AC: Squamous-cell epithelioma of the skin. Ann Surg 1921;73:141.

130. Frierson HF Jr, Cooper PH: Prognostic factors in squamous cell carcinoma of the lower lip. Hum Pathol 1986;17:346.

131. Mendenhall WM, Amdur RJ, Williams LS, et al: Carcinoma of the skin of the head and neck with perineural invasion. Head Neck 2002;24:78.

132. Luce EA: Oncologic considerations in nonmelanotic skin cancer. Clin Plast Surg 1995;22:39.

133. Abide JM, Nahai F, Bennett RG: The meaning of surgical margins. Plast Reconstr Surg 1984;73:492.

134. Freeman RG, Knox JM, Heaton CL: The treatment of skin cancer. Cancer 1964;17:535.

135. Chernosky ME: Squamous cell and basal cell carcinomas: preliminary study of 3818 primary skin cancers. South Med J 1978;71:802.

136. Dzubow L, Grossman DJ: Squamous cell carcinoma and verrucous carcinoma. In Friedman RJ, Rigel DS, Kopf AW, et al, eds: Cancer of the Skin. Philadelphia, WB Saunders, 1991:80.

137. Demian SDE, Bushkin FL, Echevarria RA: Perineural invasion and anaplastic transformation of verrucous carcinoma. Cancer 1973;32:395.

138. Moller R, Reymann F, Hou-Jensen K: Metastases in dermatological patients with squamous cell carcinoma. Arch Dermatol 1979;115:703.

139. Dinehart SM, Pollack SV: Metastases from squamous cell carcinoma of the skin and lip. J Am Acad Dermatol 1989;21:241.

140. Kwa RE, Campana K, Moy RL: Biology of cutaneous squamous cell carcinoma. J Am Acad Dermatol 1992;26:1.

141. Bessede JP, Vinh D, Khalifa N, et al: Lymph node metastases of cutaneous epidermoid carcinomas of the head and neck: prognostic factors and therapeutic strategies. Apropos of a series of 13 cases. Rev Laryngol Otol Rhinol (Bord) 2001;122:111.

142. Wagner JD, Evdokimow DZ, Weisberger E, et al: Sentinel node biopsy for high-risk nonmelanoma cutaneous malignancy. Arch Dermatol 2004;140:75.

143. Michl C, Starz H, Bachter D, Balda BR: Sentinel lymphonodectomy in nonmelanoma skin malignancies. Br J Dermatol 2003;149:763.

144. Weisberg NK, Bertagnolli MM, Becker DS: Combined sentinel lymphadenectomy and Mohs micrographic surgery for high-risk cutaneous squamous cell carcinoma. J Am Acad Dermatol 2000;43:483.

145. Werner JA, Dunne AA, Ramaswamy A, et al: The sentinel node concept in head and neck cancer: solution for the controversies in the N0 neck? Head Neck 2004;26:603.

146. Rook A, Wilkinson DS, Ebling FJB, et al: Textbook of Dermatology, 4th ed. Oxford, Blackwell, 1986.

147. Haag ML, Glass LF, Fenske NA: Merkel cell carcinoma. Dermatol Surg 1995;21:669.

148. Goepfert H, Remmler D, Silva E, et al: Merkel cell carcinoma (endocrine carcinoma of the skin) of the head and neck. Arch Otolaryngol 1984;110:707.

149. Warner TF, Uno H, Hafez GR, et al: Merkel cells and Merkel cell tumors: ultrastructure, immunocytochemistry, and review of the literature. Cancer 1983;52:238.

150. Shaw JH, Rumball E: Merkel cell tumour: clinical behaviour and treatment. Br J Surg 1991;78:138.

151. Khan Durani B, Hartschuh W: Merkel cell carcinoma. Clinical and histological differential diagnosis, diagnostic approach and therapy. Hautarzt 2003;54:1171.

152. Ott MJ, Tanabe KK, Gadd M, et al: Multimodality management of Merkel cell carcinoma. Arch Surg 1999;134:388.

153. Boyer JD, Zitelli JA, Brodland DG, D'Angelo G: Local control of primary Merkel cell carcinoma: review of 45 cases treated with Mohs micrographic surgery with and without adjuvant radiation. J Am Acad Dermatol 2002;47:885.

154. Nelson BR, Hamlet KR, Gilliard M: Sebaceous carcinoma. J Am Acad Dermatol 1995;33:1.

155. Kwitko ML, Boniuk M, Zimmerman LE: Eyelid tumors with reference to lesions confused with squamous cell carcinoma: I. Incidence and errors in diagnosis. Arch Ophthalmol 1963;69:696.

156. Bailet JW, Zimmerman MC, Arnstein DP, et al: Sebaceous carcinoma of the head and neck: case report and review of the literature. Arch Otolaryngol Head Neck Surg 1992;118:1245.

157. Ni C, Kuo PK: Meibomian gland carcinoma: a clinicopathologic study of 156 cases with long-period follow-up of 100 cases. Jpn J Ophthalmol 1979;23:388.

158. Ni C, Searl SS, Kuo PK: Sebaceous carcinomas of the ocular adnexa. Int Ophthalmol Clin 1982;22:23.

159. Wick MR, Coffin MC: Adnexal carcinomas of the skin, I. Eccrine carcinomas. Cancer 1985;56:1147.

160. Snow SN, Reizner GT: Eccrine porocarcinoma of the face. J Am Acad Dermatol 1992;27:306.

161. Mehregan AH, Hashimoto K, Rahbari H: Eccrine adenocarcinoma: clinicopathological study of 35 cases. Arch Dermatol 1983;119:104.

162. Matloub HS, Cunningham MW, Yousif NJ, et al: Eccrine porocarcinoma. Ann Plast Surg 1988;20:351.

163. Huet P, Dandurand M, Pignodel C, Guillot B: Metastasizing eccrine porocarcinoma: report of a case and review of the literature. J Am Acad Dermatol 1996;35:860.

164. Goedde TA, Bumpers H, Fiscella J, et al: Eccrine porocarcinoma. J Surg Oncol 1994;55:261.

165. El Domeiri AA, Brasfield RD, Huvos AG, et al: Sweat gland carcinoma: clinicopathologic study of 83 patients. Ann Surg 1971;173:270.

166. Gloster HM, Brodland DG: The epidemiology of skin cancer. Dermatol Surg 1996;22:217.

167. Rutgers EJ, Kroon BR, Albus-Lutter CE, et al: Dermatofibrosarcoma protuberans: treatment and prognosis. Eur J Surg Oncol 1992;18:241.

168. Mark RJ, Bailet JW, Tran LM, et al: Dermatofibrosarcoma protuberans of the head and neck: a report of 16 cases. Arch Otolaryngol Head Neck Surg 1993;119:891.

169. Waldermann F, Hagedorn M: Clinical picture and pathology of dermatofibrosarcoma protuberans. Z Hautkr 1985; 60:1886.

170. Ratner D, Thomas CO, Johnson TM, et al: Mohs micrographic surgery for the treatment of dermatofibrosarcoma protuberans. J Am Acad Dermatol 1997;37:600.

171. Mitsuyasu RT: Update on the pathogenesis and treatment of Kaposi's sarcoma. Curr Opin Oncol 2000;12:174.

172. American Cancer Society: What is Kaposi's sarcoma? Available at: http://www.cancer.org/docroot/cri/content/cri_2_4_1x_what_is_kaposis_sarcoma_21.asp?sitearea=cri.

173. Pyakurel P, Massambu C, Castanos-Velez E, et al: Human herpesvirus 8/Kaposi sarcoma herpesvirus cell association during evolution of Kaposi sarcoma. J Acquir Immune Defic Syndr 2004;36:678.

174. Levine AM, Tulpule A: Clinical aspects and management of AIDS-related Kaposi's sarcoma. Eur J Cancer 2001;37: 1288.

175. Dezube BJ: Acquired immunodeficiency syndrome-related Kaposi's sarcoma: clinical features, staging, and treatment. Semin Oncol 2000;27:424.

176. Jones GW: Total skin electron radiation in the management of mycosis fungoides: consensus of the European Organization for Research and Treatment of Cancer (EORTC) Cutaneous Lymphoma Project Group. J Am Acad Dermatol 2002;47:364.

177. Weinstock MA, Gardstein B: Twenty-year trends in the reported incidence of mycosis fungoides and associated mortality. Am J Public Health 1999;89:1240.

178. Zackheim HS, McCalmont TH: Mycosis fungoides: the great imitator. J Am Acad Dermatol 2002;47:914.

179. Lamberg SI, Green SB, Byar DP, et al: Clinical staging for cutaneous T-cell lymphoma. Ann Intern Med 1984;100:187.

180. Duvic M, Lemak NA, Redman JR, et al: Combined modality therapy for cutaneous T-cell lymphoma. J Am Acad Dermatol 1996;34:1022.

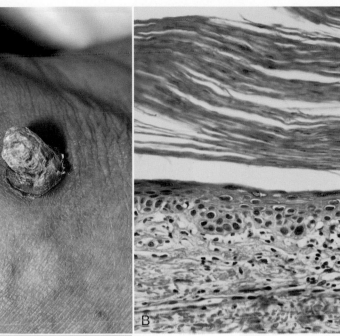

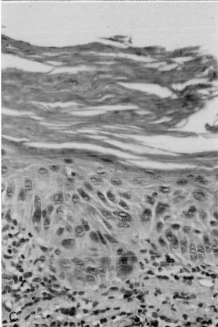

COLOR PLATE 113-1. Actinic keratosis. *A*, Excessive scale formation in this lesion has produced a "cutaneous horn." *B*, Basal cell layer atypia is associated with marked hyperkeratosis and parakeratosis. *C*, Progression to full-thickness nuclear atypia, with or without superficial epidermal maturation, heralds the development of early SCC in situ. (From Cotran RS, Kumar V, Collins T: Robbins Pathologic Basis of Disease, 6th ed. Philadelphia, WB Saunders, 1999.)

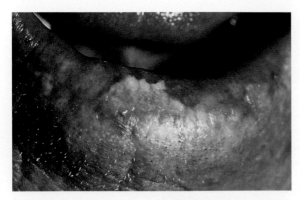

COLOR PLATE 113-2. Leukoplakia. (From Habif TP: Clinical Dermatology, 4th ed. Philadelphia, Mosby, 2004.)

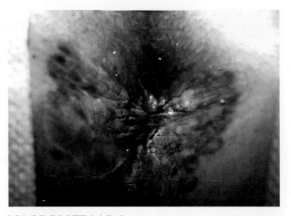

COLOR PLATE 113-4. Bowen disease of perianal skin.

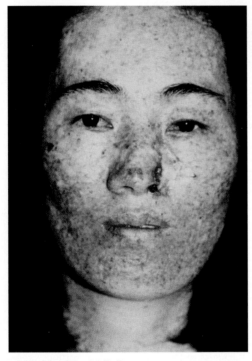

COLOR PLATE 113-3. Xeroderma pigmentosum. Typical features include poikilodermatous changes of the face. (From Wee SY, Ahn DS: Facial resurfacing in xeroderma pigmentosum with chemical peeling. Plast Reconstr Surg 1999;103:1464.)

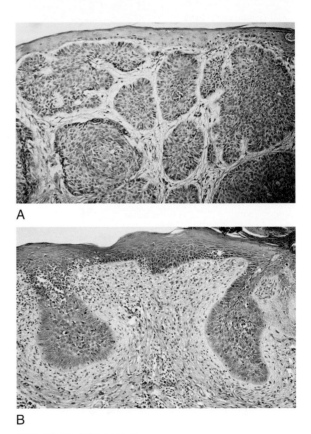

COLOR PLATE 113-5. *A,* Nodular BCC. Nests of atypical basal cells are found in the dermis. *B,* Superficial BCC. Buds of atypical cells extending from the basal layer of the epidermis. (From Habif TP: Clinical Dermatology, 4th ed. Philadelphia, Mosby, 2004.)

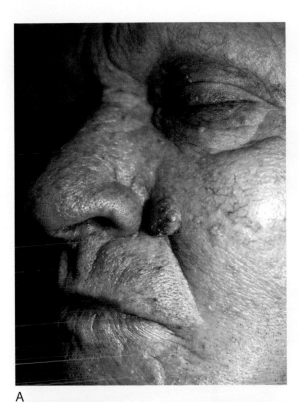

A

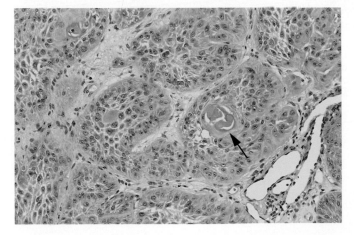

B

COLOR PLATE 113-6. *A,* Nodular BCC of the cheek.
B, Nodular BCC of the lower lip.

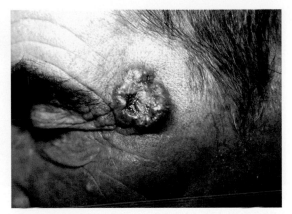

COLOR PLATE 113-7. Pigmented BCC of the temple
that can be mistaken for melanoma.

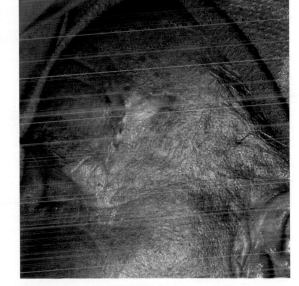

COLOR PLATE 113-8. Sclerosing BCC of the left
temple.

COLOR PLATE 113-9. Well-differentiated
SCC of the skin. The tumor cells are strikingly
similar to normal squamous epithelial cells, with
intercellular bridges and nests of keratin pearls
(arrow). (Courtesy of Dr. Trace Worrell, Department of Pathology, University of Texas South-
western Medical School, Dallas. From Cotran RS,
Kumar V, Collins T: Robbins Pathologic Basis of
Disease, 6th ed. Philadelphia, WB Saunders,
1999.)

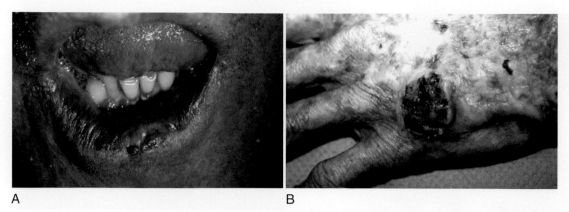

A   B

COLOR PLATE 113-10. *A,* SCC of the lower lip. *B,* SCC of dorsum of the hand.

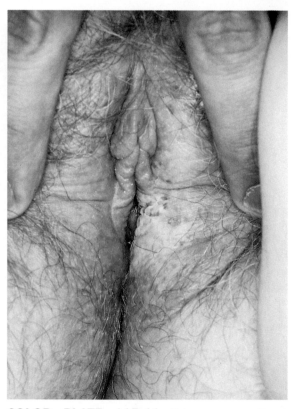

COLOR PLATE 113-11. Extramammary Paget disease. A white, eroded plaque with ill-defined borders on the labia. (From Habif TP: Clinical Dermatology, 4th ed. Philadelphia, Mosby, 2004.)

Malignant Melanoma

Stephan Ariyan, MD, MBA

Few diseases are as fascinating and as troublesome to physicians as malignant melanoma, and perhaps no other disease elicits as much fear in the patient as does this diagnosis. Although it accounts for only 4% of all malignant neoplasms, its very diagnosis suggests to some patients an aggressive, rapid progression to death. The name alone may leave some patients with a sense of hopelessness that is often unjustified. Despite some reported descriptions of rapid spread, the natural history of melanoma and its overall cure rate of 80% compare favorably with those of cancers of the breast, colon, rectum, and oropharynx and are far better than for cancer of the lung.

Epidemiologic studies of malignant melanoma have shown a steady rise in the incidence of this disease in various parts of the world in the last few decades. In the year 2000, 47,700 new cases and 9500 deaths are expected in the United States.[1] The incidence of new melanomas is the fastest growing among all cancers, now surpassing colon carcinoma, oropharyngeal carcinoma, renal carcinoma, and uterine carcinoma. Our understanding of melanoma has also increased over the years, and we can now differentiate low-risk from high-risk patients on the basis of multifactorial analyses from several series of large numbers of patients.

HISTORICAL NOTATIONS

Although Hippocrates is credited with the first reported observation of what appears to be a melanoma,

Handley[2] attributes the first clinical case of malignant melanoma reported in England to Dr. William Norris. In 1820, Norris felt compelled to report this case because of the rapid spread of the tumor, which led to his patient's death. He reported that at the autopsy, every organ except the spleen and the bladder was riddled with "black specks."[3] The patient's father had died of similar disease, and the patient's brothers and his children had "many moles on various parts of their bodies."

Handley had never himself treated a patient with a melanoma, but he did have the opportunity to make considerable observations after performing an autopsy on a 34-year-old woman who had died of disseminated metastatic melanoma. He became interested in the mechanisms of spread of melanoma after observing the spread of breast cancer along the lymphatics surrounding the primary tumor. This latter concept was well accepted at the time for breast cancer because it also had been proposed by Halsted.[4,5] In his two Hunterian Lectures, delivered before the Royal College of Surgeons in London, Handley proposed that the primary spread of melanoma was through the lymphatics and not by blood vessels. In his first lecture, he reported his observations on the autopsy that he had performed 2 years previously on a patient with melanoma. This 34-year-old woman on whom he had performed the postmortem examination had had a primary melanoma excised from her right foot over the Achilles tendon. At the autopsy, Handley had observed a large collection of tumor growths in the right groin and virtually every part of the body except the entire left leg (Fig. 114-1). Arguing incorrectly that every organ would have been involved if the tumor spread were hematogenous, he stated that the sparing of the spleen, bladder, stomach, and left leg could be explained by "lymphatic permeation." Although Handley did not discount the concept of hematogenous spread, he believed that early dissemination was by lymphatics and that invasion of the blood stream occurred later "either by local infiltration of veins from concomitant permeated lymphatics, or by malignant cells carried into the blood along the thoracic duct from invaded lymphatic glands."[2]

In his second lecture, Handley proposed that lymphatics were amenable to surgical removal with the primary melanoma.[6] He based his treatment recommendations on histologic examination not of the primary site but of the regional groin recurrence.

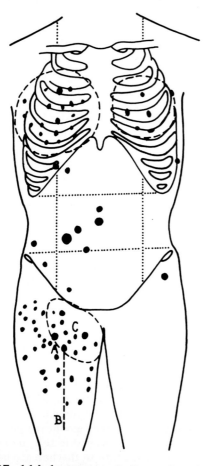

FIGURE 114-1. Autopsy findings of patient with melanoma of right ankle spreading in a centripetal manner to right groin and remainder of body while sparing the left leg. (Redrawn from Handley WS: The pathology of melanotic growths in relation to their operative treatment. Lecture I. Lancet 1907;1:927.)

Indeed, Handley had confessed that "no opportunity of investigating the spread of permeation round a primary focus of melanotic growth has fallen to me."[2]

Nevertheless, because the site of the groin recurrence had shown "permeation spreading centrifugally in the lymphatic plexus of the deep fascia and invading skin and muscle secondarily over a smaller area," he advocated a wide radical resection for a primary melanoma (Fig. 114-2):

A circular incision should be made through the skin round the tumour . . . situated as a rule about an inch from the edge of the tumour, should be just deep enough to expose the subcutaneous fat. . . . The skin with a thin attached layer of subcutaneous fat is now to be separated from the deeper structures for about two inches in all directions round the skin incision. . . . Finally, the whole mass with the growth at its centre is removed by scooping out with a knife a circular area of the muscle immediately subjacent to the growth.[6]

This approach presented a minimal excision of 2.5 cm of skin and 5 cm of subcutaneous tissue surrounding the melanoma, down to and including the muscle fascia, as well as incorporating a portion of the underlying muscle. Therefore, it is this report by Handley, in which he recommended a 5-cm margin of skin and soft tissues around a melanoma, that appears to be the first such proposal for a wide margin of resection.

Handley believed that the regional lymph nodes also should be removed as part of the first operation. Furthermore, he advised that the excision of these glands be complete, "that is to say, a larger circular area of the surrounding deep fascia must be exposed, dissected up from its circumference towards the infected glands, and removed in one piece with them."[6] He then reported the treatment of a melanoma of the thigh by a senior colleague, A.P. Gould, by resection of the primary tumor and femoral nodes in this manner, but the patient had iliac node recurrence within 2 months.

In the year after Handley's lecture, Pringle[7] described three patients with melanoma whom he treated during the previous 10 years. However, Pringle further advocated removal of all subcutaneous tissue, including the lymphatics, between the primary site and the regional nodes together with the specimen. This was the first paper to describe the technique of an in-continuity dissection. He reported that one of his patients—a young woman who was alive 9 years after surgery at the time of the report—had moved to Canada, married, and had children. Pringle concluded in his report that "all that is removed should be in one continuous strip as far as possible."

These early papers established the trends toward aggressive treatment of primary melanoma by wide excision of the tumor together with the underlying muscle and its fascia and by in-continuity lymph node

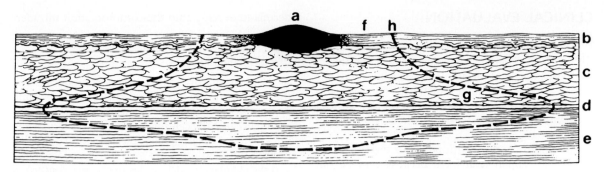

FIGURE 114-2. Handley recommended removal of melanoma (a) together with 1 inch (f) of skin (b) and 2 inches (g) of underlying subcutaneous fat (c), muscle fascia (d), and muscle (e). h, skin incision. (Redrawn from Handley WS: The pathology of melanotic growths in relation to their operative treatment. Lecture I. Lancet 1907;1:927.)

dissection in an effort to achieve better cures. As Handley stated in his Hunterian Lecture:

Nowadays the improved operation for breast cancer produces prolonged or permanent immunity in about 50 percent of cases. And upon the evidence I have laid before you I venture to predict that the application of more thorough and scientific methods to the surgery of cutaneous melanomata will produce a corresponding, though perhaps a smaller, improvement in the results of operation.[6]

However, the methods of treating melanoma changed very little during the first half of the 20th century. The various reports of cure rates after aggressive surgical treatment of melanoma remained the same: a better prognosis if the patient did not have clinically palpable nodes (80% 5-year cure rate for stage I disease) than if the nodes were palpable (40% cure rate for stage II disease).[8]

Subsequently, surgeons gained some information on prognostic factors of this tumor. Within each clinical stage, the prognosis is improved by the pathologic findings of no evidence of metastatic tumor cells on microscopic examination of the removed lymph nodes. However, the advantage of in-continuity removal of all tissues between the primary site and the regional lymph nodes, as advocated by Pringle[7] and as widely employed for decades, was challenged by Goldsmith et al,[8] who demonstrated no difference between this technique and that of discontinuous dissection of the primary tumor and the lymph nodes (Table 114-1). They, too, found no difference between immediate and delayed lymphadenectomy.

Finally, the issue regarding excision of underlying muscle and fascia was evaluated and resolved. Olsen[9] reviewed a series of 67 patients treated for melanoma in Denmark between 1949 and 1957. She found a 45% incidence of subsequent regional nodal metastases among the 31 patients who had the fascia removed during excision of the primary tumor and a 14% incidence of metastases among the 36 patients in whom this fascia was left intact. Because the patients who underwent a fasciectomy may have had more aggressive tumors, Olsen reviewed the next 51 patients treated from 1958 to 1961 who did not undergo excision of the fascia and observed only a 10% incidence of regional metastases. Kenady et al[10] reviewed their data of 202 patients treated at the M.D. Anderson Hospital, Houston, from 1961 to 1974 and found that local recurrence, regional nodal recurrence, distant metastases, and survival were not statistically different between the 107 patients who had the fascia excised and the 95 patients who did not. There appears to be no indication for removal of underlying muscle fascia unless the fascia becomes involved by contiguous tumor growth.

TABLE 114-1 ✦ OUTCOME BASED ON INTERVAL OF TIMING OF NODE DISSECTION

Clinical Stage	No. of Patients	Nodal Dissection	5-Year Cure Rate	
			Simultaneous	*Delayed*
I	296	In continuity	63 (76%)	165 (78%)
		Discontinuous	15 (75%)	53 (75%)
II	435	In continuity	53 (42%)	167 (42%)
		Discontinuous	20 (35%)	195 (41%)

Modified from Goldsmith HS, Shah JP, Kim DH: Prognostic significance of lymph node dissection in the treatment of malignant melanoma. Cancer 1970;26:606.

CLINICAL EVALUATION

Clinical Diagnosis

Although an experienced clinician should be able to diagnose malignant melanoma by its appearance, the diagnosis is often not made until the specimen is examined histologically. Therefore, a review of the various pigmented lesions is essential for making a differential diagnosis.

All infants are born with nevi, but the lesions are usually not apparent at birth because they do not produce pigment. During the following few weeks or months, melanocytes produce pigment as a response to circulating hormones. As the nevi develop, they undergo maturation, which leads to the classification of the following various forms.

JUNCTIONAL NEVUS

Junctional nevi are small flat lesions that first appear after birth and are smooth, nonpalpable, and light to dark brown or black (Fig. 114-3A). They are called junctional because the nevus cells are located at the interface of the epidermis and dermis. As the person develops and matures, the nevus cells grow and push into the

dermis to develop into the common adult intradermal nevus.

COMPOUND NEVUS

As the nevus matures, the central portion pushes into the dermis, causing this central portion to elevate and appear thicker (Fig. 114-3B). This nevus is called compound because the central portion is intradermal and thick, whereas the periphery is still junctional and flat. Compound nevi often are seen during adolescence, and the changes in such moles may cause concern to the patient, family, or primary care physician.

INTRADERMAL NEVUS

The intradermal nevus is the common adult mole of the face or trunk that is elevated because of the maturation and proliferation of the nevus in the dermis, which now pushes up the overlying epidermis (Fig. 114-3C). It may be light or dark, usually is elevated, and may be sessile or pedunculated.

BLUE NEVUS

Most nevi appear brown or black because the melanin is superficial and absorbs light. When the nevus

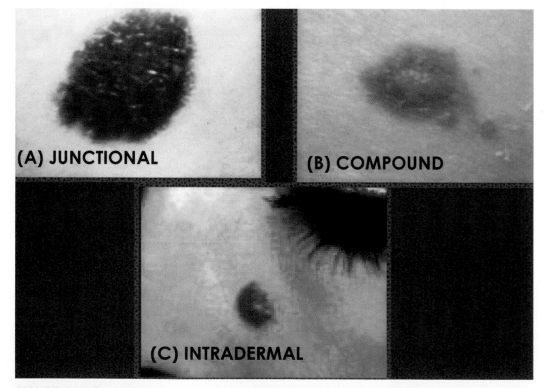

FIGURE 114-3. *A,* Junctional nevus is flat, smooth, and nonpalpable. *B,* Compound nevus is developing into mature, thicker intradermal nevus in center within a flat junctional nevus in periphery. *C,* Intradermal nevus is mature mole with elevation of the surface elements due to thickening of the layer of nevus cells.

contains melanin that is located more deeply, blue wavelengths of light pass through the less pigmented epidermis and are reflected back to the eye as a blue nevus.

CONGENITAL NEVUS

Congenital nevi differ from others in that they already produce pigment at birth (Fig. 114-4). The controversy about congenital nevi is whether they are precursors of malignant melanoma. Kaplan's review[11] of the literature reported the transformation to melanoma to occur in 2% to 42% of congenital nevi. In a retrospective study of 234 melanomas by Rhodes and Melski,[12] some of the histologic features of congenital nevi were found among 8% of the melanoma specimens. However, this percentage does not represent the true incidence of the development of melanoma within congenital nevi; rather, it is the incidence of congenital nevi associated with melanoma. The true incidence is not known because the total number of patients in the normal population who have congenital nevi but never consult a physician, or eventually undergo excision, is unknown.

On the basis of available information about the potential for malignant transformation, it is a good policy to remove congenital nevi if it can be done without much difficulty. Because malignant transformation does not usually occur before adolescence, if the lesion is to be excised, it should be done before adolescence. Because it is difficult to excise nevi from the skin of children under local anesthesia and general anesthesia is often necessary for children younger than 12 years, the risk of complications from general anesthesia should be weighed against the risk of malignant transformation before adolescence. On the other hand, patients may request removal of the lesion to improve their appearance. Despite concerns for appearance, some lesions cannot be completely removed because in doing so we may cause a greater deformity. These lesions may require staged excisions (Fig. 114-5).

DYSPLASTIC NEVUS (ATYPICAL NEVUS)

The atypical nevus is a clinical diagnosis of a nevus with melanocytes involving the epidermis and dermis that have features suggestive of malignancy. Clinically, it is large (>6 mm), with a macular surface, irregular margin, and variegated color. It may have a background of erythema (Fig. 114-6). These are benign lesions with histologic features that are abnormal. At various times, they have been called atypical nevi or dysplastic nevi. However, a National Institutes of Health Consensus Conference in 1992 recommended the descriptive term *atypical nevus* for the clinical diagnosis and the histologic term *dysplastic nevus* to describe the histologic degree of atypia and architectural disorder.[13]

Because the atypical nevus is a clinical diagnosis only, confirmation of its being a dysplastic nevus requires microscopic examination. On histologic examination, the dysplastic nevus has melanocytic hyperplasia, with the melanocytes arranged as solitary units or small elongated nests oriented parallel to the long axes of the rete ridges. The melanocytes have nuclear atypia and abundant cytoplasm with a fine "dusty pattern" of melanin deposits.[14] Dysplastic nevi are often associated with atypical melanocytic hyperplasia, lymphocytic infiltration, and some evidence of regression. As such, they are believed to be at greater risk for malignant transformation to melanomas.

DYSPLASTIC NEVUS SYNDROME

More recent studies in several institutions have found atypical nevi in association with melanoma that has no familial pattern. At the University of Pennsylvania, Elder et al[15] first described this as the dysplastic nevus syndrome in their 1980 report. In the same year, the Yale Melanoma Unit visited the Sydney Melanoma Unit in Australia and documented the presence of atypical nevi in 37% of 296 patients with melanoma who had no known family history. Similar atypical nevi were discovered in only 7% of a control population of male prison inmates without any history of melanoma. Clinically, these moles were large and resembled the dysplastic nevi of familial melanoma. Biopsies showed a 90% correlation between the histologic diagnosis of dysplastic nevi and the clinical appearance of these atypical moles.

B-K MOLE SYNDROME

Some prospective studies have shown that melanoma may be associated with a familial distribution in 10%

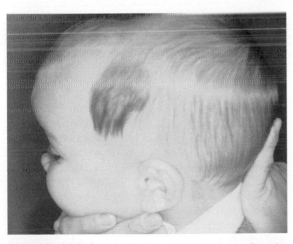

FIGURE 114-4. Congenital nevus is a large flat pigmented mole that had produced pigmentation in utero and was present as a pigmented lesion on the day of birth. It may be hairy (as in this case) or not.

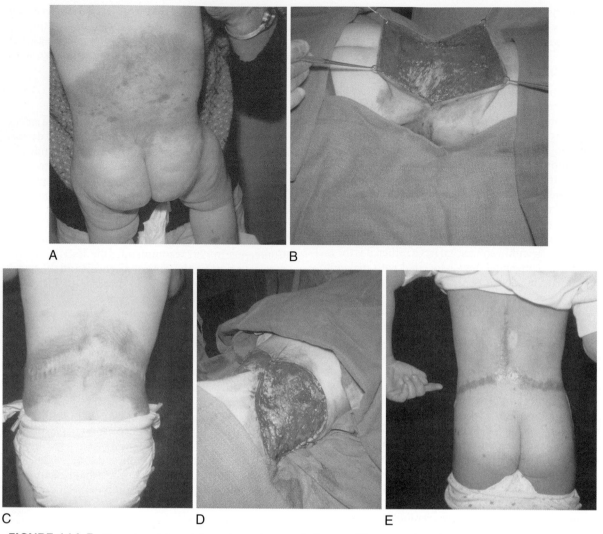

FIGURE 114-5. Staged excision. A large truncal congenital nevus *(A)* was excised from the central portion of the lesion *(B)* to reduce the size of the lesion to half after one operation *(C)*. A second procedure a year later *(D)* removed the remainder of the lesion *(E)*.

to 11% of the cases.[16] These familial melanomas tend to appear earlier and are distributed among dysplastic nevi over the body, with an excess over the trunk and a deficit over the upper extremities. Clark et al[17] and Reimer[18] suggested the role of atypical moles and dysplastic nevi in the development of hereditary melanoma when they described these moles in association with melanomas in seven families. They applied the initials of the first family, which were B. K., to name this clinical entity the B-K mole syndrome.

Differential Diagnosis

The clinician is faced with the task of differentiating the malignant melanoma from a number of other lesions that may clinically resemble melanoma, such as seborrheic keratosis (Fig. 114-7A), pyogenic granuloma (Fig. 114-7B), and pigmented basal cell carcinoma (Fig. 114-7C). This differentiation may sometimes be more difficult because of a recent growth, bleeding into a lesion, or peripheral inflammation. In these instances, only microscopic examination of the tissue provides the proper diagnosis.

Extensive or radical surgical procedures should not be performed without the proper diagnosis of a malignant melanoma because clinical impressions are not uniformly correct. Epstein et al[19] reviewed 559 patients with black lesions that they believed might be melanomas. They found that their diagnosis of melanoma was correct only a third (38.7%) of the time.

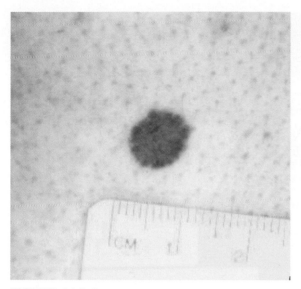

FIGURE 114-6. Dysplastic nevus is a histologic confirmation of the clinical entity called atypical nevus. This is a large (>6 mm) flat mole of varying coloration.

Indeed, the most common diagnoses were benign nevi (35%), pigmented basal cell cancer (30%), and benign angiomas or vascular lesions (13%). Only 2% of all the lesions were found to be melanoma.

HUTCHINSON FRECKLE

Hutchinson freckle is a flat, brown, macular lesion that may grow at various rates and achieve different shades of pigmentation (Fig. 114-8). This lesion occurs most commonly on the face, neck, and other sun-exposed surfaces of adults in middle age or later. On histologic examination, this lesion appears as an overgrowth of melanocytes at the epidermis dermis junction. Although lentigo maligna is an in situ melanoma, invasive melanoma may develop within a Hutchinson freckle and is then called lentigo maligna melanoma.

MALIGNANT MELANOMA

The lesions of malignant melanoma may be flat or nodular, with significant darkening, erythema, or bleeding. On histologic examination, the earliest lesions demonstrate atypical melanocytes migrating above the dermis-epidermis junction and appearing within the upper portions of hair follicles and eccrine ducts. These changes are typical of malignant melanoma in situ.[20] Special staining with S100 and HMB45 may be necessary to confirm the diagnosis in cases with histologic features that may be equivocal. However, when even a single atypical melanocyte invades from the dermis-epidermis junction down into the dermis, the diagnosis is a malignant melanoma.[21]

There are clinical features of pigmented lesions that are characteristic for melanoma. These criteria have been promoted by the American Cancer Society as the ABCD Guidelines (Fig. 114-9).

A Asymmetry of the lesion as it grows from a round or oval lesion
B Border irregularity, which is a result of irregular growth rates of different parts of the lesion
C Color changes representing pigment granules deposited at varying depths in the dermis, depending on the rate of invasion
D Diameter of the lesion becoming more than $^1/_4$ inch (>6 mm)

Perhaps the best clinical indication of malignant melanoma is intralesional depigmentation (Fig. 114-10A). This is a manifestation of immunologic regression of the tumor as a result of the destruction of the melanoma cells by the host's immune response. The histologic examination of only a section through the depigmented portion may be misread as an inflammatory reaction. However, deposits of residual melanin granules may exist in the depigmented portion (Fig. 114-10B; see also Color Plate 114-1), and histologic examination of sections through the adjacent pigmented portion may reveal the true diagnosis of the malignant melanoma.

Depigmentation does not always indicate melanoma; a halo nevus (Fig. 114-11A) is a benign lesion with a peripheral ring of depigmentation.[22] Histologic examination of the halo portion shows lymphocytic infiltration without pigment granules (Fig. 114-11B; see also Color Plate 114-2). Further evaluation of the lesion and surrounding tissue shows no evidence of cells of malignant melanoma.

MULTIPLE PRIMARY MELANOMAS

Multiple primary melanomas have been reported to occur among 3% of melanoma patients.[23] The risk for a second melanoma in a patient with one melanoma approaches 4% to 5%.[24] However, with a positive family history of melanoma, the risk for multiple primary melanomas rises to 10% or more.[25] The highest risk of all appears to be in individuals who have a family history of melanoma in one or two first-degree relatives and who have clinical evidence of dysplastic nevi, suggesting a probability approaching 100% in due time.[26]

SURGICAL BIOPSIES

Some clinicians have questioned the safety of a biopsy of a malignant melanoma (Fig. 114-12) for fear that tumor cells would be disseminated through the blood stream. To evaluate this risk, Epstein et al[19] reviewed 170 melanoma patients from the California Tumor Registry from 1950 to 1954, 115 of whom had had a biopsy

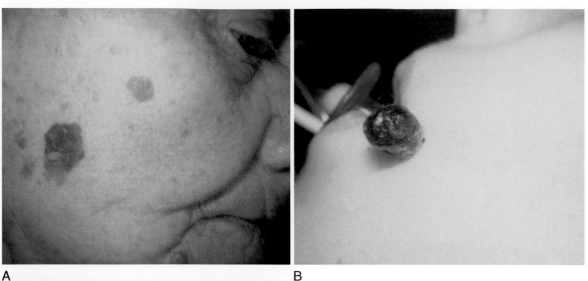

A   B

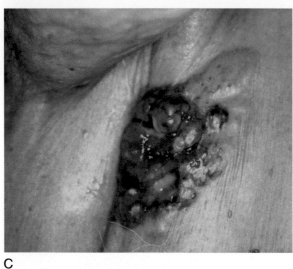

C

FIGURE 114-7. Pigmented lesions that need to be differentiated from a melanoma. *A,* Seborrheic keratosis of cheek is a velvety smooth keratosis that may turn dark brown to black with drying of the keratin layer. *B,* Pyogenic granuloma with exophytic granulation tissue and darkening due to desiccation of the blood and coagulum. *C,* Pigmented basal cell carcinoma with heaped up "pearly" margins. Pigment may represent hemosiderin or melanin granules from melanocytes that may be incorporated into the lesion.

of the melanoma before surgical treatment and 55 of whom had not. The 5- and 10-year cure rates, as well as relative cure rates by life-table analysis to eliminate differences in the age distribution of the two groups, were more favorable for those patients who had had a previous biopsy (Table 114-2). The results of this study suggest not that biopsies improve the overall cure rates but rather that an incomplete removal of a melanoma by a surgical biopsy followed by the definitive surgery does not decrease the cure rate. Two additional studies have confirmed this observation, one from the United States with 230 patients[27] and a subsequent study from Denmark[28] with 225 patients followed up for a minimum of 5 years. Clearly, the incisional or excisional biopsy of the lesion will make the diagnosis of the melanoma as well as demonstrate the aggressiveness of the lesion by the degree of invasion into the dermis, as discussed later.

TABLE 114-2 ✦ EFFECT OF INTRALESIONAL BIOPSY ON OUTCOME

Survival	Biopsy (115 patients)	No Biopsy (55 patients)
Observed rate		
5-year	79%	75%
10-year	65%	56%
Relative rate		
5-year	89%	80%
10-year	84%	67%

Modified from Epstein E, Bragg K, Linden G: Biopsy and prognosis of malignant melanoma. JAMA 1969;208:1369.

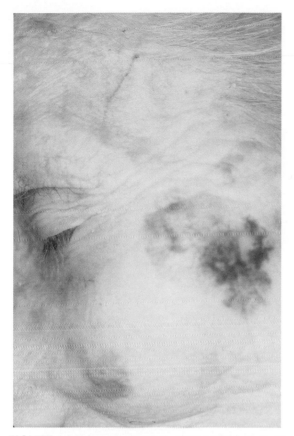

FIGURE 114-8. Hutchinson freckle is a flat lesion with various shades of pigmentation.

If the lesion is small, an excisional biopsy with a 1- to 2-mm margin is sufficient to permit the pathologist to render a diagnosis reliably and to determine the thickest depth of invasion. If the lesion is too large for a simple excision under local anesthesia, an incisional biopsy or punch biopsy is an acceptable alternative. The only drawback of such a partial biopsy is that the final therapeutic excision may show a lesion that is classified with greater depth of invasion than had been initially discovered. In some cases, the patient would have been eligible for studies (e.g., sentinel node biopsy, as discussed later) if the proper depth had been assessed before wide excision and resurfacing.

CLASSIFICATION

Melanoma is most commonly located in the skin, although it may also occur rarely in the mucosa of the oral cavity, nasopharynx, esophagus, vagina, and rectum. Because the staging systems developed for melanoma apply to lesions arising in the skin, the discussion in this chapter is limited to cutaneous melanoma.

The purpose of a classification system in malignant disease is to separate varying stages of severity to predict prognosis and to propose treatment options based on those predictions. Therefore, all classification systems have evolved from data collected over time. As such, each of these classifications needs to be re-evaluated

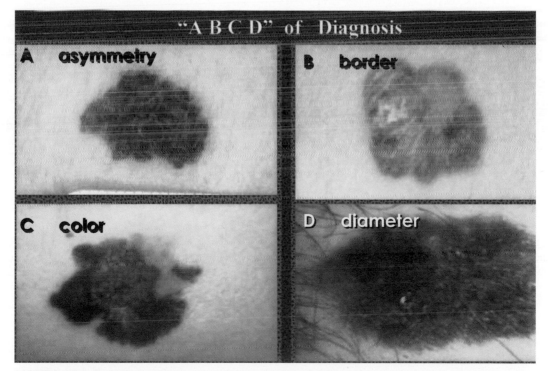

FIGURE 114-9. Melanoma with characteristic changes. *A,* Asymmetry of lesion shape. *B,* Border irregularity. *C,* Color variegation. *D,* Diameter greater than 6 mm.

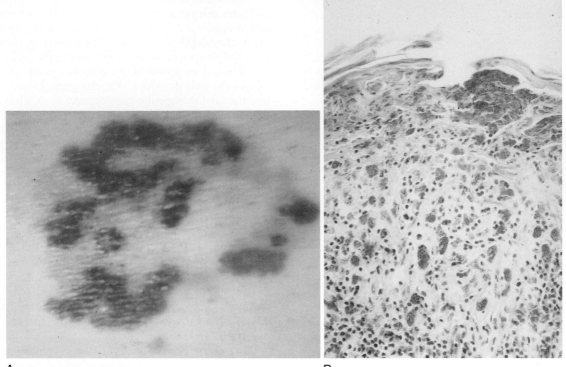

A   B

FIGURE 114-10. *A,* Melanoma with areas of depigmentation within the lesion. *B,* Histologic examination of the specimen cut through the area of depigmentation shows significant lymphocytic infiltration with disrupted pigment granules leading to the colorless patches within. (See also Color Plate 114-1.)

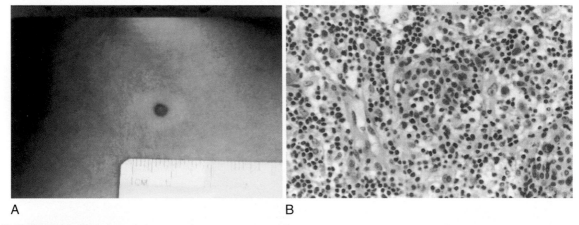

A   B

FIGURE 114-11. *A,* Halo nevus with a ring of depigmentation surrounding the lesion. *B,* Histologic examination of the depigmented portion shows infiltration with lymphocytes, but there is no evidence of pigment granules or malignant cells. (See also Color Plate 114-2.)

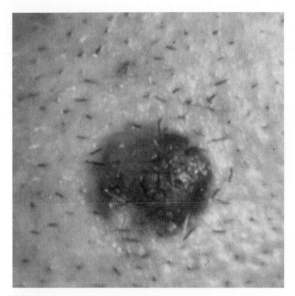

FIGURE 114-12. Punch biopsy through a lesion suspected of being a melanoma

periodically to refine the separations of the stages on the basis of changes in outcome. Historically, melanoma was first classified according to clinical findings. Subsequently, a morphologic classification and then a histologic classification were added. These need to be reviewed.

Clinical Classification

Melanoma is classified according to the extent of clinical spread of the disease. Stage I represents melanoma limited to the tumor at the site of origin alone. This is defined by the absence of signs or symptoms of spread to regional draining lymph nodes or to distant sites. A special category of stage I disease is associated with clinically or pathologically apparent satellite lesions that may extend for several centimeters from the primary tumor and confer a more ominous prognosis.[29] The 5-year cure rate of more than 80% in stage I disease is substantially better than that of stage II or stage III and has been shown to vary with morphologic features and depth of invasion, as will be further discussed later. In addition, the patient's sex and the location of the primary tumor may also affect cure rates.

Stage II represents a primary melanoma associated with palpable regional draining lymph nodes suspected of harboring metastatic disease. Patients with stage II disease have approximately a 40% 5-year survival rate, but the prognosis is influenced by the number of lymph nodes involved and whether the lymph nodes are clinically apparent and histologically found not to harbor tumor cells. The detection of tumor spread in lymph nodes may be improved by the use of new

immunohistochemistry techniques. Cochran et al[30] have shown that the use of anti-S100 antibody increases the number of lymph nodes that are identified to contain melanoma, although it does not increase the number of patients found to have metastases. Clearly, the use of immunohistochemistry is not to increase the degree of involvement of lymph nodes in patients with known metastases but to define the subset of patients who have microscopic disease in the lymph nodes that is too small to be detected by standard histologic studies.

Stage III melanoma consists of a heterogeneous group of patients who have distant spread of disease. This form of melanoma is usually not curable. Patients with melanoma metastatic to the skin and subcutaneous tissue or lymph nodes have a better prognosis than do those with visceral metastases. However, Amer et al[31] showed that even in patients with brain metastases, disease in the brain alone is associated with substantially longer median survival than in those with brain disease associated with lung involvement; this, in turn, is associated with longer survival than in those with metastases to liver or multiple viscera.

Morphologic Classification

Melanoma is also classified morphologically into lentigo maligna, superficial spreading, nodular, and acral lentiginous types (Fig. 114-13). This classification provides prognostic assessment of the melanoma based on the morphologic features of the primary tumor.[32] Superficial spreading melanoma (Fig. 114-13B) represents 50% to 80% of all the types and is characterized by growth in the radial (horizontal) phase for a period of years before evolution into the vertical growth phase. Nodular melanoma (Fig. 114-13C), on the other hand, evolves into the vertical growth phase early in its development and represents 20% to 30% of the group but in some series may compose the majority of the lesions.[33] Lentigo maligna melanoma (Fig. 114-13A) is differentiated from superficial spreading melanoma and nodular melanoma by its location on sun-exposed surfaces of the body and within preexisting lentigo maligna (Hutchinson freckle). This morphologic type of melanoma was believed to have a better prognosis than these two types by virtue of a different biologic behavior, but it has been shown to have a prognosis identical with that for superficial spreading melanoma with comparable depths of invasion.[34] It has been shown that lentigo maligna melanoma merely grows in a horizontal fashion more than in a vertical fashion, resulting in thinner lesions than superficial spreading melanoma or nodular melanoma, which is the reason for its purported better prognosis.

Acral lentiginous melanoma is a melanoma that appears on the palms of the hands, soles of the feet (Fig. 114-13D), subungual areas of the fingers and toes

316   V ◆ TUMORS OF THE HEAD, NECK, AND SKIN

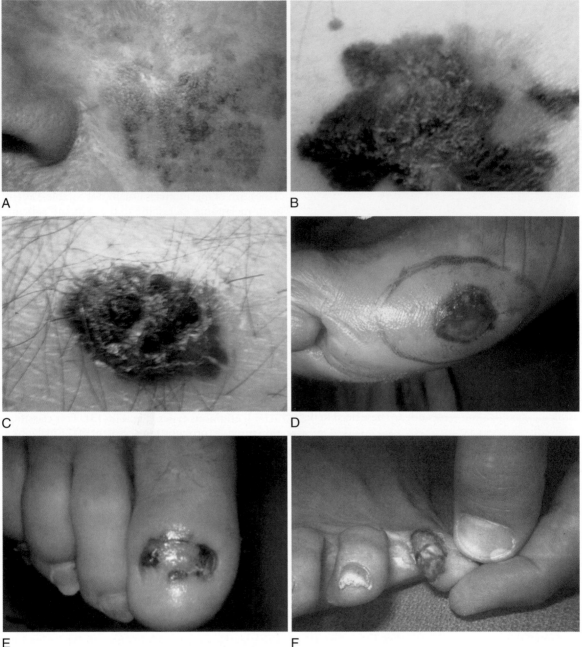

FIGURE 114-13. Various morphologic types of melanoma. *A,* Lentigo maligna melanoma—thin, flat lesion within patchy discoloration of Hutchinson freckle. *B,* Superficial spreading melanoma—flat lesion with cells proliferating in the horizontal plane. *C,* Nodular melanoma—thicker lesion growing in a vertical plane. *D to F,* Acral lentiginous melanoma of the foot, nail bed, and web space.

(Fig. 114-13E), and web spaces (Fig. 114-13F).[35] The importance of the subungual melanoma is that it is often erroneously believed to be a fungal infection, and its proper treatment may be delayed because of a delay in its diagnosis by biopsy. This type of melanoma has the lowest 5-year survival rates of all these

variants, generally found to be in the range of 10% to 20%.[16,36]

Another clinical variant of melanoma has been described that produces no pigmentation. The lesion grows on the external surfaces of the skin and has the appearance of a hypertrophic scar (Fig. 114-14A) at

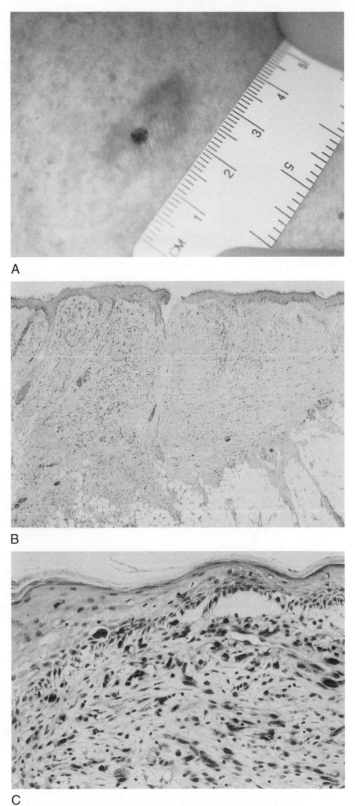

FIGURE 114-14. *A,* Desmoplastic melanoma is often nonpigmented and has the appearance of hypertrophic scar. There was a punch biopsy performed in the center of the lesion that has been inked with a marking pen. *B,* Low-power magnification of the desmoplastic melanoma shows the proliferation of the tumor in a cicatricial fashion. (See also Color Plate 114-3*A.*) *C,* High-power magnification of the lesion shows the spindle cell variant of the malignant melanocytes with the production of some pigment granules. (See also Color Plate 114-3*B.*)

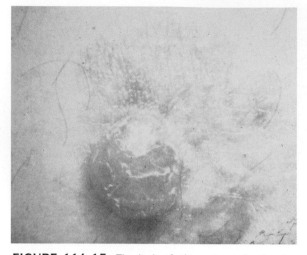

FIGURE 114-15. The lack of pigment production in this amelanotic melanoma is deceptive in a lesion that is otherwise suggestive of malignancy.

a location where the patient does not recall having had an injury to the skin. It must be differentiated clinically from a dermatofibroma and other benign or malignant tumors of the dermis. Histologic examination reveals a cicatricial growth of the lesion (Fig. 114-14B; see also Color Plate 114-3A) with spindle cell variants of malignant melanocytes (Fig. 114-14C; see also Color Plate 114-3B). Because of these features,

this clinical variant has been classified as desmoplastic melanoma.[37-39] This tumor also needs to be differentiated from amelanotic melanoma (Fig. 114-15), which is simply a variant of nodular melanoma or superficial spreading melanoma that is not producing sufficient pigment granules to appear as a pigmented lesion. In one series of melanomas, the incidence of amelanotic melanoma was found to be 1.8%.[40]

Histologic Classification

The depth of invasion of melanoma into the dermis has been shown to be the most powerful determinant of outcome of melanoma. In 1965, Mehnert and Heard[41] reported the earliest correlation of depth with prognosis. A few years later, Clark et al[42] described the following system of levels for the classification of depth of invasion into the dermis (Fig. 114-16):

Level I   In situ melanoma; limited to the dermis-epidermis junction

Level II   Invading the papillary dermis but without expansion of this layer

Level III Invading and expanding the papillary dermis but not into the reticular dermis (to the interface of the papillary-reticular dermis)

Level IV   Invading the reticular dermis, but not into the subcutaneous fat

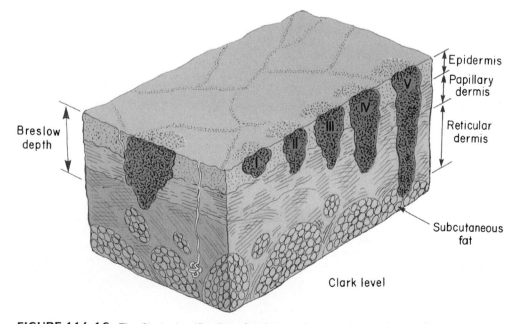

FIGURE 114-16. The Clark classification of melanoma is dependent on the qualitative determination of the extent of invasion into the various areas of the dermis or subcutaneous fat. The Breslow classification is determined by the micrometer reading of the depth of invasion into the dermis, measured in tenths of millimeters.

Level V   Invading the subcutaneous fat or the associated subreticular tissues

The difficulty with this classification system is the qualitative and subjective nature of determining the depth of invasion. Various pathologists examining a histologic slide of mid-dermal invasion often disagree as to its Clark level of invasion; some call it a level III, others call it a deep level II, and still others call it an early level IV invasion. As a result of this difficulty, Breslow[43] reported a method of quantitative measurement that employs a simple and readily reproducible system of microstaging. According to Breslow, the melanoma's depth of invasion is measured in tenths of millimeters as a thickness from the surface of the tumor in the epidermis to the deepest tumor cell identified by means of an ocular micrometer on the microscope. In a number of studies using multivariate analyses,[33] Breslow's method has been shown to be the most powerful prognostic indicator for survival in clinical stage I melanoma. Additional factors that have been shown in appropriate multivariate analyses of several thousand patients to be associated with recurrence include ulceration in the lesion, the patient's age and sex, the site of the primary lesion, and the morphologic type of melanoma.[44]

TNM STAGING

The validity of staging systems is based on scientific evidence that can then direct and assign outcome and prognosis. To support and maintain this goal, the American Joint Committee on Cancer (AJCC) developed a TNM classification that is reviewed and revised every few years to reflect the changes in prognostic separation of the characteristics of the various stages according to updated data review. The AJCC is now revising the classification for melanoma, and a preliminary staging update has been published[45] for evaluation and opinion input to the Committee by the profession (Fig. 114-17). This new version has upgraded the tumor (T)

staging to full 1-mm increments and included up-staging if there is histologic evidence of ulceration of the tumor. It has simplified the nodal (N) staging and has now incorporated local recurrences, in-transit metastases, and soft tissue metastases with the N staging. Distant metastases (M) are classified according to the various organs involved. The one real change these modifications have effected is the down-staging of tumors greater than 4.0 mm, from stage III in the former classification to stage II in this revised classification.

EVALUATION OF SYSTEMIC DISEASE

The evaluation of the patient with malignant melanoma requires a complete physical examination of the primary site and regional draining lymph nodes to detect any clinical evidence of satellite or in-transit lesions (metastases) in the skin or of metastases to lymph nodes. The abdomen needs to be examined for evidence of an enlarged liver, enlarged spleen, or abdominal masses that would suggest intra-abdominal metastases. The extent of examination and the tests ordered for such evaluations are predicated on the stage of the primary diagnosis (Table 114-3). A routine chest radiograph is indicated to look for pulmonary metastases, and computed chest tomograms may add to the detection of small and early lesions. Liver enzyme function tests are simple, sensitive, and reliable for detecting liver metastases and, when results are negative, may serve as a baseline for later annual follow-up examinations.

Computerized Scans

Although tomographic radiographs of the lungs are helpful in detecting pulmonary metastases, computed tomographic (CT) scanning of the chest and abdomen does not offer a significant advantage as an initial

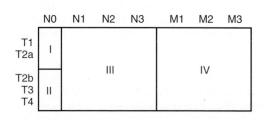

FIGURE 114-17. Proposed AJCC staging of TNM for cutaneous melanoma. (Redrawn from Balch CM, Buzaid AC, Atkins MB, et al: A new American Joint Committee on Cancer staging system for cutaneous melanoma. Cancer 2000;88:1484.)

TABLE 114-3 ✦ STAGING EVALUATION: TESTS
RECOMMENDED FOR
DETERMINATION OF
PRESENCE AND EXTENT
OF TUMOR SPREAD

Primary Tumor (no clinical evidence of other involvement)

Physical examination
Chest radiography
Liver function tests
Lymphoscintigraphy to detect sites of sentinel nodes (if
    primary tumor is 1 mm or more thick)

Local and Regional Disease (in-transit lesions or nodal involvement)

Physical examination
Liver function tests
CT scans
    of chest and abdomen (to examine lungs and liver)
    of pelvis if tumor involves lower extremities
    of neck if tumor involves the head and neck
Lymphoscintigraphy to detect sites of sentinel nodes
Additional scans as indicated by clinical signs or
    symptoms

Distant Organ Metastases

Physical examination
Liver function tests
CT scans as indicated above
MRI scans if required to detect extent of soft tissue
    invasion
PET scans to detect extent of tumor involvement of
    vital organs (lung, liver, brain)

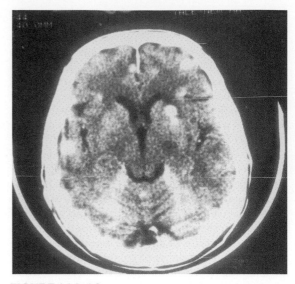

FIGURE 114-18. CT scans of the brain can detect small lesions. In this patient, several lesions are identified in both hemispheres.

abdominal viscera, soft tissues, and mediastinum.[47,48] However, gallium scans have been less useful for detecting metastases of melanoma to the lung parenchyma and brain (Table 114-4). Furthermore, because the liver excretes gallium into the intestines, use of this scan to detect liver metastases is difficult, and a good bowel preparation is essential to perform a meaningful examination of the abdomen.

On the other hand, CT scans can be helpful for staging the disease in patients who present with local or regional extension of the disease. In some patients, the extent of the disease detected from the CT scans can be elaborated by the use of magnetic resonance imaging scans (Fig. 114-20). More recently, positron emission tomography (PET) scan has been found to be valuable for evaluating the patients for extension of their disease and assigning stage.[49,50] The increased metabolism of the tumor is reflected in the increased uptake of radioactive-labeled glucose, which is represented by the brighter activity at the site of the metastases (Fig. 114-21). In the absence of infectious processes, the false-positive rate has been reported to be less than 5% with PET scans. The restrictions to the use of PET scans are the limited availability of the scanners and the greater expense for these studies.

Lymphatic Mapping

Skin is composed of the three layers of epidermis, dermis, and subcutaneous fat. As in all parts of the body, arterial blood pressure diffuses serum and nutrient material out of the vessels into the interstitial tissue to nourish the cells. The breakdown

screening test over chest radiographs and liver function tests.[46] Even though this imaging technique requires skillful interpretation for optimal use, analysis of patients demonstrates that screening chest radiographs not only are as useful as CT scans in detecting metastatic lesions at the time of the initial diagnosis but are also much more cost-effective. However, CT scans do offer the potential for superior detection of metastatic lesions in various organs, and they are quite useful for evaluating the brain (Fig. 114-18).

Whereas patients with primary melanomas thicker than 1 mm may be considered at moderate risk, those with lesions greater than 2 mm are considered at high risk for metastases. Patients with clinical stage III disease are certainly candidates for intensive surveillance. These higher risk patients should be evaluated for distant organ metastases with chest and abdominal CT scans, which enable the physician to examine the lungs, the liver, and the spleen in one test. Enhanced brain CT scans and tomographic gallium scans are valuable for detecting metastatic melanoma to a number of distant sites (Fig. 114-19), including lymph nodes,

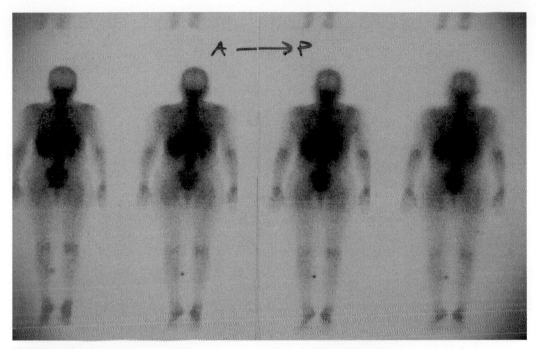

FIGURE 114-19. Tomographic gallium scans can detect small lesions at multiple sites that may escape detection by routine CT scans. (A → P , anterior to posterior cuts.)

products of metabolism are then picked up by the veins and taken back into the systemic system. Because the pressure in the arteries is greater than in the veins, more of this vascular fluid is diffused into the tissue than is taken away by the vein. To avoid the consequences of edema, lymphatic vessels (the micro sump pumps of the system) draw away this excess fluid and take it to the regional lymph nodes to filter the product before returning it to the systemic vascular system. This filtering function of the lymph nodes allows it to detect and attack foreign bacteria, antigens, and cancer cells. It was this principle that permitted

Sappey[51] to show the lymphatic patterns of the human body in 1874 by injecting mercury into the skin. Sappey's lines are a helpful guide to determine the likely directions of lymphatic spread. Subsequent experience has shown that lesions located more than 2 cm above or below a "belt line" drawn through the umbilicus usually drain to the axillary or groin nodes, respectively. Lesions more than 2 cm on either side of the midline drain to the lymph nodes on that respective side. Lesions within 4 cm of the vertical and horizontal bands may go to any one of the pairs of options (Fig. 114-22).

TABLE 114-4 ✦ ORGAN METASTASES DETECTED BY GALLIUM SCAN

	Lymph Nodes	Lung	Intra-abdominal	Bone
Number of patients	36	15	9	8
Gallium scan results negative, physical examination findings abnormal	7	3	6	2
True positive	6	3	5	1
Gallium scan results negative, physical examination findings normal	7	7	0	2
True negative	3	0	0	2
Sensitivity	90%	68%	100%	100%
Specificity	99%	100%	100%	99%

Modified from Kirkwood JM, Myers JE, Vlock DR, et al: Tomographic gallium-67 citrate scanning: useful new surveillance for metastatic melanoma. Ann Surg 1983;198:102.

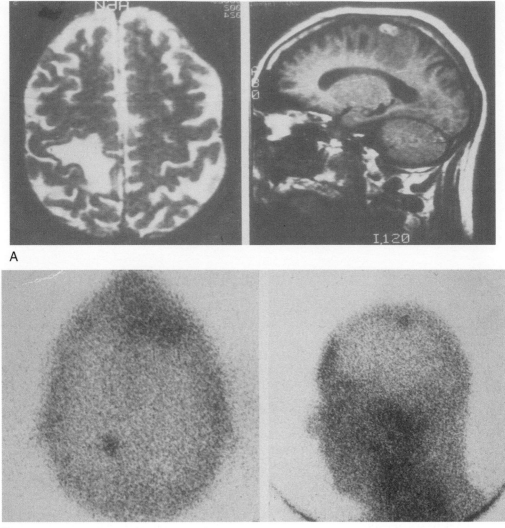

FIGURE 114-20. Magnetic resonance imaging *(A)* can give better soft tissue details than obtained by gallium scan *(B)* to determine the involvement of adjacent soft tissue by tumor extension.

Therefore, Sherman and Ter-Pogossian[52] introduced lymphoscintigraphy in 1953 to study lymphatic flow more accurately. They injected radiocolloid gold (^{198}Au) intradermally and used a gamma counter to detect the concentrated colloidal isotope in the filtering lymph nodes. This technique has since been modified with various other isotopes and colloids of various particle sizes for specific diagnostic purposes. The intent of each of these modifications is to identify the lymphatic vascular pattern in the tissue being evaluated.

The technique of lymphatic mapping is helpful for detecting metastases of melanoma of the extremities to the regional draining lymph nodes.[53] This test may be useful in patients with T2 or thicker lesions of the lower extremity for evaluation of the iliac and pelvic lymph nodes to determine the extent of lymphadenectomy that may be indicated. The iliac nodes should certainly be removed if they appear to be involved, but a pelvic lymphadenectomy is not indicated if the para-aortic lymph nodes are involved because cure is unlikely in these cases.

The sites of lymphatic spread from melanoma in these locations and in the head and neck may be evaluated by radionuclide lymphoscintigraphy.[54] Several radiocolloids have been employed for lymphoscintigraphy, including gold, sulfur, and antimony. Antimony sulfide colloid and technetium sulfur colloid have been found to be safe, and both give reliable information for determining appropriate lymph nodes for elective

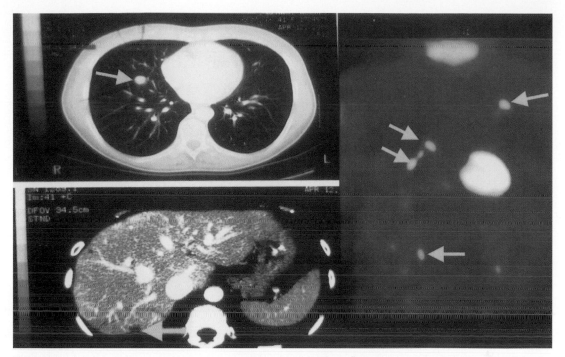

FIGURE 114-21. PET scan of the chest and abdomen *(right)* confirms the increased activity of metastatic lesions in the lung *(upper left)* and liver *(lower left)*.

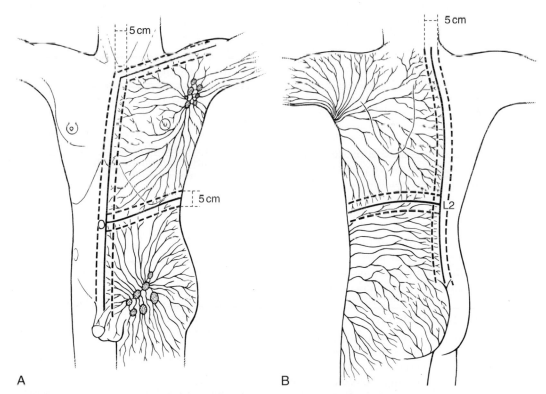

A   B

FIGURE 114-22. *A* and *B,* Lymphatic drainage as predicted by Sappey's lines. (Redrawn from Sugarbaker EV, McBride CM: Melanoma of the trunk: the results of surgical excision and anatomic guidelines for predicting nodal metastasis. Surgery 1976;80:22.)

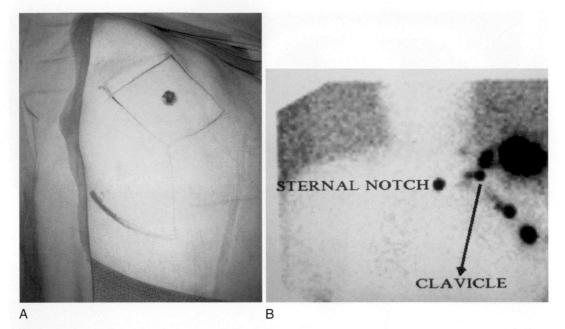

FIGURE 114-23. Lymphoscintigram of a scapular lesion *(A)* demonstrates the lymphatic drainage to the axillary nodes *(B)*.

dissection among patients with truncal or head and neck melanomas (Fig. 114-23).

A lymphoscintigram can detect the normal as well as unexpected patterns of lymph node drainage from lesions at primary sites. This test has been determined to provide a reliable predictor of the sites of nodal involvement. In a prospective study of 51 consecutive patients with primary melanomas greater than 1 mm thick and observed for a mean of 45 months, 23% of the 35 patients who chose to undergo elective lymphadenectomy were found to have micrometastases to these lymph nodes; all were in the node groups detected by the lymphoscintigram.[55] During the several years of their follow-up, 5 of the 16 patients (31%) who chose to be observed eventually developed clinical evidence of nodal metastases; in each case, the nodes that were involved with tumor were at the very sites of drainage predicted by the lymphoscintigrams that were performed at the time of initial diagnosis (Table 114-5). During the 7-year interval of follow-up, no patient in either group developed metastases to any nodes not predicted by lymphoscintigraphy.

SENTINEL LYMPH NODE BIOPSY

The concept of the sentinel lymph node is based on the principle that all lymphatic fluid from specific tissues is filtered by lymph nodes, and as such the first (or sentinel) lymph node filtering a specific site can be removed and evaluated for metastases of malignant cells. The validity of this entire principle is predicated on the tenets that

1. finite regions do drain specifically to a node;
2. the node can be found;
3. a negative biopsy finding means no other metastases;
4. a negative node is truly negative.

Morton[56] introduced the technique of detecting the sentinel lymph node with the intraoperative injection of vital blue dyes in the dermis surrounding the site of the primary melanoma. He identified the sentinel lymph node in more than 80% of the patients and reported that the false-negative rates had been about 5%. Subsequent investigators[57-59] reported that the use of preoperative lymphatic mapping and the intraoperative use of radiocolloids together with vital blue

TABLE 114-5 ✦ RELIABILITY OF LYMPHOSCINTIGRAMS

	ELND	Observe
Number of patients*	35 (70%)	16 (30%)
Lymph node metastases	8 (23%)	—
Subsequent lymph node metastases	—	5 (31%)

*51 patients with melanoma greater than 1 mm thick; 7-year follow-up (mean of 45 months).

ELND, elective lymph node dissection.

Data from Stephens PL, Ariyan S, Ocampo RJ, et al: The predictive value of lymphoscintigraphy for nodal metastases of cutaneous melanoma. Conn Med 1999;63:387.

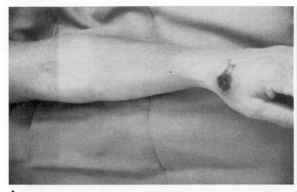

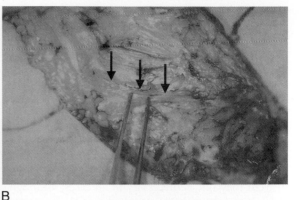

A   B

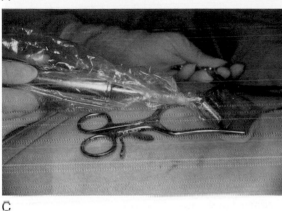

C   D

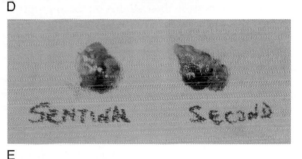

FIGURE 114-24. Sentinel node dissection. Blue dye injected into the dermis *(A)* at the site of the primary melanoma can be detected in the lymphatic vessels *(B)*. The radiocolloid injected in the dermis is detected by the hand-held gamma counter *(C)* to localize the sentinel lymph node *(D)*. A second node *(E)* was also identified adjacent to the first.

E

dyes have increased the identification and successful removal of the sentinel lymph node to the range of 98% to 99% of patients with melanoma (Fig. 114-24).

SURGICAL CONSIDERATIONS

The purpose of wide excision of melanoma is to decrease the incidence of local recurrence, reported in the literature to range from 3% to 20%. In large series, the highest risk of local recurrence has been documented with primary tumors on the hands and feet, with a recurrence rate of 11% to 12%, whereas the risk is only 5% to 6% for tumors on the face, scalp, and ear.[44]

It has generally been accepted that melanomas less than 0.76 mm thick are uniformly curable, as reported by Breslow.[43] Breslow and Macht[60] reported in a small series of 62 patients with lesions less than 0.76 mm that neither local recurrences nor metastases developed, regardless of the width of resection margin. Day et al[61] reported that although thin lesions have a good prognosis, the prognosis may be worse when the melanoma is located within the BANS area, an acronym for the upper *back,* upper posterior *arm,* posterior *neck,* and posterior *scalp.* On the other hand, Woods et al[62] reported 11 deaths among 400 patients with melanomas less than 0.76 mm treated at the Mayo Clinic; seven of the melanomas were not within the BANS area at all. In a smaller series, Briggs et al[63] reported that 10% of the patients with melanoma less than 0.76 mm died during their 10-year experience.

The World Health Organization (WHO)[64] evaluated the importance of the width of resection of the primary melanoma and the surrounding normal skin in a study of 593 patients with clinical stage I disease. Curability was not influenced by the resection margins but decreased with increasing thickness of the primary melanoma. In a large study of more than 3400 patients, Urist et al[44] noted that the recurrence rate of 146 melanomas of the neck was less than 2% even though most of the patients (84% to 87%) were treated with resection margins of only 1 to 2 cm.

These studies suggest that conventional margins of 5 cm may not be necessary in all cases; although these issues have been raised, the trials necessary to prove that narrower margins do not decrease the cure rates have yet to be completed. In a study of 598 patients with clinical stage I melanoma, the New York University–Massachusetts General Hospital Melanoma Clinical Cooperative Group noted that resection margins of 1.5 cm or less were associated with a significantly greater incidence of recurrences than were resection margins greater than 1.5 cm. However, margins greater than 3 cm did not lead to a lesser recurrence rate.[65] Indeed, for melanomas greater than 2 mm thick, retrospective data suggest that margins less than 2 cm may decrease the cure rates.[44,66-68]

At this time, it is not possible to draw any significant conclusions from these studies on the appropriate margins of resection because most of them have been retrospective and with selected patients. The answers will become available with the current WHO prospective randomized trial evaluating the differences in recurrence and death among patients who are treated by wide or narrow surgical margins.[69] In the meantime, the standard of treatment is to employ wide margins of resection for high-risk melanomas whenever feasible, as in the trunk, and a more conservative approach where such an excision will result in a deformity or functional deficit.

In determining the extent of the operation, whether on the face or on the trunk, it is important to consider the impact of the scar on the patient's self-image. The Pigment Lesion Study Group of the University of Pennsylvania evaluated the extent to which patients were distressed by scars after melanoma resections.[70] The two factors that had a negative impact were the degree of surgical depression or indentation and the patients' preoperative perception of the scar to be expected. The actual scar length did not have as much of an effect as the extent of depression of the scar. Skin grafts are acceptable for reconstructions of large resection sites, but they cause significant deformities (Fig. 114-25), which are usually avoided with flaps for coverage. The author has previously reported on the safety of coverage of these wounds with flaps.[71]

SURGICAL TREATMENT

Lesions suspected of being melanomas should be treated by excisional biopsy if they are small (<3 cm wide) and by incisional biopsy if they are larger to determine the extent of surgical excision. In situ lesions, those that have not invaded the dermis, may be treated by simple excision with a few millimeters of normal skin margins. Melanomas that invade the dermis less than 1 mm are at low risk for local recurrence and may be treated with a wide resection of 1 cm of normal skin margins. Melanomas deeper than 1 mm (and certainly lesions greater than 2 mm) are at high risk for recurrence and should be treated with a wider local excision. The question is, how wide is wide enough?

Head and Neck

High-risk melanomas of the face should be excised as just described and closed with adjacent flaps. Although resurfacing the resection site with a skin graft is possible, the cosmetic results are not as acceptable as with a flap. A local or regional skin flap covers the wound with a far more satisfactory color match to the rest of the face than a distant flap (Fig. 114-26).

A difficult area to resurface is a surgical defect over the chin because this area requires skin that firmly adheres to the mandible, soft tissue for contour, and a good match of the skin flap to the remainder of the face. A distant flap simply does not provide a satisfactory color match. A wide excision of this area can be resurfaced satisfactorily with an advancement flap of the neck.

On occasion, the melanoma forms on the upper part of the cheek, requiring removal of skin from the lower eyelids. This area cannot be resurfaced with a skin flap because it requires thin pliable covering. Resurfacing is best accomplished by employing a cheek advancement flap to cover most of the defect and a full-thickness skin graft to the eyelids. The best place to harvest this skin graft is from the ipsilateral or contralateral upper eyelid; the postauricular area may be a good second choice.

Extremities

Thin melanomas of the fingertips may be excised and the defect reconstructed with volar advancement flaps (Fig. 114-27) to provide sensate coverage. Lesions of the finger thicker than 1 mm are more safely treated with an interphalangeal joint amputation (Fig. 114-28) or a ray amputation, depending on the extent of the tumor.

Melanomas of the dorsum of the hand, the forearm, and the leg may be treated more readily with a wide excision. These surgical wounds have traditionally

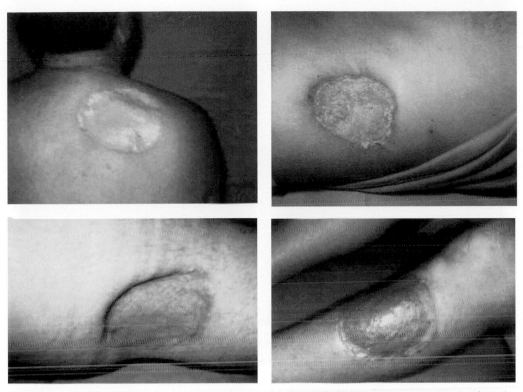

FIGURE 114-25. Skin grafts provide adequate coverage for wide resections, but they lead to significant deformities.

been covered with skin grafts with good success. However, coverage of these wide excisions with local flaps (Fig. 114-29) has been accomplished with successful control of the primary site and a more cosmetically acceptable result.[71] Furthermore, these patients do not need to have the arm immobilized, and they have a shorter hospital stay than do those who have had skin grafts.

Melanomas of the toes and feet are usually of the acral lentiginous type. These tumors spread aggressively and have a high incidence of local and regional recurrences. Therefore, they are best treated by aggressive resections (Fig. 114-30). A significant advantage to the use of flaps in the lower extremity is that patients may be able to ambulate the day after surgery and leave the hospital much sooner than patients treated with skin grafts.

Trunk

Primary melanomas of the trunk may be excised with more liberal margins (as much as 2 to 4 cm if need be) and still be closed easily. Some areas may be closed by wide undermining and large advancement flaps. Otherwise, these areas may still be closed readily by one

or more local flaps (Fig. 114-31). Deep fascia and muscle may be preserved if not involved by tumor invasion.

LYMPHADENECTOMY

The decision to perform a lymphadenectomy in a patient with malignant melanoma requires further thought. Certainly there is a uniformity of opinion among clinicians about the necessity to perform a lymphadenectomy when the regional draining lymph nodes can be detected and palpated. However, opinions differ about the efficacy of prophylactic lymphadenectomy in patients with clinical stage I disease.

In a WHO study of clinical stage I melanomas of the upper and lower extremities, delayed therapeutic lymphadenectomies (performed after the patients developed palpable regional lymph nodes) were found to be as effective as immediate prophylactic lymphadenectomies.[72] Although this was a randomized trial, the criticisms have been that the study was limited to melanomas of the extremity and might not be applicable to melanomas of the head and neck or the trunk; that a significant majority of the patients were women, who are well known to have better survival rates; and that many of the patients included in the study had

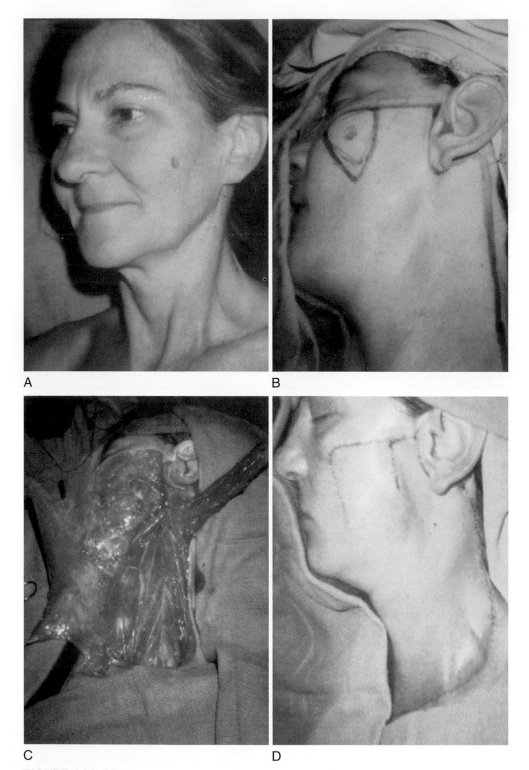

FIGURE 114-26. Melanoma of the cheek *(A)* was treated with a wide excision of the primary site *(B)*, a complete functional neck dissection *(C)*, and coverage with a large cervicofacial myocutaneous flap incorporating the platysma muscle *(D)*.

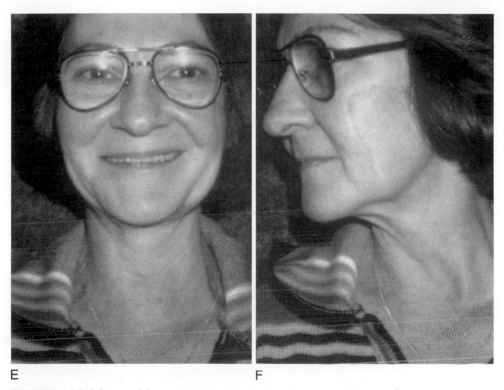

E   F

FIGURE 114-26, cont'd. *E* and *F,* One year postoperative photographs.

thin lesions and were at low risk for recurrences. Indeed, a careful review of the data reveals a subgroup of high-risk patients (with melanoma thickness of 1.6 to 4.5 mm) who did better with prophylactic immediate node dissections than with therapeutic delayed lymphadenectomies (78.5% versus 69.7%).

In a review of 206 patients with melanoma of the head and neck, Roses et al[73] reported that 31 of 73 patients who had been treated with prophylactic neck dissections had histologically positive nodes. Balch et al[74] reported that the most significant benefit of elective lymphadenectomy based on actuarial survival was for high-risk patients with melanomas in the 1.51- to 3.99-mm-thickness group. A review of additional studies from the melanoma registries in the United States and Australia has shown a benefit of elective lymph node dissections for patients with melanomas 0.76 to 3.99 mm thick.[75,76] Furthermore, these studies showed that contrary to previous beliefs, the biologic behavior of melanoma in these two parts of the world is the same, and by all variables in the multifactorial analysis, survival rates for melanoma in these two institutions are not significantly different.

The indications for prophylactic lymphadenectomy in stage I disease are further supported by the WHO Collaborating Center study of patients assigned to clinical stage I. The study showed that 20% of all patients with melanomas who underwent elective lymphadenectomy had histologically positive nodes,[77] whereas 29% of the patients who were observed showed subsequent lymph node recurrence (Table 114-6). Roses et al[78] demonstrated that 25% to 35% of their stage I patients with melanomas 1 to 3 mm thick had histologically positive nodes (Table 114-7). Therefore, the decision to perform a prophylactic lymphadenectomy in stage I melanoma patients should be based on the benefits expected and the risk of morbidity of the added procedure.

TABLE 114-6 ✦ FREQUENCY OF NODAL METASTASES

	Immediate (Elective) Lymph Node Dissections	Delayed (Therapeutic) Lymph Node Dissections
Number of patients*	173	165
Positive nodes	20%	29%

*17 WHO Collaborating Centers, 18 randomized prospective clinical trials.
Modified from Veronesi U, Adamus J, Bandiera DC, et al: Delayed regional lymph node dissection in stage I melanoma of the skin of the lower extremities. Cancer 1982;49:2420.

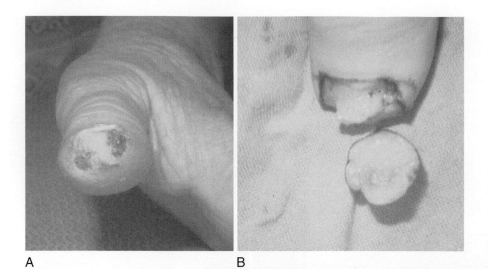

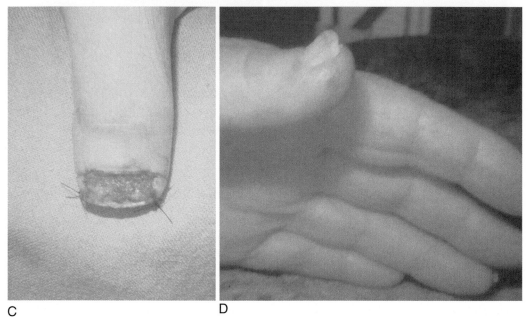

FIGURE 114-27. Melanoma of the fingertip *(A)* was excised with the nail, nail matrix, and nail bed *(B)*. The wound was covered with a volar advancement flap (*C* and *D*).

Much of this decision-making has been resolved during the past few years by the observations of a slight benefit to those patients undergoing early lymphadenectomy and the added benefit of adjuvant immunotherapy given to patients with early nodal metastases. The prospective randomized trial of more than 700 patients reported by the Intergroup Melanoma Surgical Program[79] showed a slight but significant improvement in survival rates in patients with melanoma thicknesses of 1 to 2 mm, those without tumor ulceration, and those 60 years of age or younger. In 1996, Kirkwood and associates[80] reported a higher cure rate and longer survival among patients with micrometastases to regional nodes. More recently,

this group has reported a subsequent evaluation of more than 600 patients, 25% of whom had melanomas greater than 4 mm thick; whereas they did show a significant improvement in relapse-free survival with interferon, they were unable to show any difference in overall cure rate.[81]

In regard to the patients with nodal metastases from malignant melanoma of unknown origin, Reintgen et al[82] reviewed 124 patients and demonstrated that regional lymphadenectomy resulted in a survival rate equal to that of lymphadenectomies in patients with known sites of primary melanoma. However, there is no place for the simple excision of the involved palpable lymph node alone because it is more than

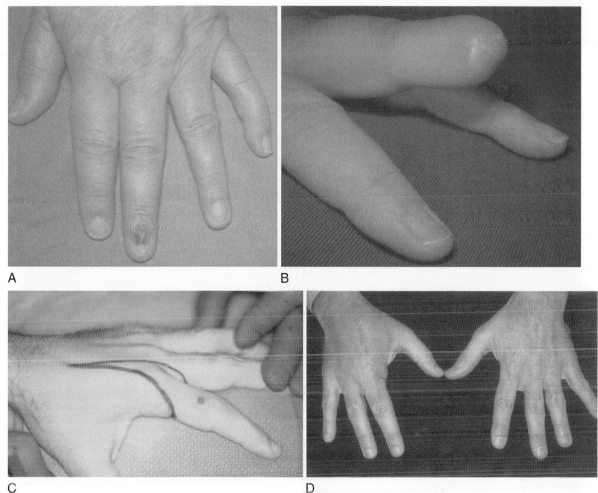

FIGURE 114-28. Thicker melanomas of fingers *(A)* need to be treated more aggressively with interphalangeal joint amputation *(B)* or ray amputation (*C* and *D*).

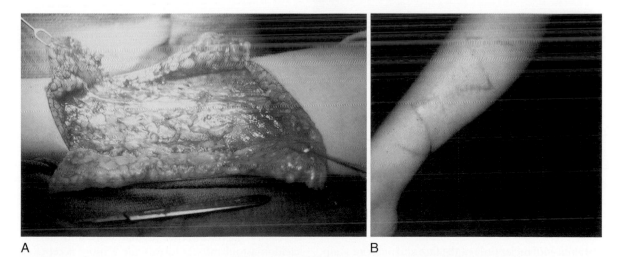

FIGURE 114-29. Wide excisions of melanomas of the hands, forearms, and legs *(A)* may be treated with local transposition flaps *(B)* to allow the patient to use the extremities early in the postoperative period.

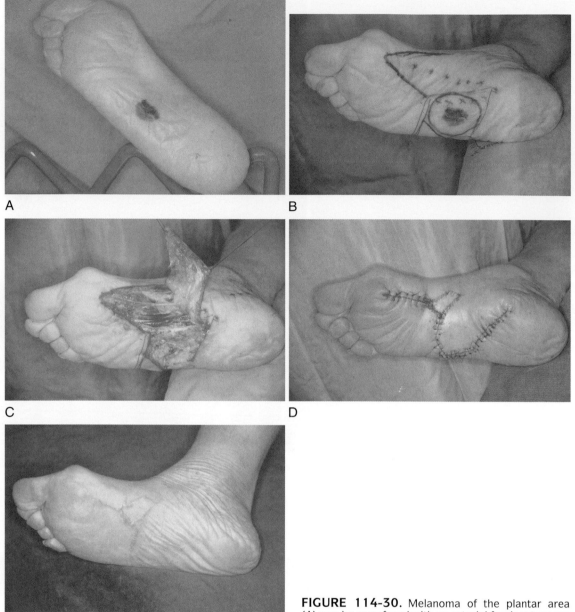

FIGURE 114-30. Melanoma of the plantar area *(A)* may be resurfaced with an arterial fasciocutaneous flap *(B to E)*.

likely that additional lymph nodes have microme-tastases. The only accepted treatment is a complete lymphadenectomy of the regional group of lymph nodes.

Cervical Lymphadenectomy

Patients with melanoma of the face and anterior scalp (Fig. 114-32) who are selected for cervical lym-phadenectomy because of the risk of micrometastases to these lymph nodes also should be treated with a superficial parotidectomy on the same side because the preparotid lymph nodes are the first echelon of nodal drainage. A cervical lymphadenec-tomy (Fig. 114-33; see also Fig. 114-26) can be per-formed with or without preservation of the spinal accessory nerve, internal jugular vein, and sterno-cleidomastoid muscle to provide a more acceptable appearance and functional neck and shoulder muscles.[83]

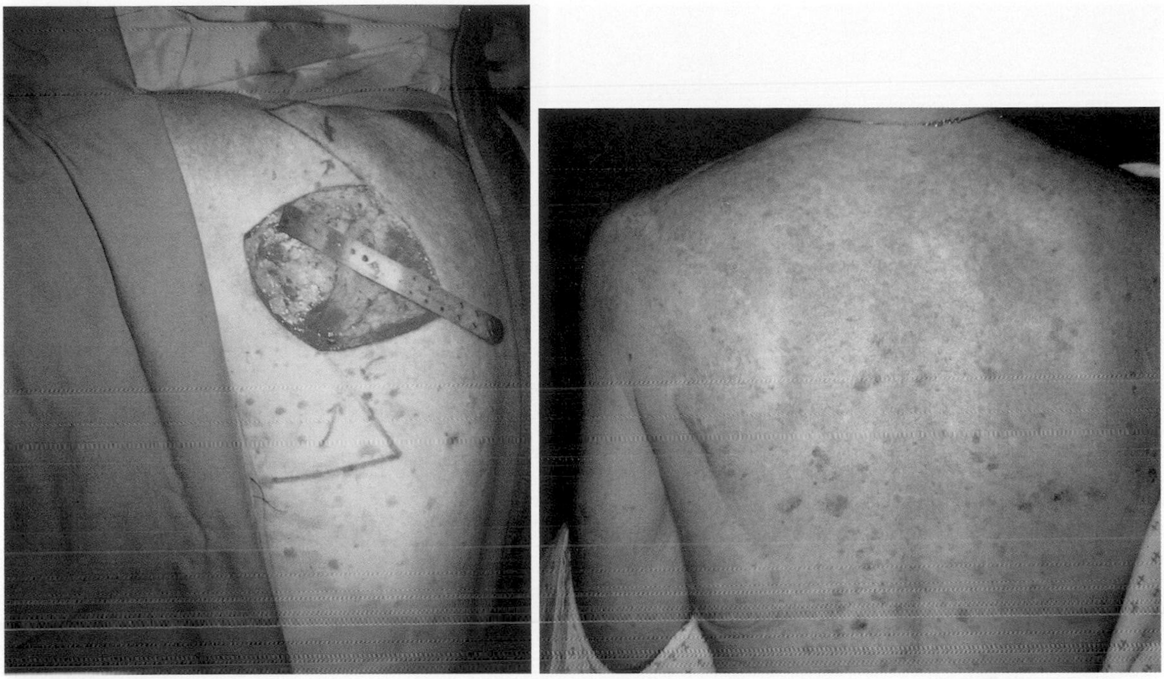

A B

FIGURE 114-31. In the truncal area, deep melanomas may be resected widely *(A)* and still be closed reliably with large transposition flaps *(B)*.

Axillary Lymphadenectomy

Place the patient in the supine position with the arm abducted and placed freely on two arm boards. The entire arm, including the hand, is prepared for surgery and draped, so that the arm can be moved as needed during the procedure. Make a prominent S-shaped incision with the midportion placed transversely across the apex of the axilla, with one limb descending behind the anterior edge of the lateral border of the pectoralis major muscle (Fig. 114-34) and the second limb descending along the posterior border of the upper arm. Elevate the two opposing skin flaps at the level of Scarpa fascia to expose the axillary contents.

Identify the brachial vein along the arm and dissect proximally to the axilla, from the anterior portion of the upper arm toward the posterior portion. Dissect the entire axillary contents in this fashion, moving in a distal to proximal direction. Ligate and transect the branches of the brachial vein; leave the thoracodorsal artery, vein, and nerve intact, however.

Dissect the axillary contents from along the lateral border of the pectoralis major muscle, leaving the muscle fascia behind with the muscle. Free the contents from the posterior surface of the pectoralis major, which is then retracted to expose the pectoralis minor. Dissect the fat and lymphatic contents from behind both the pectoralis major and minor muscles and retract this material downward. Using a surgical sponge pad, sweep the axillary contents away from the chest wall in a caudad direction. This maneuver usually exposes the long thoracic nerve along the chest wall. Preserve this nerve.

After the axillary contents are removed, reposition the skin flaps and suture them closed over large suction

TABLE 114-7 ✦ INCIDENCE OF MICROSCOPIC NODAL METASTASES IN CLINICAL STAGE I MELANOMA

Lesion Thickness (mm)	Positive Regional Nodes (%)		
	Roses[78]	*Balch*[74]	*Veronesi*[77]
<1.0	0	0	0
1.0-1.49	26	25	14
1.5-1.99	32	57	14
2.0-2.49	33	57	14
2.5-2.99	25	57	14
3.0-3.49	14	57	12
3.5-3.99	17	57	12
>4.0	50	62	40

Modified from Wanebo HJ, Harpole D, Teates D: Radionuclide lymphoscintigraphy with technetium 99m antimony sulfide colloid to identify lymphatic drainage of cutaneous melanoma at ambiguous sites in the head and neck and trunk. Cancer 1985;55:1403.

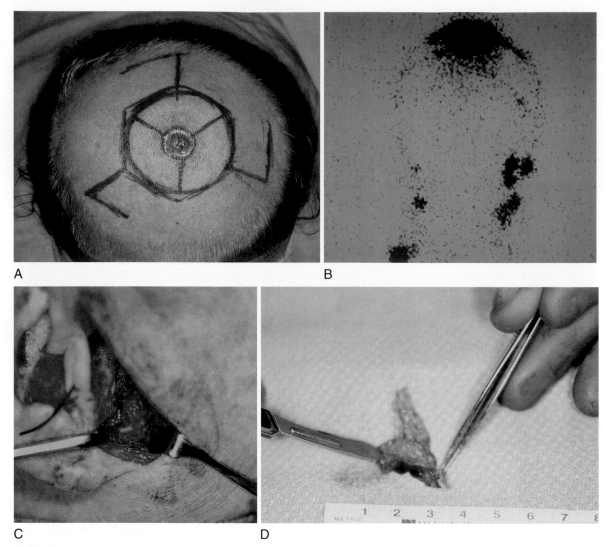

FIGURE 114-32. Melanoma of the vertex of the scalp *(A)* was found to have lymphatic drainage to bilateral parotid and cervical nodes *(B)*. The parotid sentinel node *(C)* was found to be positive *(D)*.

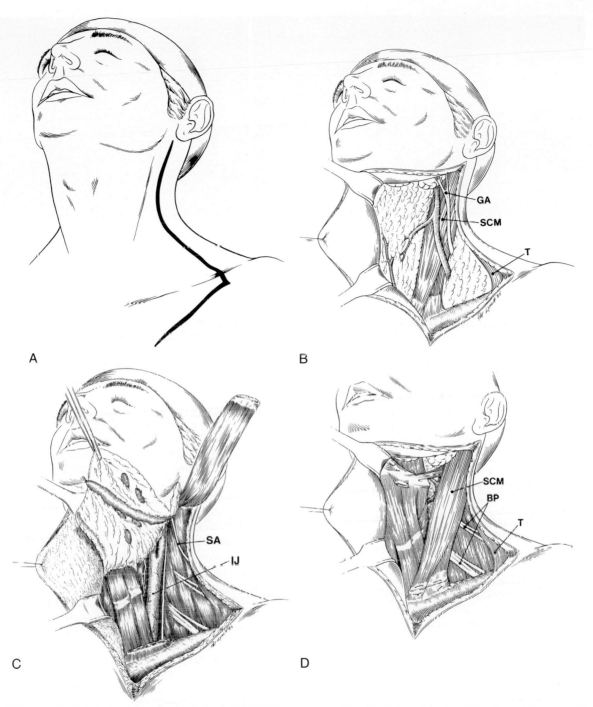

FIGURE 114-33. Functional radical neck dissection can be performed while preserving the sternocleidomastoid muscle (SCM), the internal jugular vein (IJ), and the spinal accessory nerve (SA). GA, great auricular nerve; T, trapezius; BP, brachial plexus. (Reproduced from Ariyan S: Radical neck dissection. Surg Clin North Am 1986;66:133.)

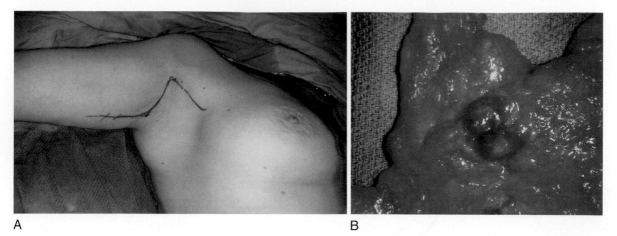

FIGURE 114-34. Axillary incision is S shaped *(A)* to provide opposing flaps for greater access to the axillary contents *(B)*. See text for details.

catheters. These catheters remain in place for 3 to 10 days, depending on the amount of 24-hour drainage accumulated. The decision to remove the drain should be based on the pattern and rate of daily decrease in the drainage rather than the actual amount. The drains are most commonly ready to be removed by the fifth or sixth day. The patient is instructed to keep the arm in a sling during waking hours to decrease shearing forces on the dissected tissues and thereby lessen the drainage.

Inguinofemoral Lymphadenectomy

Excision of inguinofemoral lymph nodes is facilitated by a horizontal incision along the skin crease 2 cm above and parallel to the inguinal region and a vertical incision over the femoral vessels, beginning in the inguinal skinfold and extending inferiorly for 8 to 10 cm. This approach results in an "interrupted" T incision (Fig. 114-35). Carry the skin incision in the inguinal area down to the fascia of the external oblique muscle and split it open to expose the internal oblique muscle. Dissect this origin of the internal oblique muscle sharply off the iliac crest to provide access to the retroperitoneal space. Pull the peritoneum away along the undersurface of the transversalis fascia from the external iliac vessels and lymph nodes. This provides an excellent view of the nodes for the lymphadenectomy.

Elevate the skin flaps on either side of the femoral incisions at the level of Scarpa fascia as well as the skin below the horizontal incision (Fig. 114-36). Elevate the skin completely from the inguinal incision to the lower end of the femoral incision. Dissect the femoral fat and lymphatic tissues down to but not including the muscle fascia. Continue the dissection cephalad on the surface of the muscle fascia until the saphenous vein and saphenous bulb are reached on the femoral vein.

Dissect the contents in the inguinal region down to the fascia of the external oblique muscle and in the caudad direction to communicate with the femoral dissection. Do not remove the muscle fascia or transpose the muscles adjacent to the femoral vessels to cover these vessels; such procedures increase the risk of lymphedema. Close the wounds over large suction catheters that remain in place for 3 to 10 days. Patients are permitted to ambulate the night of surgery or the next morning.

SURVEILLANCE

Patients treated at the Yale Melanoma Unit are initially monitored closely (Table 114-8), with increasing intervals each year. Education of the patient for early self-detection of recurrences together with interval follow-up with a physician member of our team has been most successful in maintaining an effective monitoring program.[84] Patients are examined for local or in-transit metastases at varying intervals based on the stage of the melanoma at diagnosis (Table 114-9).

COMPLICATIONS

The incidence of wound infection, wound separation, and partial skin flap losses is the same as for any other operation, ranging from 5% to 7%. Although the incidence of lymphedema of the extremities is reported in the literature to be as high as 20% to 50%, in the author's experience, this complication occurs in 10% of patients seen.[85] This low incidence of lymphedema appears to be related to the preservation of muscle fascia and avoidance of the use of local muscle flaps.

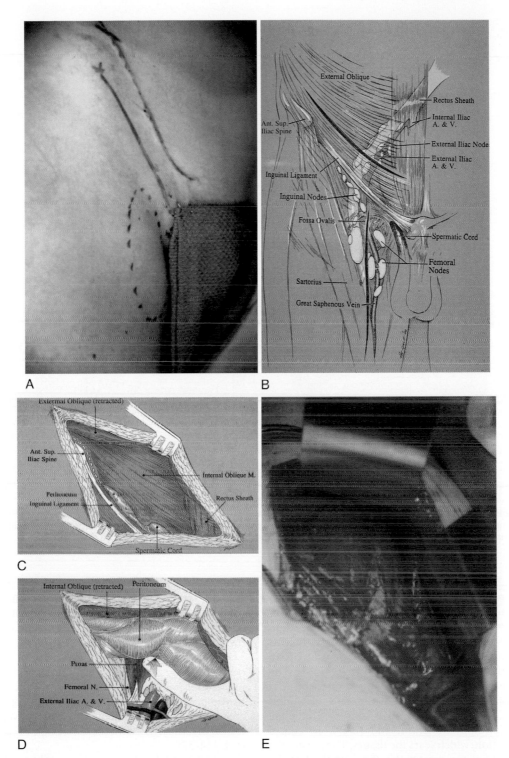

FIGURE 114-35. An "interrupted" T incision (*A* and *B*) is used for access to both the inguinal and iliac nodes. The fascia of the external oblique muscle is split *(C)*, and the internal oblique and transversalis are dissected away from the inguinal ligament and iliac crest. The peritoneum is peeled back by finger dissection *(D)* to obtain retroperitoneal access to the iliac and obturator nodes *(E)*.

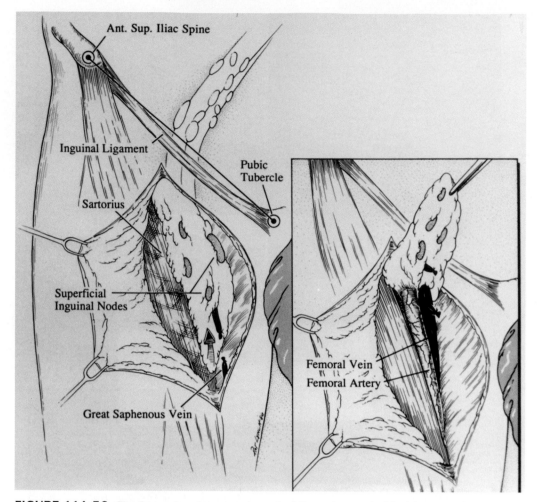

FIGURE 114-36. The femoral nodes are approached through a vertical incision over the region of the femoral vessels. After the medial and lateral flaps are elevated *(left)*, the subcutaneous fat containing the lymph nodes is dissected off the deeper muscle fascia *(right)*.

Experience with axillary lymphadenectomies for breast cancer has demonstrated that the incidence of lymphedema is lowest with surgery alone. If radiation therapy is added to the operation, the incidence of lymphedema increases. If the wound becomes infected, the incidence of lymphedema also increases. The probability of lymphedema is the greatest when the operation is followed with radiation and the wound becomes infected; the reason is that each of these (surgery, wound infection, and radiation) causes inflammation, which scars the tissues. The greater the inflammation, the greater the scar and the less the potential of lymphatic drainage over the muscle fascia.

Patients are encouraged to swim in a swimming pool as early as 2 weeks after the operation to increase the range of motion of the involved extremity. On occasion, this exercise has corrected early lymphedema of the arm. The late onset of lymphedema (several weeks or months later) is an ominous sign and usually represents a more permanent lymphedema that requires the patient to use elastic support garments.

Finally, tumor recurrences correlate with the thickness of the lesion. Between 60% and 70% of recurrences appear in the first 18 to 24 months after surgical treatments (Table 114-10).[86] The earliest recurrences are to local or regional lymph nodes, followed by in-transit metastases; distant metastases appear the latest (Fig. 114-37).

Patients with local recurrences may be treated with wider surgical resections, but extensive local recurrences or in-transit metastases are more difficult to treat. In-transit metastases of extremities are treated with isolation-perfusion of that extremity with dacarbazine (DTIC),[87] cisplatin, or hypo-osmolar perfusions

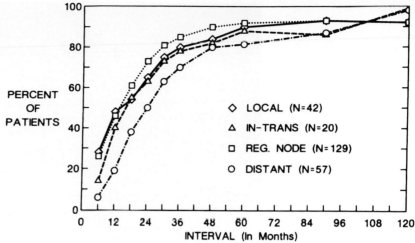

FIGURE 114-37. The curve of the timing of local recurrences precedes that of lymph node recurrences and distant organ metastases.

TABLE 114-8 ✦ SURVEILLANCE GUIDELINES

Follow-up Guidelines

Office visits and physical examination	
Stage 0	Yearly by dermatologist or primary care physician
Stage I	Every 6 months for 5 years
Stage II-IV	Every 3 months for 2 years
	Every 6 months for 3 years

Metastatic Surveillance

Lactate dehydrogenase level and complete blood cell count	At each visit, at least yearly
Chest radiograph	Every other visit, at least yearly
CT scans	With laboratory test or chest radiograph abnormality, physical findings, or symptoms

with carboplatin.[88] Carboplatin eradicated the lesions after perfusion in some patients (Fig. 114-38), whereas the control was temporary in other patients. The advantage of DTIC is its low incidence of hepatic and systemic toxicity, which is far less than that after perfusion with L-phenylalanine mustard. Indeed, we found that such perfusions were tolerated well among our elderly patients, with no greater risk of complications in this group than in our younger patients (Table 114-11).[89]

If the recurrence is a single small metastasis in the lung, liver, or brain that is accessible to surgical removal, the surgical removal of this solitary metastasis may be worthwhile (Table 114-12). However, multiple recurrences cannot be treated by surgery but need to be considered for systemic chemotherapy. Although DTIC has been approved for systemic palliation of metastatic melanoma for 15 years, it has never been demonstrated to prolong survival of the treated patients. A large collection of clinical trials[90] has demonstrated an objective response rate (regressions of all

TABLE 114-9 ✦ PROTOCOL FOR FOLLOW-UP SURVEILLANCE

	Physical Examination	Chest Radiography	Liver Function Tests	Imaging
Stage I, T1	Semiannual × 2 yr, then annually	—	—	
Stage I-II, T2-4	Every 3 months × 3 yr, then semiannually	Annual	Annual	
Stage III (lymph nodes positive)	Every 3 months × 3 yr, then semiannually	Annual	Annual	Annual or as indicated

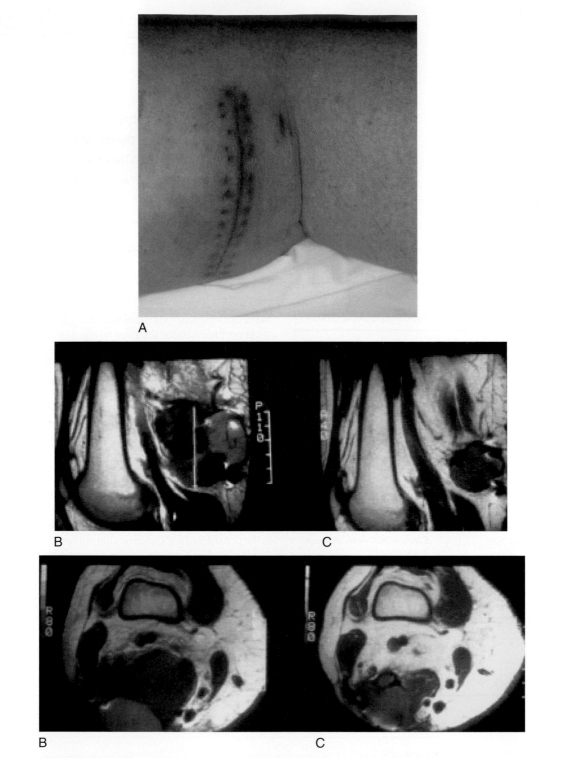

A

B   C

B   C

FIGURE 114-38. Regional isolated perfusion of a lower extremity recurrence *(A)* led to signifi-cant response and shrinking of the tumor *(B* is before perfusion at left, and *C* is after perfusion at right), permitting radical resection of the mass *(D)* without compromise to the popliteal vessels.

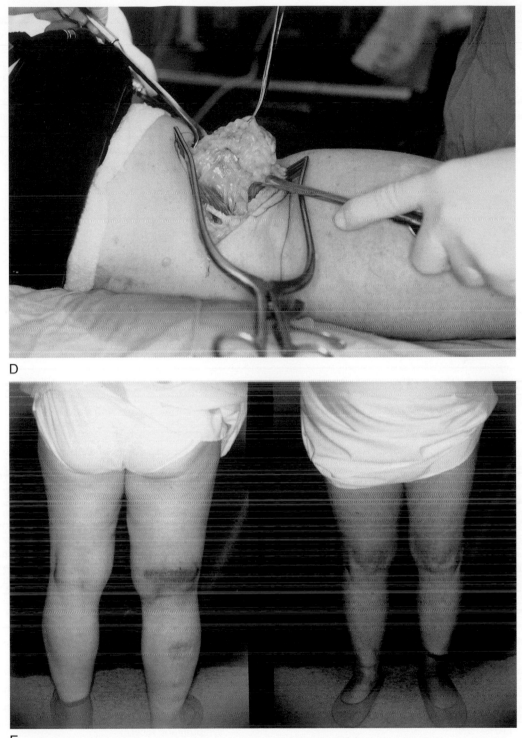

D

E

FIGURE 114-38, cont'd. At 1 year, there was no local recurrence *(E)*.

TABLE 114-10 ✦ TIMING OF RECURRENT MELANOMA AFTER SURGICAL TREATMENT

Site	18 Months	24 Months	3 Years	5 Years	10 Years
Nodal	63%	74%	86%	93%	95%
Local	55%	67%	81%	88%	95%
In-transit	55%	67%	80%	90%	97%
Systemic	40%	52%	71%	83%	95%
Overall	57%	67%	81%	90%	95%

Modified from Fusi S, Ariyan S, Sternlicht A: Data on first recurrence after treatment for malignant melanoma in a large patient population. Plast Reconstr Surg 1993;91:94.

TABLE 114-11 ✦ PERFUSION COMPLICATIONS*

Age	20s	30s	40s	50s	60s	70s	80s	Total
Number	4	7	11	9	16	14	6	67
Edema (pre/post)			1		2	2	1	6
Edema (post)	1		2		2			5
Seroma	1			1	1	1		4
Wound				1	5	1	2	9
Pulmonary embolus					1			1
Total	2	0	2	2	9	2	2	19
			15/47 (32%)			4/20 (20%)		

*67 perfusions in 60 patients, 1976-1995.
From Ariyan S, Poo WJ: The safety and efficacy of isolated perfusion of extremities for recurrent tumor in elderly patients. A 20-year experience. Surgery 1998;123:335.

the lesions by 50% or more) of 21%, but the median duration has been only 5 to 7 months.

UNSOLVED PROBLEMS

The overall cure rates for this disease have not been significantly improved during the past several decades because we are unable to treat the subclinical micrometastases that are present in systemic organs at the time of the treatment of the primary melanoma. Once these metastases become evident clinically, there is little chance of cure by further surgery, chemotherapy, radiation therapy, or combinations of these treatment modalities. Surgical adjuvant trials with chemotherapy or chemoimmunotherapy have not been successful for any meaningful time. However, employment of adjuvant immunotherapy to seek out and destroy these micrometastases combined with the

TABLE 114-12 ✦ SURGERY FOR METASTATIC MELANOMA: OUTCOME

Site of First Recurrence	Incidence	5-Year Survival	Median Survival
Skin, fat, lymph node	50%-60%	5%-40%	8-50 months
Lung	15%-35%	5%-30%	8-20 months

Gastrointestinal tract
  Small bowel (35%-65%)
  Colon (10%-15%)
  Stomach (5%)
	2%-4%	Minority of patients
		Mostly palliative for
		  symptomatic relief
			10-20 months

Brain (at autopsy, 50%-80%)	8%-15%	Unexpected (5%) 80%-90% have symptomatic relief	6-8 months
Liver (rarely single metastasis)	5%	Anecdotal cases	—

Modified from Allen PJ, Coit DG: The surgical management of metastatic melanoma. Ann Surg Oncol 2002;9:762.

surgical removal of the clinically apparent melanoma has theoretical potential. These trials are ongoing at several institutions, and there is hope that such modalities will improve cure rates in the future.

REFERENCES

1. Greenlee RT, Murray T, Bolden S, Wingo PA: Cancer statistics, 2000. CA Cancer J Clin 2000;50:7.
2. Handley WS: The pathology of melanotic growths in relation to their operative treatment. Lecture I. Lancet 1907;1:927.
3. Norris W: Case of fungoid disease. Edinburgh Med Surg 1820;16:562.
4. Halsted W: The results of operations for the cure of the breast performed at the Johns Hopkins Hospital. Ann Surg 1894;20:497.
5. Halsted W: The results of radical operations for the cure of carcinoma of the breast. Ann Surg 1907;46:1.
6. Handley WS: The pathology of melanocytic growths in relation to their operative treatment. Lecture II. Lancet 1907;1:996.
7. Pringle JH: A method of operation in cases of melanotic tumours of the skin. Edinburgh Med Surg 1908;123:496.
8. Goldsmith HS, Shah JP, Kim DH: Prognostic significance of lymph node dissection in the treatment of malignant melanoma. Cancer 1970;26:606.
9. Olsen G: The malignant melanoma of skin. Acta Chir Scand Suppl 1966;365:128.
10. Kenady DE, Brown BW, McBride CM: Excision of underlying fascia with a primary malignant melanoma: effects on recurrences and survival rates. Surgery 1982;92:615.
11. Kaplan EN: The risk of malignancy in large congenital nevi. Plast Reconstr Surg 1974;53:421.
12. Rhodes AR, Melski JW: Small congenital nevocellular nevi and the risk of cutaneous melanoma. J Pediatr 1982;100:219.
13. National Institutes of Health Development Panel on Early Melanoma: Diagnosis and treatment of early melanoma. JAMA 1992;268:1314.
14. Ackerman AB, Mihara I: Dysplasia, dysplastic melanocytes, dysplastic nevi, the dysplastic nevus syndrome, and the relation between dysplastic nevi and malignant melanomas. Hum Pathol 1985;16:87.
15. Elder DE, Goldman LI, Goldman SC, et al: Dysplastic nevus syndrome: a phenotypic association of sporadic malignant melanoma. Cancer 1980;46:1787.
16. Wallace DC, Beardmore GL, Exton LE: Familial malignant melanoma. Ann Surg 1973;177:15.
17. Clark WII, Reimer RR, Greene M, et al: Origin of familial melanoma from heritable melanocytic lesion: "B-K mole syndrome." Arch Dermatol 1978;114:732.
18. Reimer RR: Precursor lesions in familial melanoma. A new genetic pre-neoplastic syndrome. JAMA 1978;239:744.
19. Epstein E, Bragg K, Linden G: Biopsy and prognosis of malignant melanoma. JAMA 1969;208:1369.
20. Ackerman AB: Macular and patch lesions of malignant melanoma: malignant melanoma in-situ. J Dermatol Surg Oncol 1983;9:8.
21. Rywlin AM: Malignant melanoma in situ, precancerous melanosis, or atypical intraepidermal melanocytic proliferation. Am J Dermatopathol Suppl 1984;6:97.
22. Mooney MA, Barr RJ, Buxton MG: Halo nevus or halo phenomenon? A study of 142 cases. J Cutan Pathol 1995;22:342.
23. Scheiber A: Clinical features: prognosis and incidence of multiple primary melanomas. Aust N Z J Surg 1981;51:386.
24. Veronesi U, Cascinelli N, Bufalino R: Evaluation of the risk of multiple primaries in malignant cutaneous melanoma. Tumori 1976;62:127.
25. Greene MH, Fraumeni F: The hereditary variant of malignant melanoma. In Clark WH, Goldman LI, Mastrangelo MJ, eds: Human Malignant Melanoma. New York, Grune & Stratton, 1979;109.
26. Greene MH, Goldin LR, Clark WH, et al: Familial cutaneous malignant melanoma: autosomal dominant trait possibly linked to the Rh locus. Proc Natl Acad Sci USA 1983;80:6071.
27. Knutson CO, Hori JM, Spratt JS: Melanoma. Curr Probl Surg 1971;Dec:3.
28. Drzewiecki KT, Ladefoged C, Christensen HE: Biopsy and prognosis for cutaneous malignant melanomas in clinical stage I. Scand J Plast Reconstr Surg 1980;14:141.
29. Sugarbaker EV, McBride CM: Survival and regional disease control after isolation-perfusion for invasive stage I melanoma of the extremities. Cancer 1976;37:188.
30. Cochran AJ, Wen DR, Herschman HR: Occult melanoma in lymph nodes detected by antiserum to S-100 protein. Int J Cancer 1984;34:159.
31. Amer MHJ, Al-Sarraf M, Vaitkevicius VK: Clinical presentation, natural history, and prognostic factors in advanced malignant melanoma. Surg Gynecol Obstet 1979;149:687.
32. Clark WH, Elder DE, Guerry D, et al: A study of tumor progression: the precursor lesions of superficial spreading and nodular melanoma. Hum Pathol 1984;15:1147.
33. Balch CM, Murad TM, Soong SJ, et al: A multifactorial analysis of melanoma: prognostic histopathological features comparing Clark's and Breslow's staging methods. Ann Surg 1978;188:732.
34. Koh HK, Michalik E, Sober AJ, et al: Lentigo maligna melanoma has no better prognosis than other types of melanoma. J Clin Oncol 1984;2:994.
35. Taylor DR, South DA: Acral lentiginous melanoma. Cutis 1980;26:35.
36. Coleman WP, Loria PR, Reed RJ, et al: Acral lentiginous melanoma. Arch Dermatol 1980;116:773.
37. Conley J, Lattes R, Orr W: Desmoplastic malignant melanoma (a rare variant of spindle cell melanoma). Cancer 1971;28:914.
38. Egbert B, Kempson R, Sagebiel R: Desmoplastic malignant melanoma: a clinicohistopathologic study of 25 cases. Cancer 1988;62:2033.
39. Bruijn JA, Mihm MC, Barnhill RL: Desmoplastic melanoma. Histopathology 1992;20:197.
40. Giuliano AE, Cochran AJ, Morton DL: Melanoma from unknown primary site and amelanotic melanoma. Semin Oncol 1982;9:442.
41. Mehnert JH, Heard JL: Staging of malignant melanomas by depth of invasion: a proposed index to prognosis. Am J Surg 1965;110:168.
42. Clark WH, From L, Bernardino FA, et al: The histogenesis and biologic behavior of primary human malignant melanoma of the skin. Cancer Res 1969;29:705.
43. Breslow A: Thickness, cross-sectional areas and depth of invasion in the prognosis of cutaneous melanoma. Ann Surg 1970;172:902.
44. Urist MM, Balch CM, Soong SJ, et al: The involvement of surgical margins and prognostic factors predicting the risk of local recurrence in 3,445 patients with primary cutaneous melanoma. Cancer 1985;55:1398.
45. Balch CM, Buzaid AC, Atkins MB, et al: A new American Joint Committee on Cancer staging system for cutaneous melanoma. Cancer 2000;88:1484.
46. Buzaid AC, Sandler AB, Mani S, et al: Role of computed tomography in the staging of primary melanoma. J Clin Oncol 1993;11:638.
47. Kirkwood JM, Myers JE, Vlock DR, et al: Tomographic gallium-67 citrate scanning: useful new surveillance for metastatic melanoma. Ann Intern Med 1982;97:694.
48. Kirkwood JM, Myers JE, Vlock DR, et al: Tomographic gallium-67 citrate scanning. Useful new surveillance for metastatic melanoma. Ann Surg 1983;198:102.
49. Holder WD, White RL, Zuger JH, et al: Effectiveness of positron emission tomography for the detection of melanoma metastases. Ann Surg 1998;227:769.

50. Rinne D, Baum RP, Hor G, et al: Primary staging and follow-up of high risk melanoma patients with whole-body ^{18}F-fluorodeoxyglucose positron emission tomography. Results of a prospective study of 100 patients. Cancer 1998;82:1664.

51. Sappey MPC: Anatomie, physiologie, pathologie des vaisseaux lymphatiques considérés chez l'homme et les vertébrés. Paris, A Delahaye, 1874.

52. Sherman A, Ter-Pogossian M: Lymph node concentration of radioactive colloidal gold following interstitial injection. Cancer 1953;6:1238.

53. Ariyan S, Kirkwood JM, Mitchell MS, et al: Intralymphatic and regional surgical adjuvant immunotherapy in high risk melanoma of the extremities. Surgery 1982;92:459.

54. Wanebo HJ, Harpole D, Teates D: Radionuclide lymphoscintigraphy with technetium 99m antimony sulfide colloid to identify lymphatic drainage of cutaneous melanoma at ambiguous sites in the head and neck and trunk. Cancer 1985;55:1403.

55. Stephens PL, Ariyan S, Ocampo RJ, et al: The predictive value of lymphoscintigraphy for nodal metastases of cutaneous melanoma. Conn Med 1999;63:387.

56. Morton DL, Wen DR, Wong JH, et al: Technical details of intraoperative lymphatic mapping for early stage melanoma. Arch Surg 1992;127:392.

57. Reintgen D, Cruse CW, Wells K, et al: The orderly progression of melanoma nodal metastases. Ann Surg 1994;220:759.

58. Albertini JJ, Cruse CC, Rappaport D, et al: Intraoperative radiolymphoscintigraphy improves sentinel lymph node identification for patients with melanoma. Ann Surg 1996;223:217.

59. Cascinelli N, Belli F, Santinami M, et al: Sentinel lymph node biopsy in cutaneous melanoma: the WHO Melanoma Program experience. Ann Surg Oncol 2000;7:469.

60. Breslow A, Macht SD: Optimal size of resection margin for thin cutaneous melanoma. Surg Gynecol Obstet 1977;145:691.

61. Day CL, Mihm MC, Sober AJ, et al: Prognostic factors for melanoma patients with lesions 0.76 to 1.69 mm in thickness. Ann Surg 1982;195:30.

62. Woods JE, Soule EH, Creagan ET: Metastases and death in patients with thin melanomas (less than 0.76 mm). Ann Surg 1983;198:63.

63. Briggs JC, Ibrahim NB, Hastings AG, et al: Experience of thin cutaneous melanomas (0.76 and 0.85 mm thick) in a large plastic surgery unit: a 5- to 17-year followup. Br J Plast Surg 1984;37:501.

64. Cascinelli N, van der Esch A, Breslow A, et al: Stage I melanoma of the skin: the problem of resection margin. Eur J Cancer 1980;16:1079.

65. Golomb FM: Invited discussion. Plast Reconstr Surg 1983;71:76.

66. Day CL, Mihm MC, Sober AJ, et al: Narrower margins for clinical stage I malignant melanoma. N Engl J Med 1982;306:479.

67. Kirkwood JM, Ariyan S: Malignant melanoma margins. N Engl J Med 1982;307:439.

68. Roses DF, Harris MN, Rigel D, et al: Local and in-transit metastases following definitive excision for primary cutaneous melanoma. Ann Surg 1983;198:65.

69. Veronesi U, Cascinelli N, Adamus J, et al: Thin stage I primary cutaneous malignant melanoma. Comparison of excision with margins of 1 or 3 cm. N Engl J Med 1988;318:1159.

70. Cassileth BR, Lusk EJ, Tenaglia AN: Patient's perceptions of the cosmetic impact of melanoma resection. Plast Reconstr Surg 1983;71:73.

71. Cuono CB, Ariyan S: Versatility and safety of flap coverage for wide excision of cutaneous melanoma. Plast Reconstr Surg 1985;76:281.

72. Veronesi U, Adamus J, Bandiera DC, et al: Inefficiency of immediate node dissection in stage I melanoma of the limbs. N Engl J Med 1977;297:627.

73. Roses DF, Harris MN, Grunberger I, et al: Selective surgical management of cutaneous melanoma of the head and neck. Ann Surg 1980;192:692.

74. Balch CM, Soong SJ, Murad TM, et al: A multifactorial analysis of melanoma. II. Prognostic factors in patients with stage I (localized) melanoma. Surgery 1979;86:343.

75. Balch CM, Soong SJ, Milton GW, et al: A comparison of prognostic factors and surgical results in 1,786 patients with localized (stage 1) melanoma treated in Alabama, USA, and New South Wales, Australia. Ann Surg 1982;196:677.

76. Milton GW, Shaw HM, McCarthy WH, et al: Prophylactic lymph node dissection in clinical stage I cutaneous malignant melanoma: results of surgical treatment in 1,319 patients. Br J Surg 1982;69:108.

77. Veronesi U, Adamus J, Bandiera DC, et al: Delayed regional lymph node dissection in stage I melanoma of the skin of the lower extremities. Cancer 1982;49:2420.

78. Roses DF, Harris MN, Hidalgo D, et al: Primary melanoma thickness correlated with regional lymph node metastases. Arch Surg 1982;117:921.

79. Balch CM, Soong S, Bartolucci A, et al: Efficacy of an elective regional node dissection of 1- to 4-mm thick melanomas for patients 60 years of age and younger. Ann Surg 1996;224:255.

80. Kirkwood JM, Strawderman MH, Ernstoff MS, et al: Interferon alfa-2b adjuvant therapy of high-risk resected cutaneous melanoma: the Eastern Cooperative Oncology Group Trial EST 1684. J Clin Oncol 1996;14:7.

81. Kirkwood JM, Ibrahim JG, Sondak VK, et al: High- and low-dose interferon alfa-2a in high-risk melanoma: first analysis of Intergroup Trial E1690/S9111/C9190. J Clin Oncol 2000;18:2444.

82. Reintgen DS, McCarthy KS, Woodward B, et al: Metastatic malignant melanoma with unknown primary. Surg Gynecol Obstet 1983;156:335.

83. Ariyan S: Functional radical neck dissection. Plast Reconstr Surg 1980;65:768.

84. Poo-Hwu WJ, Ariyan S, Lamb L, et al: Follow-up recommendations for patients with American Joint Committee on Cancer Stages I-III malignant melanoma. Cancer 1999;86:2252.

85. Lawton G, Rasque H, Ariyan S: Preservation of muscle fascia to decrease lymphedema after complete axillary and ilioinguinofemoral lymphadenectomy for melanoma. J Am Coll Surg 2002;195:339.

86. Fusi S, Ariyan S, Sternlicht A: Data on first recurrence after treatment for malignant melanoma in a large patient population. Plast Reconstr Surg 1993;91:94.

87. Ariyan S, Mitchell MS, Kirkwood JM: Regional isolated perfusion of high-risk melanoma of the extremities with imidazole carboxamine. Surg Gynecol Obstet 1984;58:238.

88. Ariyan S, Poo WJ, Bolognia J: Regional isolated perfusion of extremities for malignant melanoma. A 20-year experience. Plast Reconstr Surg 1997;99:1023.

89. Ariyan S, Poo WJ: The safety and efficacy of isolated perfusion of extremities for recurrent tumor in elderly patients. A 20-year experience. Surgery 1998;123:335.

90. Balch CM, Reintgen DS, Kirkwood JM, et al: Cutaneous melanoma. In DeVita VT, Hellman S, Rosenberg SA, eds: Cancer: Principles and Practice of Oncology. New York, JB Lippincott, 1997:1947.

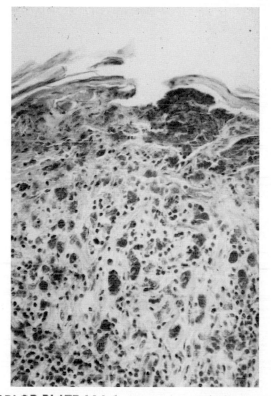

COLOR PLATE 114-1. Histologic examination of the specimen cut through the area of depigmentation shows significant lymphocytic infiltration with disrupted pigment granules leading to the colorless patches within.

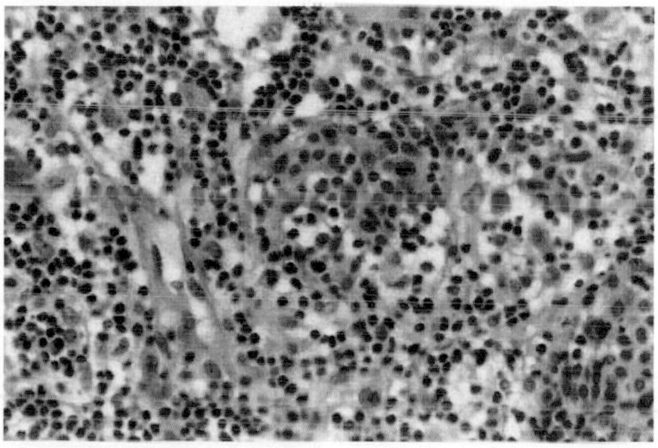

COLOR PLATE 114-2. Histologic examination of the depigmented portion shows infiltration with lymphocytes, but there is no evidence of pigment granules or malignant cells.

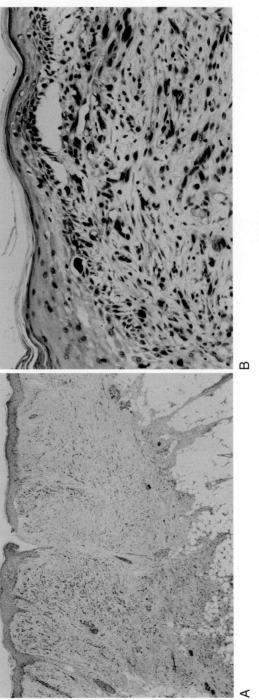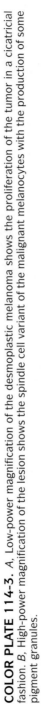

B

COLOR PLATE 114–3. *A,* Low-power magnification of the desmoplastic melanoma shows the proliferation of the tumor in a cicatricial fashion. *B,* High-power magnification of the lesion shows the spindle cell variant of the malignant melanocytes with the production of some pigment granules.

A

Local Flaps for Facial Coverage

Ian T. Jackson, MD, DSc (Hon), FRCS, FACS, FRACS (Hon)

The basic rule in facial flaps is not to choose the flap without consideration of the defect and careful examination of the possible donor sites. It is also optimal to have several reconstructive options if this is possible with the chosen donor site. Above all, especially in resection of malignant neoplasms, the excision should not be designed to fit in with the method of reconstruction. It is also important to keep in mind that complexity is frequently worse than simplicity. If reconstruction of the defect is beyond your reconstructive abilities, whether in technique or knowledge, use of a full-thickness skin graft is acceptable as long as skin color and texture are taken into consideration and function is only minimally or not at all impaired.

The rule in local flap surgery of the face is that you can rob Peter to pay Paul only if Paul is sufficiently wealthy. On the face, cosmesis is of prime importance. There is a tendency not to consider tissue expansion in local flap surgery. The surgeon should consider use of this technique when necessary. A variant of tissue expansion is used in many reconstructive efforts. When a wound is closed tightly or a flap seems too small and yet the defect is closed, the biomechanical properties of creep and stress relaxation are harnessed, and the skin elongates (Table 115-1). There is a limit to these mechanisms, and skin blood supply must also be considered. Familiarity with these principles is essential

in all flap procedures. This knowledge is a "must" for all plastic surgeons, regardless of seniority.[1-3]

Flaps on the face have many designs according to the area to be reconstructed and the size of the defect. It must not be forgotten, however, that there are only certain basic well-defined tissue manipulations; these are based on the concepts of advancement, transposition, and rotation. These manipulations can sometimes be combined when the pedicle is long and mobile enough, as in the island flap.

Among the many challenges of facial reconstruction are differences in color, texture, areas of hair-bearing skin, wrinkles, nerve supply, and function. In addition to these challenges, there are specific anatomic areas including the nose, lips, ears, eyelids, and eyebrows that require specific (and often difficult) reconstructive techniques for optimal functional and aesthetic results.[2]

Another technique to consider, although it is not used much in the local flap area, is the musculocutaneous flap. This type of flap will occasionally be considered to increase the probability for success in a skin flap transplantation.

FOREHEAD AND SCALP

The characteristics of the forehead vary with age and nationality. The smooth forehead of youth becomes

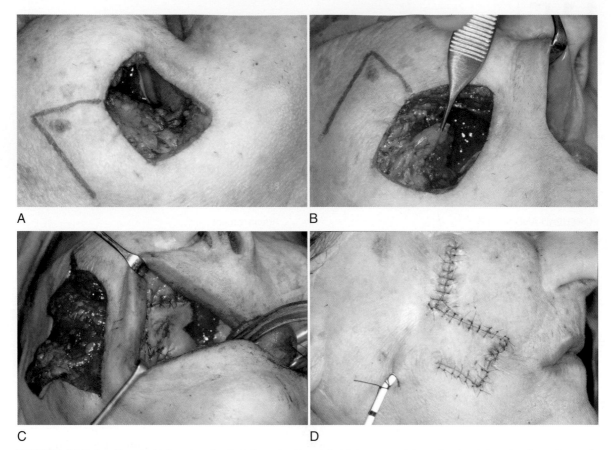

FIGURE 115-1. Rhomboid flap for cheek defect. *A,* After full-thickness excision of a cheek basal cell carcinoma in a rhomboid fashion. The rhomboid flap is drawn out, bisecting the 180-degree angle. *B,* The buccal fat pad will be used to provide volume, and a mucosal flap will be based on that. *C,* The mucosal flap is sutured in place and is viable. *D,* The rhomboid flap is transposed, and the secondary defect is closed directly.

the wrinkled forehead of seniority. The high, hair-free forehead of the white individual is different from the Indian or Arab forehead, which is small in all dimensions because of the encroachment of hair; the former makes for much easier reconstruction than the latter. All foreheads have a limited amount of spare skin

TABLE 115-1 ✦ VISCOELASTIC PROPERTIES OF THE SKIN

Creep	When a sudden load is applied and kept constant, skin will stretch.
Stress relaxation	A constant load on the skin will cause lengthening. With time, the load required to maintain the lengthening decreases. This explains why white flaps will frequently become pink with time.

available and are surrounded by a frame with distinct outlines that should not be disturbed.

Rhomboid Flap

This flap can be used, but as with all flaps, it is important to check if the tissue is available. In the forehead, vertical donor sites are preferred to horizontal, which may cause shift of the eyebrows or forehead hairline (Fig. 115-1).[3] Small rotation flaps or transposition flaps are also possibilities; however, these tend to "trap-door" because of the round or oval design.

In larger defects, a triple rhomboid may be used. This necessitates excision in a hexagonal design (Fig. 115-2). Careful planning and assessment of the availability of loose skin in all three areas of flap harvest are essential.[3-5]

In the temporal area, flaps can be used, but this must be carried out with great care to prevent too great a shift of the hairline. This applies to reconstruction of

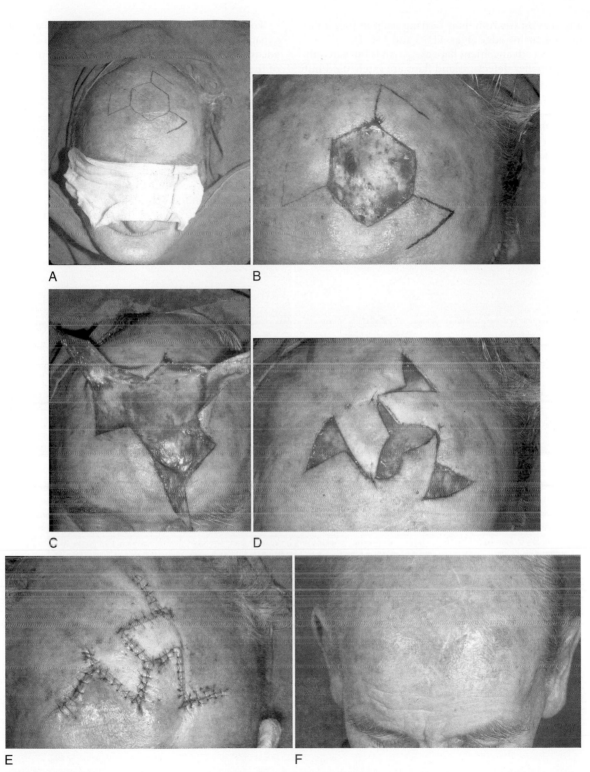

FIGURE 115-2. Triple rhomboid flap. *A,* A hexagonal excision is planned around the basal cell carcinoma of the scalp on each of the 180-degree angles. These are bisected, and the rhomboid flap is outlined on each of them. *B,* The hexagonal defect is developed. *C,* The rhomboid flaps have been elevated, and there is undermining all around the base of these flaps. *D,* The flaps are being sutured into position. *E,* Closure with a moderate degree of tension. *F,* Long-term satisfactory result.

any area on the non–hair-bearing scalp in proximity to the hairline edge (Figs. 115-3 and 115-4).

Direct advancement flaps are possible but can only close smaller defects. Island flaps are rarely used but are certainly possible. Island flaps are frequently based on subcutaneous tissue rather than on definite blood vessels.

Bilobed flaps can be used, but they tend to trap-door or pincushion and are therefore obvious in any form of indirect lighting. They are not recommended.[6,7]

A small forehead with a lot of surrounding hair encroaching onto the forehead represents a considerable problem. Hair removal by use of the laser should be considered in such a patient.

For any large forehead reconstruction, a tissue expander will be inserted to provide enough skin for adequate reconstruction by simple advancement or one of the flaps described before (Fig. 115-5).[8]

EYEBROW RECONSTRUCTION

This is an extremely difficult proposition. The anatomy of the eyebrow is complex. Hair grows according to a fixed pattern that is not uniform and is difficult to reproduce. An island flap based on the temporal blood supply can be used, but the hair must be trimmed. The hair is often too dense and does not grow in the correct manner. In spite of this, eyebrow reconstruc-

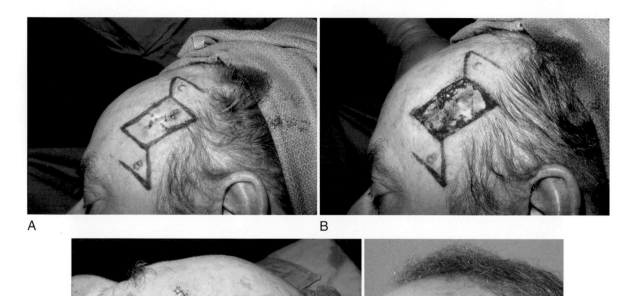

FIGURE 115-3. Double rhomboid flap for basal cell carcinoma lying just in front of the temporal hairline. *A,* The planned excision is a composite of two rhomboids. On the obtuse angle on the rhomboids above and below, rhomboid flaps are drawn out to maintain the hairline in its correct position. *B,* The lesion is excised. *C,* The flaps are being transposed, and the secondary defect is closed. *D,* End result.

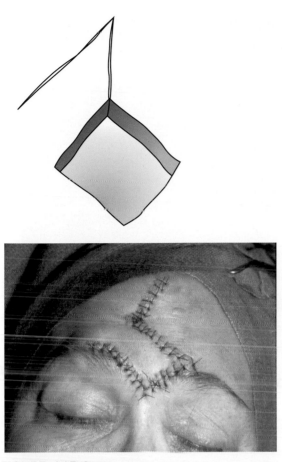

FIGURE 115-4. Rhomboid closure of defect in the glabellar area. The lesion was a basal cell carcinoma that was excised in the glabellar area, and an appropriately placed rhomboid allows the defect to be closed without disturbing the position of the medial ends of the eyebrows. The donor site is closed directly, and this of course gives a satisfactory overall result.

tion can be beneficial, especially in the burned patient, in whom both eyebrows are frequently involved. In such a patient, symmetry can be achieved. An alternative is micro-hair transplants with frequent trimming. These, unfortunately, rarely produce the unique anatomy and the density of the eyebrow hair. Eyebrow flaps must be designed with care to maintain the correct anatomic relationship (Fig. 115-6). Also, there is a paucity of material available.

NASAL RECONSTRUCTION

Many different flaps for nasal reconstruction have been described. In the bridgeline region, the glabella is the preferred donor site, and the flaps can be direct advancement (Fig. 115-7), transposition (Fig. 115-8), bilobed (Fig. 115-9), rhomboid (see Fig. 115-4), or island (Fig. 115-10). On the lateral aspect of the nose, bilobed (see Fig. 115-9), rotation (Fig. 115-11), or

transposition flaps (Fig. 115-12) will give excellent results. There is often more skin in this area than expected.

For nasal tip reconstruction, the bilobed flap is ideal. The long advancement flap of Rintala,[9] which looks unreliable, usually works nicely but can cause some apprehension on the part of the surgeon and the patient (Fig. 115-13). Another method is that of Schmidt,[10] in which the supraorbital area is tubed to a length that will reach to the nasal tip (i.e., just above the eyebrow). Laterally, a nostril is made by dissecting a skin pocket and lining it with a skin graft and cartilage for support (if necessary). Approximately 2 to 3 weeks after the initial reconstruction, this composite is brought down to reconstruct the rim and alar region (Fig. 115-14). In the author's experience, this procedure is reliable and yields good results.

A composite graft from the ear is an excellent choice when the nostril is to be reconstructed. A cutout of the planned defect is made and transferred to the ear. A portion of the rim of a satisfactory size and shape is taken full thickness; lateral to or inferior to this, a long triangular full thickness of skin is taken in continuity from the posterior surface of the ear. The ear is closed directly, resulting in a minor reduction of the ear size that rarely seems to be a problem. The nose lesion is resected with a superior skin excess. The ear graft is then sutured in place with meticulous accuracy so that raw skin edges of the graft and ear oppose exactly, and the ear rim becomes the nostril rim. In this way, revascularization of the composite graft from the full-thickness replacement area will occur with excellent results. A thin vertical forehead flap can also be used, but this must be based correctly (see next section).

When a more complex reconstruction is required (e.g., bilateral alar rims and columella), the total central forehead should be used. This area should be mapped and marked carefully to ensure that there is adequate tissue for the columella and alar rims. At this point, the flap is elevated. The key to complete survival of the flap is the position of its base; this should be at the medial canthal level or below. In this way, the vascular anastomosis on the side of the nose between the cheek and forehead vessels is used to give length to the flap. With the base correctly positioned, the midline flap will comfortably reconstruct the nasal tip and the columella without tension and with absolute safety. The reason for poor results and failures is usually anatomic placement of a flap pedicle based on the brow area. Poor results are due to a lack of understanding of the vascular anatomy (i.e., anastomosis between the facial and the forehead vascular systems in the superolateral area of the medial orbit–lateral nasal area). The forehead is closed directly, but if there is tension in the area just anterior to the hairline, it should be left to close spontaneously. The

Text continued on p. 360

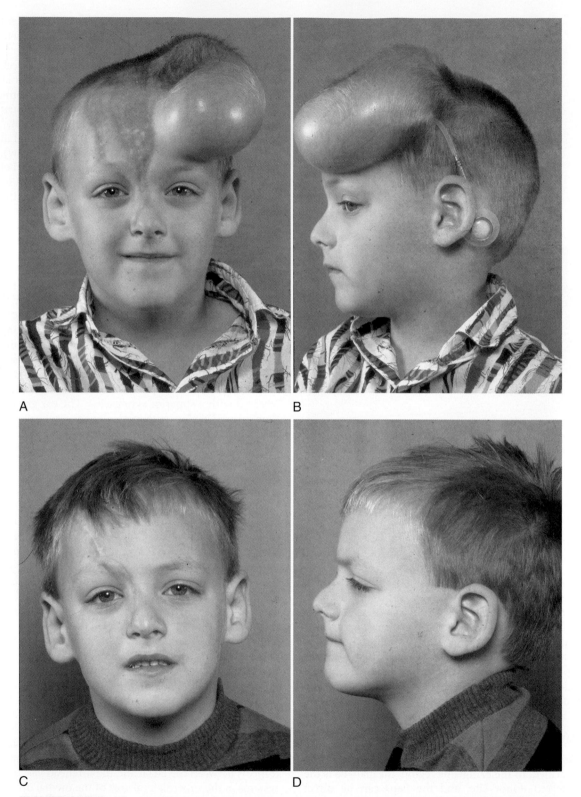

FIGURE 115-5. Tissue expansion to achieve defect closure. *A* and *B,* Right hemi-forehead deformity due to ectodermal dysplasia. The tissue expander has been placed to deal with the ensuing defect after excision. Note the external valve. *C* and *D,* Postoperative result after resection and large forehead and scalp rotation flap. No secondary defect.

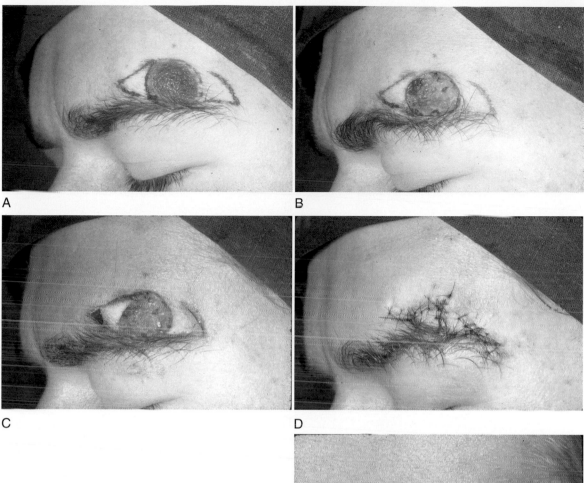

A   B

C   D

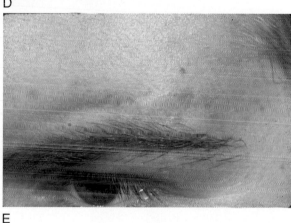

FIGURE 115-6. Nevus of left supraorbital area involving eyebrow—hatchet flap reconstruction. *A,* The planned excision has been drawn out together with bilateral hatchet flaps. *B,* Nevus has been excised. It can be seen that the flap pedicles are superior for the lateral flap and inferior for the medial flap. *C,* The flaps are elevated. *D,* The flaps are transposed, and the secondary defect is closed. *E,* Satisfactory end result with the eyebrow in a good position.

E

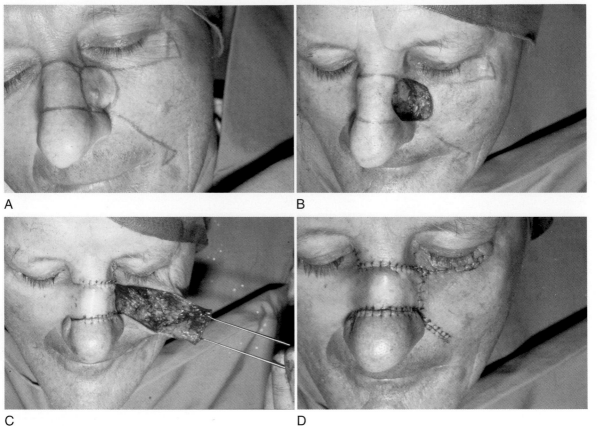

A

B

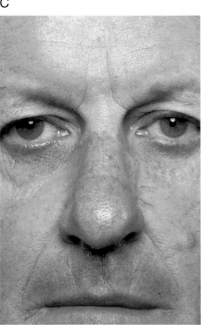

C

D

E

FIGURE 115-7. Reconstruction of nasal defect with lateral advancement flaps. *A,* Basal cell carcinoma involving the lateral aspect of the nose, extending slightly onto the left cheek. The plan is excision with reconstruction by cheek and nasal advancement flaps. *B,* The lesion is resected. *C,* Transverse advancement of right nasal flap. *D,* Advancement of left cheek flap to ensure a junction line where the nose meets the cheek. *E,* End result.

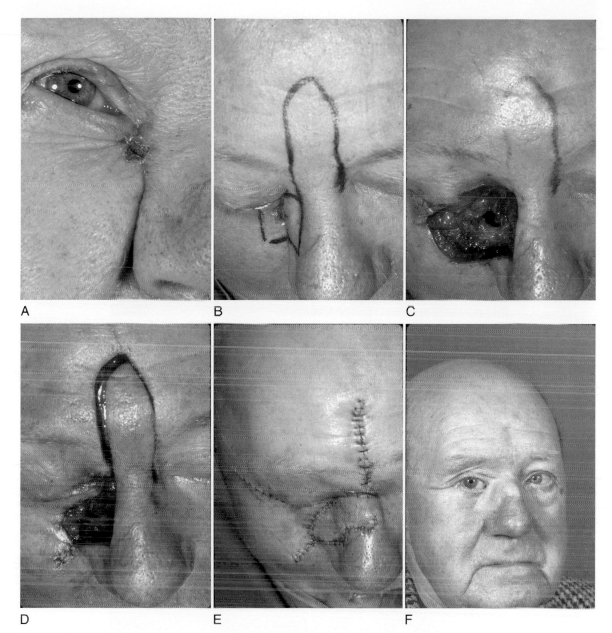

FIGURE 115-8. Reconstruction of lateral nasal defect with forehead flap. *A,* Basal cell carcinoma involving right medial canthus, right nasolablal area, and right side of nose. *B,* Plan of excision for reconstruction from central forehead flaps. *C,* Resection with underlying bone. *D,* Elevation of midline forehead flap. *E,* Closure of defect with some advancement of inferior lid skin but mainly with central midline forehead flap. *F,* End result.

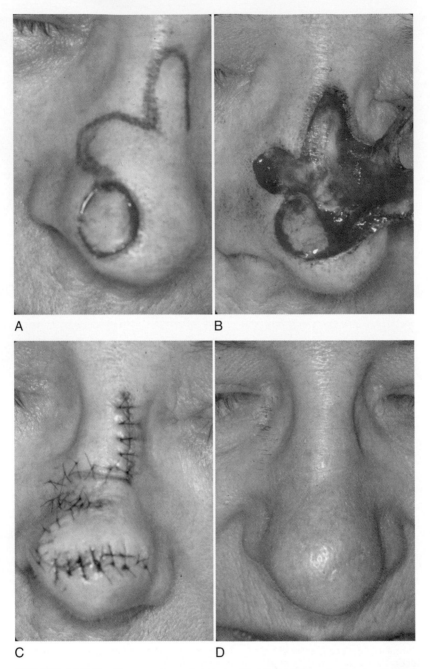

FIGURE 115-9. Closure of nasal defect with bilobed flap. *A,* Basal cell carcinoma, right side of nasal tip, excised. The plan of the reconstruction with a bilobed flap has been drawn out. *B,* Bilobed flap is widely elevated. Note dissection beyond the base of the flap on the left. *C,* Reconstruction of nasal tip defect with closure of the vertical portion of the flap defect at the nasal bridgeline. *D,* Long-term end result.

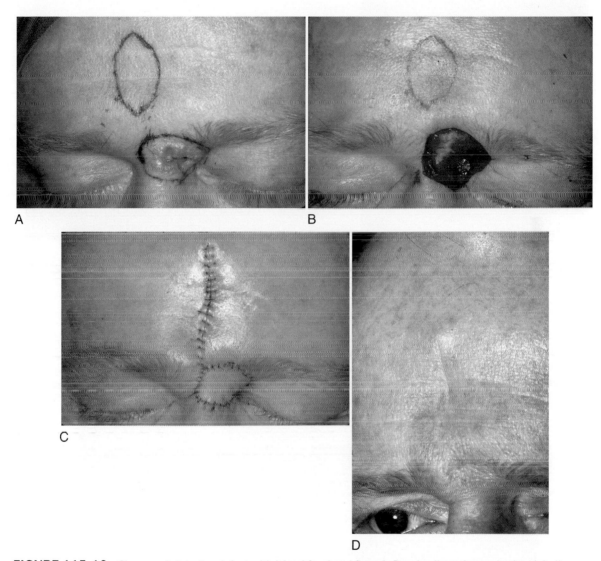

FIGURE 115-10. Closure of glabellar defect with island forehead flap. *A,* Basal cell carcinoma in the glabellar area encroaching on the medial end of the left eyebrow. *B,* Excision completed down to periosteum. *C,* Closure with forehead island flap. *D,* Long-term result.

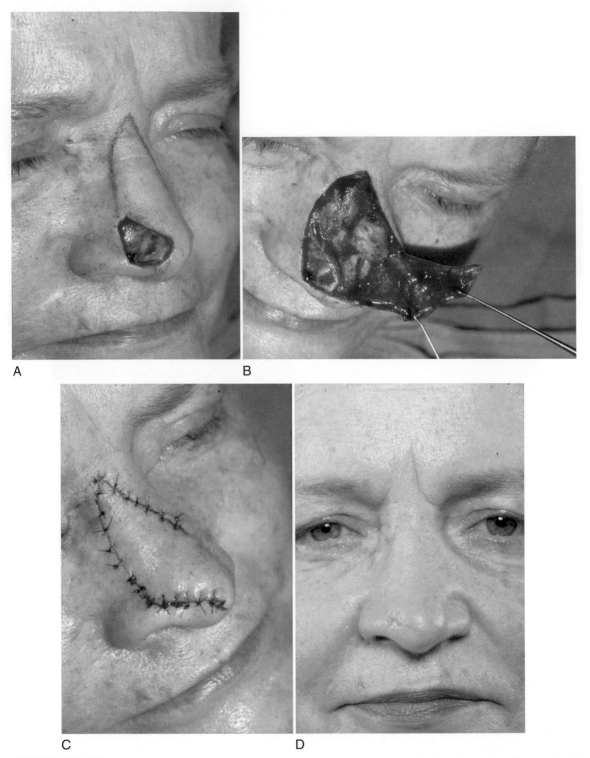

FIGURE 115-11. Nasal transposition flap to close nasal tip defect. *A,* The basal cell carcinoma has been excised; the transposition flap is drawn out. *B,* The flap is widely elevated. *C,* The flap is sutured into position. It can be seen that this is part rotation and part advancement. *D,* Long-term end result.

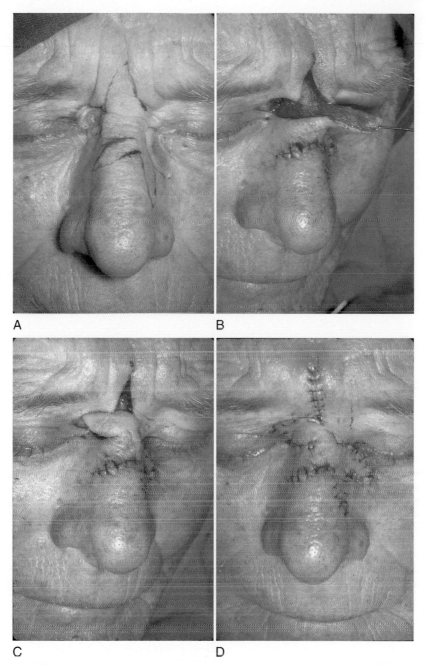

A

B

C

D

FIGURE 115-12. Transposition of a bilobed flap for closure of right nasal bridge-line defect. *A,* The glabellar flap is drawn out and the resection is outlined. There is some confusion because a bilobed flap is going to be used for the medial canthal area on the left. *B,* The glabellar flap is elevated. *C,* The glabellar flap is transposed into position. *D,* The flap is inset, and the donor site is closed without tension.

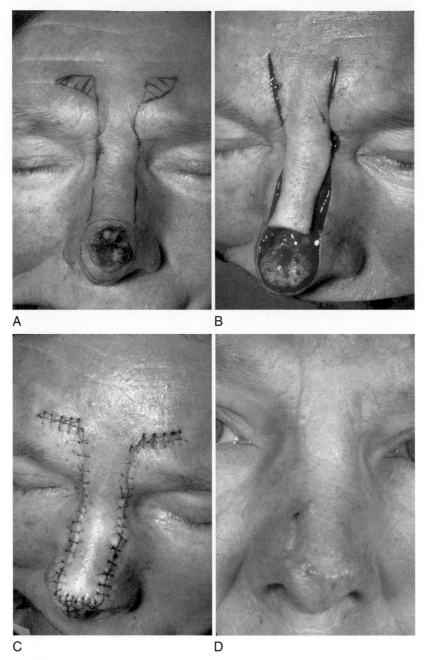

FIGURE 115-13. Rintala dorsal nasal advancement flap to close nasal tip defect. *A,* The basal cell carcinoma of the nasal tip is outlined, and the Rintala flap has been drawn out. The area of Burow triangle resection is crosshatched on the forehead. *B,* The excision is completed and the flap is elevated. *C,* The flap is advanced after excision of the Burow triangles. The flap is pale, but this is due to epinephrine having been injected with the local anesthetic. *D,* End result with slight scarring to the right of the nasal tip that settled uneventfully.

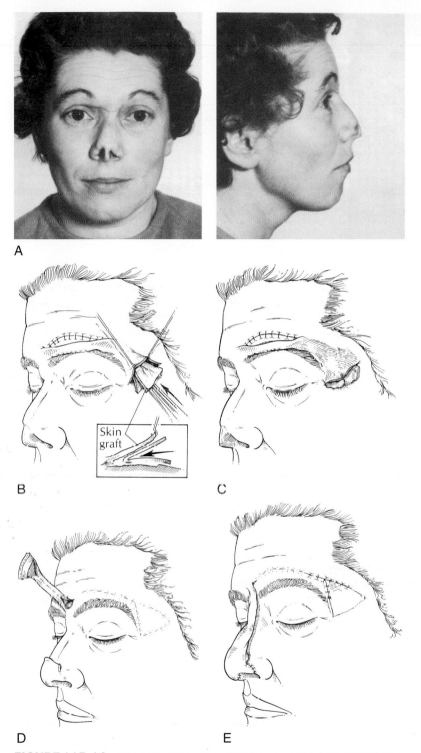

FIGURE 115-14. Nasal reconstruction—transverse pedicle (Schmidt). *A*, Preoperative appearance. *B* and *C*, Tube pedicle is designed above the eyebrow. Split skin graft inserted into the lateral subcutaneous pocket. *D* and *E*, Pedicle elevated between 3 and 4 weeks and transferred to nasal tip.   *Continued*

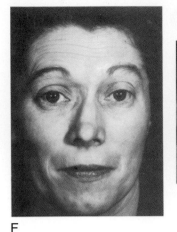

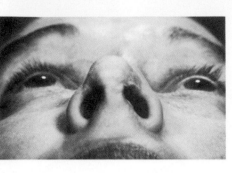

F

FIGURE 115-14, cont'd. *F,* End result.

scar resulting from this rarely if ever requires any modification. The pedicle is divided at 2 to 3 weeks, depending on the inset, and the nasal tip is fashioned. Apart from thinning, it is unusual to have to make any further adjustments (Figs. 115-15 and 115-16). If there is any concern about vascularity, the base of the flap may be delayed.

If a total nasal reconstruction is required, a larger amount of forehead skin is harvested in the transverse dimension, but again, the base should be positioned at or below the medial canthal ligament. The septal mucosa is used for lining. For closure of the midline forehead defect, the skin can frequently be advanced. If there is concern, a tissue expander can be inserted to expand the whole forehead, but this is rarely necessary. If support is required, a cranial bone graft from the outer table is taken from an area where the curvature is similar to that required for the defect reconstruction.[11] This may be done at the same time, but it is safer to delay this to the time of division or to a third procedure. A less common method to reconstruct the tip of the nose is to use a donor site from the neck. A long, transverse tube pedicle is raised transversely after 2 to 3 weeks; one end is delayed, and this end is taken up 10 days later to reconstruct the tip. After another 2 to 3 weeks, the flap is divided and inset (Fig. 115-17).

Noses may be prefabricated elsewhere (e.g., on the forearm by a radial flap) and subsequently transferred by microvascular techniques. At present, only a few surgeons are able to achieve good results with this technique.

EYELIDS
Partial Lower Lid Defects

Frequently, defects excised in a V fashion can be carefully closed in layers. If this is not possible, the lower portion of the lateral canthal ligament can be divided through a small lateral canthal incision. This allows the lid to move medially, and closure can be obtained without tension. If there is too much tension, the incision and dissection are taken further laterally onto the cheek. Closure can then be obtained without difficulty. The lateral incision is usually closed with a Z-plasty to reduce any tension that may be present (see Fig. 115-22*B*).[12]

If the defect is extensive, a portion of nasal septum, with the mucosa attached on one side, is inserted with the mucosa toward the globe to form an internal lamella.[13] A portion of ear cartilage, with perichondrium in place of the mucosa, can also be used. Mucosalization of the inner surface occurs fairly rapidly. A cheek rotation flap of the required size then provides external cover (Fig. 115-18). If the cheek skin is insufficient, prior expansion of the lateral cheek can be performed, or a narrow midline forehead flap can be used.

Partial Upper Lid Defects

Reconstruction of the upper lid is a more difficult problem because it is needed for protection of the eye. It is best for the surgeon to sit at the head of the operating table and think of the upper lid as the lower lid and use the same techniques described for the lower lid modified to the required shape of the upper lid. Any failure of reconstruction, particularly in the vertical dimension, may impair vision. Without an adequate upper lid, the eye will be at risk for exposure, scarring, and loss of vision.

ADVANCEMENT FLAP

For a triangular defect in the upper lid (e.g., after tumor resection), an incision is made horizontally from the lateral canthus, with division of the superior limb of

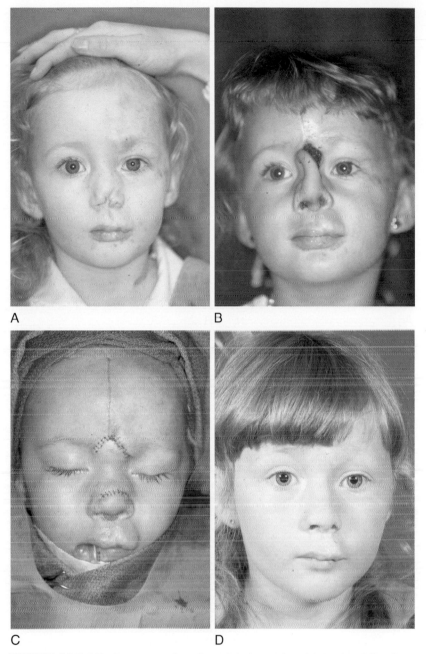

FIGURE 115-15. Reconstruction of nasal tip in a child with forehead flap for a defect resulting from resolving hemangioma. *A,* The size of the nasal deformity can be noted. This involves the nasal tip, the columella, and the lateral aspect of the nose bilaterally. *B,* The scarred area is resected, and a forehead flap is brought down to reconstruct the columella and nasal tip. *C,* The tip has been reconstructed with inset of the flap; excess of flap is removed, and the glabellar area is reconstructed. *D,* Long-term result.

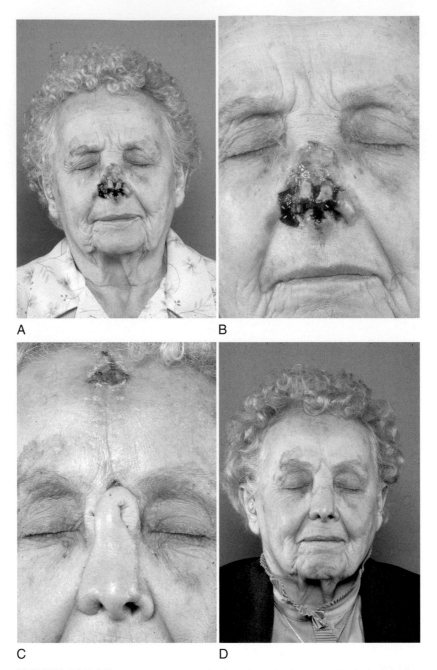

FIGURE 115-16. Reconstruction of nasal tip and dorsum with forehead flap after resection of basal cell carcinoma. *A* and *B,* Extent of excision after Mohs resection of basal cell carcinoma. Further wide resection was carried out. *C,* Reconstruction with midline forehead flap. Note the low position of the base of the flap. The pre-hairline defect was allowed to close spontaneously. *D,* Long-term result.

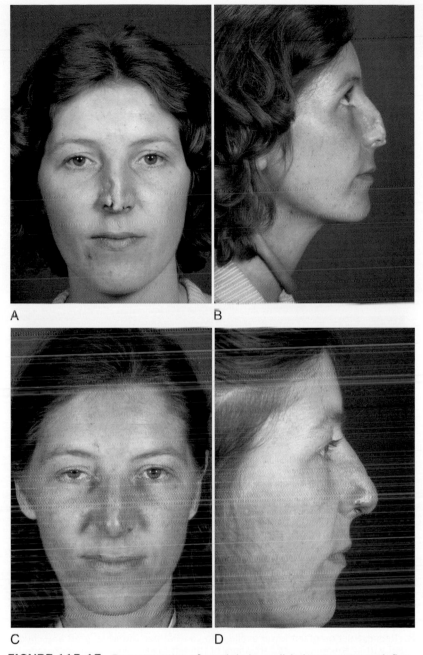

A

B

C

D

FIGURE 115-17. Reconstruction of nasal tip by pedicled transverse neck flap.
A, The defect on the tip of the nose can be seen. *B,* The defect is more clearly
appreciated in this view, and reconstruction of the nasal tip has been raised on the
neck. *C* and *D,* End result after a two-staged procedure: first, to take the pedicle
onto the tip of the nose; and second, to divide the pedicle and contour the nasal
tip.

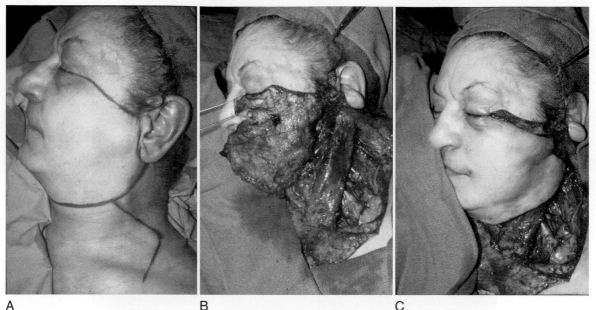

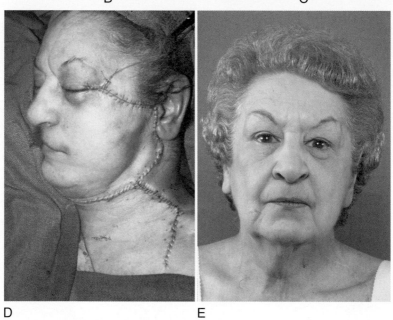

FIGURE 115-18. Reconstruction of left lower eyelid with conchal-perichondrial graft and cheek advancement flap. This patient presented with a squamous cell carcinoma of the left lower eyelid with neck node involvement. *A,* Skin operative plan drawn out. *B,* After excision of lower eyelid and modified radical neck dissection with preservation of facial nerve. The lower eyelid is reconstructed with conchal cartilage with perichondrium facing toward the globe. *C* and *D,* Advancement of cheek flap to reconstruct the lower eyelid. *E,* Long-term result.

the lateral canthal ligament.[14] An incision is also made in the conjunctiva of the superior fornix. This alone will allow small defects to be closed. For the best result to be obtained laterally at the end of the horizontal incision, an unequal Z-plasty can be performed to deal with the dog-ear. As in the lower lid, accurate suturing of the gray line, the lash line, and the rim-conjunctiva junction is essential (Fig. 115-19).

LID-SWITCH FLAP (ABBE FLAP)

By the same principle as the Abbe flap on the lip, a similar reconstruction can be used for defects on the upper lid (Fig. 115-20).[15] There are marginal vessels in the lid, and a full-thickness V flap (the defect of which can be closed easily) can be taken from the lower lid, swung up, and sutured into the upper lid in layers.

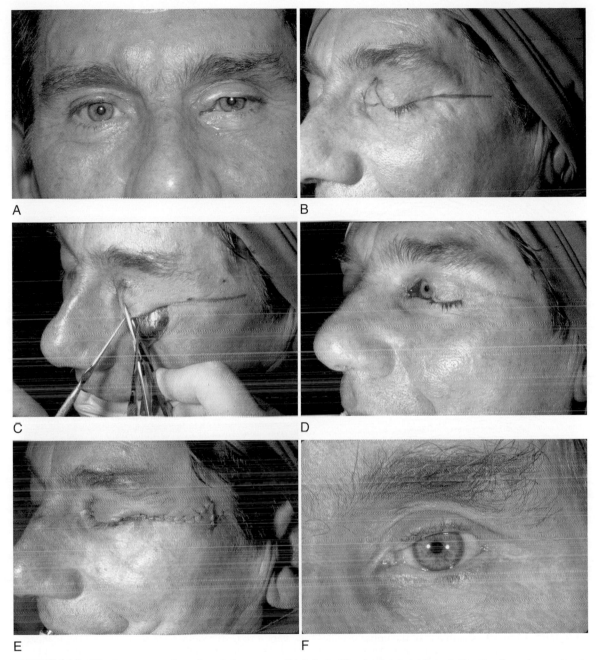

FIGURE 115-19. Reconstruction of partial upper eyelid defect with advancement flap. *A,* Basal cell carcinoma involving medial end of upper eyelid. *B,* Operative plan of excision and rotation and advancement of the upper lid. *C,* Excision of upper lid basal cell carcinoma. Note spoon to protect eye and the use of sharp pointed scissors to resect the lid. *D,* Defect after excision of medial portion of the upper eyelid. *E,* Lateral canthotomy performed superiorly. The lid is advanced with lateral Z-plasty in the temporal region. *F,* End result.

To close the lower lid defect, the edges frequently come together directly without tension. If this does not occur, a small lateral canthal incision can be made, and the inferior limb of the lateral canthal tendon is divided. If this is not sufficient, a lateral transverse incision from the canthus out to the temporal skin (incorporating a Z-plasty if necessary) will suffice to obtain tensionless closure.

FREE GRAFTS

For larger defects, free, full-thickness lid replacements as composite grafts have been considered. This is

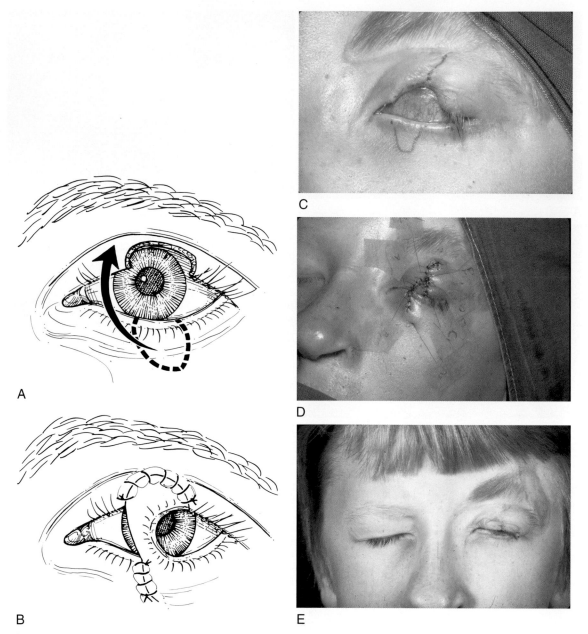

FIGURE 115-20. Coloboma of the upper eyelid—Abbe flap. *A to C,* The defect can be seen, and the planned Abbe flap from the lower to the upper eyelid is outlined and shown in diagrammatic form. *D,* The flap is in position. *E,* The patient can close his eye satisfactorily.

hazardous if it is performed in the standard fashion. It is possible to use a full-thickness lid replacement as a composite graft if a portion of conjunctiva and subconjunctival tissue can be preserved. With use of the methods previously described, a small vertical defect will need to be reconstructed. A full-thickness graft can be taken from the lower lid, and the conjunctiva is excised from the graft, leaving just enough for the full-thickness defect. The full-thickness skin portion

remaining will be enough to allow the graft to survive; however, meticulous reconstructive technique is imperative. The lower lid defect is closed as described previously.

Large and Total Upper Lid Defects

For larger defects, the lower lid is used and the subsequent lower lid defect is reconstructed. For this type of reconstruction, a large full-thickness portion of lower lid is moved up on its vascular pedicle. This means that a partial lower lid reconstruction is necessary. As the portion of lower lid is turned up, the full thickness of the cheek is advanced and grafted with nasal septum on its inner surface (Fig. 115-21).[14]

When a total upper lid is to be reconstructed, the whole lower lid is turned up. The lower lid reconstruction is based on an advancement cheek flap lined with nasal septum, cartilage, and mucosa. These pedicled lid reconstructions are left attached for 2 to 3 weeks, depending on the vascularity of the upturned flaps. Once the upper lid reconstruction is in position, small adjustments are often necessary on one or both lids. Adjustments are usually required for the lateral canthus and occasionally to the edge of the lower lid or height variation of the lower lid. With

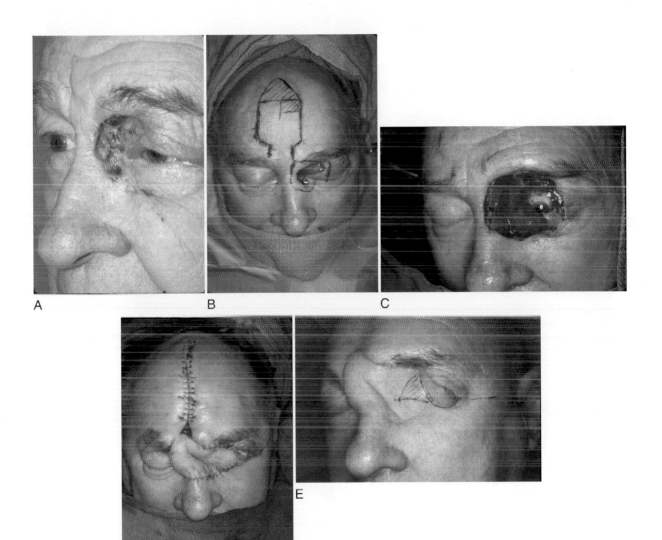

FIGURE 115-21. Reconstruction of upper and lower eyelid defect with a forehead flap after resection of medial canthal and upper and lower eyelid basal cell carcinoma. *A,* Extent of the lesion can be seen. *B,* The planned excision and the planned reconstruction with a forehead flap for the upper and lower lids and the medial canthal area. *C,* Excision completed. Note large defect of upper and lower eyelids, medial canthal area, and nasal area. *D,* Reconstruction with a forehead flap. *E,* Forehead flap sitting well in position. Reconstruction is performed by trimming of the forehead flap, harvesting of a chondromucosal flap from the septum, and elevating a cheek flap. *Continued*

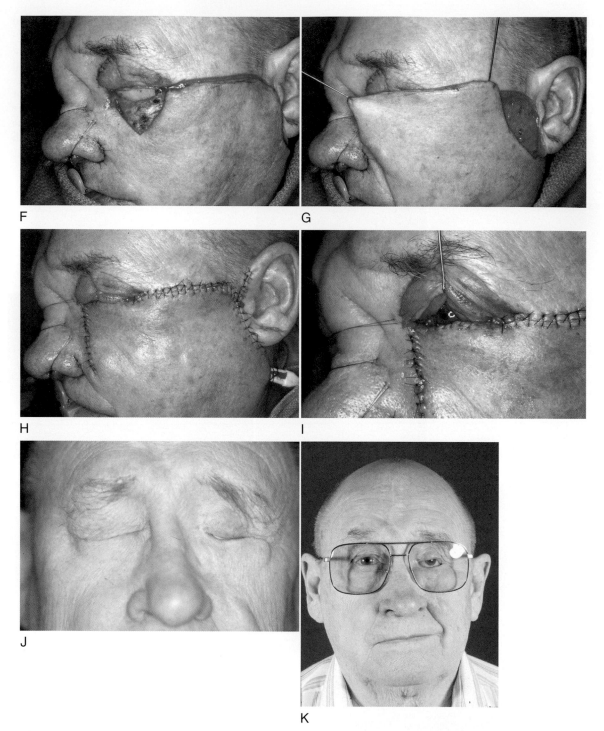

FIGURE 115-21, cont'd. *F* and *G,* Cheek flap advanced and sutured into position. The eye has now been opened up. *H* and *I,* Reconstruction complete. *J,* Closure of lids. *K,* Opening of lids.

meticulous technique, a good cosmetic and functional result can be obtained (Fig. 115-22).[15]

When a healthy eye is present, a lid can be prefabricated on the forehead. A pocket the size of the lid is designed and a mucosal graft is inserted. When this reconstruction is complete, it is brought down on a vascular pedicle to replace the lid. The pedicle is divided at 3 weeks. This protects the eye, but movement is minimal unless there is some orbicularis remaining to use at a later date (Fig. 115-23).

Total Lower Lid Defects

These occur from tumor resection, from trauma, or when the lower lid is used to reconstruct the upper lid (see Fig. 115-22). Reconstruction of the total lower lid is primarily performed for cosmesis.

The lower lid can be reconstructed by a cheek rotation flap lined with oral mucosa or more satisfactorily with nasal septal cartilage with its perichondrium intact (see Fig. 115-23). In other instances, a forehead flap may be necessary.

Medial Canthal Defects

In most instances, forehead flaps provide a reliable and reasonably good method of reconstruction. It is

necessary to line these flaps with mucosa; however, additional support is not required because of the inherent rigidity. It is important to place a flap of sufficient size into the canthal area (Figs. 115-24 to 115-26).

CHEEK

Skin tumors are common in this area. The whole range of flaps can be used—rotation, advancement, transposition, and island—with many variations for each type of reconstruction.[16]

Rotation

Because the cheek is relatively large in area, rotation flaps may be designed in many sizes, depending on the position of the defect to be reconstructed. Small flaps may simply be rotated around the circle to close the defect. The area to be excised is triangulated. The design of rotation can be calculated by placing one end of a thread on the angle apex and the other at the edge of the defect. By rotating the outer end of the flap on the skin, the required circumference can be marked. In some instances, however, the flap edge may fall short. It is preferable to use the point to be closed as the length of the flap edge. By obtaining this

Text continued on p. 375

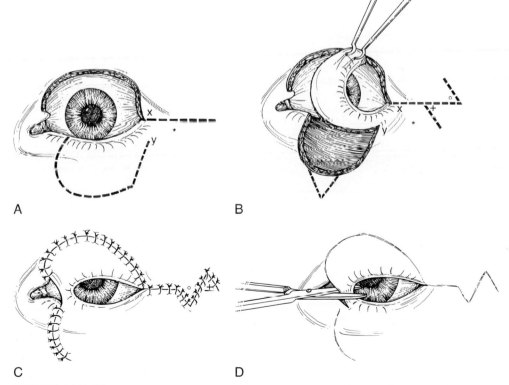

A   B

C   D

FIGURE 115-22. Reconstruction of total upper eyelid defect with lower lid transposition. *A* to *D,* Illustration of planned reconstruction of an upper eyelid defect with lower lid transposition.

Continued

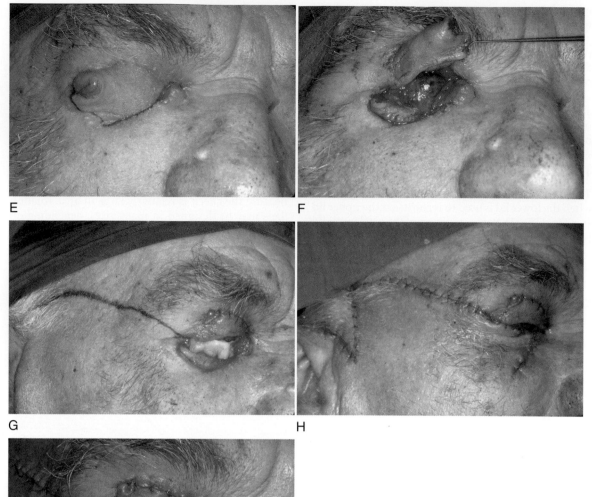

FIGURE 115-22, cont'd. *E,* Preoperative markings indicate the upper eyelid area to be resected. *F,* The total upper eyelid is resected; the lower eyelid will be rotated up to reconstruct the upper eyelid with use of a medial pedicle. *G,* The medial pedicle is divided, and the medial end of the lower lid is inset into the defect of the medial side of the upper lid. *H* and *I,* A nasal septal chondromucosal graft is placed in position, and the cartilage is scored to make it bend as favorably as possible. A lateral cheek rotation flap is performed. Note the lateral Z-plasty to give as much medial movement as possible. This will give a good end result.

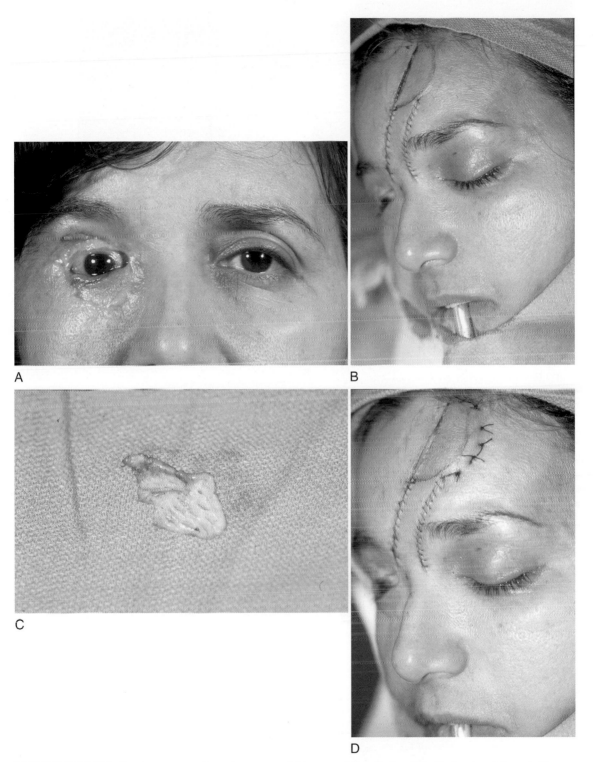

FIGURE 115-23. Total reconstruction of upper eyelid by a prefabricated composite forehead flap. *A,* The pre-operative appearance with no upper eyelid whatsoever. The lower eyelid is intact. *B,* An upper eyelid is delayed vertically on the forehead with a bucket being designed under the forehead skin and subcutaneous tissue. *C,* A mucosal graft is harvested, and holes are made in it to stretch it. *D,* The mucosal graft is placed, mucosal side down, into the pocket in the center of the forehead with a small pack. Sutures are holding the mucosa in position.

Continued

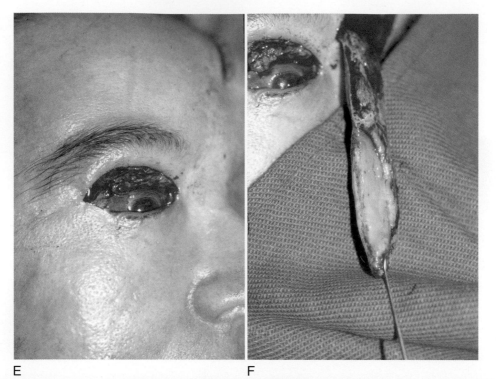

E

F

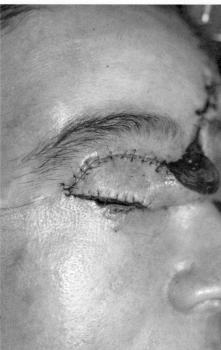

G

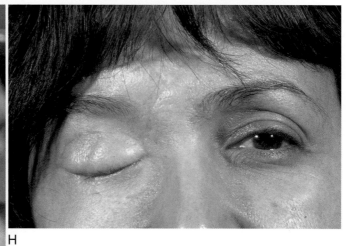

H

FIGURE 115-23, cont'd. *E,* Upper eyelid is released as much as possible. *F,* Upper eyelid reconstruction being brought down to reconstruct the upper lid. Note the mucosa on the undersurface of the flap. *G,* The lid is inset. *H,* The lid reconstruction is complete and ready for levator muscle repositioning.

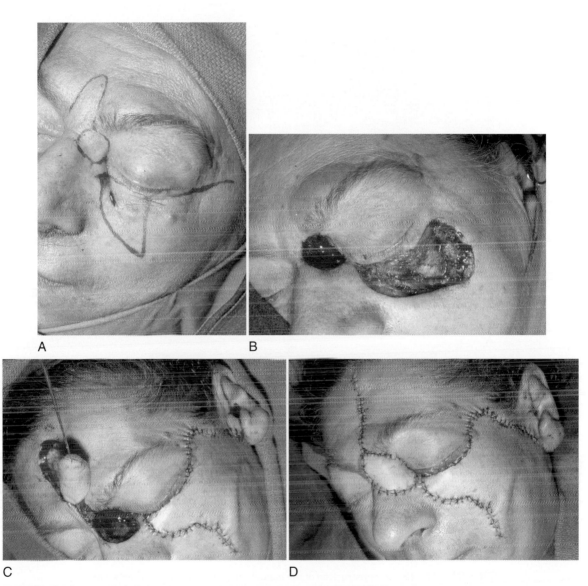

FIGURE 115-24. Reconstruction of medial canthal area with island flap. *A*, Basal cell carcinoma of the medial canthus. *B*, Resection and proposed reconstruction outlined. *C*, Island flap to reconstruct the medial canthal area together with transposition flap. *D*, End result.

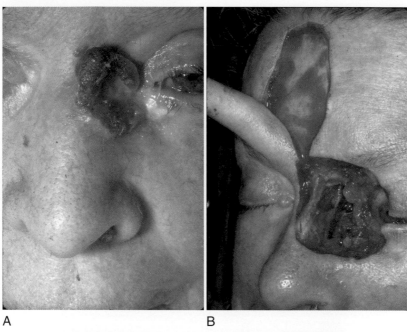

A

B

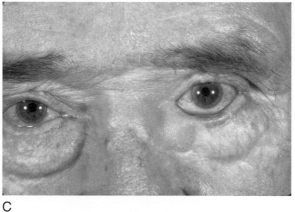

C

FIGURE 115-25. Reconstruction of the medial canthal area and lid defects with forehead flaps. *A,* Extensive basal cell carcinoma of left medial canthus. *B,* Midline forehead flap elevated to reconstruct large post-resection defect of upper and lower lids, medial canthal area, and nose. *C,* End result.

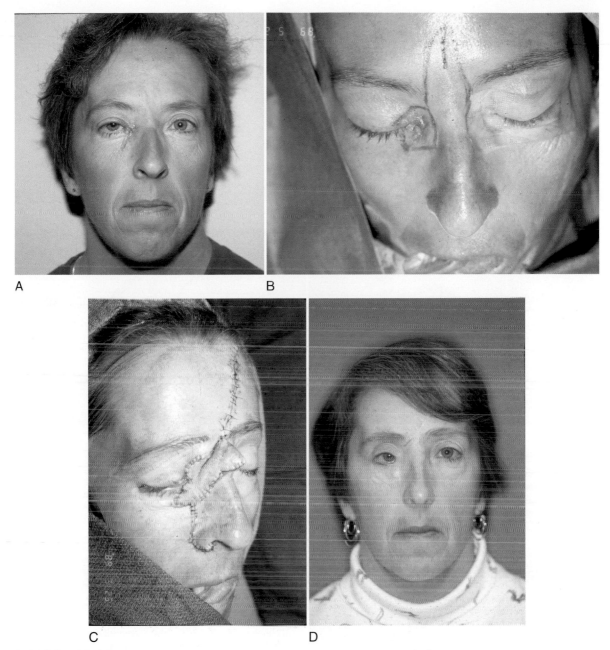

FIGURE 115-26. Forehead flap to medial canthus and lower lid defect. *A*, Penetrating basal cell carcinoma. *B*, Planned excision and tailored forehead flap. *C*, Excision completed and flap in place. *D*, End result.

measurement and rotating back to the donor area of the flap, adequate flap dimensions are achieved. It may be necessary to make adjustments along the line of the flap (Figs. 115-27 and 115-28).

Advancement

Advancement flaps can be applied at any location on the cheek. Like the rotation flap, the advancement flap can be of any size. It is best to use natural lines, even if they diverge away from the defect, because this will still give a better and more natural cosmetic result. The defect is outlined and resected, usually as a square or a rectangle. The flap is raised from one edge and dissected backward until there is enough skin and subcutaneous tissue to allow the distal portion to advance and close the defect. Trimming may be necessary. In some patients, when the advancement is used to close

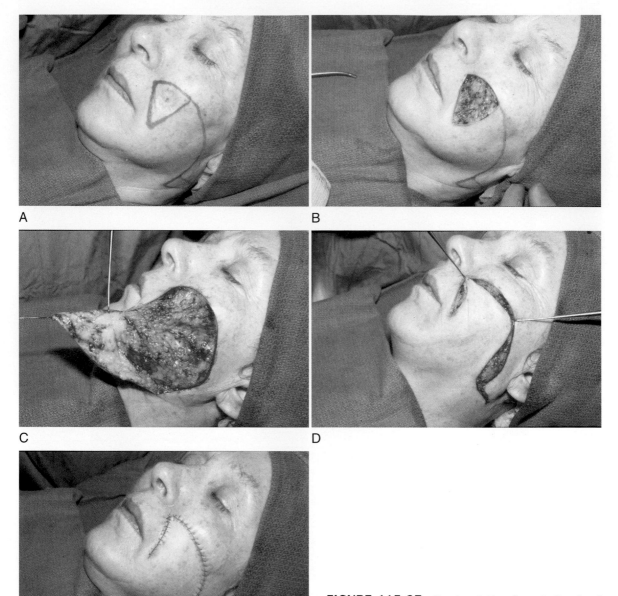

FIGURE 115-27. Cheek rotation flap. *A,* Basal cell carcinoma of the right cheek. The rotation flap is outlined. *B,* Resection of basal cell carcinoma. *C,* Elevation of cheek rotation flap. *D,* Trial of flap rotation. Note Burow triangle excised just below the ear. *E,* Closure of defect with cheek rotation flap.

a relatively large defect, there is an accumulation of excess skin on either side of the base of the flap. This excess is lateral to the base and can be excised as bilateral triangles. This excess skin has been termed Burow triangles. In composite defects of the cheek and nose, a composite reconstruction is effective. The nose is resurfaced with a full-thickness skin graft, and an advancement flap with excision of Burow triangles is used to reconstruct the cheek (Figs. 115-29 to 115-31; see also Fig. 115-7).

Transposition

A transposition flap is elevated from a nearby area and moved to close a defect while the base of the flap remains intact. This technique lends itself to geometric flap planning. The best and most satisfactory example of this is the rhomboid flap. The lesion is resected in a rhomboid design. Before this reconstruction, it is necessary to determine the location of

Text continued on p. 381

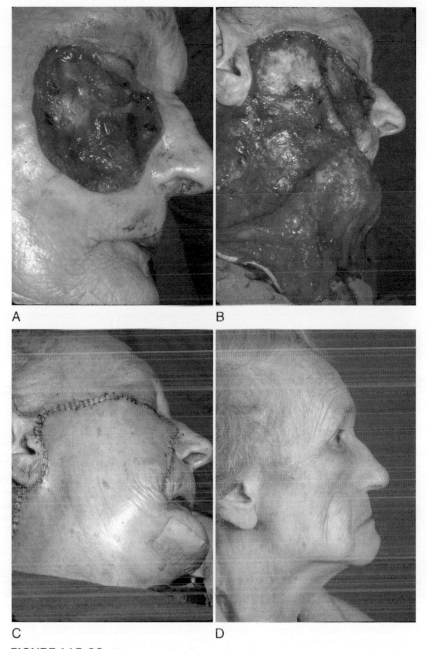

FIGURE 115-28. Cheek rotation flap to close large cheek and paranasal defect. *A,* Defect established after resection of squamous cell carcinoma. *B,* Large cheek rotation flap elevated. *C,* Rotation flap to close defect with medial suture line in nasolabial area. *D,* End result.

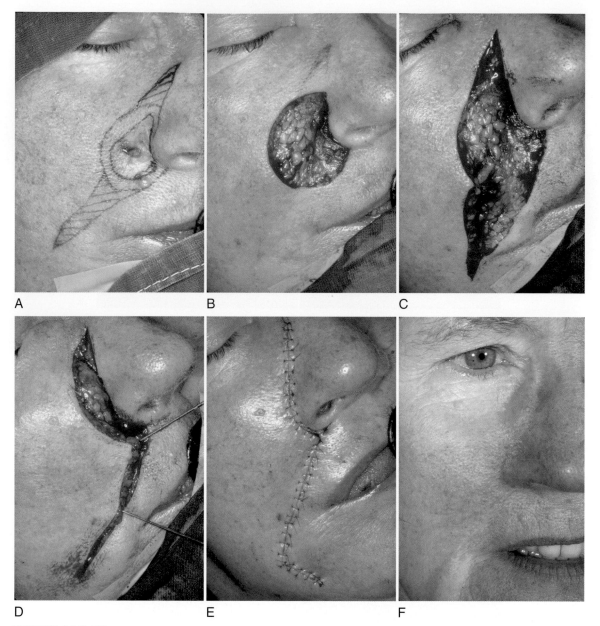

FIGURE 115-29. Extended perialar crescentic advancement flap for medial check defect. *A,* Outline of resection of basal cell carcinoma with ellipse from nasal area and nasolabial area. *B,* Excision of lesion. *C,* Extended perialar crescentic area excised. *D,* Advancement of cheek. *E,* Closure of defect. *F,* Long-term result.

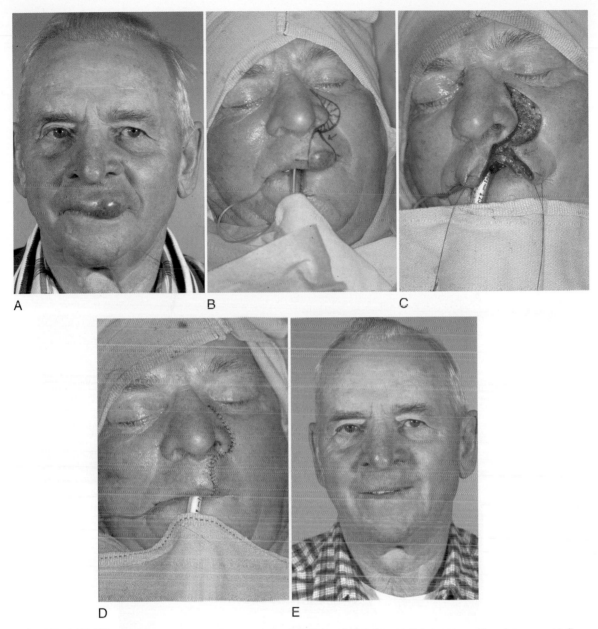

FIGURE 115-30. Excision of hemangioma on the left side of the lip—perialar crescentic advancement flap. *A*, Hemangioma. *B*, Perialar crescentic advancement and excision of lower lip. *C*, Excision completed. *D*, Closure of defect. *E*, Long-term result.

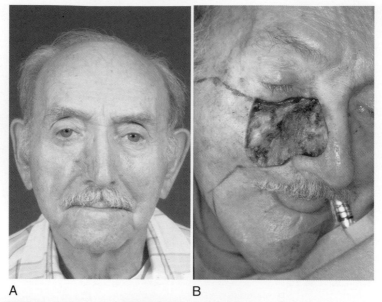

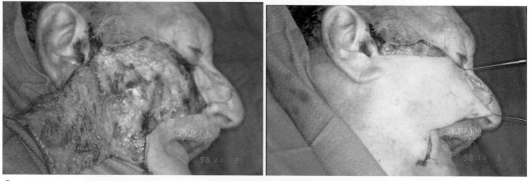

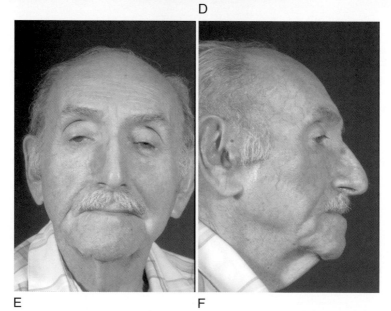

FIGURE 115-31. Resection of basal cell carcinoma, right paranasal area—check advancement flap. *A,* Basal cell carcinoma, right paranasal area. *B,* Wide resection of medial aspect of cheek and right side of nose. *C,* Elevation of a large cheek advancement flap. *D,* Cheek advancement flap to close defect. *E* and *F,* End result.

excess skin by pinching the area between the thumb and index finger and determining the location of a 120-degree angle opposite this. The flap can then be taken from the area with the most available skin. The flap is rhomboid and should fit perfectly into the defect. Because it has corners, pincushioning rarely if ever occurs. The donor site can be closed directly (see Figs. 115-1 and 115-4).

Finger Flap

The finger flap is similar to the rhomboid flap with removal of the corners, although it is usually longer and narrower (see Fig. 115-8). The finger flap is easy to design and use, but there tends to be shortening of the scar around its oval edge. The flap becomes elevated within the scar and forms a surface irregularity, referred to as an island or pincushion. Because the cosmetic result is not optimal, it is not advisable to use this flap for facial reconstruction.

Island

The island technique can be used for advancement or transposition, but it must be employed with care because of the tendency to pincushion. It is similar to the flaps mentioned previously without the skin pedicle. The island flaps tend to be round or triangular; the triangular flap is less likely to pincushion. It is better to keep the dermis intact, but unfortunately this is not always possible. The advantage of this variety of flap is that it is a one-stage procedure, and it is probably more flexible than the standard flap. On the other hand, if care is not taken, these flaps can be devascularized more easily than pedicled flaps. This can occur by traction on or twisting of the pedicle or with a tunnel that is too narrow and constricts the pedicle, compromising flap survival (see Fig. 115-10).

Large Cheek Defects

When large areas of the cheek require removal, it is possible to lift the inferior skin of the cheek and neck. This large amount of skin can be moved upward and medially, a combination of advancement and rotation. This will allow significant defects to be closed with the correct skin match and a tension-free manner. The scar can be hidden in the preauricular and prehairline area. The results from this technique can be excellent. It may be necessary to remove a lateral triangle of excess skin that results from the rotation (see Figs. 115-28 and 115-31).

LIPS

The upper lip and lower lip must be considered individually because the methods used for reconstruction are not always applicable to both locations.

Upper Lip

The Cupid's bow, the position of the base of the nose, and the oral commissure are the areas to be considered in upper lip reconstruction. Any method that compromises the symmetry of these areas is not satisfactory. Unfortunately, when the defect is large, an optimal result may not be obtainable.

DIRECT CLOSURE

Direct closure is used whenever possible, but care should be taken to realign the mucocutaneous margin and the white roll. In some instances, to prevent a notch on the free margin, a mucosal Z-plasty may be employed. This must be done with care. Dry (external) mucosa should be extraoral, and wet (internal) mucosa should be intraoral. If it is exposed, wet mucosa will be obvious because it is red and shiny and tends to crust. The Cupid's bow should always be considered, and its symmetry should not be compromised unless this is unavoidable. In full-thickness defects, careful muscle reconstruction is mandatory.

Lateral and central defects can be closed directly, but judgment must be used. Any degree of asymmetry should be minimal.

Orbicularis oris repair has previously been a neglected area. The muscle must be dissected out from the mucosa and the skin. The muscle topography is then examined and reconstructed with accuracy. Magnification helps greatly. In lip repair, there should be equal emphasis on aesthetics and function.

LARGER DEFECTS

In the lateral and central areas of the upper lip, the perialar crescentic flap can be used (see Fig. 115-30). To allow the lip to advance without tension, a crescent of skin and deep subcutaneous tissue is removed from around the lateral area of the alar base. It is important to construct the lower part of the crescent end at the alar base. This maintains the correct vertical height of the lip. In addition, the mucosa is incised transversely in the upper buccal sulcus. This allows the whole lip segment to move, and closure can be performed without tension. When there are large midline defects, these can sometimes be closed with bilateral perialar crescentic advancement flaps. The problem with this reconstruction is that it may result in a tight lip. In addition, Cupid's bow may, more than likely, be compromised.

Abbe Flap

The Abbe flap is a full-thickness flap taken from the lower lip to the upper (Fig. 115-32).[17] The advantage of this flap is that in a central defect of the upper lip, a full-thickness segment of lip is inserted. The structure of the central portion of the lower lip also allows

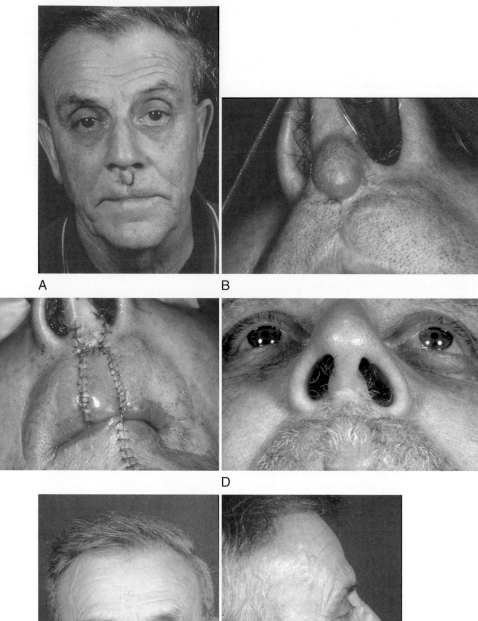

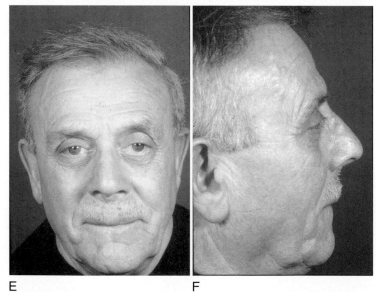

FIGURE 115-32. Reconstruction of central portion of upper lip—Abbe flap. *A* and *B*, Midline deformity of upper lip in patient with bilateral cleft. *C*, Resection of deformity of upper lip and closure with Abbe flap. *D*, Base of columella reconstructed with residual prolabium. *E* and *F*, Full-face and profile end result.

a Cupid's bow to be fashioned. If it is possible to reconstruct the upper lip muscles directly, the sandwich concept can be used. To employ the sandwich concept, the skin, mucosa, and lip margin can be taken from the lower lip on the marginal vessels and inserted into the upper lip to provide skin and muscle cover together with a lip margin of correct bulk. Because this is almost a full-thickness graft, the pedicle can be divided at 2 to 5 days, earlier than with the conventional flap.[18] This flap is applicable to the cleft patient, particularly for reconstruction of the secondary bilateral cleft lip deformity.

In the traditional flap, all layers are carefully sutured. The pedicle should be left intact for 2 to 3 weeks before division. Division is performed under local anesthesia.

These flaps are well tolerated, and patients can eat any type of food they can comfortably consume. This food may be solid or puréed, depending on the patient's preference.

At the second-stage procedure, it will be necessary to rearrange the mucocutaneous junction with additional trimming of the flap.

Fan Flaps

Fan flaps can be used for hemilip or total upper lip defects. These defects may be skin only or a full-thickness lip defect. Fan flaps can be standard or full thickness and are based on the perioral vasculature. The commissures are maintained and the flaps are rotated around them; thus, the anatomy of the mouth is maintained. However, fan flaps yield a much better result on the lower lip. This type of reconstruction has largely been overtaken by the perialar crescentic advancement flap (see Fig. 115-30).

Lower Lip

In the lower lip, skin defects can be reconstructed with nasolabial flaps. These can be transferred as a two-stage procedure or in one stage as island flaps. Pincushioning is a problem whether the flaps are round or square.

FULL-THICKNESS DEFECTS

In the lower lip, as opposed to the upper lip, larger defects can be closed directly because of the greater laxity. The closure should be performed in a careful, layered fashion in the following order: mucosa, muscle, and skin.

Karapandzic Technique

By use of the Karapandzic technique, three quarters of the lower lip can be reconstructed without difficulty (Fig. 115-33).[19] It has some resemblance to the perialar crescentic advancement flap, but it is a superior method. The reconstruction should replace the full thickness and depth of the lip. The skin is incised in a transverse direction to just beyond the nasolabial fold. Laterally, the vessels and nerves are dissected out and carefully preserved. The orbicularis muscle fibers are spread apart as far laterally as necessary. After this, it should be possible to move the leading edge to the midline or beyond, if necessary.

It is best to use bilateral flaps and to perform a layered closure where they meet. In this way, a loose and symmetric lip is obtained, and the blood and nerve supply are maintained. Also, a properly functioning lip with a virtually normal anatomy is formed. The scars settle well and are acceptable from a cosmetic viewpoint.

Gillies Fan Flap

Until the Karapandzic procedure was published, the Gillies fan flap was considered the method of choice.[20] Full-thickness nasolabial flaps based on the labial vessels are swung around the commissure into the lower lip defect. These flaps can be unilateral or bilateral.

Comparison Between Karapandzic and Gillies Techniques

In the Karapandzic technique, the commissures are maintained and the width of the commissure is satisfactory. There is no need to supply lower lip mucosa. The flaps are neurotized and result in function and sensation in the lower lip. In the Gillies reconstruction, the mouth is narrowed, and there is no mucosal cover of the flaps at the lip margin. Mucosal cover is supplied by advancing intraoral mucosa. Unfortunately, mucosa from this area is always red and shiny and frequently has a tendency to crust when it is exposed to the air. The nerves are not kept intact, and lip function and sensation are compromised. In spite of this, the function may be better than expected, especially in hemilip reconstruction.

Tongue Flaps

Tongue flaps are used to replace the red margin in reconstructions that do not supply the mucosa required. Tongue flaps are also used in patients with advanced and extensive leukoplakial involvement of the lip mucosa. The traditional method is to use the dorsum of the tongue, but its color and surface irregularity make it unsuitable as a lip mucosal substitute. The undersurface of the tongue is smooth, may have good color, and can easily be transferred in a staged procedure (Fig. 115-34).

The flap is based anteriorly. It should be of a sufficient length and width. It is sutured into the lip defect. In 10 days, under local anesthesia, the flap is divided and inset. The tongue defect is closed directly. The mucosa tends to be a deeper shade of red and shinier than normal. Because of its tendency to crust,

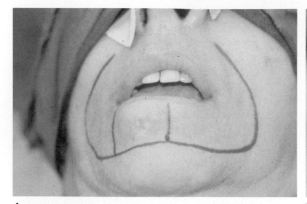

A

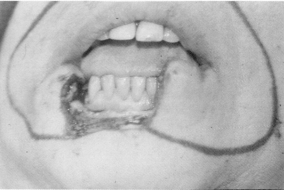

B

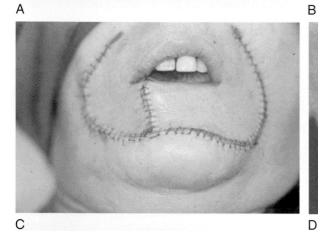

C

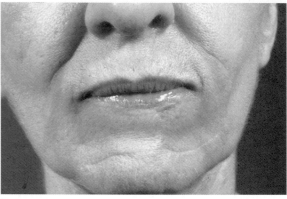

D

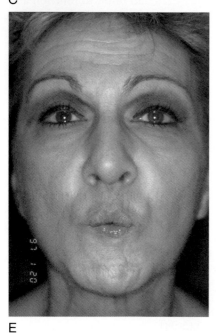

E

FIGURE 115-33. Reconstruction of partial defect of lower lip with Karapandzic rotation-advancement flaps. *A,* Flaps drawn out. The area to be excised in the lower lip is drawn out. *B,* Defect is developed. *C,* Defect closed with little deformity of lower lip. *D,* Lower lip reconstruction. *E,* Long-term function of lips.

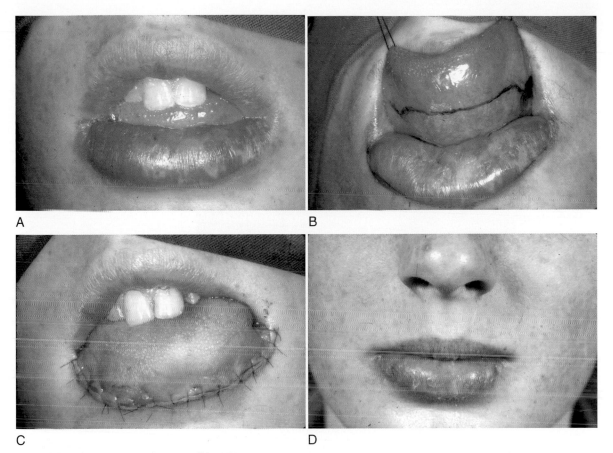

FIGURE 115-34. Resurfacing of the lower lip with a tongue flap. *A*, Vascular malformation of the lower lip. *B*, Tongue flap planned from undersurface of tongue. *C*, Flap sutured to lip. *D*, Result after 2 years.

the patient must apply petroleum jelly frequently. Sensation is reduced as with any free transplant on the lip.

TOTAL LOWER LIP RECONSTRUCTION

The Karapandzic technique can be used for total lower lip reconstruction, but the reconstructed lip is frequently too tight. The method of choice is bilateral fan flaps with inferior tongue flap resurfacing.[21]

The Webster advancement technique, in which bilateral full-thickness horizontal advancement cheek flaps can be brought into place by excision of bilateral upper and lower vertical triangles at their bases, is another possibility. The mucosa is again supplied from the undersurface of the tongue. The scars in the nasolabial lines and around the chin heal well. The main problem is that the reconstructed lip is flat and tight and tends to trap-door. On occasion, two Abbe flaps from either side of the prolabial segment of the lip can be turned down to increase lip volume, but the end result is not particularly satisfactory from a cosmetic point of view. Function (e.g., drooling) may be improved.

COMMISSURE RECONSTRUCTION

The commissure mucosa occasionally requires reconstruction. When analyzed, this can be divided into two rhomboids, one for each lip. Rhomboid flaps from the intraoral cheek area can resurface the defects without difficulty, and the donor sites close directly. However, this is wet mucosa and is redder than the normal lip.

Another method for larger defects (e.g., electrical burns) is to develop a large triangular mucosal island flap, advance its base to the commissure, and then use the considerable amount of tissue obtained as required. The donor site is closed directly. Later rearrangement of the mucosa is always required, but a sufficient supply is available after the procedure.

Finally, in some instances, lateral tongue flaps can be used to cover the upper and lower lip region at the commissure. These are divided after 10 days. These flaps are not widely used because anteriorly based flaps have proved to be more satisfactory in terms of position and the patient's comfort.

EAR

The areas of the ear most often requiring excision and reconstruction are the rim and the conchal area.

Rim Defects

It is frequently possible to excise a rim lesion and advance the rim by incising full thickness down to the lobule. There is no residual defect with this method (Fig. 115-35). If there is concern about the viability of the tip of this flap or if the defect is larger, the posterior skin is dissected up and may be included with the rim. A larger flap with a large base has a better blood supply and is more likely to survive. It does not result in any ear deformity.

In some instances, superior and inferior rim flaps will be used in conjunction with one another. Even larger defects are better reconstructed by postauricular flaps (Fig. 115-36). The flap is elevated and sutured to the anterior edge of the defect. After 3 weeks, a large flap is incised in the postauricular area, dissected up

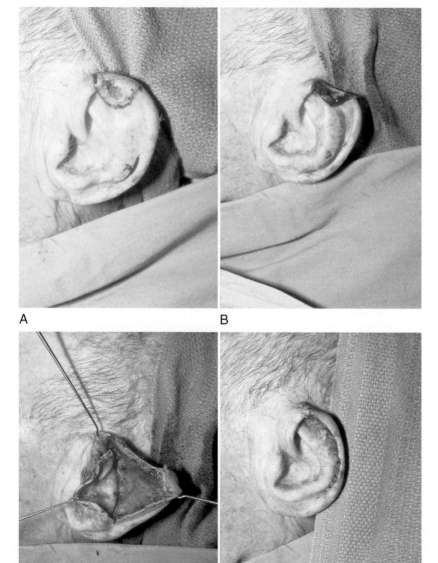

A

B

C

D

FIGURE 115-35. Reconstruction of ear defect with advancement of rim and posterior skin. *A,* Defect of left ear outlined. *B,* Defect excised. *C,* Flap of rim and posterior skin elevated. *D,* Rotation of flap to close defect, resulting in an ear that looks relatively normal.

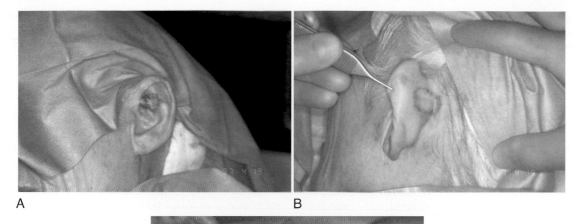

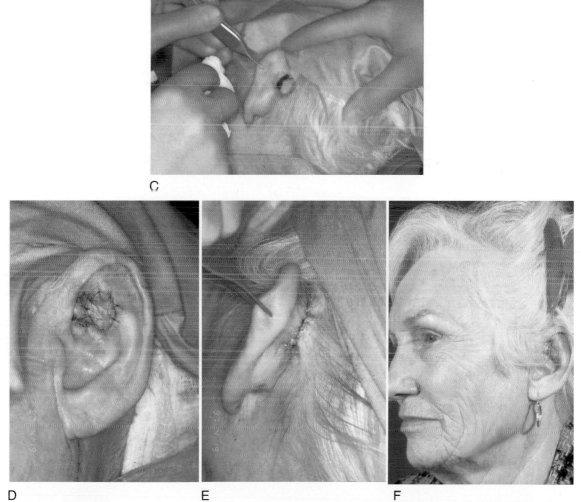

FIGURE 115–36. Revolving door flap to close anterior ear defect. *A,* Defect on the anterior aspect of the upper portion of the antihelical fold is outlined. *B,* The area of postauricular skin to be taken is outlined. *C,* The skin is totally incised around. *D,* The postauricular skin is revolved around the central pedicle and then comes to lie on the anterior aspect of the ear. It is sutured in position. *E,* The posterior defect is closed directly. *F,* End result.

to provide laxity, and brought to the ear rim to provide more tissue. It is trimmed as necessary and sutured in place. Further adjustments will most likely be necessary.

Anterior Concha

If a lesion of significant size occurs in the anterior concha, resurfacing will be required. To achieve this, the lesion is resected together with the underlying conchal cartilage. The ear is then distracted forward, and a flap is designed with a central vertical pedicle based on the ear mastoid groove. The skin anterior and posterior to the groove is elevated, with some division of the subcutaneous hinge superiorly and inferiorly, and rotated into the ear defect. The posterior edge of the postauricular island is sutured to the posterior edge of the defect, and the anterior edge of the island is sutured to the anterior edge of the defect. The posterior defect is closed directly. This will give an excellent result both on the anterior aspect of the concha and in the postauricular groove.[22]

In large deglovings of the ear, a temporal fascial flap is used to cover the ear. The flap is then covered with a full-thickness skin graft. This is a rare injury, but this technique can also be used in reconstruction of the congenitally absent ear. The end result is suboptimal because of the poor color of the skin graft. It may also have a shiny surface, especially if a split-thickness graft is used.

SKIN EXPANSION

Skin expansion for facial coverage is somewhat limited because it requires time for the expansion to be achieved. In some instances, immediate reconstruction may be required. In addition, the process of skin expansion is often uncomfortable and undesirable to the patient. However, if the time is available and only extra skin is required to reconstruct a defect, it is a good idea to gain some extra skin by this technique. The author favors expansion by use of external ports with inflation performed by the patient or relatives. This method leads to safe, efficient, and relatively comfortable expansion, particularly in children. This technique is especially useful when large amounts of skin are necessary (Fig. 115-37; see also Fig. 115-5).[23]

CONCLUSION

The use of facial tissue to close facial defects requires experience, artistry, and knowledge of skin

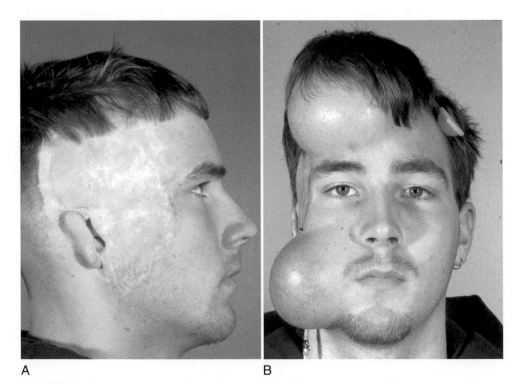

A   B

FIGURE 115-37. Closure of large cheek and scalp defect with expanded skin flaps. *A,* Post-traumatic defect reconstructed with split skin grafts. This involves the temporal, frontal, and cheek area. *B and C,* Tissue expanders inserted in frontal area, cheek, and scalp. Note position of external valves.

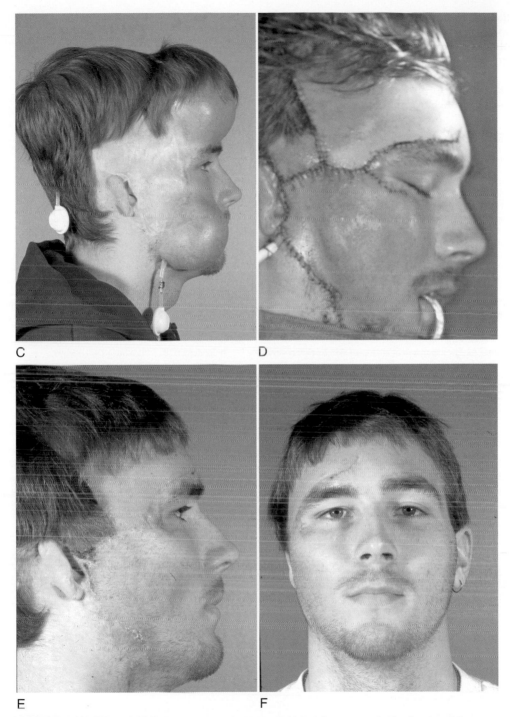

FIGURE 115-37, cont'd. *D,* Area excised and expanded flaps moved. The forehead flap was moved posteriorly. The scalp was moved to form a sideburn and the posterior cheek. *E* and *F,* End result of reconstruction in two stages.

biomechanics. The ability to close defects, large and small, and to produce cosmetically acceptable results is one of the great challenges of plastic surgery. It is important that plastic surgeons equip themselves with the knowledge and techniques required to meet this challenge and to provide patients with optimal functional and aesthetic results.

REFERENCES

1. Gibson T, Kenedi RM: Biomechanical properties of the skin. Surg Clin North Am 1967;47:279.
2. Borges AF, Alexander SE: Relaxed skin tension lines, Z-plasties on scars, and fusiform excision of lesions. Br J Plast Surg 1962;15:242.
3. Jackson IT: Local Flaps in Head and Neck Reconstruction. St. Louis, CV Mosby, 1985.
4. Limberg AA: Mathematical Principles of Local Plastic Procedures on the Surface of the Human Body. Leningrad, Government Publicity House for Medical Literature (MEDGIZ), 1946.
5. Dufourmentel C: Le fermeture des pertes de substance cutanée laitées. Le lambeau de rotation en L pour losange dit LLL. Ann Chir Plast 1962;7:61.
6. Zimany A: The bilobed flap. Plast Reconstr Surg 1953;11:424.
7. McGregor JC, Soutar DS: A critical assessment of the bilobed flap. Br J Plast Surg 1981;34:197.
8. Neumann CG: The expansion of an area of skin by progressive distention of a subcutaneous balloon. Plast Reconstr Surg 1957;19:124.
9. Rintala AE, Asko-Seljavaara S: Reconstruction of midline skin defects of the nose. Scand J Plast Reconstr Surg 1969;3:105.
10. Schmidt E: Nasal reconstruction. In Gibson T, ed: Modern Trends in Plastic Surgery. London, Butterworth, 1964.
11. Jackson IT, Clay R, Choi HY, et al: Long-term survival of cranial bone grafts in nasal reconstruction. Plast Reconstr Surg 1998;102:1869.
12. McGregor IA: Eyelid reconstruction following subtotal resection of the upper or lower lid. Br J Plast Surg 1973;26:346.
13. Mustardé JC: Eyelid repairs with costochondral grafts. Plast Reconstr Surg 1962;30:267.
14. McCoy FJ, Chow ML: Adoption of the "switch flap" to eyelid reconstruction. Plast Reconstr Surg 1965;35:633.
15. Mustardé JC: Repair and Reconstruction in the Orbital Region. Edinburgh, Churchill Livingstone, 1980.
16. Garrett WS, Giblin TR, Hoffman GW: Closure of skin defects of the face and neck by rotation and advancement by cervicopectoral flaps. Plast Reconstr Surg 1966;38:342.
17. Abbe R: A new operation for the relief of deformity due to double harelip. Med Rec N Y 1898;53:477.
18. Jackson IT, Soutar DS: The sandwich Abbe flap in secondary cleft lip deformity. Plast Reconstr Surg 1980;66:38.
19. Karapandzic M: Reconstruction of lip defects by local arterial flaps. Br J Plast Surg 1974;27:93.
20. Gillies HD: Plastic Surgery of the Face. London, Frowde, 1920.
21. Jackson IT: Use of tongue flaps to resurface lip defects and close palatal fistulae in children. Plast Reconstr Surg 1972;49:537.
22. Masson JK: A simple island flap for reconstruction of concha-helix defects. Br J Plast Surg 1972;25:399.
23. Jackson IT: Update on tissue expansion using external ports. Perspect Plast Surg 1990;4:129.

CHAPTER 116

Management of Nonmelanoma Skin Cancer

KEITH DENKLER, MD ◆ WILLIAM F. KIVETT, MD

Although nonmelanoma skin cancers (NMSCs) are multivariate in presentation, the majority of these tumors and their precursors are benign. However, one should never underestimate the potential for growth and the slow but progressive course of these lesions. These tumors grow by spreading into tissue planes of minimal resistance. Of course, less well differentiated tumors and those in immunocompromised individuals routinely behave otherwise.

Commonly, in the early stages of growth of either a tumor or its precursor, the patient more frequently and the physician less frequently underappreciate the growth potential. The standard assumption is that a biologically aggressive lesion grows rapidly. However, a less common tumor, such as Merkel cell carcinoma or a morpheaform basal cell carcinoma masquerading as a scar, may well not present to the physician until it is far advanced, with the accompanying morbidity or even mortality associated with this tumor type. Clearly, the effect of our nearest star, the sun, plays a major role in the development of most NMSCs. A patient's melanocytic endowment, lifestyle, chronic-

ity of ultraviolet irradiation, inherited DNA repair defects, and acquired immunosuppression all play a role in solar-induced tumor incipience and progression. In addition, certain human papillomaviruses have been highly implicated in the development of skin cancers.[1,2]

More leisure time and air transportation have enabled individuals with lighter skin on the Fitzpatrick scale of skin types[3,4] to acquire more actinic (sun-induced) damage with migration south toward the equator (Table 116-1). Such population migration, temporary or permanent, has resulted in development of skin cancer in a greater proportion of that group and in increasingly younger individuals. The additional effects of marketing pressures to tan and unclothe and self-indulgent lifestyles promoted by the media have resulted in purposeful cutaneous radiation injury.

In the 1700s and 1800s, the great majority of the U.S. population was forced by economics and social status to labor outdoors, therefore consigned to a life of solar radiation exposure and the expected cutaneous tumors. Sunlight as cause of skin cancers was first

TABLE 116-1 ✦ FITZPATRICK SKIN TYPES[3,4]

Code	Description
I	Always burns easily, never tans (very white or freckled skin)
II	Always burns easily, tans minimally (white skin)
III	Burns occasionally and tans gradually (olive or light brown skin)
IV	Burns rarely and tans very well (moderate brown skin)
V	Rarely burns, tans easily (dark brown skin)
VI	Never burns, darkly pigmented (black skin)

postulated by Thiersch in 1875 and Unna in 1894.[5] During those times, wealthier, more highly educated individuals worked inside; laborers working in the fields developed cutaneous cancers. It was fashionable to sport an alabaster complexion. In fact, it was in fashion for some time to apply arsenic to the skin to induce the highly desired pallor, which bespoke wealth and therefore higher social status even though arsenic was first noted to be a cause of skin cancers in 1887.[6]

It was not until the earlier part of the 20th century that fashionable skin color began to change from pale skin to a tanned appearance. This skin tone change came in part from the appearance of darker-skinned French models brought by Coco Chanel into the salons of haute couture sporting skimpier clothing fit for the beach more than for daily wear. At the same time, improved transportation methods allowed migration of wealthier individuals to climates previously deemed inaccessible. Naturally, the warmer lower latitude climates were sought. Thus, a generation of individuals never previously exposed to the sun became more susceptible to cutaneous tumors. Large numbers of military troops deployed for long periods outdoors, including to the South Pacific, where humidity and temperatures forced skimpy clothing, exacerbated the problem. As increasing entitlement to instant gratification was perceived by the public, the increasing use of convertible automobiles, the propagation of tanning parlors, and the migration of U.S. populations to southern, western, and coastal states were seen. Increasing rates of radiation-induced cutaneous injury followed. Only now, as public awareness grows about the influence of the diminishing protective ozone layer and the greater incidence of skin cancers, do we see a slight but perceptible interest in pallid complexions in the popular media and the use of hats, long sleeves, higher sun protection factor (SPF) sunscreens, and temporary spray-on and lotion tanning mimics.

A greater sense of hope has emerged as additional developments in the treatment of skin cancer have evolved away from the early painful hot-poker destructions leaving scars and remnants of tumor. Physicians have developed better tumor control, less tissue loss, and less scar acceptance. At the same time, recognition of greater virulence of tumors has led to a more aggressive approach to tumor management.

A separate science dealing with cutaneous oncology has grown up within the shadow of several medical sciences. A number of generalists and specialists have become involved in the treatment of lesions originally routinely treated by the family practitioners and general surgeons. Out of this multidimensional group has grown improvement in diagnostic and treatment techniques. Physicians with like interests have contributed to the field. Plastic surgeons, dermatologists, otolaryngologists, pathologists, general surgeons, gynecologists, urologists, and others have contributed within their areas of expertise. One example of a cross-specialty collaboration is that seen in the evolution of the work of Frederic Mohs, who as a general surgery–trained physician beginning in the 1930s brought his technique of horizontal section tumor control to a high level of effectiveness. In 1974, dermatologists Tromovitch, Stegman, and others recognized the value of frozen section processing of tissue as equal to that of the painful zinc chloride paste application.[7,8] Dr. Mohs retired in the 1990s, having seen his technique endorsed by several specialties after his personal demonstration of it in more than 100,000 patients.

Treatment of cutaneous malignant neoplasia requires skills in diagnosis, extirpation, and often reconstruction. The physician wears many hats in dealing with cutaneous cancer. Not all specialties can develop and maintain an expertise in all aspects relative to cutaneous oncology. Those clinicians weak in diagnostics and strong in therapeutics may, in the course of consultation, overlook or overdiagnose the presence or extent of cutaneous cancers. Those physicians who extirpate tumors in unfamiliar anatomic territory may fail to excise margins adequately in the "interest of tissue preservation" because of concerns about reconstructive necessities. This may lead to higher rates of intraoperative positive margins, recurrence, or persistence of tumor. These issues can be addressed with additional concurrent or proactive education of physicians as well as partial or complete referral to the appropriate specialist who can best meet the patient's requirements. Attention to outcomes of patients should be driven by the unwavering algorithm of the following priorities: tumor elimination, preservation of function, and finally cosmetic considerations.

The ascendancy of nonsurgical treatment of NMSCs and their precursors and recognition of the value of prevention by proactive education of patients and stimulation of compliance remain as challenges. The adoption of diagnostic and treatment methods perfected by multiple disciplines will benefit both patients and physicians alike.

ETIOLOGY

At our current level of understanding, the fact of induction of NMSC by solar radiation is irrefutable.[9] The question is, What is the exact nature of sunlight exposure necessary to induce NMSC growth and how do we reverse or prevent it? The answer is still not clearly known.

There is an incomplete correlation between the incidence of basal cell carcinoma (BCC) and cumulative exposure to ultraviolet B sunlight (290- to 320-nm wavelength). However, squamous cell carcinoma (SCC) exhibits a strong correlation with such exposure.[10,11]

Harbingers of SCC are solar actinic (sun-induced) keratoses (which have been referred to as SCC grade $1/_2$), keratinocytic intraepidermal neoplasia, and intraepidermal SCC.[12] Actinic keratoses appear to be more sensitive than invasive neoplasia as an indicator of chronic sunlight exposure. Actinic keratoses change in appearance over time. Only late in their course do they slowly convert to frank clinical and histologic carcinomas.[13] It has been calculated that in a person with the average number of actinic keratoses (measured in a series of patients to be 7.7), SCC would develop at a rate of 10.2% during 10 years[14]; other series suggest a range up to 20%.[14,15] One study noted that 60% of SCCs (10 of 17) arose from a lesion diagnosed as an actinic keratosis in the previous year.[16] Some have surmised that most untreated actinic keratoses would progress to frank SCCs during 20 to 30 years, but because of their appearance in the elderly, the limits of lifetime do not allow observation of such transformation.[17]

Because not all actinic keratoses become SCCs, we must look at postulated steps in the pathogenesis of SCCs induced by ultraviolet radiation. The *p53* gene is the most commonly mutated tumor suppressor gene. It is found in more than 90% of SCCs and in most BCCs and actinic keratoses.[9] This negative regulator serves like a brake in a car; in the normal state, it prevents the cell from proliferating without control. During this negative control, cells divide continuously, and those detected to be genetically defective are destroyed through a process of controlled cell suicide called apoptosis. This process ensures that abnormal cells do not survive to replicate. Because replication is an imperfect process, and many millions of mitoses take place on an hourly basis, the mechanism of apoptosis eliminates abnormally growing or dividing cells. However, if the *p53* gene becomes mutated and dysfunctional, the cell's self-monitoring process goes awry and uncontrolled growth ensues. Multiple areas of mutation in the *p53* gene may be present in the same tumor (Color Plate 116-1).[18]

Ultraviolet radiation causes mutations of *p53* genes. As more than one mutation in a given location takes place, the capacity for apoptosis decreases and the irregular cell clones expand into the lesion of actinic keratosis. It has been postulated that the initial development of an actinic keratosis may not be clinically detectable until the lesion presents as SCC.[9] This may explain why many SCCs become visible seemingly de novo. Equally minimally understood is the process by which most SCCs do not metastasize, whereas others do so or extend regionally. Indeed, there is no relationship yet known between *p53* mutation and tumor size, histologic subtype, or recurrence.[19]

Actinic keratoses are brown-red macules (flat areas of color change), papules (1- to 3-mm-diameter, minimally raised hemispheres), or plaques (elevated wider surface area macules with sharp step-off borders) with dry scales. The borders are frequently ill defined. It is common to be able to feel them with the examining fingertip before they can be seen. Examination is first carried out by lightly running the examining hand over the skin surface and then marking the lesions in question. They may be as large as several centimeters in diameter.[20,21] Less commonly seen is an obvious tall, hard cutaneous horn. Actinic keratoses are most frequently seen in areas normally exposed to sun, those being face, forehead, balding scalp, upper limb dorsum, lateral and superior ears, and neck wherever it is uncovered by the collar.[22] It is not unusual to have three to ten times more subclinical lesions than visible ones.[23] This presumes the presence of a sea of actinoelastotic change (the field effect), namely, thin, pale, telangiectatic, friable, scaly, variously pigmented skin.

Clinical changes that hint of the evolution of an actinic keratosis to SCC include new-onset erythema, pain, ulceration, induration, hyperkeratotic thickening with a history of temporary removal of the thickening by trauma, and increasing size or formation of a frank cutaneous horn (Fig. 116-1).[24-26]

In contrast to precursors for SCC, there are no precursors for BCC.[27] However, the same *p53* gene mutation in SCC has been demonstrated in BCC.[28-30]

PREVENTION

One clear factor in tumor induction is sunlight exposure early in life. The chronicity of sun-induced damage has a significant effect on the development of NMSCs. The majority of NMSCs arise from solar damage incurred in the first 18 years of life, thus making NMSC a pediatric prevention problem. For an infant born in 1994, the lifetime risk for development of BCC and SCC is 33% and 11%.[31] Because 80% of lifetime ultraviolet exposure occurs before the age of 20 years, preventive measures should be stressed to parents and children.[31]

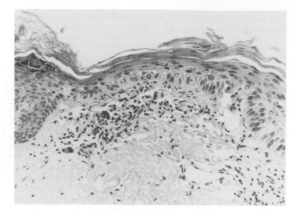

FIGURE 116-1. Histologic appearance of actinic keratosis. Dermal changes include dilated blood vessels with perivascular inflammatory cells. Epidermal changes include dysplastic keratinocytes and flattening of rete ridges. Stratum corneum changes include nuclei (parakeratosis), thickening, and small spicules of scale. (From Marks VJ: Actinic keratosis. A premalignant skin lesion. Otolaryngol Clin North Am 1993;26:23-35.)

The largest unknown is in transforming the behaviors of patients and parents of children. There must be a system to convince these individuals that prevention is important; this may appeal to fear of pain and disfigurement or death, intellectual sensibility, economics of time or money, or altruism.

Emphasis on prevention as a daily way of life will demand some behavior transformation for most individuals. A simple summary "to do" list may be taped to the bathroom cabinet. It should list the following:

- Apply sunscreen (SPF 15 or, better, SPF 30) by 8 AM every day to allow adequate penetration before stronger sun exposure at 9 AM.
- Apply sunscreen every day of the year no matter what the weather, including the presence of fog, active snow or rain, and overcast. (Ultraviolet rays penetrate nearly equally well in summer and winter and through moisture in the air.) Men prefer gel forms to lotions because gels are more reminiscent of shaving lotion.
- Reapply sunscreen for every 2 cumulative solar hours realized.
- Be aware of the boosting effect of ultraviolet light injury near reflective surfaces of water or walls.
- Use sunglasses when appropriate, with lenses capable of dispersion of ultraviolet A and B rays, to protect the thin-skinned periorbita.
- Schedule more activities when possible outside the 9:00 AM to 4:00 PM time slot when the sun's rays are the most direct.
- Avoid deliberate tanning activities, including tanning salons that administer ultraviolet A light. Substitute high-quality, relatively inexpensive skin tanners ("brown in a bottle") made up of

dihydroxyacetone, a component of sugar, which looks real and fades naturally during 5 days but does not confer photoprotection. Some salons now have relatively inexpensive tanning showers called Mystic Tan or Mist-On Tan. Thus, the patient will have less motivation for obtaining a true tan through sun exposure.

- Avoid tobacco use. The nurses' study shows a 50% increase in relative risk of SCC in cigarette smokers.[32]

For oncologically predisposed or concerned individuals, a one-time photographic session with a good camera and a ruler in each photograph, visually recording the cutaneous surface by region, is indispensable in monitoring for new lesions or changes in old ones. No patient, spouse, or physician can hope to remember a given lesion's appearance or presence. Around 25 photographs are required to record the whole body surface. The photographs should be printed on acid-free paper, stored in library-quality archiving envelopes in a dresser drawer, and pulled out for comparison by the patient once a year on his or her birthday as a reminder. Any new, larger, or changed lesions can then be systematically analyzed by a qualified physician.

Chemopreventive agents including 5-fluorouracil, retinoids, interferon, imiquimod, and aminolevulinic acid are discussed in detail in a later section.

BASAL AND SQUAMOUS CELL CARCINOMA

Incidence, Epidemiology, and Risk

BASAL CELL CARCINOMA

BCC is the most common malignant tumor in humans and the most common skin cancer in white individuals. The reported incidence of BCC in white persons in the United States ranges from 185 to 422 per 100,000 (Table 116-2).[33-35] Skin cancers occur in black patients with much less prevalence than in white patients.[36,37] The incidence of BCC in African Americans is 3.4 per 100,000.[38] Light-skinned African Americans are more susceptible to the development of skin cancer than are more darkly pigmented individuals, and the anatomic locations for development of BCC are similar to those of whites.[39] African blacks are also at risk for BCC but at an extremely low incidence of 0.65 per 100,000.[40] In fact, light-skinned people of all races are at the most risk for development of skin cancers.[41] The most common skin cancer in blacks is SCC as opposed to the more common BCC found in whites.[39,42]

Sunlight exposure during childhood, especially a history of sunburns, is the most significant host factor in the development of skin cancers.[43] Other host factors significantly increasing the risk of skin cancers include hazel or blue eyes, blond or red hair, freckling, facial

TABLE 116-2 ◆ INCIDENCE RATES PER YEAR (PER 100,000) OF BASAL CELL CARCINOMA AND SQUAMOUS CELL CARCINOMA BY GEOGRAPHIC LOCATION

Geographic Location	Basal Cell Carcinoma (men/women)	Squamous Cell Carcinoma (men/women)
Finland	49/45	9/5
Switzerland	52/38	16/8
The Netherlands	53/38	—
United Kingdom	112/54	32/6
New Hampshire	159/87	32/8
Rochester, Minnesota	175/124	63/23
United States	247/150	65/24
Hawaii	576/298	153/92
Nambour, Australia	2074/1579	1035/472

From Miller SJ, Moresi M: Actinic keratosis, basal cell carcinoma and squamous cell carcinoma. In Bolognia JL, Jorizzo JL, Rapini RP, eds: Dermatology. London, Mosby, 2003:1677-1696.

telangiectasias, outdoor occupations, and radiation exposure (Table 116-3).[44,45] The risks seem to be higher in light-skinned individuals and are related to the cumulative total exposure to radiation.[41,46]

The average age of patients with BCC is older than 60 years, although this age is far lower in tropical climates.[47,48] BCC is more common in men, but that trend is reversing, particularly in the younger sports-minded female population.[49-51] A 10-year study in England of BCC patients 15 to 34 years of age revealed an incidence of 1.2% in the targeted cohort.[52,53] This study excluded those with inherited disorders with predisposition to BCC. Of the 150 patients completing 5-year follow-up, 39 (21%) had incomplete excision requiring further early treatment, later local recurrence, metastasis, or another primary tumor subsequently.[50]

Australian studies note higher incidence figures. Australia has a high proportion of people from Celtic descent who have a higher propensity for skin cancers because of their light skin and poor ability to tan compared with those of southern European descent.[54,55] The incidence in Australia ranges from 672 to 760 per

TABLE 116-3 ◆ RISK FACTORS FOR DEVELOPMENT OF BASAL CELL AND SQUAMOUS CELL CARCINOMAS

	Squamous Cell Carcinoma	Basal Cell Carcinoma
Ultraviolet light (UV, PUVA, tanning beds)	+	+
Ionizing radiation	+	+
Chemicals (arsenic)	+	+
Human papillomavirus	+	(+)
Cigarette smoking	+	
Genetic Syndromes		
Xeroderma pigmentosum	+	+
Oculocutaneous albinism	+	
Epidermodysplasia verruciformis	+	
Dystrophic epidermolysis bullosa	+	
Ferguson-Smith syndrome	+	
Muir-Torre syndrome	+	
Nevoid basal cell carcinoma syndrome		+
Bazex syndrome		+
Predisposing Clinical Settings		
Rombo syndrome		+
Chronic nonhealing wounds and ulcers	+	
Discoid lupus erythematosus, lichen planus, lichen sclerosus	+	
Porokeratosis	+	
Unilateral basal cell nevus		(+)
Nevus sebaceus		(+)
Immunosuppression		
Organ transplantation		(+)
AIDS	(+)	(+)
Other	+	

From Miller SJ, Moresi M: Actinic keratosis, basal cell carcinoma and squamous cell carcinoma. In Bolognia JL, Jorizzo JL, Rapini RP, eds: Dermatology. London, Mosby, 2003:1677-1696.

100,000.[47,48] In recent population-based studies, Australia noted an incidence rate of more than 2% for BCC and 1% for SCC in males.[56] Another Australian study revealed an age-adjusted incidence rate for BCC of 2074 per 100,000 per year, one of the highest incidence rates of a specific cancer ever reported, except in heart transplant recipients.[57] A history of repeated sunburns combined with an examination noting nonmalignant solar skin damage was strongly associated with the development of cancers.[58,59] In these Australian studies, those patients who lived the longest in Australia had a much higher risk than did those who moved to Australia in later life.[44] Those patients with a previous skin cancer have perhaps a 10- to 15-fold risk for development of another skin cancer.[60]

In the United States, an Arizona study of 918 adults with significant sun damage but without a prior history of skin cancer revealed overall incidence in both men and women, with a mean age of 61 years, of 4106 per 100,000 person-years.[58] The 9-year study of skin cancer rates in southeastern Arizona revealed a plateau and even a slight decline effect during the study period. The incidence rates in Arizona, although among the highest in the world, do not appear to be increasing as rapidly as has been predicted for other locations.[61]

A prospective 5-year population-based study in Kauai, Hawaii, from 1983 to 1987 demonstrated a BCC incidence rate of 30 per 100,000 Japanese ethnic Hawaiians with an average age of 75 years, with 80% localized to the head and neck.[51] Another 5-year population study[62] in the same region identified an average annual incidence rate per 100,000 residents of 174 for men and 115 for women, with a combined rate of 142. The incidence increased in older groups with a mean age of 65.2 years. The most common anatomic site was on the extremities, and concurrent skin cancers on lesion presentation were noted in 36.6%.[62] There was no increased incidence of internal malignant disease in spite of an occurrence rate of 11.3% of Bowen disease.[62]

In the United States, there are now about 100,000 individuals living with organ transplants.[63] The frequency of skin cancer in organ transplant recipients is high, up to 15%.[57] A heart transplant recipient group numbering 111 was studied for a 9-year period, and either BCC or SCC developed in 15.2% of patients.[57] This represented an overall incidence of 45.3 per 1000 post-transplantation person-years with an incidence of 25.8 for BCC. Most cancers developed between 2 and 3 years after transplantation; most of the recipients had been exposed to significant ultraviolet radiation chronically, and most were of Fitzpatrick skin type II or III.[57] There was no significant association between skin cancer and haplotypes. The investigators emphasized the need for photoprotection and regular screening examinations after transplantation.[57]

On the other hand, BCC rates are much lower in Canada, noted in one study to be 171 per 100,000 men and 120 per 100,000 women.[49] A study of residents of Rochester, Minnesota, during an 8-year period cited an incidence of 175 per 100,000 men, 124 per 100,000 women, and 146 per 100,000 combined.[50] Recurrent or subsequent BCC was noted in 30% of those patients during a 4.5-year follow-up, and no metastases occurred.[50]

The risk of BCC in Malmö, Sweden, increased rapidly with age older than 55 years. Two thirds of the tumors were present in the head and neck region. The age-standardized incidence of BCC doubled from 1970 to 1986.[53]

A prospective study for more than 29 years of 80,000 cohort members through the population-based Hiroshima and Nagasaki, Japan, tumor registries demonstrated an excess risk for BCC that decreased markedly as the age increased at the time of atomic blast exposure.[64] There was no evidence for damage interaction between atomic bomb ionizing radiation and solar ultraviolet radiation. The conclusion was that the basal layer of the epidermis appears to be quite sensitive to radiation carcinogenesis, particularly at a young age, whereas the suprabasal layer is more resistant, as shown by the lack of an association for SCCs in the same population. In a related study, follow-up of 66,276 Nagasaki atomic bomb survivors revealed a high correlation between the incidence of skin cancer and distance from the blast center. Additional data revealed an increasing incidence of skin cancer with distance from the central point of the blast.[65]

The incidence of BCC is always greater than that of SCC, varying by latitude and exhibiting BCC-to-SCC ratio ranges of 10:1 to 2.5:1. The incidence of NMSC has been increasing 2% to 3% per year in the United States.[66]

SQUAMOUS CELL CARCINOMA

Approximately 200,000 SCCs of the skin are diagnosed every year in the United States. This figure is extrapolated from information that approximately 1.2 million NMSCs are diagnosed yearly in the United States, and approximately 20% to 30% of these are SCCs.[67] The quoted figures taken from cancer registries and other sources are expectedly understated because most cutaneous carcinomas are treated in an outpatient setting, thereby excluding these myriad cases from hospital-based cancer registries.[68] The frequency of cutaneous SCC is increasing as well. During a 17-year study period, the incidence of SCC increased 15-fold in women and 4-fold in men.[67] A large retrospective case-controlled study in Canada revealed average onset at 68 years in men and at 72 years in women. Less than 3% of the patients with primary SCC were in the 30- to 39-year age group. In spite of the more rapid increase of SCC in the female population, its prevalence in men is still twice that in women.[69-72]

Solar radiation exposure is the major risk factor for this condition.[13,72] Additional factors playing roles in skin cancer development are exposure to ionizing radiation, petroleum distillates, and arsenic and the presence of chronic irritation in long-standing scars, ulcerations, areas of previous burns, or infected cutaneous sinuses.[27,72] Ionizing radiation was commonly used to treat acne and hemangiomas in the 1950s, and fluoroscopy had widespread use until the 1960s.[41,46,73] Another iatrogenic risk is that seen in psoriasis patients treated with ultraviolet A light (320- to 400-nm wavelength) and an oral light sensitizer, the combination known as PUVA.[41,74-76]

The highest incidence of SCC in the world is in Queensland, Australia.[48] In this region, during a 5-year period, there was a 51% increase in SCCs.[77] In Rochester, Minnesota, during an 8-year period, the age-standardized incidence was 39 per 100,000, with 63 in men and 23 in women.[78] Metastasis occurred in 3.6% during an average of nearly 4 years of follow-up; recurrence was seen in 3.6% and subsequent new lesions in 12%.[78]

Mortality rates from SCC are decreasing, in spite of the increasing incidence. Mortality has decreased by as much as 30% for men and women.[79] The number of deaths per year in the United States (1200) has not changed appreciably in spite of the decreasing rate of mortality because of the increasing incidence of the tumor. A study of nearly 3000 cases of NMSC in Denmark noted 40 deaths caused by NMSCs, of which 25 were from SCC. This represents an estimated lethality of 4.3% for SCC.[80]

The role of immunosuppression in the development of SCCs is well known. Immunosuppressed organ transplant recipients are at high risk for development of skin cancers.[74,81,82] However, the patient's age, skin type, and sunlight exposure may be more important than the immunosuppressive regimen.[83] In the organ transplant group, SCCs are the most frequent skin cancers.[82] Increased risk for skin cancers after transplantation is associated with duration of immunosuppression, male sex, presence of actinic keratosis, advanced age at transplantation, outdoor occupation, and smoking tobacco.[84] Patients with AIDS also have an increased risk for both BCC and SCC; SCCs are the most common type.[85] Studies in organ transplant recipients show increase in the incidence of both premalignant and malignant epithelial lesions, which may be from human papillomavirus.[86] A comparative study of heart transplant recipients demonstrated a higher incidence of SCC, which by the nature of their illness yielded an older population of patients.[87] In addition, the SCCs in the transplant population are more aggressive. Rowe[88] found the rate of metastasis of SCC in the immunosuppressed to be 13%. Penn[89] and Euvrard[90] also reported aggressive SCC in transplant recipients.

Those patients with immune conditions such as discoid lupus erythematosus, lichen sclerosus, lichen planus, dystrophic epidermolysis bullosa, and lupus vulgaris have increased risks for development of NMSC.[91-100] Those who received immunosuppressive medications for connective tissue diseases had an increased risk for development of SCC about five times above that of the general population.[101]

Darker-skinned individuals have fewer SCCs (Table 116-4).[34,35,37,39,74,102-106] Among Japanese residents of Kauai, Hawaii, the incidence of SCC was 23 per 100,000; the average age of patients was 80 years. The rates are at least 45 times higher among Japanese living

TABLE 116-4 ✦ INFLUENCE OF SKIN COLOR ON EPIDEMIOLOGY OF NONMELANOMA SKIN CANCER

Characteristic	Lightly Pigmented Skin	Darkly Pigmented Skin
NMSC incidence	232.6[39]	3.4[39]
BCC-to-SCC ratio	4:1[102]	1:1[37]
BCC male-to-female ratio	1.5:1[35]	1.3:1[104]
SCC male-to-female ratio	2:1[35]	1.3:1[104]
% of BCCs developing in the head and neck	60[55]-80	89[104]
% of SCCs developing in the head and neck	67[103]	35[104]
% of SCCs developing in scars and ulcers	Less than 2[74]	28-39[37]
NMSC incidence rates	Increasing[103]	?
NMSC mortality rates	Decreasing[105]	Decreasing[105]
% of skin cancer deaths due to NMSC in persons younger than 50 years	10[105]	65[105]
% of skin cancer deaths due to NMSC in persons older than 85 years	56[106]	65[106]

NMSC, nonmelanoma skin cancer; BCC, basal cell carcinoma; SCC, squamous cell carcinoma.
From Miller SJ, Moresi M: Actinic keratosis, basal cell carcinoma and squamous cell carcinoma. In Bolognia JL, Jorizzo JL, Rapini RP, eds: Dermatology. London, Mosby, 2003:1677-1696.

in Kauai than among those living in Japan. This difference in SCC rates has been attributed to Kauai's intense ultraviolet radiation and emphasis on outdoor activities.[51]

In a New Mexico study of more than 10,000 tumors in nearly 5000 people during a 28-year period, incidence rates were much lower in Hispanics, in part because of the protection afforded by their darker skin.[107] A Danish study of nearly 3000 cases of NMSCs estimated lethality of BCC at 0.12%.[80]

Genetic and Predisposing Syndromes

BASAL CELL CARCINOMA

Genetic syndromes are nevoid BCC syndrome, Bazex syndrome, and Rombo syndrome. Predisposing skin lesions are nevus sebaceus of Jadassohn, linear basal cell nevus, and dermatofibroma.

Nevoid BCC syndrome, also known as Gorlin syndrome or Gorlin-Goltz syndrome, is autosomal dominant and has more than 100 associated anomalies.[108,109] Its incidence is estimated a 1:57,000; most of the cases arise from spontaneous genetic development.[110] The most common findings are of palmar or plantar pits (a pathognomonic feature); frontoparietal bossing; multiple BCCs; odontogenic keratocysts of the jaws; cutaneous epidermal cysts; high-arched palate; rib anomalies, such as fused, partially missing, or bifid; spina bifida occulta of the cervical or thoracic vertebrae, calcified falx cerebri, and diaphragma sellae; and hyperpneumatization of the paranasal sinuses (Table 116-5). In one series of 105 patients, 80% of white patients and 38% of black patients had at least one BCC; the first tumors occurred at a median age of 23 years.[111] Palmar and plantar pits were found in 87% of patients, and jaw cysts occurred in 74% of patients. Kimonis et al[111] proposed that Gorlin syndrome require the presence of two major or one major and two minor criteria (Table 116-6).

Curiously, in Gorlin syndrome, BCCs occur about 35% of the time on the trunk, in contradistinction to the normal ratio of 10% of BCCs occurring on the trunk.[112] The chromosome 9q23.1-q31 has been implicated as being defective in Gorlin syndrome.[111,113]

Of patients with BCC who present before the age of 19 years, 22% have this disorder.[114] There is no predilection for either gender, and it occurs most commonly in the white race. In spite of the large numbers of BCCs that have developed (occasionally into the hundreds), only rarely have they become invasive tumors and even more rarely fatally metastasized. Prophylactic management includes meticulous attention to sun protection and visits to a qualified cutaneous examiner every 3 months.

There is a particular sensitivity in these individuals to ionizing radiation in that hundreds of

TABLE 116-5 ✦ THE MAJOR CLINICAL FEATURES OF NEVOID BASAL CELL CARCINOMA SYNDROME

65% or greater frequency

Odontogenic keratocysts
Calcified falx cerebri
Relative macrocephaly/frontal bossing
Palmar/plantar pits

50% or greater frequency

Multiple basal cell carcinomas
Facial milia
Cutaneous epidermoid cysts of skin
High-arched palate
Rib anomalies
Spina bifida occulta (cervical, thoracic vertebrae)
Calcified diaphragma sellae
Hyperpneumatization of paranasal sinuses

Less than 50% frequency

Ventricular asymmetry (central nervous system)
Calcified ovarian fibromas
Calcified tentorium cerebelli
Short fourth metacarpals
Kyphoscoliosis/lumbarization of sacrum
Narrow sloping shoulders/prognathism
Strabismus
Pectus excavatum or carinatum
Hamartomas
Syndactyly/synophrys
Medulloblastoma
Cardiac fibroma
Cleft lip/palate

From Miller SJ, Moresi M: Actinic keratosis, basal cell carcinoma and squamous cell carcinoma. In Bolognia JL, Jorizzo JL, Rapini RP, eds: Dermatology. London, Mosby, 2003:1677-1696.

BCCs may develop in response to radiation delivered to the cutaneous surface for reasons such as internal malignant neoplasia.[115,116] Therefore, radiation therapy is contraindicated for treatment in patients with Gorlin syndrome because new cancers may be induced.

A rarer autosomal dominant condition described by Bazex[117] includes multiple BCCs, anhidrosis, hypotrichosis, and atrophoderma in a follicular pattern, frequently the presenting sign, with an appearance of ice pick defects of the foot and hand dorsum. BCCs are present early in childhood and classically involve the face.[118] Prognosis improves with earlier treatment.[119,120]

Rombo syndrome may be a variant of Bazex syndrome in that it is autosomal dominant with facial trichoepitheliomas from which BCCs may develop as well.[121,122] Hypotrichosis supports this relative mimicry of Bazex syndrome.[123,124]

TABLE 116-6 ◆ CRITERIA FOR DIAGNOSIS OF GORLIN SYNDROME

Major Criteria	Two or more basal cell carcinomas in a person younger than 20 years	Odontogenic keratocysts of the upper or lower jaw	The presence of three or more palmar or plantar pits	Calcification of the falx cerebri	Bifid or fused ribs	First-degree relative with Gorlin syndrome
Minor Criteria	Macrocephaly	Congenital malformations, such as cleft lip/palate, hypertelorism, or frontal bossing	Skeletal deformities, such as pectus excavatum, syndactyly, or Sprengel deformity	Radiographic findings of hemivertebrae, elongation or fusion of the vertebral bodies, bridging of the sella turcica, or lucencies in the hands or feet	Ovarian fibroma	Medulloblastoma

Diagnosis of Gorlin syndrome requires the presence of two major criteria or one major and two minor criteria.

Nevus sebaceus of Jadassohn is found at birth as a yellow-orange plaque or papule most often on the scalp and sometimes on the face and neck.[125,126] Ectopic apocrine glands are present microscopically along with localized malformations of the epidermis and pilosebaceous units.[127,128] This lesion will develop into BCC 5% to 20% of the time in younger patients,[129,130] although others disagree.[131] Growth of other neoplasms within the nevus sebaceus also supports the proposition that BCC development in these lesions is not malignant degeneration but rather a lessened primary germ cell differentiation with resultant increased proliferation.[132] Cancers arising in this condition show no aggressive features or tendency to metastasize.[133]

Dermatofibromas are common benign, papulonodular lesions on the extremities in adults. They are composed of spindle cells, histiocytes, and blood vessels in varying proportion.[134] BCC transformation takes place in up to 8% of these lesions.[135,136] Immunohistochemical studies demonstrate findings identical to those of sporadically occurring BCCs.[137]

A linear unilateral basal cell nevus, foreshadowing an extensive unilateral linear eruption of BCCs, is usually noted at birth.[138] This rare disorder includes scoliosis, heart problems, and abnormal bone mineralization.[139] The histologic changes are the same as those seen with routine BCCs, that is, features of benign basaloid proliferation.[139]

SQUAMOUS CELL CARCINOMA

Several conditions result in a relatively selective predisposition for SCC development. Such genetic syndromes include xeroderma pigmentosum; oculocutaneous albinism; epidermodysplasia verruciformis; epidermolysis bullosa dystrophica; poikiloderma congenitale (Rothmund-Thomson syndrome); dyskeratosis congenita; keratitis, ichthyosis, and deafness

(KID) syndrome; Werner syndrome; chronic mucocutaneous candidiasis; Fanconi anemia; and multiple self-healing squamous epitheliomas (Ferguson-Smith syndrome).

Predisposing skin conditions are consistent with a history of alterations in repair of wound healing observed by burns, nonhealing cutaneous ulcers, and sinus tracks of the skin as well as scars. Noninfectious scarring dermatoses and infectious scarring dermatoses also clearly play a role.[140]

Common to several of the syndromes is impairment of the repair process for DNA damage induced by ultraviolet light. The classic syndrome in this regard is xeroderma pigmentosum, an autosomal recessive genodermatosis (Fig. 116-2). The defective step is the initial endonucleolytic portion of repair of pyrimidine dimers or photoproducts induced by ultraviolet light.[141-144] Freckles, hyperpigmentation, diffuse erythema, and scaling, all in sun-exposed areas, develop as early as the age of 1 or 2 years. Soon thereafter, skin atrophy, additional pigmentation irregularities, and telangiectasias are followed by cutaneous BCC, SCC, and melanoma at a median age of 8 years, approximately 50 years earlier than in the general population in the white race.[141,143] BCC or SCC occurs in 57% and melanoma in 22%. There is a 70% probability of survival to age 40 years, a reduction from the general population, attributed to the increased incidence of melanoma. Progressive neurologic degeneration including mental retardation and sensorineural deafness and associated dwarfism and immature sexual development are seen in approximately 20%.[141] Abnormalities of the eyelids, conjunctivae, and cornea have been reported in 40% of patients.[145]

Oculocutaneous albinism is autosomal recessive with hypomelanosis of the skin, hair, and eyes.[146] This form of albinism is divided into two types: type I, tyrosinase-related oculocutaneous albinism with afflicted activity of tyrosinase; and type II,

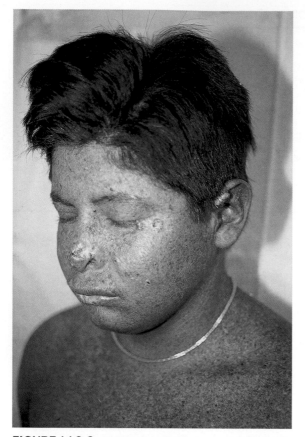

FIGURE 116-2. Xeroderma pigmentosum. Multiple skin cancers on the face of a 12-year-old Hispanic boy. (From Miller SJ, Moresi M: Actinic keratosis, basal cell carcinoma and squamous cell carcinoma. In Bolognia JL, Jorizzo JL, Rapini RP, eds: Dermatology. London, Mosby, 2003:1677-1696.)

tyrosinase-positive oculocutaneous albinism, with normal tyrosinase activity.[147] Several types remain unclassified. Actinic keratoses occur in 91% of oculocutaneous albinism patients older than 20 years.[148] SCC is the most common malignant neoplasm in this group.[149,150] Those affected in the tropical populations have higher rates of metastatic lesions.[151]

Epidermodysplasia verruciformis has a rare, mostly autosomal recessive susceptibility to cutaneous infection with specific strains of human papillomaviruses, most commonly type 5.[152-155] Impaired cellular immunity and T-cell responses have been described, but B-cell responses are normal.[156,157] In early childhood, widespread flat warts appear.[158] SCC develops in 30% to 50%, especially in uncovered areas.[152,158] SCC develops in the average patient at the age of 27 years, approximately 40 years earlier than in the general population.[159] The mean age for metastasis is 34 years, although metastasis and death are rare.[159]

Epidermolysis bullosa dystrophica has several categories including simplex, junctional, and dystrophic or scarring type. All three categories have both autosomal dominant and recessive forms.[160,161] They are generally classified by significant skin fragility and blister formation of the skin and mucous membranes with minor trauma. In the most severe form of epidermolysis bullosa dystrophica, this generalized condition presents shortly after birth with repeated blistering over joints that leads to severe scarring and acral mutilation, joint contracture, and upper gastrointestinal tract scarring and strictures.[162] SCCs arise in the scarred areas most commonly on the arms and legs in up to 95% of patients.[97,163] Other more localized forms of epidermolysis bullosa are not as severe and account for far fewer cases of SCC.[164] Abnormalities in the anchoring fibrils involving type 7 collagen in the dermis attaching to the basement membrane of the epidermis have been identified as one cause of this condition.[165,166] A number of chromosomal and collagenous irregularities have been speculated to have a role in the SCCs resulting from this condition.[167,168]

A syndrome of rare autosomal dominance is multiple self-healing squamous epitheliomas (Ferguson-Smith syndrome), in which keratoacanthoma-like tumors of the face and other sun-exposed areas rapidly develop in the late teens.[169,170] This syndrome is different from the familial multiple keratoacanthoma syndromes. The lesions are histologically indistinguishable from SCC.[171,172] Rarely, metastasis takes place.[173] Chromosome 9q22-q31 has been identified with a possible genetic locus that is in the same region as the genetic defect in nevoid BCC syndrome.[174]

Poikiloderma congenitale (Rothmund-Thomson syndrome), an autosomal recessive condition, presents with facial erythema and blistering, spreading to the dorsum of the hands, feet, and proximal extremities shortly after birth.[175] The skin changes evolve into pigmentary irregularities, telangiectasias, and poikiloderma with atrophy, particularly on the sun-exposed areas. Photosensitivity is common.[176] The hair thins slightly or full alopecia develops frequently. The nails thin and deform, and hypoplastic teeth are present. Skeletal abnormalities and short stature are the rule. By the age of 13 years, cataracts develop in 50%. Delayed sexual development is noted less commonly.[176] In photosensitive individuals and in sun-exposed areas, SCC develops.[177] However, the most common malignant neoplasm in these patients is osteosarcoma.[178,179] The cause of this syndrome is thought to be a defect in DNA repair mechanisms,[180-182] although others disagree.[183,184]

Dyskeratosis congenita is a rare X-linked, recessive ectodermal dysplasia.[185] Leukoplakia of the oral or anal mucosa, dystrophic nails, and extensive reticulated hyperpigmentation demonstrating atrophy and telangiectasias are notable.[186] Aplastic anemia develops in approximately 50%.[186] A number of other organ systems are involved as well. SCC develops in the areas of leukoplakia between the ages of 6 and 15 years.[187,188] The majority of these occur in the oropharynx. Cutaneous SCC is rare. Median survival is 33 years of age; death is caused by aplastic anemia and its complications.[185]

Keratitis, ichthyosis, and deafness (KID) syndrome is variably inherited. It is associated with cutaneous ichthyosis (fish-like skin) and neurosensory deafness, vascularizing keratitis of the eyes, and impaired physical and mental development.[185,189] Frequent bacterial and fungal infections grow in the dry and thickened skin with early childhood development of SCCs, occasionally fatal.[190-192]

Werner syndrome involves striking premature aging of all organ systems, especially of the face.[193,194] This accelerated aging syndrome leads to early atherosclerotic coronary heart disease and malignant degeneration with mostly sarcomas.[195-198] Cutaneous SCC and melanomas occur in these patients in addition to other cancers.[196,199] Japanese individuals with this syndrome have a high prevalence of melanoma.[199] This premature aging syndrome has demonstrated a mutation in the gene coding for DNA helicase.[200,201]

Chronic mucocutaneous candidiasis is a genetic syndrome with associated immunodeficiency.[185,202,203] Several familial and nonfamilial types have been described.[185] In the late-onset group associated with malignant neoplasms, most commonly thymomas, oral mucosal SCC develops commonly during young adulthood and is commonly fatal.[204]

Fanconi anemia results in acute myelogenous leukemia in up to 52% of patients by the age of 40 years, along with progressive bone marrow failure.[205,206] This autosomal recessive disorder is also a disorder of DNA repair and involves a number of organ systems.[207] Multiple, variously pigmented macules are seen along with dystrophic nail changes.[206,208] The most common cutaneous cancer is carcinoma of the tongue.[206,209-211] Frequent clinical examination and biopsy of all chronic nonhealing wounds are necessary.

Apart from the genodermatoses noted and beyond the well-known actinic keratoses and nevus sebaceus of Jadassohn, SCC may develop in linear epidermal nevi that present at birth as a linear collection of verrucous scaly papules.[212,213] Another condition, porokeratosis of Mibelli, presents with raised borders and central keratotic debris. It is associated with immunosuppression and may become malignant.[214-217] Another form of porokeratosis, disseminated superficial actinic porokeratosis, presents as many smaller papules mostly on sun-exposed areas, appearing and disappearing with sun exposure.[218] Invasive SCCs arise in both types of porokeratosis,[215,219,220] which represent mutant clones of keratinocytes by way of abnormal DNA ploidy.[221]

Diagnosis

BASAL CELL CARCINOMA

Several clinical variants of BCC are known, but 60% are noduloulcerative, referred to in the older literature as rodent ulcer, a term coined by Jacob[222] in 1827. The classic presentation is a pearly or translucent mass with or without a pebbly appearance or texture and with telangiectatic strands. A superficial scale or crust can develop that may suggest a diagnosis of SCC.[223] Melanin pigment may be present as a brown, black, or blue coloration of the tumor, resulting in confusion with a melanocytic lesion. Pigmented BCC represents less than 10% of clinical presentations.[224]

Although a number of histologic variations of BCC are known, there is not a great deal of predictability in use of the features of a clinical lesion to estimate the histologic diagnosis. For example, there are no unique clinical features distinguishing a nodular BCC from a micronodular one, not to mention the complicating factor of pigmentation.

A superficial BCC (Fig. 116-3) subtype is characterized as an erythematous macule with slight scaling, atrophy, hypopigmentation, or scar. There may be some confusion with this condition and other more common inflammatory skin conditions including eczema, tinea corporis, and psoriasis.[223] Their chronicity and nonresponse to or worsening with application of topical corticosteroids may be the only indicators that there is an error in diagnosis.

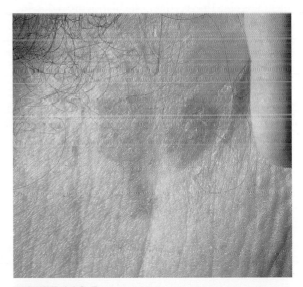

FIGURE 116-3. Superficial spreading basal cell carcinoma. Erythematous plaques of superficial basal cell carcinoma can resemble eczematous or papulosquamous diseases and can be difficult to distinguish from Bowen disease and lichenoid keratosis. (From Miller SJ, Moresi M: Actinic keratosis, basal cell carcinoma and squamous cell carcinoma. In Bolognia JL, Jorizzo JL, Rapini RP, eds: Dermatology. London, Mosby, 2003:1677-1696.)

Infiltrating tumors may not have distinguishing clinical characteristics. They may be nodular or flat. Employment of the examining hand to palpate a lesion, in an attempt to displace it back and forth, may give a hint of infiltration by its superficial inflexibility but without true fixation to the deeper tissues.

Morpheaform BCCs, also known as fibrosing, sclerosing, and desmoplastic subtypes, resemble localized scar tissue or scleroderma. They are frequently slow growing, present as ivory-colored flat to slightly raised areas, and have variable telangiectasias. The historical report of very slow growth with perhaps a history of minor trauma may lull the unsuspecting examiner into complacence in diagnosis. Tumor borders are frequently indistinct and subtly blend into the surrounding skin. The lesions may be depressed. Only late in their course do they ulcerate. Rarely, they are pigmented. A condition known as fibroepithelioma of Pinkus represents strands of basal cells tracking along eccrine gland ducts.[225]

A nodular BCC has large islands of basophilic uniform cells with separation artifact from the stroma by uniformly aligned nuclei (palisading) within the outermost row of basal cells (Figs. 116-4 and 116-5).[226,227] The clear zone adjacent to the palisaded cells results from loss of mucin during tissue processing. Strands of tumor in nests or individual cells in a row ("Indian filing") are frequently present. Several histologic subtypes are frequently seen. These include but are not limited to adenoid, pigmented, pleomorphic, and basosquamous, with a variety of differentiations including apocrine, eccrine, follicular, neuroendocrine, and sebaceous.

One notable exception to these patterns of differentiation is the morpheaform BCC, which commonly appears microscopically to be scar tissue, with narrow strands and finger-like projections of basophilic cells

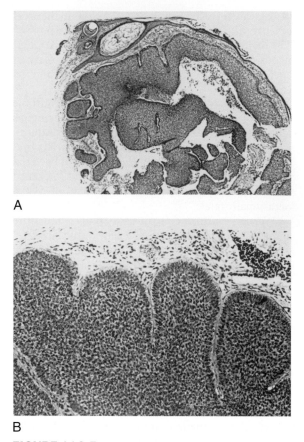

A

B

FIGURE 116-5. *A,* Low-power view of a nodular basal cell carcinoma. Note the round, well-circumscribed mass of neoplastic cells. *B,* In the high-power view, peripheral palisading of cells and retraction clefts are apparent (hematoxylin-eosin). (From Goldberg DP: Assessment and surgical treatment of basal cell skin cancer. Clin Plast Surg 1997;24:673-686.)

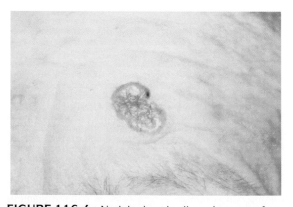

FIGURE 116-4. Nodular basal cell carcinoma on forehead characterized by pearly, telangiectatic nodule with an elevated, rolled border. (From Nguyen AV, Whitaker DC, Frodel J: Differentiation of basal cell carcinoma. Otolaryngol Clin North Am 1993;26:37-56.)

one- to two-cell layers thick, without peripheral nuclear palisading and without retraction of the tumor from the surrounding stroma on which the tumor depends for growth. Indeed, close intermingling of the cells of BCCs in general, with or without morpheaform differentiation, bespeaks the increased potential for infiltrative aggressive growth and thus difficulty in extirpation and elevated frequency of recurrence.

There are a number of histologic mimics of BCC, and confusion may arise because these mimics may also have nodular or infiltrative basaloid tumor islands with nuclear palisading. Expert opinion, including special stain techniques by a qualified dermatologic histopathologist, may be necessary to sort out the confusion. These mimics include but are not limited to adenoid cystic carcinoma, desmoplastic trichoepithelioma, eccrine carcinoma, Merkel cell carcinoma, metastatic breast carcinoma, microcystic adnexal carcinoma, mucinous carcinoma, and sebaceous carcinoma.[228,229]

Although the ideal situation is that biopsy of BCCs is performed before definitive therapy is carried out, the practicality of this approach is questionable. If a lesion is diagnosed clinically (visually), the treatment method itself will result, in many instances, in a specimen that should be submitted for pathologic confirmation of both diagnosis and excision margins. A situation frequently arises in which a wider area of the skin appears affected, and a diagnosis cannot practically be made by wide excision of such an area without significant morbidity of function or cosmesis. In that case, selective small shave or punch biopsies of the areas most potentially productive are valuable, with minimal morbidity. These specimens may be submitted with color labeling and geographically marked with anatomic stamps.*,[230] Curettage of specimens purely as a diagnostic method is less valuable with respect to diagnosis and has no value at all with respect to margin determination.

There is significant value in having a close relationship with one or more histopathologists and an understanding with them that diagnosis of BCC is more valuable with detailed subtypes and differentiation. It is good practice for the plastic surgeon to encourage the clinical-histologic connection by review of the permanent slides (permanent histologic sections) or the micrographic or frozen sections with the pathologist at the time of extirpation. This gives the histopathologist an opportunity to describe key points of the tumor under the microscope. This helps maintain surgeon-pathologist communication to ensure appropriate decisions in regard to diagnosis and tumor margins.

SQUAMOUS CELL CARCINOMA

There is no pathognomonic lesion that distinguishes primary cutaneous SCC from other skin lesions. These tumors normally present as nodules or plaques with a variable degree of scale, crust, erosion, or ulceration. They differ from BCC in clinical appearance by the absence of a pearly, translucent aspect, much less telangiectasis. The lesion is usually pink, tan, or a combination thereof. In moist anatomic sites such as skinfolds and mucosa, if hyperkeratosis is present, the lesions appear white. The diagnosis is best confirmed by histologic examination to help rule out keratoacanthoma, skin adnexal tumor, hypertrophic actinic keratosis, Bowen disease, inflammatory or infectious disorders, and reactive disease processes such as psoriasis and pseudoepitheliomatous hyperplasia.

---

*Available from Delasco, Council Bluffs, Iowa; www.delasco.com.

MEDICAL TREATMENT: CHEMOPREVENTIVE AND CHEMOTHERAPEUTIC AGENTS

Chemopreventive and chemotherapeutic agents, delivered both topically and systemically, may be incorporated into skin tumor management (Table 116-7). Well-established agents include 5-fluorouracil (5-FU) and retinoids. Newer chemopreventive and chemotherapeutic agents include aminolevulinic acid, interferon alfa, selenium, imiquimod, and diclofenac, which may be useful in *initial* tumor management.

5-Fluorouracil

The long-proven chemotherapeutic agent 5-FU also serves as a chemopreventive agent. SCC precursors that are not visible are destroyed along with the visible lesions for which the chemotherapy was originally prescribed. The compound's value in cutaneous eruptions was discovered when a woman with cancer of the reproductive tract was receiving intravenous 5-FU. The patient had an inflammatory skin reaction at several sites on the face and on other sun-exposed areas. Investigation soon led to recognition that the compound was interacting in a salutary fashion with the patient's visible and invisible tumor precursors.

Topical 5-FU is known commercially as Efudex. It works as a pyrimidine analogue (mimic) that serves as an antimetabolite by direct inhibition of thymidine and thus of DNA synthesis.[231,232] This antimetabolite competes with normal metabolites for specific enzymes, thereby preventing their function. With the exception of a substitution of the fluorine atom at the 5-position, 5-FU is identical to both uracil and thymine. The molecule, with a van der Waals radius similar to that of uracil, thus fits perfectly into the DNA synthesis pathway. Thymine deficiency results in the prevention of DNA replication, leading to cell death. The arrest of cell growth in the S phase causes the cells to undergo apoptosis with the production of proinflammatory mediators that induce an inflammatory response facilitating the removal of dead and dying cells.

The inflammatory response represents the value of the agent; however, it is antagonistic in use by patients from a cosmetic, economic, and socially acceptable point of view. Compliance of patients is difficult to maintain because of induced symptoms of itching, burning, and sleeplessness. Residual erythema and hyperpigmentation frequently last 1 to 8 months.[233]

The value of this medication in nodular BCC treatment is limited. One study noted 50% complete resolution without evidence of recurrence during a 3-year observation period, concluding that this medication is not indicated for the routine treatment of solitary nodular BCC.[233] Another study with superficial

TABLE 116-7 ✦ MEDICAL TREATMENTS FOR ACTINIC KERATOSIS, KERATOACANTHOMAS, AND NONMELANOMA SKIN CANCERS

Technique	Mechanism of Action	Indications	Dosage	Complications	Effectiveness
5-Fluorouracil (5-FU)	Antimetabolite inhibits DNA synthesis	Actinic keratoses, keratoacanthoma	0.5%, 1%, and 5% cream	Poor penetration into nodular or deep tumors; inflammatory	Good for actinic keratoses or superficial BCCs
Retinoids	Modulation of cell differentiation	Actinic keratoses, photoaging, chemoprevention	Topical or oral forms	Inflammatory; poor results on active lesions	Poor results for active tumors
Imiquimod (Aldara)	Localized stimulation of immune modifiers	Chemoprevention, treatment	5% cream	Localized ulceration	Excellent for actinic keratoses or superficial BCCs
Interferons	Nuclear cellular modifiers	BCC and SCC, experimental	Varies	Inflammation, influenza-like symptoms	Remission 50%-80%
Diclofenac	Inhibition of the cyclooxygenase pathway	Actinic keratoses	3%	Inflammation	Fair to good for actinic keratoses; remission about 60%-70%
Photodynamic therapy	Topical application of precursor to protoporphyrin, then fluorescent light exposure	Actinic keratoses approved BCC? SCC?	20% aminolevulinic acid topically to each lesion or other photosensitizer	Painful, limited penetration	Good for actinic keratoses; remission 80%-90%

BCC, basal cell carcinoma; SCC, squamous cell carcinoma.

BCCs that used a variety of concentrations from 0.005% to 20% gave inconsistent results with one exception—the 5% and 20% concentrations resolved at least 80% of the tumors. The cure rate was the same with either concentration, but the 20% concentration produced an intense inflammatory reaction resulting in scarring.[234] Combination of 5-FU with topical tretinoin, a retinoid, has increased the efficacy of the medication beyond that expected with 5-FU alone.[235-237]

Actinic keratoses have become the main target of 5-FU. Several series have demonstrated good clinical efficacy with 2 to 6 weeks of therapy (Color Plate 116-2).[238-242] Studies have also demonstrated between 70% and 98% resolution. Actinic keratoses should be observed for persistence. If a superficial lesion persists to the end of the treatment period, SCC should be suspected, and biopsy should be performed for confirmation of diagnosis. Repeated biopsy of the site may be necessary.

Attempts to reduce the inflammatory component and thereby increase tolerability have been made. Some practitioners treat with frequent or intermittent applications of topical steroids, such as triamcinolone 0.1% cream. This "rescue cream" is valuable for brief periods

for treatment of intolerable inflammation of a few individual sites. Widespread use of this cream for more than a day or two essentially defeats the purpose of the 5-FU treatment. Some patients do well with systemic antihistamines, such as diphenhydramine (Benadryl), 25 to 50 mg at bedtime and once during the day. It is still necessary to have the patient return frequently in an attempt to ensure compliance.

One study has evaluated the use of weekly pulse dosing. Follow-up at 9 months noted an 86% cure rate.[243] Another study published 7 years later refuted the value of intermittent topical 5-FU therapy. Inflammation, erythema, edema, erosion, and ulceration were deemed likely to be necessary for full efficacy of 5-FU.[244] Thus, as it currently stands, older, retired patients are ideal candidates if they have multiple widespread actinic keratoses and are willing to tolerate some minor to moderate erythema and itchy inflammation for approximately 4 weeks to help eliminate disease. 5-FU is available as Efudex 2% and 5% solutions and 5% cream. There is minimal systemic absorption with the 5% cream preparation. Toxic effect has been associated with use of the medication in only 1 of 1,949,288 cases.[245] As a way to avoid systemic absorption, handwashing immediately after application is valuable.

Minimizing exposure to ultraviolet rays between 9 AM and 4 PM each day immediately during and after the treatment sessions helps. There should be no application to the eyelids or onto mucous membranes. Increased absorption may occur if the skin is inflamed or ulcerated. Pregnant women or women attempting pregnancy should not use 5-FU.

Retinoids

Retinoids are a group of naturally occurring and synthetic vitamin A analogues and related compounds that bind to nuclear retinoid receptors and are intimately involved in the proliferation and differentiation of various tissues, including skin. The two main clinical agents are all-*trans* retinoic acid (tretinoin) and 13-*cis* retinoic acid (isotretinoin).[246] Retinoids suppress the proliferation and regulate the differentiation of normal skin and skin cancer cells.[246-252] The chemopreventive effect of oral retinoids is demonstrated by the prevention of development of new lesions.[248] A chemotherapeutic rather than a chemopreventive effect is seen in the resolution of new lesions in patients with multiple advanced SCCs. Oral isotretinoin treatment of xeroderma pigmentosum results in reduction of new cancer development.[253-255]

Retinoids bind to intracellular retinoic acid receptors and modify gene transcription and epidermal differentiation.[248,256] However, systemic doses of isotretinoin (0.4 to 2.0 mg/kg per day) or etretinate (1 mg/kg per day) have been attempted to prevent the appearance of new BCCs and SCCs in those with excessive irradiation of a solar or ionizing nature, nevoid BCC syndrome, or xeroderma pigmentosum and in immunosuppressed organ transplant recipients.[257-259] Such significant adverse side effects were sustained in these patients as to make the employment of retinoids in these situations less attractive. Common adverse side effects include relatively severe cheilitis, nasal mucosal dryness and nosebleeds, eye irritation secondary to reduction in tear production, alopecia, peeling of the fingernails, very dry skin, and eczema. Also seen are elevated liver enzyme and triglyceride levels, myalgias, arthralgias, and, in some patients, calcification of the spinal ligaments and vertebral hyperostosis. Because therapeutic responses are dose dependent, the practitioner needs to be assured of a therapeutic response with minimal symptoms to foster compliance of the patient.[260]

Isotretinoin (Accutane) has teratogenic potential, but because the majority of NMSCs are present in the population beyond childbearing years, this is not particularly a problem. There is still some controversy as to the role isotretinoin plays in depressive and suicidal reactions.[261-263] The role of systemic retinoids in post-organ transplantation patients is currently under study.[264-266]

In studies with isotretinoin used directly on existing BCCs, approximately 10% of tumors underwent complete clinical and histologic remission, indicating there are better methods for treatment of existing BCCs.[267] Studies with acitretin (Soriatane) have demonstrated a significant reduction in the total number of tumors excised during the long-term period of acitretin therapy compared with an equivalent immediate pretreatment interval in immunocompromised renal transplant recipients.[112] Approximately 50% of patients remained free of both BCCs and SCCs while receiving acitretin without hematologic or liver function changes. All patients experienced cutaneous drying effects that were generally well tolerated. The study took place during a 4-year period.[112]

Systemic retinoids have been used in patients with multiple actinic keratoses. These improved significantly, both in and out of the immunosuppressed state.[268-270]

Topical retinoic acids (tretinoin, known as Retin-A and Renova) have been used for more than 30 years as chemopreventive and chemotherapeutic agents. These have also been used to enhance 5-FU therapy.[271] The histologic changes resulting from such therapy include increase in epidermal thickness, increase in stratum granulosum thickness, reduction of a more compact stratum corneum, increase in collagen synthesis, increase in skin elasticity, formation of new vessels, and reversal of epidermal dysplasia.[272] In essence, the use of topical retinoids returns the skin to a younger era with the effect of reduction of fine wrinkling, skin atrophy, pigmentary irregularity, and sallow (whitish yellow discoloration) appearance. Also, there is significant reduction in the small areas of fine scaling found with actinic keratoses. As an additional measure, the keratin plugs (solar comedones) around the eyes and nose, not resulting from acne and seen in older, Mediterranean area individuals (known as Favre-Racouchot syndrome), are reduced.

Retin-A has had an overwhelming public acceptance as a cosmetic "youthening agent" and in the treatment of acne with the expected low- to medium-grade dryness associated with its use. In response, Ortho Pharmaceutical Corporation developed the emollient form of tretinoin called Renova and received approval by the Food and Drug Administration for the treatment of fine wrinkling.[273] Renova has also received significant acceptance by the public in the search for maintenance of younger skin and the regression of sun damage.

Interferons

Three newer chemopreventive and chemotherapeutic agents are now available for clinical application.

The interferons bind to cell surface receptors for transmission of a signal that activates multiple gene transcriptions, although the mechanisms are not completely understood.[274] This behavior allows interferons to play multiple roles in cell proliferation and differentiation.[260,275] Of the three major groups of interferons—alfa, beta, and gamma—the alfa form has been used in conjunction with the retinoids for advanced cutaneous SCC or regional and distant metastases of cutaneous SCC in an attempt to reduce the dose and systemic toxicity of the retinoids.[276] In one study, 68% of patients had major responses. Slightly less than a third of these were complete responses, including one in a patient with distant metastasis.[260] Intralesional injections of interferons hold promise, and response rates have varied from about 50% to 80%.[277-281] Other studies are currently under way to assess the value of other modifications of the protocols to include the integration of cisplatin.[282]

Imiquimod

Imiquimod (Aldara), an immune response modifier, has been used to treat BCCs, Bowen disease, and SCCs.[283-287] It has a salutary effect on macrophages and Langerhans cells. Its mechanism of action seems to be binding of imiquimod to the cell wall, causing a release of localized cytokines and an activation of macrophages.[288,289] Proinflammatory cytokines produced by these and other cells have been studied in cutaneous cancers. The localized cytokines and chemokines released include interferons, interleukin-12, and tumor necrosis factor-α.[288,289] In a study of patients with BCC-confirmed biopsies, the BCCs cleared in 100% of patients with the imiquimod applied twice daily, once daily, or three times weekly.[290] Other studies have shown similar results.[291-293] This immune modulator has also been used in conjunction with 5-FU for the treatment of Bowen disease as well as of anal and perianal SCC in situ in an HIV-positive patient. The results have been favorable.[285,294,295]

Diclofenac

Solaraze (3% gel) is a topical nonsteroidal anti-inflammatory drug similar to Voltaren. The complete mechanism of its favorable treatment in actinic keratoses is unknown. However, the nonsteroidal anti-inflammatory drugs work in part by inhibition of the cyclooxygenase pathway, resulting in a reduction in prostaglandin E_2 synthesis.[296-298] Diclofenac demonstrated complete clearance of actinic keratoses in up to 64% of patients in one study.[299] Other studies report similar results.[300,301] Side effects are minor.[299] As with other nonsteroidal anti-inflammatory medications, aspirin sensitivity represents a contraindication to use of this medication.

PHOTODYNAMIC THERAPY

Photodynamic therapy (PDT) is based on the administration of a photosensitizer, more readily maintained in tumor than in normal tissue, followed by illumination of the tumor with light in a wavelength matching the absorption spectrum of the photosensitizer (Fig. 116-6).[302,303] PDT is a minimally invasive treatment for skin cancers and may be used before or after surgery and with or without chemotherapy or radiotherapy. It was first demonstrated in 1905 when topical eosin plus sunlight was used to destroy skin cancers.[304] PDT may be repeated multiple times.[305] Unfortunately, PDT is still in clinical testing in the United States for skin cancers. PDT is approved in the United States for use in esophageal and lung cancers.

Aminolevulinic acid is a precursor of protoporphyrin IX, which is synthesized in the actinic keratosis when it is treated with aminolevulinic acid. The protoporphyrin IX photosensitizes the actinic keratosis so that fluorescent blue light exposure can lead to its destruction.[306] Aminolevulinic acid is applied to each actinic keratosis lesion followed by exposure to the fluorescent blue light for about 15 minutes the next day. Jeffes et al[307] reported an 88% complete clearance of actinic keratosis after a single treatment. The resulting redness and inflammation with PDT are less than with a treatment of 5-FU. Drawbacks include lack of histologic confirmation of destruction and limited penetration into deep tumors, and the treatments can be painful.[308,309]

Results after treatment with PDT for skin cancers have been good. However, the comparison treatments of surgery, Mohs excision, and radiotherapy have cure rates above 90%, so it may be some time before PDT moves out of clinical trials. Reported results on NMSCs of the head and neck range from 50% to 92%.[310-312] Repeated treatment in a time interval of 1 week improves results.[313]

There are potential future applications of PDT in premalignant conditions or carcinoma in situ.[314,315] For cancers, PDT may be more effective after curettage of tumors.[305,312,316] It has been used with success in patients who develop multiple malignant neoplasms.[317,318] PDT in conjunction with topical 20% aminolevulinic acid has been approved by the Food and Drug Administration for use in facial and scalp actinic keratosis.[319]

SURGICAL TREATMENT

The surgical modalities for treatment of BCC and SCC are curettage and electrodesiccation, cryosurgery, shave excision, and full-thickness excision including Mohs micrographic surgery (Tables 116-8 and 116-9). Each has its advantages, disadvantages, and frank contraindications. A number of factors must be taken

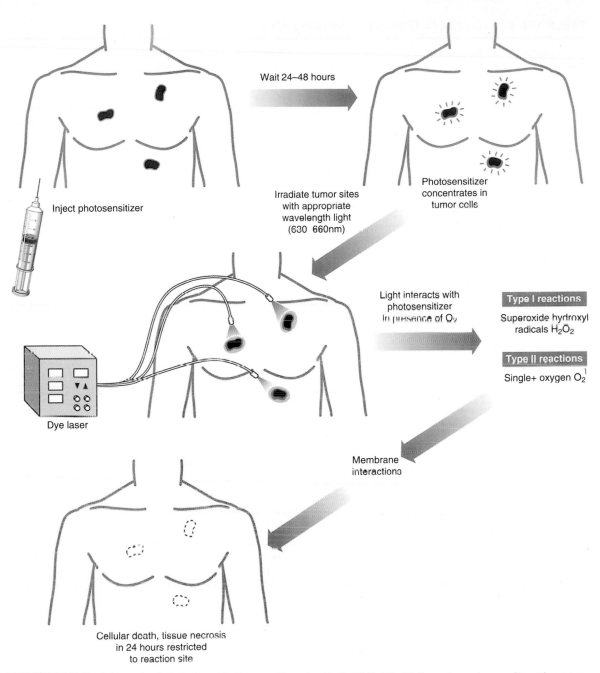

FIGURE 116-6. Schematic of photodynamic therapy. (From Leshin B, White WL: Malignant neoplasms of keratinocytes. In Arndt KA, LeBoit PE, Robinson JK, Wintroub BU: Cutaneous Medicine and Surgery: An Integrated Program in Dermatology. Philadelphia, WB Saunders, 1996:1378-1391.)

into consideration, including (but not limited to) the tumor's location, histologic subtype, size, and known recurrence; the background of ionizing radiation and solar radiation; the skin color; and the patient's overall health, age, gender, and aesthetic target. Although the treatment plan will be based on individual tumor types and surgical modalities, treatment is highly individualized for each patient and is based on both the

surgeon's experience and functional and cosmetic considerations.

Preoperative Considerations

Part of the approach to surgical treatment of skin cancer involves adequate assessment of the patient as a candidate for surgical care. Complete review of the

TABLE 116-8 ✦ SURGICAL TREATMENT OPTIONS AND RADIOTHERAPY

Treatment Options	Recurrence Rate	Side Effects	Effects on Future Treatment	Length of Treatment	Cost
Surgery	5%-10%	Scarring, infection, bleeding	Minimal unless flaps or grafts are used	Fast	Inexpensive, but requires additional laboratory costs; flaps, grafts are extra
Mohs excision	<5%	Scarring, infection, bleeding	Minimal unless flaps or grafts are used	Fairly fast	More expensive; flaps, grafts are extra
Radiotherapy	5%-10%	Radiodermatitis	Cannot be repeated; damages tissue	Slow	Very expensive
Curettage and electrodesiccation or cryotherapy	Varies with experience and depth of tumor; can be less than 5%	Scarring and hypopigmentation	Can be repeated, but works less effectively for recurrent tumors	Fast	Inexpensive

patient's health status is paramount. All organ systems must be cleared for the patient's tolerance of advised surgical interventions. Basic criteria include the ability to withstand the procedure psychologically and to be compliant with perioperative instructions; adequate cardiopulmonary, renal, and gastroenterologic status; adequate hematologic and coagulation dynamics; and ability to tolerate the procedure. Accurate assessment is important of the history of drug effects; prior operative interventions; anesthesia tolerance; concurrent and previous medical diseases; allergies; nicotine, alcohol, and recreational drug use; and vitamins, supplements, hormones, and dietary intake.

In today's medicolegal world, the nature, goals, course, prognosis, alternatives, risks, and complications need to be discussed fully with the patient and informed consent obtained. All questions must be answered, and the patient must be fully willing to proceed with the operative interventions. Most important, the patient must be able to remain in a monitored setting with the surgeon or a reliable substitute during a protracted postoperative time. Oncologic disease demands a coordinated follow-up by the treating physician, patient, and other physicians including the primary physician.

Decision about nonsurgical versus surgical intervention relies on the treating physician's experience and knowledge base. If clinical acumen allows a visual diagnosis of a given lesion as BCC, biopsy as a preliminary step is unnecessary. If there is question about the diagnosis of the tumor or if the margins are poorly defined, a biopsy specimen of the tumor or samples (color coded for further tracking) from various portions of the tumor must be taken before final decision-making. Fortunately, these lesions grow relatively slowly, so time may be taken for additional biopsies, consultation with colleagues, referral of the patient to another setting, and repeated examinations if required. Accumulated and persistent acquisition of information about the tumor or tumors takes precedence over rapid diagnosis and treatment decision-making.

Shave Biopsies Versus Removal

For BCCs with an aggressive growth pattern or recurrent tumors, the findings of a shave biopsy may be negative if the shave is shallow. A repeated, deeper shave biopsy or a punch biopsy is then necessary.

Shave (tangential) excision is best reserved for biopsy of lesions or removal of clinically superficial tumors.[301,320] Traditionally, a No. 15 or No. 10 surgical blade on or off the handle is employed with the dominant hand in a deliberate stroking to-and-fro motion to achieve an adequate scooped specimen; the nondominant hand squeezes and raises the site, thus stabilizing it for the angle of attack of the blade. Others have used flexible blades for biopsies (Fig. 116-7).[320] These are best purchased as double-sided blades, split longitudinally, and sterilized before use. The advantage of this is the ability to squeeze the flexible blade between the dominant thumb and index finger to adjust the angle of the incision around the lesion. Once shave excision is complete, the site may be cauterized for additional tumor destruction and hemostasis. Hemostatic solutions include but are not limited to aluminum chloride, ferric subsulfate (Monsel solution), and trichloroacetic acid 10% solution.[321] As opposed to curettage and electrodesiccation, this technique allows a cursory glance at margins for tumor clearance. One disadvantage is in an overly

TABLE 116-9 ✦ SURGICAL TREATMENT TABLE

Treatment	Curettage and Electrodesiccation	Cryosurgery	Shave Excision	Surgical Excision	Mohs Excision	Radiotherapy
In situ disease	+	+	+	++	++	−
Lesions < 2 cm, face	++	++	+	++	++	+ depending on location
Lesions > 2 cm, face	−	−	+	++	++	++
Lesions < 2 cm, trunk	+	+	+	+	+	−
Lesion > 2 cm, trunk	+	+	+	++	++	+
Recurrent disease, face	−	−	−	++	+++	+
Recurrent disease, trunk	−	−	−	+++	+++	+
Advantages	Fast, fair cosmetic results; excellent for small nodular or superficial tumors	Excellent for superficial tumors; a rapid treatment, good cosmetic result	Excellent for superficial tumors; inexpensive; may be performed with scalpel or razor blade; allows margin control	Excellent for many tumors; excellent cosmetic result as incisions may be planned; good margin control	Cosmetic results can be excellent	Excellent for recurrent, ill-defined, or sclerosing tumors; excellent margin control; requires special training and is time-consuming
Disadvantages	Slow healing, no margin evaluation	Hypopigmentation slow healing; no margin control; requires special equipment	Depressed scar may be a problem; not for deep tumors	Surgical complications such as bleeding, infection, scarring	Surgical complications; higher cost; not indicated for small tumors	Expensive; special equipment needed over extended sessions, plus chronic irradiation damage

− is poor; + is better.

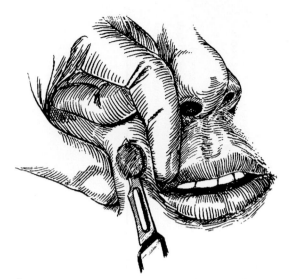

FIGURE 116-7. *A,* Shave biopsies are highly useful in diagnosis of nonmelanoma skin cancers, and specimens may be taken with a scalpel. (From Limmer BL, Clark D: Nonsurgical management of primary skin malignancies. Otolaryngol Clin North Am 1993;26:167-183.) *B* and *C,* Double-edged razor blades are flexible, inexpensive, and very sharp. They are excellent for office shave biopsies and easily sterilized.

A

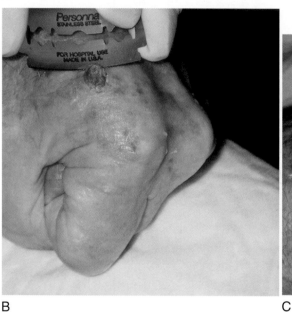

B

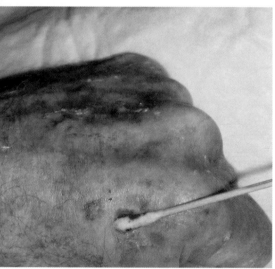

C

conservative excision resulting in a layer of tissue not optimal for full histologic verification of the diagnosis. Healing is relatively uneventful as long as post-shave electrical or hot-point destruction is conservative. Healing is by secondary intention and usually results in minimal scarring and pigmentation change. The information obtained from a biopsy with permanent or frozen sections allows delayed or immediate action. If a biopsy specimen has positive margins before surgery, with the patient's permission, the tumor can then be extirpated by a deeper shave, full-thickness excision (with or without micrographic excision), curettage and electrodesiccation, or cryosurgery. Should the histologic interpretation of a benign process be confirmed on frozen or permanent section, the patient will have had no additional exposure to more invasive methods of treatment.

Curettage and Electrodesiccation

The technique of curettage and electrodesiccation is commonly used to treat BCCs and SCCs.[321-328] The tumor is scraped with a sharp, open, spoon-like handled instrument by the dominant hand while the skin is stretched in two dimensions by the nondominant hand. Tumors will frequently have a mushy or gritty consistency. Once the firmer, more normal peripheral borders are encountered, the hand will feel a firmer resistance in many cases, indicating the tumor border. A heat element, usually electrical more than direct heat, is then applied to the site. Further curettage of the burn eschar is then performed until it is clear. This process is frequently carried out through three scrape-and-burn cycles. Advantages are ease and speed of employment in addition to an aggressive treatment. The disadvantages include the unavailability of tissue for margins, the pure white scar, the contour deformity, an occasional hypertrophic scar or keloid, and the higher recurrence rate in low- and high-risk tumors. Such a technique also presupposes the patient's ability to heal wounds readily by secondary intention, which may be a problem in the distal lower extremities in elderly patients.

On occasion, the curet—especially a smaller "bucky" curet—encounters a narrow-diameter, deep nest of tumor cells and falls through into the deep dermis or subcutaneous fat. At this point, the procedure needs to be stopped and the extirpation choice redirected toward a deeper and possibly wider excision.[379] This technique should not be used for recurrent tumors, large tumors, and infiltrative, morpheaform, sclerosing, or deeply penetrating tumors.[379]

Cryosurgery

Cryosurgery is a widely used technique for destruction of superficial precancerous lesions, especially actinic keratoses, and superficial BCCs and SCCs. It works by boiling heat transfer when the cryogenic substance (liquid nitrogen at −196°C) results in tissue necrosis and vascular stasis.[330-333] Tumor destruction occurs most efficiently when the tissue is frozen rapidly.[334] A 1-second application is usually sufficient for selective destruction of an actinic keratosis; longer applications are required for superficial BCCs and SCCs (Figs. 116-8 and 116-9).[335]

As the tissue thaws, vascular stasis ensues from thrombosis of microvasculature. Additional immediate freezing and thawing applications naturally destroy

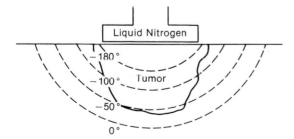

FIGURE 116-8. Cryosurgery is most effective at the surface. Deeper tumor treatment requires a deep thermocouple for best results. (From Limmer BL, Clark D: Nonsurgical management of primary skin malignancies. Otolaryngol Clin North Am 1993;26:167-183.)

tissue.[331,336] Keratinocytes frozen to −40°C display destructive nuclear changes within minutes.[337] Temperature ranges necessary for tissue destruction are −15°C to −60°C. Current temperature recommendations range from −50°C to −60°C for all tumor regions.[332,338,339] In general, collagen and cartilage resist freezing injuries, and therefore freezing is effective in the ear and the nose. Although epidermal healing is adequate after freezing, the melanocytes are lost with resultant hypopigmentation of an otherwise well-healed wound.[340]

A second phenomenon, conduction heat transfer, takes place when a superchilled piece of metal is applied to the skin. The cryoprobe may be designed with a liquid nitrogen–frozen forceps handle that is applied to a skin lesion with a padded gloved hand. Several more elaborate cryoprobes are available to facilitate direct application. A thermocouple needle is often implanted within the tumor substance to accomplish freezing. Adequate freezing of BCCs or SCCs requires a temperature of −50°C within the tissue.[332,339,341] Open-spray systems, such as the CRY-AC, are extremely popular. Additional modification of the open-spray, boiling heat transfer technique involves use of a cone, within which the spray is confined to the site, with the vapor venting peripherally; in the closed cone technique, a trap confines the spray solely to the lesion, thus further concentrating the spray.[342,343] Both the open-spray and the cone technique are used by different practitioners. Both are effective in experienced hands. The cone technique involves the use of a plastic cone with the tip slightly larger than the lesion to confine the spray to restricted areas.

Residual permanent hypopigmentation or complete depigmentation of the treated area is common.[331] Unlike the localized edema, persistent erythema, and hyperpigmentation visualized early, the later hypopigmentation is permanent. Hypertrophic scarring may be temporary or permanent and may be treated with cryotherapy.[344] Infectious sequelae are rare but may occur during prolonged healing, especially in the lower extremity.[345] Wound healing problems are not usually seen unless there is decreased vascularity to the area from peripheral vascular disease or a systemic metabolic problem such as steroid intake, diabetes, chemotherapy, or venous stasis. In the eyelids, specific complications include notching, corneal ulcers, and trichiasis.[346]

The advantage of cryosurgery is its cost-effectiveness and ease of use. It is safe with minimal restriction of activity, and the cosmetic result is usually acceptable. Most clinicians use the hand-held open-spray technique without a cone. Few clinicians use a cone with the open or closed technique or the cryoprobe with a thermocouple needle. Liquid nitrogen costs little and is easily obtainable from any local gas supplier. It has been used to treat virtually any part of

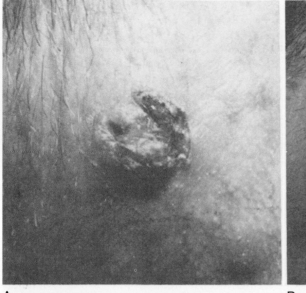
A

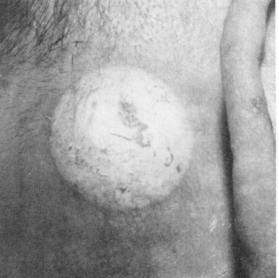
B

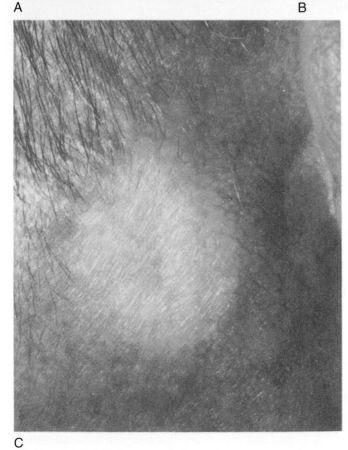
C

FIGURE 116-9. A patient with nodular basal cell carcinoma in the right postauricular position. *A,* Before cryosurgery. *B,* Immediately after cryotherapy with an intact iceball. *C,* A hypopigmented atrophic scar 8 months after cryosurgery. (From Limmer BL, Clark D: Nonsurgical management of primary skin malignancies. Otolaryngol Clin North Am 1993;26:167-183.)

the cutaneous surface. Those tumors most appropriate for treatment have well-delineated borders. The technique is suitable for patients with multiple lesions as well as elderly or debilitated persons with a limited tolerance for other surgical intervention. Indeed,

liquid nitrogen is taken into nursing homes in the standard carrier of the hand-held cryosurgical unit, the most popular being the CRY-AC. Cryosurgery can be used in pregnancy, for anticoagulation with cardiac and vascular disorders, and for elderly, demented patients. It is contraindicated for tumors with indistinct clinical borders; for recurrent lesions; for aggressive or deeply infiltrating primary tumors; and in patients with cold intolerance, cryofibrinogenemia, cryoglobulinemia, and cold urticaria.[331,332,347,348] Tumors in hair-bearing areas of skin that are susceptible to cryotherapy-induced alopecia are also a contraindication.[348]

For BCCs, cure rates from an older series of patients, depending on anatomic location, were noted from 95.3% to 100%. In a newer series by the same practitioner with a lower number of study patients, the cure rates in general rose for each anatomic location except one and ranged from 94.4% to 100%.[332,349] These high cure rates have been echoed in other series.[347,350]

For SCCs, the same practitioner in an older, larger series had cure rates, depending on anatomic location, of 95.3% to 100%. A later series with far fewer patients showed an increase in 5-year cure rates (with the exception of three anatomic locations) ranging from 88% to 100%.[349] Other practitioners report positive results with cryosurgery for SCC.[347,351]

Full-Thickness Excision

Regardless of the etiology of tumor recurrence near a scar, positive margins result in recurrence in as many as 76% of patients.[352] Although it is perceived that lymphohistiocytic infiltration of a healing wound may have a salutary effect against remnant tumor, tumor-positive surgical margins should not be observed for recurrence. As a counter to arguments that it is cost-effective to monitor for recurrence, the additional expense incurred with recurrent tumors neutralizes the argument as the recurrence rate is approximately one in three when surgical margins are positive.[353-358] For this reason, full-thickness excision remains the procedure of choice for skin cancer management. Only through pathologic examination of the tumor and its surrounding tissue can margins be determined and complete tumor excision accomplished.

Most BCCs recur within 3 years of initial treatment, but 18% recur 6 to 10 years after treatment.[359] Recurrences become apparent when circulating T-cell levels decrease, indicating that immune dysfunction plays a role in tumor surveillance.[360] Recurrences are delayed if involved deep margins are covered by a flap because the tumor may grow undetected under the flap for a prolonged period.[361]

BCCs recur variably after different types of treatment. After curettage and electrodesiccation, the recurrence rate is about 7%.[328,359,362,363] However, if the tumor is already recurrent, it recurs 36% of the time.[359,363] With cryosurgery, BCCs recur at a rate of approximately 5%.[347,359,363,364] Of course, the rates of recurrence are different for primary versus recurrent lesions (4.0% and 13.0%, respectively).[359,363]

Surgical excision of BCC has been evaluated for recurrence rates in a number of combined studies. The combined rate is 4.8% to 5.2% for primary BCCs and 11.6% to 14.6% for recurrent BCCs.[352,365-369] The recurrence rate for micrographic surgery is reported as 1% for primary BCCs and 5% for recurrent BCCs.[7,359,363,370,371] Comparison of the result of micrographic excision with the results of other modalities, such as surgical excision, cryotherapy, and radiation therapy, is difficult because of the different structures inherent in each study that make true comparisons challenging.[372]

Full-thickness excision is chosen from a variety of alternative therapies on the basis of risk assessment for recurrence of the tumor. Full-thickness excision is applied to lesions with higher recurrence risk based on clinical and pathologic risk factors. Clinical risk factors include location, size, borders, primary versus recurrent status, and prior radiation therapy. In the case of SCC only, additional clinical risk factors are tumor at a site of a chronic inflammatory process; a rapidly growing tumor; and symptoms of pain, paresthesia, or paralysis. Pathologic risk factors include perineural involvement and, in the case of BCC, subtype. In the case of SCC, additional pathologic risk factors are degree of differentiation; adenoid, adenosquamous, or desmoplastic changes; and depth (Clark level or thickness).

Recurrence is defined as regrowth of a previously treated tumor in the same location. However, continuing persistence of an established tumor is different from the disappearance and eventual return (recurrence) of a tumor. Persistence is favored by factors different from those favoring the development of a new primary. Also, new primaries in the same vicinity and even at the scar margin from an old excision do not necessarily imply tumor recurrence or persistence. The field effect (diffuse solar radiation–induced precancerous and early cancerous clones) is ripe for growth of new primaries. Factors favoring a persistent BCC are a history of multiple recurrences in the same area, histologic subtype similar to the original BCC subtype, evidence of previous inadequate margins, and extensive BCC. Factors favoring a new primary BCC are multiple BCCs, all histologically separate in the same area, with no histologic connection to the previous treatment scar; new histologic subtype in the face of adequate previous treatment; small BCC; and BCC arising in immunocompromised patients or those with BCC-related genodermatosis.[373]

Clearly, tumors in sun-damaged skin are more common and need to be dealt with aggressively. Because of the radiation damage field effect, excessively wide excisions of tumors, irrespective of functional and cosmetic importance, do not necessarily ensure a long-term tumor-free presence in that region and impart no additional cure advantage for that specific tumor. Even less advantage is present in the use of excessively wide margins where recurrence is unlikely or easily treated (see specific information in the next section, "Tumor Margins").

SCCs recur variably, depending on initial presenting size, differentiation, location, and treatment method. The largest review compiled data on local recurrence from 71 prior studies and metastases from 95 prior studies.[88] This landmark study found that a multitude of factors cause recurrence. At less than 5 years of follow-up, there were 15.0% and 17.3% recurrences after micrographic surgery and surgical excision, respectively. At more than 5 years of follow-up, the rates of recurrence widened to 10.0% and 23.3%, respectively.[88] Rates of recurrence at more than 5 years based on treatment modality were 3.1% with micrographic surgery, 3.7% with curettage and electrodesiccation, 8.1% with surgical excision, and 10.0% with radiation therapy.[88] These data may seem to imply that curettage-electrodesiccation is typically used for lesions of smaller diameter and thickness, for which recurrence rates would be expected to be lower anyway. Although some practitioners submit curettage scrapings for histopathologic tumor confirmation, little information is known about the base of the tumor in these cases unless curettage is a prelude to standard or Mohs excision techniques. Thus, study of the recurrence or persistence of tumor in these instances is less reliable. Compared with a thickness of more than 4 mm, the differences were 5.3% versus 17.2%. For well-differentiated versus poorly differentiated tumors, the differences were, respectively, 13.6% and 20.6%. On the basis of tumor site, local recurrence varied as follows: ear, lip, and other sun-exposed areas. Localized recurrence rate was 18.7% in the ear, 10.5% in the lip, and 7.9% on sun-exposed skin. When perineural involvement was noted, the local recurrence was 47.2%. Well-differentiated versus poorly differentiated tumors metastasized 13.6% and 20.6%, respectively. When the lesions were less than 4 mm versus more than 4 mm thick, the metastasis rate was 6.7% versus 45.7%. When the initial presenting diameters were less than 2 cm versus more than 2 cm, the initial report was 9.1% versus 30.3% (Tables 116-10 to 116-12).[88]

TUMOR MARGINS

The techniques for surgical excision are well understood. However, the aspects that deal with removal of

TABLE 116-10 ✦ NCCN RISK FACTORS FOR RECURRENCE OF NONMELANOMA SKIN CANCERS

	Low Risk	High Risk
Clinical Risk Factors		
Location/size	Area L < 20 mm Area M < 10 mm Area H < 6 mm	Area L ≥ 20 mm Area M ≥ 10 mm Area H ≥ 6 mm
Borders	Well defined	Poorly defined
Primary vs. recurrent	Primary	Recurrent
Immunosuppression	Negative	Positive
Tumor at site of prior radiation therapy	Negative	Positive
Tumor at site of chronic inflammatory process (SCC only)	Negative	Positive
Rapidly growing tumor (SCC only)	Negative	Positive
Neurologic symptoms: pain, paresthesia, paralysis (SCC only)	Negative	Positive
Pathologic Risk Factors		
Perineural involvement	Negative	Positive
Subtype (BCC only)	Nodular, superficial	Micronodular, infiltrating, sclerosing
Degree of differentiation (SCC only)	Well differentiated	Moderately or poorly differentiated
Adenoid, adenosquamous, or desmoplastic (SCC only)	Negative	Positive
Depth: Clark level or thickness (SCC only)	I, II, III or <4 mm	IV, V or ≥4 mm

Area L: low risk for recurrence: trunk, extremities.
Area M: middle risk for recurrence: cheeks, forehead, neck, scalp.
Area H: high risk for recurrence: "mask areas" of face (central face, eyelids, eyebrows, periorbita, nose, lips, chin, mandible, preauricular and postauricular skin/sulci, ear, temple), genitalia, hands, and feet.
BCC, basal cell carcinoma; SCC, squamous cell carcinoma.
Note: All recommendations are category 2A unless otherwise indicated.
Clinical trials: NCCN believes that the best management of any cancer patient is in a clinical trial. Participation in clinical trials is especially encouraged.
Version 1.2004, 01-05-04. © 2004 National Comprehensive Cancer Network, Inc. All rights reserved. These guidelines and this illustration may not be reproduced in any form without the express written permission of NCCN. See disclaimer at end of chapter.

TABLE 116-11 ◆ RECURRENCE AND INFLUENCE OF CLINICAL FACTORS

Influence	Basal Cell Carcinoma	Reference	Squamous Cell Carcinoma	Reference
Location	Increased on scalp, ear, eye, nose, mouth, nasal vestibule, auditory meatus, rectum	373, 375, 387, 733	Increased on ear, auditory meatus, lip, eyelid, columella	41, 88, 734-736
Age < 35 years	Increased	373		
Size (irrespective of treatment method of excision, curettage and electrodesiccation, micrographic excision, radiation therapy)	Increased	328, 366, 367, 370, 373, 430, 447, 470, 737-746	<2 cm: recurrence 7.4% >2 cm: recurrence 15.2%	88
Repair method	Full-thickness skin graft: most recurrences within first year Split-thickness skin graft: most within second year Skin flap: most within fourth year	361		
Borders	Increased inversely proportional to clear definition	379	Increased inversely proportional to clear definition	74, 701, 708
Primary	Most within 3 yr	359, 442, 747	Most (75%) within 2 yr	484
	18% of recurrences in 6-10 yr	359	3.1%-8.1% over the long term (meta-analysis)	88
	Longest interval after treatment known: 20 yr	359		
Recurrent lesions (singly or multiply recurrent)	Increased	358, 359, 361, 363, 365, 367, 411, 737, 739, 746, 748, 749	Increased (composite rate of 23%)	88
Immunosuppression	Increased	704, 705, 750, 751	Increased	509, 752, 753
Site of chronic inflammation, trauma	Not increased	681, 752	Increased	41, 88, 163, 509, 752-755
Neurologic symptoms (pain, paresthesia, paralysis)	Not applicable	379	Increased	379
Rapid growth	Not applicable	379	Increased	379

margins of tumor are not so clear. To perform a surgical extirpation, one must identify the borders. When a lesion has clearly identifiable borders by virtue of visibility with color change, topographic variability, or palpability, border recognition is reliable. However, when the border is less well defined or nonuniform, this task is more challenging. Before beginning the operation and injecting local anesthetic, one must identify the border by one or more of a variety of methods. One method involves use of a laterally angulated light to see a semblance of shadow where the topographic elevation of the tumor edges ends. In conjunction with light use, a marker then demarcates where shadow is

noted. Solutions of trichloroacetic acid of 5% to 10% may also be applied to alcohol-prepared skin. Frequently, the trichloroacetic acid will demonstrate differential staining quality by virtue of lightening the subtle hyperkeratosis that may be present within the tumor. A marker is then employed to delineate the borders.

Palpability of the tumor may be helpful in determination of its edges. Palpation is carried out subsequent to visual inspection to prevent the development of hyperemia, which could confuse the native anatomic micro-landmarks helpful in identification of borders and subtleties of infiltration. Wetting the fingers first

TABLE 116-12 ✦ RECURRENCE AND INFLUENCE OF HISTOPATHOLOGIC FACTORS

Influence	Basal Cell Carcinoma	Reference	Squamous Cell Carcinoma	Reference
Depth	Increased (when microstage is measured in Mohs excision)	352, 353, 356, 361, 382, 737, 756-759	Increased (although microstage is rarely measured)	41, 88, 380, 592, 707, 708, 718, 720
Perineural involvement	Increased within fats, muscle, or bone	373, 756, 760, 761	Increased (average incidence of perineural invasion: 4%)	41, 74, 88, 455, 456, 592, 708, 720, 756, 762-765
Differentiation degree	Not applicable	379	Increased inversely proportional to differentiation	88, 380, 707, 718, 720, 766, 767
Subtype: Micronodular, infiltrative, morpheaform	Increased (up to 95% if positive margin on initial treatment)	383, 405, 440, 739, 768, 769	Not applicable	379
Adenoid, adenosquamous, desmoplastic	Not applicable	379	Increased	379

with water may allow the examiner to palpate the edges more readily. Some examiners use a Wood's (ultraviolet) light to see subtle changes in color. Application of ultraviolet light is performed before injection of a vasoconstricting substance such as epinephrine, which may affect the Wood's light absorption. Only after examination with a sidelight, palpation, perhaps use of dilute trichloroacetic acid solution, and marking of the clinical lesion borders is the local anesthetic with epinephrine injected into and around the lesion. After an appropriate wait—12 minutes or more for epinephrine vasoconstriction to take place—the prepared and draped site is readied for operative intervention. As part of a further attempt to delineate tumor margins before formal extirpation, one may also use a 2- to 4-mm curet after the skin is prepared and injected. Scraping with the curet will elicit a particularly mushy or firm sensation. Friable tumor can then be débrided to the limits of curet-detected tumor palpability. With obvious gross clinical tumor removed, the surgical margin is marked peripheral to the resultant defect edges to ensure that areas of tumor growth are removed by a scalpel in the performance of permanent, frozen, or Mohs sections.

BCCs less than 2 cm in diameter are excised with a 4-mm margin of normal-appearing skin peripheral to the clinical edge of the tumor.[374] Other authors have recommended 2 to 10 mm.[369,374-378] BCCs greater than 2 cm in diameter are excised with 10-mm margins or with micrographic technique (Fig. 116-10 and Tables 116-13 to 116-15). This recommendation is taken from the National Comprehensive Cancer Network's Guidelines for Care of Nonmelanoma Skins Cancers.[379] The National Comprehensive Cancer

Network is a 17-institution consortium; clinical experts make recommendations from the literature and update treatment algorithms annually. For very small BCC less than 6 mm in diameter with clear borders, 3-mm margins may be taken. Recommended margins for SCC depend on the tumor diameter. If diameter is less than 2 cm, a 4-mm border will generally be adequate. With respect to SCCs, a 4- to 6-mm border of nontumorous tissue should be excised around low-risk SCCs, defined as being in a low-risk location, well differentiated, and less than 2 cm in diameter. For high-risk SCCs, recommendations for margins of 6 mm[357] to 10 mm exist (Fig. 116-11 and Tables 116-16 to 116-19). The high-risk SCCs are those greater than 2 cm, located in the scalp, ears, nose, and lips, and with poor differentiation.[380] One helpful technique in making a decision about the extent of tumor presence is not widely practiced because it adds another step to the process. It is the same step initially used in many Mohs cases and involves 30 seconds of effort. Curettage of the SCC may assist in initial delineation of the tumor margins. One may note that the curet may suddenly fall into deeper levels as a nest of tumor is encountered and débrided. It is useful to monitor the texture as crunchy or softer than surrounding normal or inflamed edematous skin. The main specimen of the tumor is débrided in this fashion, with or without submission of the débrided material for confirmation of tumor identity by frozen or permanent section. If the curet reaches subcutaneous fat at any time, the curettage is discontinued because the textural difference between fat and tumor is so minimal. Thus, the diagnostic advantage of the curet is lost. Armed with this

Text continued on p. 425

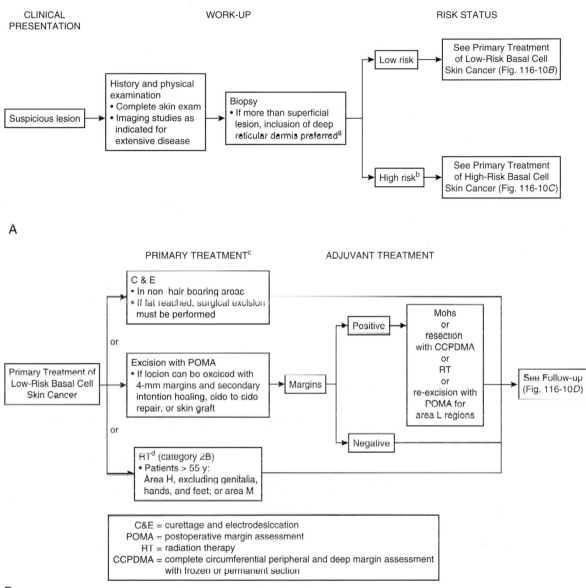

CLINICAL
PRESENTATION

WORK-UP

RISK STATUS

Suspicious lesion

History and physical
examination
• Complete skin exam
• Imaging studies as
  indicated for
  extensive disease

Biopsy
• If more than superficial
  lesion, inclusion of deep
  reticular dermis preferred[a]

Low risk → See Primary Treatment
of Low-Risk Basal Cell
Skin Cancer (Fig. 116-10*B*)

High risk[b] → See Primary Treatment
of High-Risk Basal Cell
Skin Cancer (Fig. 116-10*C*)

A

PRIMARY TREATMENT[c]

ADJUVANT TREATMENT

C & E
• In non hair bearing area
• If fat reached, surgical excision
  must be performed

or

Primary Treatment of
Low-Risk Basal Cell
Skin Cancer

Excision with POMA
• If lesion can be excised with
  4-mm margins and secondary
  intention healing, side to side
  repair, or skin graft

or

RT[d] (category 2B)
• Patients > 55 y:
  Area H, excluding genitalia,
  hands, and feet; or area M

Margins

Positive → Mohs
or
resection
with CCPDMA
or
RT
or
re-excision with
POMA for
area L regions

Negative

See Follow-up
(Fig. 116-10*D*)

C&E = curettage and electrodesiccation
POMA = postoperative margin assessment
RT = radiation therapy
CCPDMA = complete circumferential peripheral and deep margin assessment
with frozen or permanent section

B

FIGURE 116-10. *A to D,* Basal cell skin cancer management algorithm. National Comprehensive Cancer Network (NCCN) Practice Guidelines in Oncology v.1.2004. [a]See Table 116-13. [b]Any high-risk factor places the patient in the high-risk category. [c]See Table 116-14. [d]See Table 116-15. Note: All recommendations are category 2A unless otherwise indicated. Clinical trials: NCCN believes that the best management of any cancer patient is in a clinical trial. Participation in clinical trials is especially encouraged. (© 2004 National Comprehensive Cancer Network, Inc. All rights reserved. See disclaimer at end of chapter.)   *Continued*

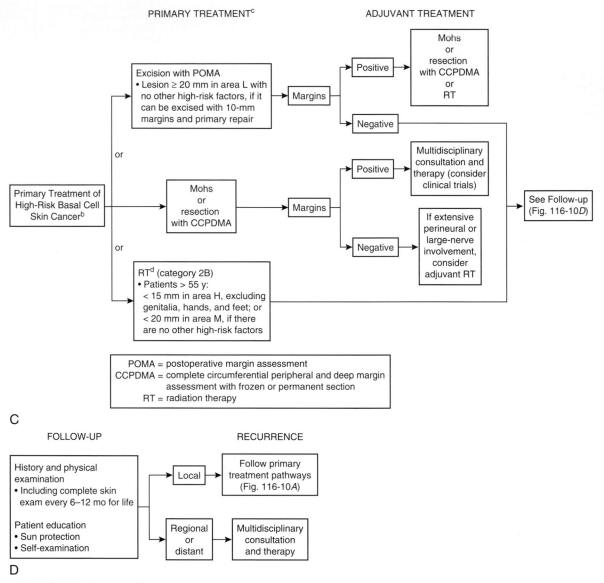

PRIMARY TREATMENT^c

ADJUVANT TREATMENT

Primary Treatment of High-Risk Basal Cell Skin Cancer^b

or

Excision with POMA
• Lesion ≥ 20 mm in area L with no other high-risk factors, if it can be excised with 10-mm margins and primary repair

Margins

Positive → Mohs or resection with CCPDMA or RT

Negative

Mohs or resection with CCPDMA

Margins

Positive → Multidisciplinary consultation and therapy (consider clinical trials)

Negative → If extensive perineural or large-nerve involvement, consider adjuvant RT

or

RT^d (category 2B)
• Patients > 55 y: < 15 mm in area H, excluding genitalia, hands, and feet; or < 20 mm in area M, if there are no other high-risk factors

See Follow-up (Fig. 116-10D)

POMA = postoperative margin assessment
CCPDMA = complete circumferential peripheral and deep margin assessment with frozen or permanent section
RT = radiation therapy

C

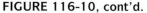

FOLLOW-UP

RECURRENCE

History and physical examination
• Including complete skin exam every 6–12 mo for life

Patient education
• Sun protection
• Self-examination

Local → Follow primary treatment pathways (Fig. 116-10A)

Regional or distant → Multidisciplinary consultation and therapy

D

FIGURE 116-10, cont'd.

TABLE 116-13 ♦ NCCN RISK FACTORS FOR RECURRENCE OF BASAL CELL SKIN CANCER

	Low Risk	High Risk
History and Physical Examination		
Location/size	Area L < 20 mm Area M < 10 mm Area H < 6 mm[a]	Area L ≥ 20 mm Area M ≥ 10 mm Area H ≥ 6 mm[a]
Borders	Well defined	Poorly defined
Primary vs. recurrent	Primary	Recurrent
Immunosuppression	(−)	(+)
Site of prior radiation therapy	(−)	(+)
Pathology		
Subtype	Nodular, superficial	Aggressive growth pattern[b]
Perineural involvement	(−)	(+)

[a] Location independent of size may constitute high risk in certain clinical settings.

[b] Having morpheaform, sclerosing, mixed infiltrative, or micronodular features in any portion of the tumor.

Area H: "mask areas" of face (central face, eyelids, eyebrows, periorbita, nose, lips [cutaneous and vermilion], chin, mandible, preauricular and postauricular skin/sulci, temple, ear), genitalia, hands, and feet.

Area M: cheeks, forehead, scalp, and neck.

Area L: trunk and extremities.

Note: All recommendations are category 2A unless otherwise indicated.

Clinical trials: NCCN believes that the best management of any cancer patient is in a clinical trial. Participation in clinical trials is especially encouraged. Version 1. 2004, 01-05-04. © 2004 National Comprehensive Cancer Network, Inc. All rights reserved. These guidelines and this illustration may not be reproduced in any form without the express written permission of NCCN. See disclaimer at end of chapter.

TABLE 116-14 ♦ NCCN PRINCIPLES OF TREATMENT FOR BASAL CELL SKIN CANCER

The goal of primary treatment of basal cell skin cancer is the cure of the tumor and the maximal preservation of function and cosmesis. All treatment decisions should be customized to account for the particular factors present in the individual case and for patient's preference. Customary age and size parameters may have to be modified.

Surgical approaches often offer the most effective and efficient means for accomplishing cure, but considerations of function, cosmesis, and patient preference may lead to choosing radiation therapy as primary treatment in order to achieve optimal overall results.

In certain patients at high risk for multiple primary tumors, increased surveillance and consideration of prophylactic measures may be indicated.

Note: All recommendations are category 2A unless otherwise indicated.

Clinical trials: NCCN believes that the best management of any cancer patient is in a clinical trial. Participation in clinical trials is especially encouraged. Version 1. 2004, 01-05-04. © 2004 National Comprehensive Cancer Network, Inc. All rights reserved. These guidelines and this illustration may not be reproduced in any form without the express written permission of NCCN. See disclaimer at end of chapter.

TABLE 116-15 ♦ RADIOTHERAPY FOR BASAL CELL SKIN CANCER (NCCN GUIDELINES)

	Dose and Field Size	
Tumor Size	*Margins*	*Orthovoltage Dose and Fractions*
<20 mm	5-10 mm	Total of 4500-5000 cGy in 250-300 cGy fractions
≥20 mm	15-20 mm	Total of 6000-6600 cGy in 200 cGy fractions or Total of 5000-6000 cGy in 250 cGy fractions

Varying energies of orthovoltage or electron-beam equipment should be available.

Add 10% to 15% to total and daily doses if using electron beam and add bolus for low-energy electrons.

Maximize fractions to maximize cosmesis.

Radiation therapy is contraindicated in genetic conditions predisposing to skin cancer (e.g., nevoid basal cell carcinoma, xeroderma pigmentosum) and connective tissue diseases (e.g., lupus, scleroderma).

Note: All recommendations are category 2A unless otherwise indicated.

Clinical trials: NCCN believes that the best management of any cancer patient is in a clinical trial. Participation in clinical trials is especially encouraged. Version 1. 2004, 01-05-04. © 2004 National Comprehensive Cancer Network, Inc. All rights reserved. These guidelines and this illustration may not be reproduced in any form without the express written permission of NCCN. See disclaimer at end of chapter.

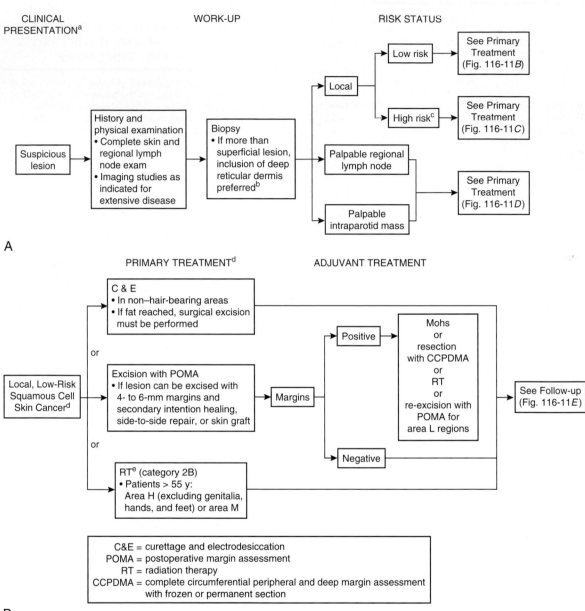

FIGURE 116-11. *A* to *E,* Squamous cell skin cancer management algorithm. National Comprehensive Cancer Network (NCCN) Practice Guidelines in Oncology v.1.2004. [a]Including basosquamous carcinoma and squamous cell skin cancer in situ (showing full-thickness epidermal atypia, excluding actinic keratoses). [b]See Table 116-16. [c]Any high-risk factor places the patient in the high-risk category. [d]See Table 116-17. [e]See Table 116-18. [f]In certain high-risk lesions, consider sentinel lymph node mapping, although the benefit of this technique has yet to be proved. [g]If invasion to parotid fascia, superficial parotidectomy. [h]Including complete skin and regional lymph node examination. [i]Consider clinical trials. Note: All recommendations are category 2A unless otherwise indicated. Clinical trials: NCCN believes that the best management of any cancer patient is in a clinical trial. Participation in clinical trials is especially encouraged. (© 2004 National Comprehensive Cancer Network, Inc. All rights reserved. See disclaimer at end of chapter.)

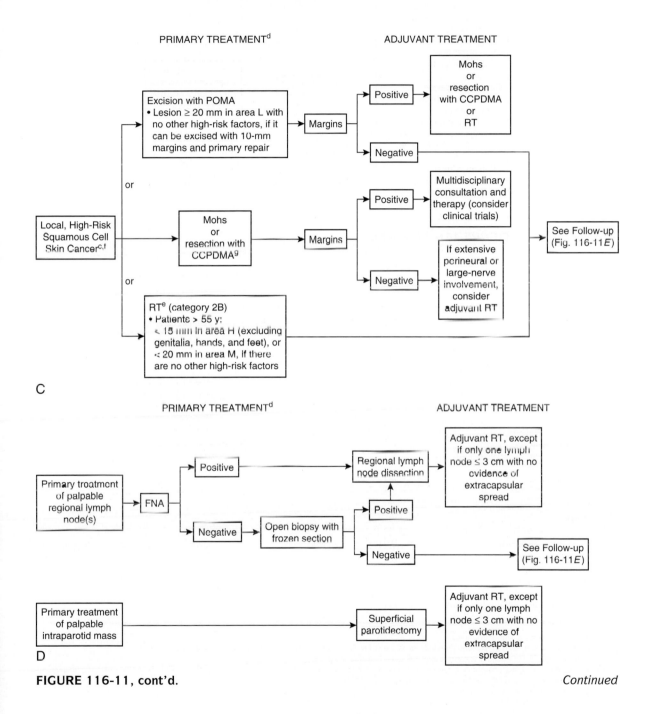

FIGURE 116-11, cont'd.   *Continued*

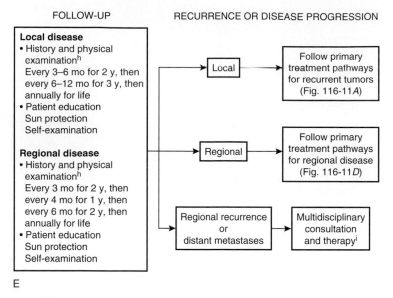

FIGURE 116-11, cont'd.

TABLE 116-16 ✦ NCCN RISK FACTORS FOR RECURRENCE OF SQUAMOUS CELL SKIN CANCER

	Low Risk	High Risk
History and Physical Examination		
Location/size[a]	Area L < 20 mm	Area L ≥ 20 mm
	Area M < 10 mm	Area M ≥ 10 mm
	Area H < 6 mm[c]	Area H ≥ 6 mm[c]
Borders	Well defined	Poorly defined
Primary vs. recurrent	Primary	Recurrent
Immunosuppression	(−)	(+)
Site of prior radiation therapy or chronic inflammatory process	(−)	(+)
Rapidly growing tumor	(−)	(+)
Neurologic symptoms	(−)	(+)
Pathology		
Degree of differentiation	Well differentiated	Moderately or poorly differentiated
Adenoid (acantholytic), adenosquamous (showing mucin production), or desmoplastic subtypes	(−)	(+)
Depth: Clark level or thickness[b]	I, II, III, or <4 mm	IV, V, or ≥4 mm
Perineural or vascular involvement	(−)	(+)

[a] Must include peripheral rim of erythema.

[b] A modified Breslow measurement should exclude parakeratosis or scale/crust and should be made from base of ulcer if present.

[c] Location independent of size may constitute high risk in certain clinical settings.

Area H: "mask areas" of face (central face, eyelids, eyebrows, periorbita, nose, lips [cutaneous and vermilion], chin, mandible, preauricular and postauricular skin/sulci, temple, ear), genitalia, hands, and feet.

Area M: cheeks, forehead, scalp, and neck.

Area L: trunk and extremities.

Note: All recommendations are category 2A unless otherwise indicated.

Clinical trials: NCCN believes that the best management of any cancer patient is in a clinical trial. Participation in clinical trials is especially encouraged.

TABLE 116-17 ✦ NCCN PRINCIPLES OF TREATMENT FOR SQUAMOUS CELL SKIN CANCER

The goal of primary treatment of squamous cell skin cancer is the cure of the tumor and the maximal preservation of function and cosmesis. All treatment decisions should be customized to account for the particular factors present in the individual case and for patient's preference. Customary age and size parameters may have to be modified.

Surgical approaches often offer the most effective and efficient means for accomplishing cure, but considerations of function, cosmesis, and patient preference may lead to choosing radiation therapy as primary treatment in order to achieve optimal overall results.

In certain patients at high risk for multiple primary tumors, increased surveillance and consideration of prophylactic measures may be indicated. (See Identification and Management of High-Risk Patients, Table 116-19.)

Note: All recommendations are category 2A unless otherwise indicated.
  Clinical trials: NCCN believes that the best management of any cancer patient is in a clinical trial. Participation in clinical trials is especially encouraged. Version 1. 2004, 01-05-04. © 2004 National Comprehensive Cancer Network, Inc. All rights reserved. These guidelines and this illustration may not be reproduced in any form without the express written permission of NCCN. See disclaimer at end of chapter.

TABLE 116-18 ✦ RADIOTHERAPY FOR SQUAMOUS CELL SKIN CANCER (NCCN GUIDELINES)

Dose and Field Size		
Tumor Size	*Margins*	*Orthovoltage Dose and Fractions*
<20 mm	5-10 mm	Total of 4500-5000 cGy in 250-300 cGy fraction
≥20 mm	15-20 mm	Total of 6000-6600 cGy in 200 cGy fractions or Total of 5000-6000 cGy in 250 cGy fractions

Varying energies of orthovoltage or electron-beam equipment should be available.
Add 10% to 15% to total and daily doses if using electron beam and add bolus for low-energy electrons.
Maximize fractions to maximize cosmesis.
Radiation therapy is contraindicated in genetic conditions predisposing to skin cancer (e.g., xeroderma pigmentosum), connective tissue diseases (e.g., lupus, scleroderma), and verrucous carcinomas.

Note: All recommendations are category 2A unless otherwise indicated.
  Clinical trials: NCCN believes that the best management of any cancer patient is in a clinical trial. Participation in clinical trials is especially encouraged. Version 1. 2004, 01-05-04. © 2004 National Comprehensive Cancer Network, Inc. All rights reserved. These guidelines and this illustration may not be reproduced in any form without the express written permission of NCCN. See disclaimer at end of chapter.

TABLE 116-19 ✦ NCCN IDENTIFICATION AND MANAGEMENT OF HIGH-RISK PATIENTS

Definition

Certain patient groups are at high risk for developing multiple squamous cell skin cancers and tumors that can behave aggressively. These include:
- Organ transplant recipients
- Other settings of immunosuppression (lymphoma, drug-induced, HIV, etc.)
- Xeroderma pigmentosum

Within these high-risk groups, individual high-risk patients should be identified for closer follow-up.

Important individual risk factors include:
- Total number of tumors
- Frequency of development
- Occurrence of aggressive tumors (e.g., extension beyond cutaneous structures, perineural involvement, large and poorly differentiated, having ≥3 risk factors for recurrence [see Table 116-16])

In these patients, urgent diagnosis and treatment of lesions is important.

Diagnosis

Skin lesions in these high-risk populations may be difficult to assess clinically. Therefore, a low threshold for performing skin biopsies of suspect lesions is necessary.

Treatment of Pre-Cancers

Actinic keratoses should be treated aggressively at first development.
- Accepted treatment modalities include cryosurgery, topical 5-fluorouracil, and curettage and electrodesiccation.
- Favorable but still experimental modalities include topical imiquimod, photodynamic therapy, chemical peel (trichloroacetic acid), and ablative skin resurfacing (laser, dermabrasion).

Actinic keratoses which have an atypical clinical appearance or do not respond to appropriate therapy should be biopsied for histologic evaluation.

CO_2 laser vermilionectomy may be of value in the treatment of extensive actinic cheilitis.

Treatment of Skin Cancers

Because patients in high-risk groups may develop multiple lesions in short periods of time, destructive therapies (curettage and electrodesiccation, cryosurgery) may be a preferred treatment for clinically low-risk tumors, because of the ability to treat multiple lesions at a single patient visit.

In patients who develop multiple adjacent tumors in close proximity, surgical excision of invasive disease sometimes does not include surrounding in situ disease, and tissue rearrangement is minimized. In situ disease may then be treated with secondary approaches.

In patients with multiple adjacent tumors of the dorsal hands and forearms, en bloc excision and split-thickness skin grafting has been used with efficacy. However, healing is prolonged and morbidity is significant.

Compared to the normal population, radiation therapy is often used more frequently as an adjuvant therapy and for perineural disease, and less frequently for the treatment of primary tumors.

Satellite lesions (in-transit cutaneous metastases) may occur more frequently in this population. They must be treated aggressively with strong consideration of radiation therapy as the primary therapy.

In organ transplant recipients, decreasing the level of immunosuppressive therapy may be considered in cases of life-threatening skin cancer or the rapid development of multiple tumors.

Follow-up

Follow-up schedules should be titrated to the frequency of tumor development, and in rare cases may be as frequently as weekly.

Patient Education

Individual risk assessment is necessary and should be discussed.

Both extensive and repetitive patient education regarding sun avoidance and protection is required.

Sun avoidance and protection methods must be stringent.

Monthly self-examination of all skin surfaces is recommended. With a history of invasive skin cancer, self-examination of the lymph nodes should be taught and performed.

Rapid entrance into the health delivery system at the onset of tumor development is critical.

Patient education should begin, in the case of organ transplant recipients, at transplantation, and in the case of xeroderma pigmentosum, at birth or diagnosis.

Prevention

Use of oral retinoids (acitretin, etretinate, isotretinoin) has been effective in reducing the development of pre-cancers and skin cancers in some high-risk patients. Side effects may be significant. Therapeutic effects disappear shortly after cessation of the drug. Oral retinoids are teratogenic and must be used with extreme caution in women of childbearing potential.

Aggressive treatment of pre-cancers can prevent the development of subsequent invasive tumors.

additional visual and palpable confirmation of tumor extent, the extirpating surgeon then proceeds with full-thickness vertical or Mohs resection technique, using tumor size and type and the edge of the curetted defect to dictate margin clearance.[329,381]

With primary excision, one must decide as to its depth. On the basis of histologic features and with three-dimensional visualization, armed with the knowledge that tumors extend periarterially and perineurally and can extend into cartilage, bone, nerve, sinuses, and cranial and oral cavities, the extirpating surgeon must balance clinical aggressiveness and biologic prudence. Although there is a frequently quoted necessity for excision of fascia along with the cutaneous tumor, studies documenting such necessity do not exist. Authors who support this state that since there are no defined depths of predictable tumor extension, there are no existing uniform standards to validate the depth of excision.[233,250,382-384] Depth of tumor growth and therefore implied requirement for resection to or beyond that depth are determined by tumor size, histologic subtype, location, previous treatment, and growth behavior. Tumors classified as high risk, as described elsewhere in this chapter, require deeper and wider resection. Such decisions are made preoperatively, with allowance for potential of more aggressive resection if intraoperative findings of tumor extension so dictate. Preoperative informed consent by the patient requires inclusion of such a possibility. With traditional or micrographic surgery approaches, it may be necessary to include in the frozen section a sample of an adjacent structure that grossly appears normal. This is particularly true in infiltrative or morpheaform BCCs, less well differentiated SCCs, recurrent or persistent tumors mixed with scar, tumors more than 2 cm in diameter, rapidly growing tumors, and those extending into subcutaneous fat, bone, cartilage,

epimysium, or embryonic fusion planes. In tumors of these types, the potential for recurrence is higher and explains in part the recurrence seen with micrographic technique.[34,379,385-387]

Frozen Versus Permanent Sections

When excision is chosen as the treatment method, choice of margins to be submitted will depend on recurrence risk. Low-risk lesions and locations (as discussed elsewhere in this chapter) do well with permanent section margins and immediate repair. High-risk lesions require frozen section control (traditional or micrographic) and either immediate or delayed repair. Delayed repair is indicated either when traditional negative frozen section margins may be expected to have positive permanent ones (in as many as 4%) or when the micrographic approach will require additional stages. The patient's status—from infirmity, immunocompromise, minimal compliance, or origin in a distant setting for which reconstruction is unavailable—will in part determine timing of repair. However, it should not determine the choice of method of assurance of tumor control. Only risk of recurrence determines that choice.

Pathology Techniques

Pathologists employ different techniques for processing specimens. One is a simple cross section technique; another is the breadloaf sectioning technique (Fig. 116-12). Another combines both by cross sectioning in an *xy* axis and taking slices in a breadloaf orientation (Fig. 116-13).[388] These techniques do not evaluate 100% of the margins for tumor!

Involvement of the margins has been correlated with incidence of recurrence of tumor. Risk of recurrence has been investigated with the following data: recurrence rate for primary BCC was 30% to 41%[361,384,389]

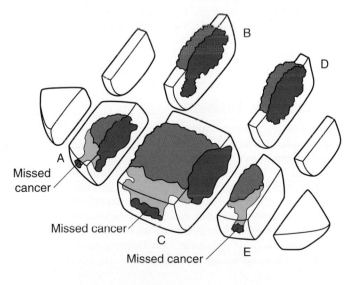

FIGURE 116-12. Breadloaf tissue section. The standard "breadloafing" technique of checking surgical margins can lead to a false sense of security and a high incidence of false-negative margins. For example, the surgical sections B and D would be interpreted as negative or clear margins, but in fact there may actually be positive margins (see sections A, C, and E). (From Nelson BR, Railan D, Cohen S: Mohs' micrographic surgery for nonmelanoma skin cancers. Clin Plast Surg 1997;24:705-718.)

Missed cancer

Missed cancer

Missed cancer

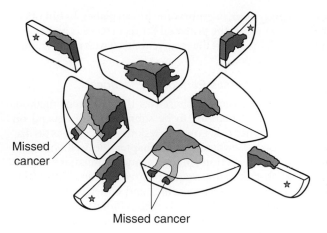

Missed
cancer

Missed cancer

FIGURE 116-13. Four-quadrant tissue section. Some of the sections will have clear margins *(stars)*, but it is clear that this method of processing excised surgical specimens can easily miss tumor at the margins of the specimen (missed cancer). (From Nelson BR, Railan D, Cohen S: Mohs' micrographic surgery for nonmelanoma skin cancers. Clin Plast Surg 1997;24:705-718.)

if margins were involved and 12% if tumor was within 1/400× field of the margin.[390] A pathology report noting a "close margin" is difficult to interpret, however; a study determined eight separate definitions from 11 pathologists.[378] One excellent recommendation is for the pathologist to note whether tumor is within 1 mm of the margins.[391] The site where the incomplete excision rate tends to be the highest is the scalp, followed by the ear, canthi, eyebrows, and nose.[392] The periorbital area, including the canthi, and recurrent tumors also have a high incidence of pathology specimens with involved margins.[393] Nodular and superficial BCCs have a low incidence of involved margins compared with infiltrative or morpheic BCCs.[394] Recurrent tumor excisions that have involved margins are more likely to recur.[361] Visual marking is 91% accurate in excision of tumors without involvement of margins.[393] Tumors excised with inadequate deep margins are more worrisome than tumors excised with a positive lateral margin.[395] A decision for early re-excision versus watchful waiting depends on the nearness to important anatomic structures and the temperament of the patient and the surgeon.[389] A precise knowledge of the pathologist's specimen evaluation will allow the surgeon to make appropriate decisions in regard to requirements for re-excision if margins are involved.

Micrographic Excision

Frederic Mohs, a general surgeon, originally described a technique in which the skin tumor is sequentially excised from superficial to deep with each section examined for tumor margins.[396] Initially, Mohs was experimenting with mouse tumors. After determining that zinc chloride solution could simultaneously necrose and fixate tissue while retaining its microscopic structure, he began to experiment with excision of tumors as a way to delineate their borders microscopically. He sectioned layers horizontally so the entire

undersurface of the tumor could be examined and traced more deeply and laterally until the tumor was extirpated. Subsequently, this technique was applied to tumor management in humans with successful extirpation of both recurrent and primary skin cancers. Eventually, Dr. Mohs established a Division of Chemosurgery at the University of Wisconsin.

The technique had a major drawback in that the application of zinc chloride, having evolved from an injectable solution to a topically applied paste, resulted in tissue necrosis of an almost intolerably painful level for approximately 48 hours. During that time, many patients required hospitalization and morphine maintenance. Periorbital lesions were treated with resultant severe keratitis or conjunctivitis. Because of these complications, Mohs used frozen section technique along with analysis of the tumors in horizontally oriented fashion. This fresh tissue technique was used infrequently.

In the early 1970s, dermatologists Tromovitch and Stegman recognized that the cure rates with fresh tissue technique were equal to those with fixation with the zinc paste. In addition, the pain was no more than would be expected with any standard excision under local anesthesia. At the same time, improved techniques for staining, sectioning, and examining the slides eventuated in the technique that evolved from chemosurgery to micrographic excision. During his career, which spanned from 1930 to 1990, Dr. Mohs applied his technique to more than 100,000 patients. Until his retirement, it was not unusual for his chemosurgery unit to treat 70 or more patients per day with as many as four histology technicians working alongside and several associate physicians moving from room to room to map and extirpate the tumors.[396] Presently, micrographic excision offers advantages over direct excision when tumor margins are indistinct, for recurrent tumors, and in areas where tissue preservation is required to preserve function (medial eye, nose).

However, it is not effective in tracking tumors that spread through lymphatics and offers no advantage over direct excision with appropriate margins for melanoma, sarcoma, and other similar cutaneous tumors.

Micrographic excision also may not obtain clear margins. One must qualify the accuracy of the term *margins*. In a study examining pathology reports with respect to margins, it was estimated, assuming 7-μm-thick sections, that true serial sectioning of a surgical specimen in an unbroken sequence would require as many as 1500 sections per centimeter of tissue; anything resembling this is rarely seen.[397,398] Thus, margins must be correlated with physical findings and the surgeon's understanding of tumor pathophysiology.

Plastic surgeons, with some training directed particularly at BCC and SCC pathology, can perform Mohs technique on their patients. More commonly, plastic surgeons perform repairs on skin defects or where extensive disease involves extirpation of tumor in or repair of deeper underlying structures, such as bone or parotid gland. The micrographic surgeon (usually a dermatologist) frequently requests care coordination with a plastic surgeon based on the limits of the extirpating surgeon's expertise and comfort level. Also, elderly, ill patients requiring hospital-level monitoring will be cared for by plastic surgeons with privileges to do so.

TECHNIQUE

Micrographic excision technique is relatively straightforward. The traditional micrographic technique was first described by Mohs (Fig. 116-14).[399] The frozen section micrographic technique can be performed on the same day with use of frozen sections to evaluate excised tumor and the margins of the tumor (Fig. 116-15).[400] Two fundamental principles represent the basis for use of this technique for tumor removal: NMSCs (unlike melanomas with skip areas of lymphangitic extension) spread mostly by contiguous growth, and all tumor cells must be removed to produce a cure. The technique begins with the clinically apparent edges of the tumor being lightly marked with gentian violet or other color (Davidson reagents). Initially, the tumor is debulked with a curet. The curet thus debulks the tumor and delineates roughly the inner edge of the margins.[329] The curet assists in clearly defining the true margins because with the curet, the tumor has a different palpable texture compared with the surrounding tissue. Once the tumor is grossly removed, the harvested tissue is not routinely examined unless there is a question about the initial diagnosis. With the blade placed approximately 1 mm from the clinical margin at a 45-degree angle to the skin, a 1- to 3-mm-thick layer of epidermis and its contiguous dermis is excised. The nondominant hand stretch stabilizes the surrounding tissue or tethers the specimen with a forceps or hook to allow the dominant hand to maneuver the blade for excision of the surrounding tumor site. The peripheral tissue is then marked with tiny epidermal nicks for orientation should another stage of resection be necessary.

After color marking of the borders and orientation on the carrier paper bearing a sketched orientation map of that tumor stage, the excised tissue is flipped over to expose the undersurface of the layer, which represents the deep margin of the current layer of tumor excision. The specimen is frozen and sliced thinly with the cryostat, and the slices are placed on a glass slide and stained. The map of the surgical site accompanies the slides to the microscope. Microscopic examination of these slides for tumor presence within 15 minutes after extirpation is routine. The slide examination initially involves viewing at lower power for potentially positive areas. Sites of significant basophilic inflammatory change frequently point to tumor presence. Where appropriate (i.e., in earlier, more superficial stages), the epidermis is used for orientation. Any positive or negative tumor areas are noted on the map sketch, and where they occur in relation to the color markings on the specimen is noted. These positive areas direct the extirpator to take further tissue stages from those areas bearing tumor. When all margins are histologically free of tumor cells, tumor excision is complete and defect management is now appropriate.

The BCCs stain more hypochromatically and thus are easier to examine than are SCC specimens. SCCs are more difficult to examine by the micrographic technique when certain histologic findings are observed, such as predominance of spindle cells, poor differentiation, and lymphohistiocytic infiltration. In these cases, the original tissue biopsy diagnosis is first established, and the specimen is best examined immediately before the slides from the micrographic excision are examined. If the original biopsy specimen is not available or if the diagnosis is still questionable, the surgeon can first obtain a specimen for establishment of a diagnosis or histologic subtype before doing the curettage and beginning the first stage. A curetted fragment specimen, if it is uninterpretable as to diagnosis, can be followed by a narrow full-thickness excision subjected to standard frozen staining to make a diagnosis before proceeding. Some surgeons insist on beginning with a 2- to 3-mm margin of normal skin, especially in dealing with SCCs, because individual SCC cells, perhaps unrecognizable under the microscope, may be left behind. Other surgeons prefer to remove an extra section of tissue wherever significant lymphohistiocytic infiltrate is obscuring the field in both BCCs and SCCs because tumor may be more likely to occur in these areas and cellular morphologic features may be obscured by the infiltrate. Some

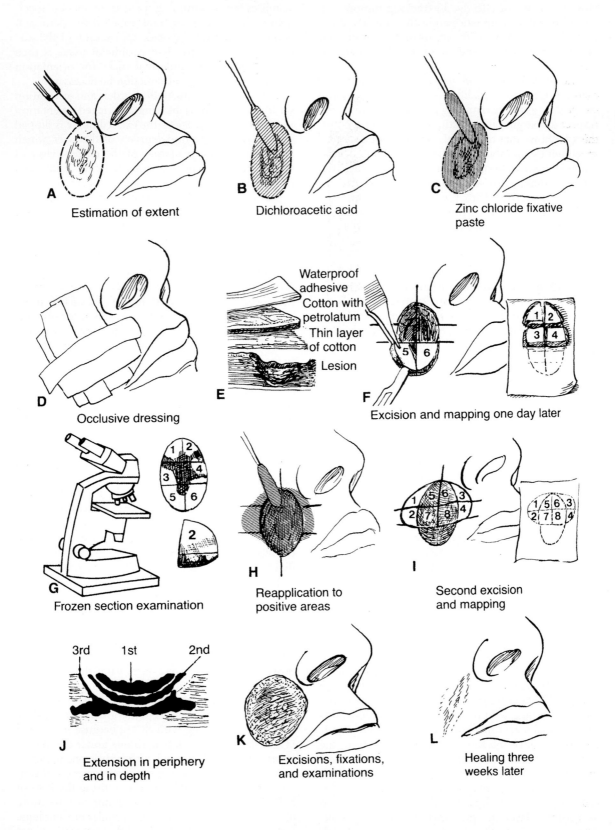

A Estimation of extent

B Dichloroacetic acid

C Zinc chloride fixative paste

D Occlusive dressing

E Waterproof adhesive
Cotton with petrolatum
Thin layer of cotton
Lesion

F Excision and mapping one day later

G Frozen section examination

H Reapplication to positive areas

I Second excision and mapping

J 3rd 1st 2nd
Extension in periphery and in depth

K Excisions, fixations, and examinations

L Healing three weeks later

FIGURE 116-14. Mohs micrographic surgery. *A,* The clinical extent of the tumor is first measured and evaluated by gross examination. *B,* Dichloroacetic acid is applied to the surface of the entire area. *C,* Zinc chloride paste fixes tissue to a depth that depends on the thickness of the layer of paste applied and the length of time it is permitted to act. *D* and *E,* The treated area is covered with an occlusive dressing in an effort to decrease absorption of water by the hydroscopic paste. *F,* After an interval of several hours to 1 day, sections of tissue approximately 1 cm^2 in area and 2 mm in thickness are surgically excised in a saucer-like shape. A map of the lesion site with a number assigned to each section is drawn at the time of excision. *G,* Each section, as it is removed, is identified by its corresponding number. Two intersecting edges are colored with red and blue dyes. These indelible marks are preserved during the histochemical staining process and allow the chemosurgeon to locate the exact position of any remaining malignant change visualized microscopically. The microscopic survey is done on frozen sections that have been cut horizontally from the undersurface of each excised tissue section and stained by hematoxylin and eosin. The location of the malignant change is marked on the original map of numbered sections and oriented exactly by the red and blue color coding. *H,* Zinc chloride paste is reapplied only to those areas of the previously treated site where residual tumor was found by microscopic survey. *I* to *L,* The procedure of fixation with zinc chloride paste, surgical excision of fixed tissue, color coding, and microscopic survey is repeated until all surgical specimens are found to be free of tumor. (From Robins P: Mohs micrographic surgery. In McCarthy JG, ed: Plastic Surgery. Philadelphia, WB Saunders, 1990:3652-3662.)

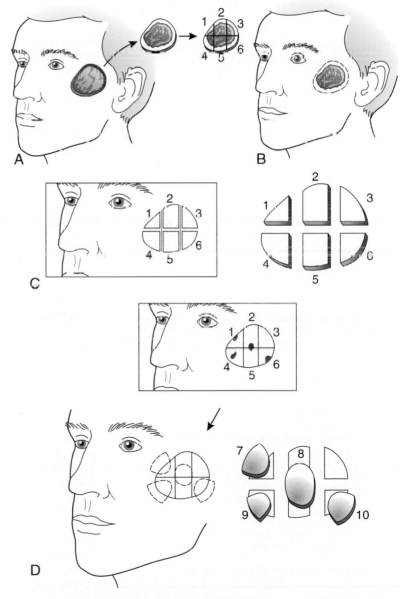

FIGURE 116-15. *A,* The patient's lesion is delineated and debulked. *B,* The thin specimen is removed and divided into easily processed portions. *C,* A tissue map is constructed, noting the exact orientation of the specimen and the tissue dyes applied to each individual portion. *D,* Finally, if tumor is found to be present in the first stage (noted with dark marker in sections 1, 4, 6, and between 2 and 5), the process is repeated until a tumor-free plane is obtained. (From Clark D: Cutaneous micrographic surgery. Otolaryngol Clin North Am 1993;26:185-202.)

surgeons have noted the value of the rapid cytokeratin stain to rule out residual tumor.[401]

INDICATIONS FOR MICROGRAPHIC EXCISION

Micrographic technique is especially useful for excision of tumors at high risk for recurrence, including recurrent tumors, incompletely excised tumors, and a number of primary tumors (Tables 116-20 and 116-21). Tumors at high risk for recurrence or metastasis include those with ill-defined clinical borders; those at anatomic sites of embryonal fusion planes, including the temporal and periorbital area, especially the medial canthus, less so the lateral canthus; and those in the columella–upper lip junction, the periauricular and tragal areas, the postauricular sulcus, the melolabial groove, the ala-cheek-lip junction, and the paranasal sites. Tumors in these locations have been demonstrated to exhibit tumor extension beyond what is clinically apparent. Other high-risk tumors are those with a history of previous ionizing irradiation, a size greater than 2 cm in diameter, and a history of significant recurrence. By tumor type, the morpheaform, infiltrating, and poorly differentiated SCCs or BCCs would qualify.[402-409] Perineural, periarterial, and perivenular extension and deep tissue or bone involvement aid decision-making toward aggressive treatment. Tissue preservation is important in the perioral and periorbital area, hands, feet, and genitalia.

TABLE 116-20 ✦ TUMORS TREATABLE WITH MICROGRAPHIC SURGERY[770]

Basal cell carcinoma
Squamous cell carcinoma
Malignant melanoma[771,772]
Tumors arising in basal cell nevus syndrome[773]
Bowen tumors of genitalia[774]
Dermatofibrosarcoma protuberans[775]
Recurrent, aggressive, or mutilating keratoacanthomas[776]
Malignant fibrous histiocytoma[777,778]
Atypical fibroxanthoma[777]
Verrucous carcinoma[778]
Microcystic adnexal carcinoma[779]
Sebaceous carcinoma[780,781]
Extramammary Paget disease[782,783]
Leiomyosarcoma[778]
Adenoid cystic carcinoma of eccrine glands[784]
Merkel cell carcinoma[785,786]
Apocrine carcinoma of the skin[787]
Oral and central facial, paranasal sinus neoplasms
Aerodigestive tract head and neck tumors[788]
Dermatofibrosarcoma protuberans[775]
Sebaceous carcinoma[780,781]
Tumors arising in basal cell nevus syndrome[773]
Malignant fibrous histiocytoma[777,778]
Microcystic adnexal carcinoma[779]
Paget disease[782,783]
Adenoid cystic carcinoma of eccrine glands[784]

TABLE 116-21 ✦ PRIMARY TUMORS AND OTHER SITUATIONS IN WHICH MICROGRAPHIC TECHNIQUE IS INDICATED

Morpheaform basal cell carcinoma
Squamous cell carcinoma of an undifferentiated, poorly differentiated, spindle cell, or acantholytic type
Locations with high recurrence or metastatic potential
Locations requiring maximal tissue sparing
Young patients, especially on the face of young women
Tumors with a diameter > 2 cm
Lesions neglected for many years
Tumors with indistinct clinical margins
Tumors with rapid or aggressive growth behavior
Tumors arising in previously non–solar-irradiated skin
Tumors in immunosuppressed patients
Patients with basal cell nevus syndrome

Tumors in immunosuppressed and young patients and patients with a high aesthetic target may benefit from micrographic excision as well.

ADVANTAGES

The micrographic surgical technique has the highest cure rate compared with other techniques for the same tumor type, location, and other characteristics.[410,411] Other advantages include potential tissue conservation, coordination of surgery with pathology, tracing of perineural or infiltrating tumors, local anesthesia safety, and lower cost relative to surgery in a hospital operating room.[412] The high cure rate is due to the theoretical evaluation of nearly 100% of tumor margins, compared with peripheral and deep margin evaluations performed by most pathologists. When the extirpating micrographic surgeon is also the margin evaluator, the improved potential for tissue orientation, true positives, and fewer false-negatives is apparent. Even if the extirpating surgeon is different from the repairing surgeon, having the surgeon performing the repair involved in the tissue examinations benefits the patient.

DISADVANTAGES

There are disadvantages to micrographic excision that are mostly due to slide preparation and interpretation points, but other issues also exist (Fig. 116-16 and Table 116-22).[412,413] The procedure costs are higher in both dollars and time (one may counter this point with data on decreased recurrence rates). Thus, Mohs surgery is performed under local anesthesia most of the time in offices not billing hourly operating room time. The problem then arises as to where to do the extirpation in usually elderly, unhealthy patients. The second problem then in larger defects requiring more than simple repair is how to transfer the patient to an

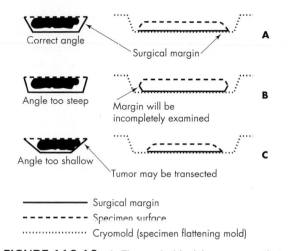

FIGURE 116-16. *A,* The angled incision ensures that the specimen's beveled edges can be pressed flat, in a contiguous plane with the deeper surgical margin. *B,* Too steep an angle precludes complete wound edge analysis. *C,* Too shallow an angle risks unnecessarily transecting tumor. (From Steinman HK: Mohs surgical techniques. In Gross GA, Steinman HK, Rapini RP, eds: Mohs Surgery: Fundamentals and Techniques. St. Louis, Mosby, 1999:49-72.)

appropriate setting in which to carry out the repair. Because some multiple-stage extirpations performed intermittently during several hours consume the greater part of a working day, the logistic implications for repair, venue, and timing become apparent. In answer to the situation, many Mohs patients sustain a wound defect on one day and have a preplanned repair scheduled for one or two days later.

Another consideration is that as the defect size increases, the cure rate begins to plateau (Fig. 116-17).[412] Thus, the diminishing cure return of large defects and the reduced potential for regional functional rehabilitation and cosmetic restoration make a reasonable argument against micrographic technique to "cure at all cost." Large defects may result from over-aggressive tumor debulking, unapparent tumor borders, peripheral actinic changes, infection or inflammation, or a number of technical points relative to slide preparation and interpretation of margins.[412]

Creation of an infrastructure to administer care for micrographic surgery patients requires the time, energy, finances, personnel, and education to do so. Tissue preparation materials and technicians require incorporation into an altered clinical schedule. Indeed, many Mohs surgeons block out a full or half "Mohs day" to extirpate tumors and another full or half day to repair the defects (if sufficiently complex).

There is no question that a significant potential for abuse of the technique exists (Table 116-23). Some of these abuses are inherent pitfalls in the technique itself rather than an unethical deliberate attempt at deception. However, unfortunately, the latter does exist as well, as motivated by treatment aggressiveness, compulsivity, and economic gain.

TABLE 116-22 ✦ PITFALLS OF MOHS SURGERY

Frozen section quality
  Thick sections with poor cellular detail
  Folds in the sections cover tumor
  Poor staining quality
Interpretation of frozen sections
  Adnexal structures mistaken for BCC
  Keratin granulomas indicating nearby SCC
  Inflammatory cell aggregates: near or obscuring tumor
  Sun-damaged skin resembling lentigo maligna in margin
  Pseudocarcinomatous hyperplasia misinterpreted as SCC
  Tangential epidermis misinterpreted as tumor
  Healing fibrotic wounds resembling spindle cell tumors
  Floaters of tumor found in margin
Incomplete tissue margins
  Holes in the dermis or adipose
  Incomplete epidermal edge
Misoriented tissue margins
  Excessive facing of the block
  Ink runs or applied to wrong place
  Insufficient ink applied
  Misnumbered blocks or slides
  Incorrectly drawn map
  Returning to re-excise wrong area
  Cutting the wrong side of the tissue
Excessively wide or narrow margins
  Usually due to other problems (listed earlier)
  Inadequate or excessive debulking before first stage
  Aggressive surgeon or patient demanding 100% cure
  Timid surgeon or patient wanting no scar
  Ill-defined tumor causes misleading apparent tumor size
  Dermatitis around tumor exaggerates apparent tumor size
  Actinic damage or infection misleads tumor size
Tumor seeding
  Cutting into tumor may (theoretically) spread it
Multifocal tumor
  Recurrent discontinuous foci in scar
  Tumor deep or lateral to scar or excised layer
  Paget, Bowen, Merkel, angiosarcoma, lentigo maligna
  Sebaceous carcinoma, superficial "multifocal" BCC
Tedious, complex, time-consuming procedure
  Anesthesia wears off
  Patient grows weary
  Many steps for potential errors
  Returning next day for extensive cases
  Repair by second person with delay and increased costs

From Rapini RP: Potential pitfalls and abuses of Mohs surgery. In Gross GA, Steinman HK, Rapini RP, eds: Mohs Surgery: Fundamentals and Techniques. St. Louis, Mosby, 1999:221-229.

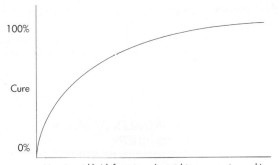

100%

Cure

0%

Margin width (defect size, diminishing cosmetic result)

FIGURE 116-17. Relationship between cure rate and defect size. As defect sizes become excessive, the cure rate does not increase very much, so "cure at all cost" may not be reasonable for basal cell carcinoma. However, Mohs surgery should theoretically result in "just the right amount" of tissue excised. (From Rapini RP: Potential pitfalls and abuses of Mohs surgery. In Gross GA, Steinman HK, Rapini RP, eds: Mohs Surgery: Fundamentals and Techniques. St. Louis, Mosby, 1999:221-229.)

Tracking multiple tumor locations on one or more body parts may be confusing. One may choose to employ anatomic rubber stamp diagrams to maintain organization of tumor data and records.[230] Rubber stamps hold basic anatomic topographic outline drawings. The stamped image in a chart allows orientation marks to be placed on the pertinent site. Additional data with respect to stage number, section number, orientation, and tumor positivity and negativity can also be drawn adjacent to the image. It may be helpful to place a rough line drawing adjacent to these, representing the corresponding facial profile of a basic rubber stamp image.

Patients may also have unrealistic expectations about the outcome of excision with the micrographic

technique.[414] Although many practices have the infrastructure and trained staff to perform the micrographic excision, standard excisional surgery with permanent sections offers a great deal of reliability. To date, no controlled prospective studies exist to prove the superiority of micrographic excision over standard excision with adequate margins. However, there has been difficulty in establishing the definition of an adequate margin.[227,398,415]

Finally, to gain expertise in micrographic excision, exposure to surgeons or pathologists willing to teach and explain the procedure as well as to review cutaneous cancer cases and slides is extremely important.[416] Physicians would do well to begin such a practice in their residency training, with short periods of rotation to a Mohs and pathology service.[321,416]

RADIOTHERAPY

Because radiation therapy is used as a component of treatment in one half to two thirds of all types of cancers (not just the skin), it is estimated that more than 10% of the population will at some time receive radiation therapy (Fig. 116-18).[417,418] Radiotherapy is less commonly used for skin cancers, but it has been used in the treatment of cancer for almost 100 years. Its effectiveness in skin cancers must be judged by the frequency of local-regional tumor control in relation to the incidence and severity of treatment-induced morbidity.[417]

BCCs and SCCs are moderately radiosensitive tumors; however, radiation therapy is infrequently used in their treatment even though the cure rate is similar between surgical excision and radiotherapy. Radiotherapy is painless, with no anesthesia necessary; it is a good treatment for medically ill or debilitated patients, and radiotherapy is free of systemic toxic effects. Disadvantages of radiotherapy are the need for

TABLE 116-23 ✦ TEN POTENTIAL ABUSES OF MOHS SURGERY

Counting the debulking excision as a stage
Flapophilia or flapophobia
Overuse of the procedure
Double billing by surgeon and pathologist
Mohs non-frozen (slow Mohs without using frozen sections)
Frozen non-Mohs (cutting corners on margin evaluations)
Underestimating lesion size, resulting in too many stages
Overestimating lesion size, resulting in large defect
Failure to use multidisciplinary approach
Use of the technique by the inadequately trained

From Rapini RP: Potential pitfalls and abuses of Mohs surgery. In Gross GA, Steinman HK, Rapini RP, eds: Mohs Surgery: Fundamentals and Techniques. St. Louis, Mosby, 1999:221-229.

FIGURE 116-18. *A,* This 37-year-old man neglected a basal cell carcinoma for 6 years. He presented with a tumor centered in his left cheek and extending into the medial canthus of his eye and the embryologic fusion plane of his lower nose. *B,* The treatment field was drawn around the tumor, and a shield was inserted below the eyelids. *C,* A lead mask was fabricated to collimate the beam. He initially received 42 Gy in 21 fractions with use of 250-kV x-rays and lead eye shields. Tungsten eye shields first became available in August 1994, and he was given another 22 Gy with use of a 9-MeV electron beam and tungsten shields. *D,* The patient 4 months later, without disease and with a functioning eyelid. He was free of disease at the time of his follow-up in January 1997. (From Morrison WH, Garden AS, Ang KK: Radiation therapy for nonmelanoma skin carcinomas. Clin Plast Surg 1997;24: 719-729.)

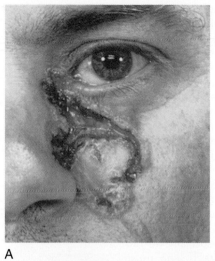

A

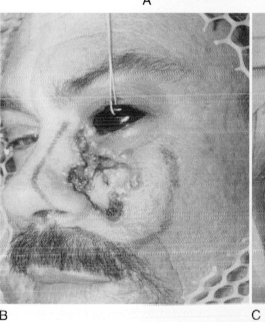

B

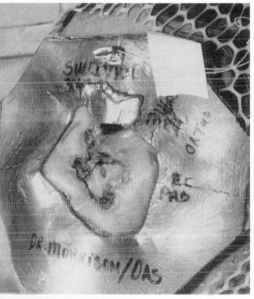

C

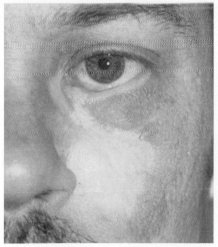

D

special skills and equipment, the high cost of treatment, the need for multiple visits, skin atrophy, and the risk of bone or cartilage necrosis.

Mammals have enzymatic repair systems available to combat radiation exposure. Radiation therapy takes advantage of the differences in repair and recovery capabilities between normal and cancerous tissues. Radiation therapy methods take advantage of different penetration rates of photons and electrons into living tissue. In certain areas such as the eyelid, lips, and ears, effective shielding mechanisms prevent damage to underlying structures. Radiation therapy is most effective when the number of tumor cells is limited, requiring only modest doses, and when the tumor has not destroyed adjacent normal tissues.[417]

Radiation exposure is considered a risk factor for the development of skin cancers, especially on the hands of dentists and radiologists.[419] The most common tumor arising after radiation therapy is BCC in the head, neck, and trunk or SCC in the hands (Fig. 116-19).[420,421] Shore et al[422] studied 22,000 children treated for tinea capitis with x-rays, and BCC developed in only one patient in 26 years of follow-up. African Americans represented 25% of the study group, and no skin cancers developed in them, emphasizing the fact that light-skinned individuals are more susceptible to skin cancers from ultraviolet light and irradiation.[422,423] The risk for development of skin cancers goes up with time after radiotherapy and the presence of radiodermatitis.[424,425] The estimated incidence of cancer development in patients with chronic radiation dermatitis is less than 5%.[426] Therefore, the overall risk of cancer development after therapeutic irradiation is small, especially if its use is restricted to the elderly.[427,428]

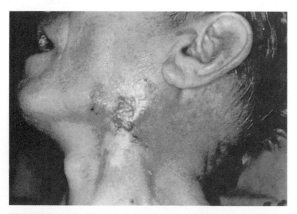

FIGURE 116-19. Radiation-induced squamous cell carcinoma of the neck in a 68-year-old man treated by irradiation for carcinoma of the larynx 16 years previously. (From Casson PR, Robins P: Malignant tumors of the skin. In McCarthy JG, ed: Plastic Surgery. Philadelphia, WB Saunders, 1990:3614-3662.)

TABLE 116-24 ✦ CONTRAINDICATIONS TO RADIATION THERAPY FOR SKIN CANCERS

Lesions arising in damaged skin, such as thermal burns, scars, and radiation dermatitis
Lesions of the palms and soles
Relative contraindications include small lesions that can be excised without deformity, especially in the trunk and extremities or in the scalp, where alopecia would result; lesions in young people and those patients with xeroderma pigmentosum, lupus vulgaris, and scleroderma
Recurrences after radiotherapy are a relative contraindication unless excellent previous treatment records are available
Patients with basal cell nevus syndrome, xeroderma pigmentosum, or epidermodysplasia verruciformis

From Westgate SJ: Radiation therapy for skin tumors. Otolaryngol Clin North Am 1993;26:295-309.

The general indications for radiation therapy are poor general health, advanced age, medical conditions that preclude surgery, and tumor size between 1 and 5 cm.[429] Radiation therapy is expensive. A standard treatment for a 1.0-cm lesion of the face would cost between $3,000 and $5,000 versus $100 to $400 dollars for cryotherapy or simple excision.[335] However, in younger patients, the cosmetic disfigurements from radiation therapy, such as pigmentation, telangiectasias, and atrophy, worsen over time.[418] In addition, the effects of radiation are permanent, and only after careful consideration and planning may it be used again, and then only in limited doses. Any future surgery in an irradiated field has the additional risk of poor healing. Therefore, it is better if radiation therapy is reserved for patients older than 55 years.[418] The overall cosmetic results to achieve tumor control were estimated to be good or excellent in 63% of patients, which is less than the good to excellent results of 91% with curettage-electrodesiccation and 84% with surgical excision.[430] These long-term cosmetic results with radiation therapy have been seen in other studies.[431]

Radiotherapy can be used for primary treatment, for the prophylactic treatment of lymph nodes, or for the treatment of advanced skin cancers. Multiple visits are necessary because increased fractionation of the radiation doses is associated with more successful treatment.[85] Radiation therapy is contraindicated in some instances (Table 116-24).[432]

Skin changes after therapeutic irradiation include hyperpigmentation and hypopigmentation, telangiectasias, fibrosis, burns, and alopecia. Radiotherapy-induced subsequent cancers occur but are rare.[427,433-436]

There are four main reasons for tumor recurrence after radiotherapy: underestimation of the size of the tumor or geographic miss; inadequate dosimetry reaching the depth of the tumor; inadequate treatment schedule; and lack of radiosensitivity of the tumor. Geographic miss is the main reason for treatment failures.[437]

BCCs that recur after radiotherapy are a distinct subgroup that demands special attention. These tumors are large, aggressive, and invasive.[438] Many metastatic BCCs are from failures after initial radiotherapy. It is unknown whether the radiation changes the tumor or alters the host response. Treatment by surgical excision is complicated by failure rates of 15% to 20%.[439-441] Attempted treatment by further radiotherapy has a failure rate of about 50%,[442,443] although intensity-modulated radiotherapy has been attempted.[444] Micrographic excision may be the best modality for treatment with a failure rate of 7%.[438] Lesions that recur after initial treatment by modalities other than radiotherapy may be successfully treated with radiotherapy with a failure rate of 17%.[445]

Radiotherapy remains a powerful tool in the treatment of skin cancers. In breast cancer, surgeries have become smaller as lumpectomy and radiation therapy have become routine. Treatment of NMSC may follow a similar path.

Primary Tumor Radiotherapy

Radiation therapy can treat skin cancers with cure rates similar to those of surgery.[88,418,432,446] It is a valuable treatment for many patients, although there is a gradual reduction in the numbers of patients referred for irradiation.[429] Head and neck skin tolerates radiation therapy well. Excellent choices for primary radiotherapy are those areas where lead shielding is easy to mold, such as the outer ear, eyelids, and lip areas. In addition, the nasal vestibule is an excellent anatomic choice because of the major reconstruction that is necessary after surgical excision. Because of alopecia risk, radiation therapy is used infrequently in the scalp.

Local control rates for basal cancers are above 90%.[447-450] Local control is correlated with the size and histologic features of the lesions.[448,449,451] In one study, small BCCs less than 1 cm had a cure rate of 97%.[447] For tumors 1 to 5 cm, the local control rate dropped to 87%, although the local control rate remained at 87% for BCCs larger than 5 cm.[447] Knox et al[450] found cure rates of 96.4% for BCCs less than 2 cm treated with radiation, although this was similar to the results with surgical excision or curettage and electrodesiccation. Sclerosing or morpheaform BCCs should not usually undergo radiation therapy.[452] The radiation field borders are indistinct, and the cosmetic results are poor.[453]

Local control rates of SCCs are around 85% to 90%.[446,448] Lesion size correlates with results. Better cure rates are achieved with the smaller lesion and the absence of previous treatment.[449] For tumors less than 1 cm, the recurrence rate is 91%; for tumors 1 to 5 cm, the recurrence rate is 87%; and for tumors greater than 5 cm, the recurrence rate is 56%.[447] Results in the eyelid have been 93%.[454]

Perineural invasive cancers may be treated primarily or adjunctively with radiation therapy.[455] This finding was noted in 14% of SCCs, and these tumors should be treated aggressively with surgery and radiotherapy.[456] Perineural invasion in the periorbital area is a grave concern because periorbital recurrence may be devastating, and radiotherapy is valuable in gaining local control.[457-459] Altered sensation in the periorbital nerves is a key in this diagnosis, especially with a history of previous cancer removal.[460]

Large or deeply invading cancers into cartilage or bone may be an excellent choice for radiation therapy; the cure rate with radiation therapy alone is 80%.[461,462] Imaging studies such as computed tomographic scanning and magnetic resonance imaging are useful to evaluate the magnitude of tumor spread. Contrast-enhanced helical computed tomography is also useful in evaluation of extremity tumors.[463] Surgical excision is key for most instances of deeply invasive tumors, but postoperative radiotherapy and palliative radiotherapy are supplemental considerations.[464]

Primary Nodal Radiotherapy

Nodal spread in skin cancer is a grave finding. The 5-year survival rate of patients with SCC and nodal spread is about 25% to 30% even with treatment.[465,466] Surgical lymph node dissection followed by radiotherapy is recommended for those patients with multiple palpable nodal metastases, nodes of 3 cm or more in diameter, or nodes with extracapsular spread.[467,468] The more difficult problem is the presence of single metastatic nodes. There is disagreement as to the method of treatment. Many would choose to excise surgically, then irradiate the field. Others think that either surgery alone or radiotherapy alone will suffice.[469]

Adjuvant Radiotherapy

Adjuvant radiotherapy is performed after surgery if the pathologic examination reveals tumors with positive or close margins or invasion of nerves, cartilage, or bone. Margin involvement in high-risk areas or high-risk tumors demands immediate re-treatment by re-excision, radiotherapy, or both.

Recurrent skin cancers from techniques other than radiotherapy have been successfully treated with irradiation with an overall 5-year cure rate of 84%.[445] The results in smaller lesions are more favorable.[470]

Prophylactic Radiotherapy

There is no standard as to which high-risk lesions require further irradiation of the primary site or nodal area. Practitioners will vary treatment regimens according to the type and location of the cancer. Some choose to wait and see, whereas others may proceed with sentinel node dissection or supraomohyoid dissection to gain more information.[471] Tumors at high risk for recurrence include tumors of large size; tumors with positive margins of excision, perineural spread, and invasion of cartilage or bone; and recurrent tumors.[458,459,461,462,472] If the risk of recurrence to lymph nodes is more than 20%, further treatment with radiation therapy or a neck dissection will provide equivalent control.[473] Mucosal SCCs that have multiple risk factors and clinically negative nodes should be considered for prophylactic lymph node irradiation.

Tumors that have spread to the parotid gland by metastasis or local extension need surgical excision followed by postoperative irradiation for the best prognosis.[474] Total parotidectomy is probably not necessary for this circumstance because it does not prolong survival.[475]

Brachytherapy

Brachytherapy (from Greek *brachys,* meaning short) is a type of radiation treatment. It involves the placement of radioactive seeds in or around a tumor, giving a high dose of radiation locally and minimizing damage to deeper tissues. Three-dimensional planning is necessary by the radiation team to optimize local treatment and to minimize distant irradiation. The technique of brachytherapy is in contradistinction to electron-beam therapy, which penetrates deeply through tissue and therefore affects tissues along the path of the beam. Historically, brachytherapy has been used effectively in the treatment of skin cancers, and newer techniques and planning have made it more effective.[476] Precise molds to fit and direct the radioactive seeds have been used with success.[476,477]

FOLLOW-UP AFTER TREATMENT

The onset of cutaneous malignant neoplasia in a patient often indicates that the sun-exposed skin has received a cumulative dose of excessive ultraviolet radiation. Therefore, the patient is at risk on a lifelong basis for cutaneous malignant neoplasia.[60,478]

Follow-up for patients with BCC and SCC is necessary because of the possibility of recurrence, metastasis, and development of other cutaneous lesions. Extended follow-up is the most valuable. Initially, the physician should see the patient twice in the first year and then yearly for at least 5 years. If new cancers continue to develop during this time, the visit frequency should be increased to every 3 to 4 months.

Physical examination involves not only a visual examination but also a palpation examination of the treated area to detect induration otherwise unnoticed by the examiner's eye. Palpation of lymph nodes and the parotid gland as potential sites of tumor extension is of value. An examination of the complete cutaneous surface from scalp to plantar surfaces should be carried out with particular emphasis on sun-exposed areas and with a view of non–sun-exposed areas and tissue folds. Any encountered lesions of unclear diagnosis require biopsy of a shave or punch type. If there is any suspicion of recurrent tumor, deeper tissue specimens requiring full-thickness excision should be obtained. This information simply cannot be obtained by a shave or more superficial punch excision.

Self-examination by the patient will allow him or her to come in with suspicious lesions that might not be seen until far later in their course. It is particularly helpful to have a single set of photographs taken on only one occasion by the patient with a good-quality camera; these photographs are printed on and archived in acid-free paper. Each photograph should have a ruler in it. Normally, 25 to 30 photographs are required to obtain a complete recording of the cutaneous surface. No patient, spouse, partner, or busy physician will remember the specifics of individual lesions. Each year, on the patient's birthday, the photographs should be pulled from the dresser drawer and a full comparison made to the photographs. If enlargement of a lesion is suspected, comparison with the ruler in the photograph helps decide whether it has in fact enlarged. Any new, suspicious, or symptomatic lesions can thus receive scrutiny in the physician's office. In this way, the cutaneous surface can be monitored over the years in a highly efficient fashion.

From an ideal point of view, patients should have lifelong follow-up for both BCCs and SCCs. Eighteen percent of BCC recurrences are noted more than 5 years after initial treatment.[359,479] Patients with previous cutaneous cancer have a higher risk for new BCCs on a lifelong basis.[480] The total body surface should be examined because nearly half of new BCCs are found on anatomic sites distinct from the initial tumor occurrence.[481] Many specialists will discontinue follow-up of their patients with BCC after approximately 4 years because of the identified lower risk of recurrence of the original tumor.[328,482,483] However, from a public health monitoring point of view, development of a new BCC in a cancer-prone patient will be a lifelong reality. Physicians who are simply uninterested in carrying out this long-term treatment relationship should refer the patient to another setting for such monitoring.

SCC follow-up is as important as BCC follow-up, if not more so, given the problems with regional spread and distant metastasis. More than 70% of SCC recurrences and metastases develop within 2 years of treatment of the primary tumor; the majority are detected within the first year.[88,484] In such cases, follow-up examination should be carried out every 3 months for the first 2 years after treatment, although the value of this is unproved. At the very least, for SCC precursors such as actinic keratoses, the examination interval may be 6 months. Clearly, new skin cancers in a patient having previously had a cancer can be expected with a risk approaching 50% at 5 years. Particular attention should be given to patients with severe actinic radiation changes even with development of only a single cancer, those who are immunosuppressed, and those with a particularly invasive tissue type of cancer originally.

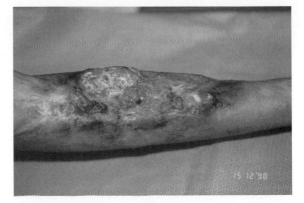

FIGURE 116-20. Large, invasive Marjolin ulcer that developed 40 years after a severe burn. The tumor invaded to bone and required microvascular surgery with a latissimus flap for reconstruction. (Photograph courtesy of Dr. R. Minami.)

VARIANTS OF SQUAMOUS CELL CARCINOMA

SCCs of the skin can present in a variety of forms. There are unusual variants, such as scar carcinomas, keratoacanthomas, Bowen disease, and other unrelated but dangerous skin tumors such as Merkel cell carcinoma (Table 116-25).

Marjolin Ulcers or Scar Carcinoma

The potential for burn scars to degenerate into neoplasia was originally noted by Celsus.[485] Jean Marjolin in 1828 described a tumor arising in burn scars.[486] De Costa gave the eponym Marjolin to scar cancer in 1903.[487] Steffen[488] and Nancarrow[489] dispute the fact that Marjolin recognized these ulcers as scar cancer. However, his name is now synonymous with cancers arising in scar tissue, burns, and wounds (Fig. 116-20). Many skin cancers, including SCCs but also BCCs, melanomas, and sarcomas, may arise in scar tissue.[490-492] SCCs are the most common type of scar cancers, followed by BCCs. Chronic irradiation

dermatitis, a cause of scar cancers, degenerates more commonly into BCC rather than SCC.[493]

Various types of chronic irritation may produce these cancers, including chronic dermatitis, chronic ulcers, chronic radiodermatitis, chronic osteomyelitis, burn scars, discoid lupus erythematosus, and even operative scars.[494] Other types of injuries causing scar carcinomas have included nonhealing ulcers, chronic fistulas, gunshot injuries, knife wounds, puncture wounds, crush injuries, vaccination scars, pressure sores, and animal bites.[495-497]

ETIOLOGY

The reasons for the malignant degeneration are unknown. Virchow thought that chronic irritation was a factor in the development of carcinoma.[485] One study reported previous trauma in 7.3% of patients with BCC.[198] Possible mechanisms include release of

TABLE 116-25 ✦ SQUAMOUS CELL CARCINOMA VARIANTS

	Bowen Disease	Keratoacanthomas	Marjolin or Scar Cancer	Merkel Cell Carcinoma
Incidence	15 per 100,000 annually in whites in Minnesota[789]	104 per 100,000 annually in whites in Kauai[530]	Unusual	Rare
Pathology	SCC in situ	Hair follicle tumor; resembles SCC	Extensive scar with aggressive SCC	Neuroendocrine tumor
Clinical picture	Slowly enlarging superficial cancer	Rapid growth, then slow regression	New growth in old area of trauma	Pink-red nodule in head and neck area
Treatment	Surgery, 5-FU, superficial ablation	Excision, watch and wait, 5-FU, curettage and electrodesiccation	Wide excision plus lymph node evaluation	Wide excision plus lymph node evaluation

injury-associated toxins, induction of dormant neo-plastic cells, and activation of injury-induced preneo-plastic cells by a co-carcinogen.[495] Others believe there is depressed immunity in the areas of scars.[499,500] Recent work has centered on breakdown of the Fas ligand, a protein induced by ultraviolet light damage, which regulates skin homeostasis.[501,502]

INCIDENCE

Marjolin ulcers occur at any age and in all races.[493,495,503] Men are more commonly afflicted than are women in a ratio of about 3:1.[494,504] These cancers usually occur in adults with an average age at onset of 58 years and a range from 18 to 84 years.[493]

The lag time from the injury to the onset of the cancer (the latent period) varies from 8 months to 60 years.[485,494,504-507] The median seems to be about 31 years. The lag time is inversely proportional to the age of the patient at the time of the injury.[489,506] Elderly patients with burns have a short latency period before scar cancers appear. Children with chronic scarring will generally have a long latency period before cancers.

Scar carcinoma is rare and the incidence is varied. Bostwick[499] noted its occurrence in 2% of SCCs. Treves and Pack[485] noted its incidence in 0.5% of BCCs. Castillo and Goldsmith[500] noted scar cancers occurring in 1.2% of all skin cancer cases. The incidence of scar cancer is much higher in Asia and Africa. These areas are inhabited by darker-skinned individuals not prone to solar skin cancers, and there are more burn injuries and healing by secondary intention. In Kashmir, the incidence of scar cancer is 7.6% of all skin cancers.[508] It is estimated that 1% of patients with chronic osteomyelitis will develop this problem.[497]

Slow healing and chronic instability of the scar are key factors in the development of scar carcinomas.[485] Most burn scar carcinomas occur in patients who were not grafted or in areas of graft failure.[506,507] There is less frequent malignant degeneration in burns that have been excised and grafted,[493] but even areas successfully grafted may develop neoplasia.[504]

CLINICAL FINDINGS

The key clinical finding is a change in sensation or appearance of the scar.[92,509] The most common initial symptoms are increased pain (74%), discharge with a foul odor (68%), and bleeding (58%).[510] The most common location is the lower extremity (40%), fol-lowed by the head and neck (30%), the extremities (20%), and the trunk (10%).[493,511,512] The lower extrem-ity carries the gravest prognosis. Scar cancers have a predilection for flexion creases of the extremities, where there is constant trauma to the scar contractures and decreased blood supply.[493] Radiographic findings are usually apparent on plain films, which will show bone destruction, soft tissue mass, and periosteal reaction.[513]

Magnetic resonance imaging and computed tomo-graphic scans are useful but not essential to clinical management.[513]

PATHOLOGY

The risk of metastases is highly correlated with the degree of differentiation of the tumor.[514] The more anaplastic the tumor, the higher the metastasis rate.[515] The most significant factor in predicting the outcome is the grade of the tumor: for grade I lesions (low grade), the incidence of metastasis is 10%; for grade II lesions (moderately well differentiated), 59%; and for grade III lesions (poorly differentiated), 86%.[514]

TREATMENT

Scar cancers should be treated with 1 to 2 cm of lateral margins around the tumor. Lateral and deep margins around a scar cancer depend on the histologic fea-tures, the location of the tumor, the size of the cancer, the depth of the cancer, whether the cancer is primary or recurrent, and the surrounding presence of scar or irradiation. Surgical judgment is necessary to deter-mine the margins of resection. A large burn scar may have a central area of cancer, and it may be practical to excise the central area with a 1- to 2-cm margin and leave some superficial scar. Other cancers may have ill-defined borders of scar and cancer, and a larger 2-cm resection may be necessary. All specimens must be evaluated by the pathologist for clear peripheral and deep margins. Sufficient deep margins may require resection of involved muscle groups, bone, fascia, or vascular structures if the tumor is fixed to bone or when bone involvement is noted on preoperative imaging. In a more superficial lesion that does not extend below dermis, the deep margin may be the sub-cutaneous fat. Deeper invasion into the subcutaneous fat requires excision to a deep margin of the under-lying fascia. Frozen sections are necessary, and after the tumor is resected, the area may be covered by a skin graft or flap.[493,503,506]

Amputations may be necessary for difficult cancers or recurrent tumors.[508,509] Some authors recommend prophylactic regional dissection, especially in the lower extremities, because lymph node metastasis is noted in about 50% of cases.[493,499] Other authors rec-ommend lymph node dissection only in the presence of clinically positive nodes.[489,495,503,515,516] Lym-phadenectomy should be followed by radiation therapy to the nodal basin.[515] Primary radiotherapy has had some success in those patients who refuse surgery.[515] Clinically negative nodes require close follow-up or prophylactic radiation therapy.[517]

PROGNOSIS

Scar carcinomas have a metastatic rate as high as 38% to 49%.[494,514] Patients with depressed immune systems may be at higher risk.[518] The treatment of choice is wide local excision and removal of clinically involved lymph nodes.[515] Recurrence is almost always to the local area or regional node and usually occurs in the first 3 years.[509,515] Survival rates are significantly better in the face, neck, and upper extremities compared with the lower extremities. Five-year survival is 52% to 70%.[492,509] Poorly differentiated tumors have a 5-year survival of less than 10%.[492] Patients with nodal metastasis have a 5-year survival of 35%.[515]

Keratoacanthoma

Keratoacanthoma is a common tumor that seems to arise from the hair follicles in sun-exposed areas of light-skinned older individuals.[519] Keratoacanthoma was first noted by Sir Jonathan Hutchinson in 1889.[520] Keratoacanthoma clinically and microscopically resembles SCC, yet keratoacanthomas spontaneously regress after a rapid growth phase (Fig. 116-21 and Table 116-26).[521]

EPIDEMIOLOGY

Solitary keratoacanthomas, the most common type, generally occur on sun-exposed areas of the body, such as the cheeks, nose, and dorsal hands. They have also been reported in mucosal regions, palms, and subungual areas.[522]

ETIOLOGY

A viral cause from human papillomavirus has been implicated but remains unproven.[31,86,523,524] Some authors consider these lesions to be strictly benign[525]; others consider these lesions to be low-grade malignant neoplasms.[526-528] It is uncertain whether they are a variant of SCC or a different lesion.[529]

INCIDENCE

The incidence of keratoacanthoma is unknown, but one study has estimated an incidence of 144 per 100,000 men, 73 per 100,000 women, and a combined rate of 104 per 100,000 individuals.[530] This incidence was the same as that of SCC. Keratoacanthoma was less likely to occur in ethnic Japanese, Filipino, and Hawaiian populations with an incidence of 22, 7, and 6 per 100,000.[530] There is an increased incidence in immunosuppressed patients.[531] Workers in tar refineries have an increased incidence of keratoacanthomas and SCC; sunlight is an important cofactor.[532]

CLINICAL FINDINGS (Table 116-27)

Keratoacanthoma occurs mainly on the face, forearms, and hands.[519] There is no genetic predisposition except for unusual variants. There are three distinct stages—proliferation, maturation, and involution—during a period of around 6 months. This may reflect the

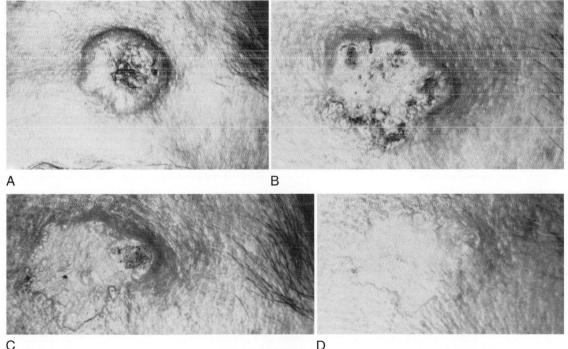

FIGURE 116-21. *A,* Keratoacanthoma. *B,* Clinical picture several weeks after incisional biopsy. *C,* Two months after biopsy. *D,* Healed scar. (From Popkin GL: Tumors of the skin: a dermatologist's viewpoint. In McCarthy JG, ed: Plastic Surgery. Philadelphia, WB Saunders, 1990:3560-3613.)

TABLE 116-26 ✦ CLINICAL DIFFERENTIATION BETWEEN KERATOACANTHOMA AND SQUAMOUS CELL CARCINOMA

Factor	Keratoacanthoma	Squamous Cell Carcinoma
Growth rate	Weeks (relatively faster)	Months (relatively slower)
Course	Rapid growth, followed by a stationary phase and then spontaneous involution	Tends to progress indefinitely
Relative size (for duration)	Large	Small
Shape	Crateriform	Irregular
Central portion of tumor	Keratotic plug	Necrotic ulcer with crust
Metastasis possible	Usually not (see text)	Yes
Response to nonsurgical treatment	Yes	No
Average age at onset	55 years	70 years
Induration of tumor and surrounding skin	Rarely	Commonly
Borders	Well circumscribed	Often ill-defined
Resemblance to molluscum contagiosum	Often	Seldom
Origin on mucosa	Rare	Not uncommon

From Hamm JC, DeFranzo AJ, Argenta LC, White W: Keratoacanthoma necessitating metacarpal amputation. J Hand Surg Am 1990;15:980-986.

anagen, catagen, and telogen phases of growth of hair, from which keratoacanthoma may arise.[519] The proliferative phase occurs during 2 to 4 weeks with rapid growth to about 2 cm and rarely to massive sizes. During the maturation phase, which lasts several months, the lesion appears stable, with little change. During involution, the central keratotic plug is expelled and the lesion is resorbed, leaving a depressed hypopigmented scar. Keratoacanthoma arising under the fingernails can erode the distal phalanx.[533]

HISTOLOGY

The histologic features of keratoacanthoma echo its clinical appearance as a crateriform squamous proliferation with a central core of compact hyperkeratosis

(Fig. 116-22).[34] There exist both follicular and nonfollicular (subungual and mucosal) types.[34] Most authorities now consider keratoacanthoma to be a variant of SCC because of its capacity for local destruction and metastasis.[34]

The problem remains that it is difficult to differentiate keratoacanthoma from SCC on the basis of histologic appearance alone.[534] Aggressive perineural invasion is not associated with metastases or recurrence.[535]

SPECIFIC KERATOACANTHOMAS
Giant Keratoacanthoma

A keratoacanthoma larger than 2 to 3 cm is considered a giant keratoacanthoma.[536] These lesions are

TABLE 116-27 ✦ CLINICAL CHARACTERISTICS OF KERATOACANTHOMA IN VARIOUS STAGES OF DEVELOPMENT

Characteristic	Rapid Growth	Maturation	Resolution
Type of lesion	Papule	Nodule	Scar
Growth pattern	Rapid growth and proliferation	Lesion ceases growth and remains stationary	Spontaneous involution
Average size	Reaches size of 10-25 mm in 6-8 weeks	10-25 mm in diameter, 5-10 mm in height	—
Time frame	2-8 weeks	2-8 weeks	2-8 weeks, although may persist for several years
Characteristic morphology	A small red macule becomes a firm, smooth, slightly dome-shaped papule, which enlarges rapidly to form the typical mature keratoacanthoma with a central keratinous core	Bud- or dome-shaped, skin-colored or slightly erythematous hemispheric mass on a smooth, round, sloping base with a central keratin plug that is firmly embedded	Expulsion of corneous plug and resorption of tumor mass occur, resulting in an atrophic, hyperpigmented, crenellated, puckered, or pitted scar

From Hamm JC, DeFranzo AJ, Argenta LC, White W: Keratoacanthoma necessitating metacarpal amputation. J Hand Surg Am 1990;15:980-986.

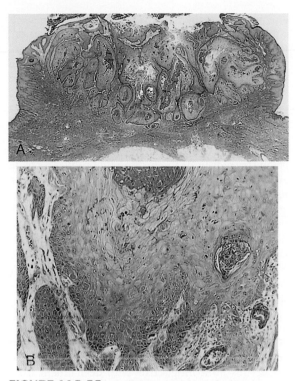

FIGURE 116-22. *A,* A scanning view of a keratoacanthoma demonstrates the characteristic architectural features of a relatively symmetric exoendophytic proliferation of cornifying squamous cells. A central crater is framed by epithelial buttresses. *B,* Aggregations of squamous cells show abundant pale-staining "glassy" cytoplasm, producing keratin without an intervening granular layer. Cytologic atypia is confined to the periphery of the aggregations, and microabscesses are present. (From Leshin B, White WL: Malignant neoplasms of keratinocytes. In Arndt KA, LeBoit PE, Robinson JK, Wintroub BU: Cutaneous Medicine and Surgery: An Integrated Program in Dermatology. Philadelphia, WB Saunders, 1996:1378-1391.)

destructive to surrounding tissue and centrally and may heal with significant scarring despite their ability to involute spontaneously.[537,538] Metastatic giant keratoacanthomas have been reported.[527] Biopsies are useful, and the histologic examination can suggest keratoacanthoma rather than SCC.[538] Because of the large size of these lesions, it is useful to think of keratoacanthoma as a potentially regressing SCC. Therefore, surgical therapy remains the mainstay of treatment because it allows histologic analysis.[539,540] Radiotherapy is useful for recurrences after surgery.[541,542] Giant keratoacanthomas have been treated successfully with oral retinoids, intralesional methotrexate, and intralesional interferon.[543-545]

Subungual Keratoacanthoma

Keratoacanthomas may occur in the subungual region.[531] They are usually fast growing, and this is important in the differentiation from SCCs because both may involve bone.[533] Subungual keratoacanthoma usually presents as a painful eruptive growth with bone invasion in middle-aged individuals.[546,547] Metastatic organ cancers may also present in the subungual region. These are usually from the lung (41%) or kidney (11%).[548] SCCs from these origins may confuse the diagnosis of keratoacanthoma. Local excision or curettage of the keratoacanthoma is the recommended treatment.[549] Difficult or recurrent cases may require amputation.[522,549]

Muir-Torre Keratoacanthoma

This autosomal dominant condition was first reported in 1967 by Muir[550] and 1968 by Torre.[551] In this syndrome, keratoacanthomas and sebaceous neoplasms can herald the existence of internal cancers, especially of the right colon.[118,552] The etiology is a genetic mutation of DNA repair genes, and it is considered a hereditary colon cancer syndrome.[553] Oral isotretinoin has been used with success in treatment of the keratoacanthomas, but there must be vigilance concerning possible internal cancers.[551]

Grzybowski-type Keratoacanthoma

This rare variant of keratoacanthoma was first described by Grzybowski in 1950; only 28 cases have been reported in the literature.[555] These keratoacanthomas may number into the thousands, do not typically involute, and are associated with pruritus.[520,555,556] Generalized treatment with acitretin has been unsuccessful, but there are reports of successful treatment of patients with cyclophosphamide or oral isotretinoin.[556,557]

Ferguson-Smith Keratoacanthoma

The existence of a genetic, autosomal dominant type of multiple self-healing keratoacanthomas was first reported in 1934 by Ferguson-Smith.[169] This is the most common type of multiple keratoacanthoma syndrome.[172] It affects males and females equally and occurs in sun-exposed areas of the skin. The patients reported in Scotland have been traced to a genetic mutation in 1790.[170] Treatment with oral retinoids has had mixed success.[558,559]

TREATMENT

Perhaps 25% of keratoacanthomas become malignant,[560] and many authorities consider keratoacanthomas to be a mild form of SCC.[34,561,562] Surgical excision is a mainstay of treatment. It avoids a potential period of watchful waiting, it avoids further enlargement of the lesion, and it avoids the potential scarring problems with involution. Watchful waiting, retrospectively, may turn out to be the best approach. However, prospectively, some sort of treatment is usually warranted. Medical treatments include topical Efudex or Aldara cream.[563-566] More aggressive medical treatments include injections with 5-FU, bleomycin, interferon, or methotrexate.[280,567-574] 5-FU is injected twice weekly in a dose of 50 mg for 2 to 3 weeks.[575] Invasive treatments available for keratoacanthoma include curettage and electrodesiccation, cryosurgery, and carbon dioxide laser therapy.[575,576] Surgical excision is the standard treatment because it allows a complete pathologic specimen with evaluation of margins. The margins should be conservative, in the range of 2 to 3 mm. Incomplete excision may lead to recurrences, either single or multiple, in the scar.

Bowen Disease

Bowen disease typically appears as a plaque or multiple plaques with scaling, with or without pigmentation. On histologic examination, these lesions are diagnosed by uniform, full epidermal thickness changes of keratinocytic atypia (Fig. 116-23). The keratinocytes lose their normal polarity. There is frequent hyperkeratosis clinically and histologically.[577] Bowen plaques enlarge quite slowly. Eventually, the epidermal basal layer is violated by downward growth, indicating the onset of invasive SCC, albeit in a small percentage of cases. Patients who have undergone light therapy for skin diseases and those with exposure to arsenic, either iatrogenically or from industrial and farm sources, may develop Bowen disease.[578-580]

Several years ago, a controversy about whether Bowen disease is associated with an increased incidence of gastrointestinal and other cancers was raised.[74,581] This controversy was resolved several years later when no true association between Bowen disease

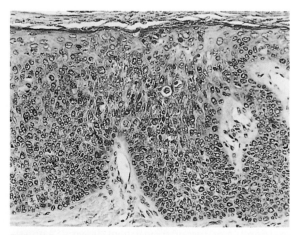

FIGURE 116-23. Bowen disease is squamous cell carcinoma in situ demonstrating markedly atypical keratinocytes throughout the epidermis that replace the granular layer and produce parakeratosis but, in early lesions, spare the basal layer. (From Leshin B, White WL: Malignant neoplasms of keratinocytes. In Arndt KA, LeBoit PE, Robinson JK, Wintroub BU: Cutaneous Medicine and Surgery: An Integrated Program in Dermatology. Philadelphia, WB Saunders, 1996:1378-1391.)

and internal malignant disease was noted in well-controlled studies.[582-584] On histologic evaluation, there is a spectrum of keratinocytic changes characteristic of actinic keratosis (see earlier description) to findings associated with SCC. The changes of SCC in situ include bowenoid actinic keratosis, bowenoid papulosis, Paget disease, extramammary Paget disease, and melanoma in situ.[585]

Beyond standard histopathology microscopic examination, increasing employment of immunohistochemistry aids in distinguishing Bowen disease from SCC. Bowen disease and SCC share the common immunohistochemical feature of a positive cytokeratin stain.[585] The differentiation must take place with the histopathologic findings. Paget disease has a positive carcinoembryonic antigen and a positive cytokeratin stain,[586,587] whereas mature SCC does not. Melanoma in situ can be differentiated by its negative carcinoembryonic antigen and negative cytokeratin stains but positive S100 stain.[588-591]

One example of this value of immunohistochemical staining is in cases of the spindle cell variant of SCC. A fully developed SCC, such as a malignant keratinocytic neoplasm, has cells that have invaded the dermis noncontiguously with detachment from the overlying epidermis. These areas of dermal invasion occur as islands and infiltrating strands alone or in combination. An infiltrating tumor has varying degrees of atypia. Minimal cellular atypia denotes a well-differentiated SCC; a poorly differentiated tumor has a few cells resembling mature keratinocytes. Spindle cells are frequently present in this situation. Beyond nuclear irregularities of varying degrees, differentiation of the tumor proceeds to keratinization, and the degree of keratinization aids in the determination of the level of differentiation of the tumor.[592] If, in this instance, there is a great deal of spindle morphology and the differential diagnosis includes spindleoid melanoma, the S100, cytokeratin, and carcinoembryonic antigen stains are the keys to the diagnosis and ultimately the determination of prognosis and therapeutic intervention.

TREATMENT

Because of its superficial nature, Bowen disease is responsive to a variety of treatments. Medical treatments with various creams has had a high success rate, and areas of failure can easily be re-treated. The standard and time-honored cream is 5-FU cream.[239,593-595] A new approach using 5% imiquimod cream has become available.[283,294,314,596-600] There may be a benefit to use of them both together.[285] More invasive semi-surgical techniques include cryotherapy and curettage-electrodesiccation.[325,345,351] There may be a higher response rate and faster time to healing with curettage and electrodesiccation versus cryotherapy.[345]

Carbon dioxide laser treatments and photodynamic therapy have also been used with success.[308,314,315,601-606] The concern with many of these treatments is that there is no pathologic specimen and that in hair-bearing areas, where involvement of the hair follicle may extend into the subcutis, these more superficial treatments may leave behind residual disease.[575,607] Surgical excision or micrographic surgical excision is the treatment of choice for many because the disease may be excised, the margins evaluated, and deeper extension of disease also treated.[608-613] Control of margins may be difficult to assess clinically, and micrographic excision may be needed.[614] Alternative therapies include radiotherapy,[615] intralesional 5-FU,[567] and interferon.[616] The most cost-effective treatments for small lesions are surgical excision and curettage-electrodesiccation; photodynamic therapy is the most expensive.[617]

Merkel Cell Carcinoma of the Skin

Merkel cell carcinoma of the skin is an aggressive tumor first described in 1972 and named trabecular carcinoma (Fig. 116-24).[618,619] It is currently believed that trabecular cancer originates from the cutaneous mechanoreceptor of the skin, the Merkel cell, although the true cell of origin is unknown.[620] Because of the presence of neurosecretory granules in these tumors, it is also called small cell carcinoma of the skin.[621,622] Merkel cell cancers have both neuroendocrine and epithelial features.[623,624] This tumor is unusual, and only about 2000 have been reported in the literature.[625]

CLINICAL AND HISTOLOGIC FEATURES

These unusual tumors present about 50% of the time in sun-exposed areas in the head and neck region, 40% in the trunk, and 10% in multiple other locations.[620] The male-to-female ratio is equal, and these patients are usually elderly, but it has affected a variety of ages.[620,623,626] It usually presents as a rapidly growing, reddish or bluish nodule.[620] Ulceration is not usually seen. It occurs more frequently in immunosuppressed patients.[627,628] In rare circumstances, Merkel cell carcinoma will present as a metastatic lymph node with no known primary.[626] Because of its nonspecific appearance, diagnosis is not usually established until biopsy. Merkel cell cancers are difficult to differentiate on light microscopy alone, and electron microscopy or immunohistochemistry is frequently required to differentiate these tumors from melanomas, metastatic small cell tumors, or lymphomas (Fig. 116-25).[629,630]

TREATMENT

It has been difficult to randomize treatment pathways for this rare disease; therefore, treatment relies heavily on opinions.[631] Multimodality treatment is necessary for these aggressive cancers.[626,632] Wide surgical excision with 2- to 3-cm margins is the traditional mainstay of treatment.[633] These wide excision margins may be difficult to achieve in the head and neck area, and wide field radiotherapy to the primary site and draining lymph nodes is an excellent supplement to surgery.[418,634] Micrographic excision has also been used for this cancer.[635,636]

Lymphadenectomy is necessary for clinically involved nodes, which are present about 15% of the time on initial diagnosis, followed by postoperative radiotherapy.[31,637] Adjuvant radiation of the tumor site is associated with diminished local recurrence.[626] Patients with inoperable disease or who refuse treatment may be treated with radiotherapy alone because this tumor is quite radiosensitive.[634]

Lymphoscintigraphy, lymphatic mapping, and sentinel node biopsy are alternatives to lymphadenectomy in node-negative individuals. Preoperative lymphoscintigraphy will usually demonstrate the lymph nodes at risk for metastases.[638] Technetium Tc 99m is injected intradermally at the cancerous site. Gamma camera photographs of the drainage area localize the sentinel nodes, and the skin over these nodes is

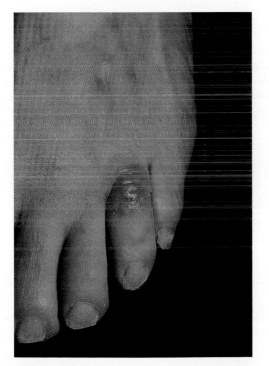

FIGURE 116-24. Merkel cell carcinoma (primary neuroendocrine carcinoma) presenting as a rapidly growing, violaceous nodule on the toe. (From Argenyi ZB: Neural and neuroendocrine neoplasms [other than neurofibromatosis]. In Bolognia JL, Jorizzo JL, Rapini RP, eds: Dermatology. London, Mosby, 2003:1843-1861.)

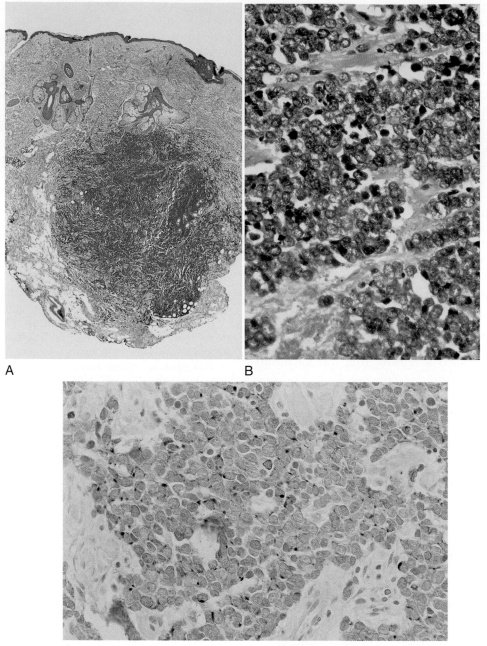

FIGURE 116-25. Primary neuroendocrine carcinoma of the skin (Merkel cell carcinoma). *A,* Dermal nodule with infiltrating borders. *B,* Anaplastic tumor cells with round to ovoid shape, scant nuclei, and fine chromatin pattern. *C,* Biopsy specimens of Merkel cell carcinoma stained for certain keratins, such as keratin 20, have a characteristic perinuclear dot pattern. (From Argenyi ZB: Neural and neuroendocrine neoplasms [other than neurofibromatosis]. In Bolognia JL, Jorizzo JL, Rapini RP, eds: Dermatology. London, Mosby, 2003:1843-1861.)

marked. At surgery, 1% isosulfan blue dye is injected into the tumor area; the blue-stained node is usually under the skin marked at lymphoscintigraphy, or a gamma probe can identify residual [99m]Tc. The nodes are excised and submitted for specimen examination.

Node-negative patients may be observed for further radiotherapy to the primary site. Node-positive patients require a lymphadenectomy plus further radiotherapy.[637] Multiple centers are reporting success with these types of treatments.[633,639-642]

RESULTS

Overall 5-year survival is 34% to 68%.[620,643] Lymph node metastasis found at initial presentation reduces survival by 50%.[644] Metastatic disease is a poor prognostic factor, but there have been cases of spontaneous regression.[636] Localized disease has a median survival of 97 months; the presence of lymph node metastasis decreases survival to 15 months.[626]

Local recurrence after primary excision occurs in 24% to 44% of patients.[620] Local recurrences should be managed aggressively because up to 50% may remain disease free. Overall 5-year survival rate is 74%.[645] Two thirds of patients with recurrent local or regional disease do not survive.[31]

Large tumors with high mitotic rates and small cell size are associated with worse prognosis.[646] Tumors of the trunk do worse than tumors of the head and neck.[632,634] Because of its similarity to small cell cancer of the lung, adjuvant chemotherapy is recommended.[647,648] Response rate of metastatic disease to chemotherapy is high but transient in nature and with no clear improvement in survival.[633,648,649]

Other Variants of Squamous Cell Carcinoma of the Skin

Carcinoma of the lip is the most common form of cancer of the mucous membranes. SCCs of the lip, beyond sun exposure, are caused by chronic nicotine exposure, poor dental hygiene, chronic heat exposure, and immunosuppression. Leukoplakia is a predisposing lesion.[650,651] Leukoplakia is a flat, whitish, micronodular or smooth plaque that develops ulceration only when the base of the mucosa is violated by growth and thus transformation to an invasive SCC. Erythroplakia is bright red oral plaques of a velvet texture. These have a higher risk of malignant transformation than does leukoplakia.[652,653]

Cervical lymph node involvement is usually 10% at the time of presentation with an increase to 20% if the SCC involves the oral commissure. Increasing size and anaplasia of lip cancers are correlated with an increased incidence of metastases.[654,655] For lower lip SCCs more than 2 cm in diameter, sentinel node evaluation is a strong consideration.[654] After tumor resection, subsequent cervical extension may occur in up to 16% of patients.[654]

SCCs also grow in the periungual and subungual areas, the latter possibly representing transformation of a papillomavirus wart. Multiple biopsies may be necessary for correct diagnosis of the condition.[656]

Verrucous carcinoma most commonly appears on the plantar surface as a plaque-like wart (Figs. 116-26 and 116-27). Because of its slow growth and benign warty appearance, the mean duration of lesions was 13 years in one series.[657] These tumors rarely metastasize[658] but are locally invasive.

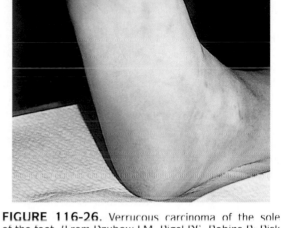

FIGURE 116-26. Verrucous carcinoma of the sole of the foot. (From Dzubow LM, Rigel DS, Robins P: Risk factors for local recurrence of primary cutaneous squamous cell carcinomas. Treatment by microscopically controlled excision. Arch Dermatol 1982;118:900-902.)

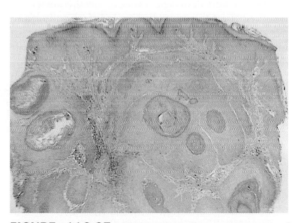

FIGURE 116-27. Histopathologic appearance of verrucous carcinoma showing the characteristic papillomatosis, hyperkeratosis, and acanthosis of the epidermis. This is a low-grade, well-differentiated neoplasm. (From Dzubow LM, Rigel DS, Robins P: Risk factors for local recurrence of primary cutaneous squamous cell carcinomas. Treatment by microscopically controlled excision. Arch Dermatol 1982;118:900-902.)

Detection of tumor cells within a thick hyperkeratotic layer may be difficult. Because of the hyperkeratosis, these tumors are resistant to cryotherapy or desiccation and curettage. The use of radiotherapy for these tumors may cause anaplastic transformation.[659] Others disagree, and radiation therapy is currently more widely used.[660-665] The other areas susceptible to verrucous carcinomas are the oral cavity and genitalia.[666] In the mouth, they may present as blisters, ulcers, or leukoplakia.[667] These variants of SCC are locally invasive but rarely metastasize.[668] Verrucous carcinoma is thought to be triggered by the human papillomavirus.[669]

Giant condylomas of the genital regions are called Buschke-Löwenstein tumors. These lesions form a continuum from condyloma acuminatum to full-blown SCC.[670] Excision of these tumors reveals carcinoma or carcinoma in situ in approximately 30% to 50% of cases.[670,671] These tumors may represent transformation into SCCs of viral warts, especially human papillomavirus types 16 and 18.[672,673] These tumors grow slowly, invade deeply, and may require extensive scalpel extirpation.[670,674]

Particular location of SCCs in areas of embryonal fusion planes demonstrates increased aggressive growth potential in such planes and a higher potential for metastasis. These areas include periauricular, nasal alar–cheek junctions, medial canthus, periorbital areas, and others.[675]

As previously discussed, actinic keratoses may lead to the development of SCCs. Within the subgroup of actinic keratoses, there are variants. Actinic cheilitis represents sun-damaged mucosa of the lower lip (pointedly not the upper lip) with diffuse scaling and hyperkeratosis, fissuring, and varying degrees of inflammation. This lesion may be mistaken for chronic dermatitis and warrants, during the course of surveillance, multiple shave or small punch biopsies to rule out invasive SCC. Treatment of actinic cheilitis should include scalpel vermilionectomy, carbon dioxide laser therapy, cryotherapy, or application of 5-FU.[676]

Disseminated superficial actinic porokeratoses are circumscribed, slightly keratotic papules appearing more commonly in women on the sun-exposed areas of the legs.[677] On histologic examination, focal dysplasia develops a column of parakeratosis (retention of the nuclei) in the stratum corneum characteristically called the coronoid lamella. This lesion is rarely associated with SCC.[219]

Lichenoid keratoses are precancerous red solitary lesions that are related to prolonged sun exposure. They most frequently occur on the extremities and may mimic BCCs. Clinically, they look much like actinic keratosis, but the histologic features are characteristic of lichen planus.[577]

These lesions may have a great deal of epidermal dysplasia with a pronounced lymphohistiocytic inflammatory infiltrate impinging on the basal and lower spiny layer of the epidermis. Lichenoid keratosis may involute spontaneously.[678]

METASTATIC BASAL AND SQUAMOUS CELL CANCERS

Both basal cell and squamous cell cancers have the potential to metastasize. It is exceedingly rare for BCCs to metastasize. Fewer than 300 are reported in the literature. The reasons for this are unknown. The accepted criteria for diagnosis of metastatic BCCs were first proposed by Lattes and Kessler[679]: the primary tumor arises from the skin; metastasis must be at a distant site and not due to tumor extension; histologic similarity between the primary and metastatic tumors must exist; and the metastasis must contain BCC.

Basal Cell Metastasis

Large studies show that the risk for BCC metastasis is about 0.1%.[680] However, many small lesions treated in private practice are never reported or referred. Even though BCCs are the most common malignant neoplasms in humans, metastatic BCC is exceedingly rare. The existence of areas of squamous differentiation in 15% of both primary and metastatic lesions of BCC compounds the problem of the true metastatic BCC.[681] Even giant BCC (>8 cm) present for years rarely metastasizes, although overall survival in these patients, even with surgery, is only 31 months.[464]

INCIDENCE AND CLINICAL FINDINGS

Several factors contribute to the incidence of metastatic BCC. Previous radiation therapy is the most significant factor in metastatic BCCs.[682] In addition, these tumors tend to be large and have proved to be refractory to previous treatment.

The primary tumor tends to arise from the head and neck area consistent with the normal locations for BCCs. Unusual locations for BCCs may have a higher risk.[683-688] Patients with metastatic BCCs tend to be men (2:1 ratio over women) with a median age at presentation of 45 years. The median interval between the onset of original tumor and the first metastasis is 9 years. Survival after diagnosis is only about 8 months after the first sign of metastasis.[681] Tumors that metastasize arise in locations similar to other BCCs.[681]

Syndromes and conditions associated with metastatic BCC include basal cell nevus syndrome, immunosuppression, and systemic amyloidosis.[689-693] An analysis of four metastatic BCCs identified trisomy 6 in all of them.[694]

TREATMENT

Treatment is surgery or radiation therapy. Chemotherapy has a poor prognosis, but cisplatin-based combination chemotherapy is the usual modality of treatment.[695]

Squamous Cell Metastasis

SCCs of the head, neck, or mucous membranes frequently metastasize if they are left untreated. However, pure SCCs of the skin metastasize at a low frequency, depending on the reporting and referral patterns of the study. The risk for metastasis of SCC depends on whether it arises from skin or mucous membranes. For primary skin SCCs, the metastatic risk is about 1% to 3%[88,696]; for primary mucosal SCCs, such as on the lip, the risk is about 8%.[697]

INCIDENCE AND CLINICAL FINDINGS

The overall incidence varies between 0.5% and 7%.[698-700] Czarnecki,[69] in a prospective study, found a 5.8% metastasis risk for SCCs of the skin. Metastatic risk from mucosal SCCs of the lip, a high-risk location, varies between 7.2% and 13.7%,[698] with an average of 8%.[697] Lund[701] studied SCC metastasis in dermatologists' offices and noted a rate of metastasis of 1.2%.

Potential risk factors for metastasis are multiple. These "high-risk" factors have been examined and outlined by multiple authors.[78,102,465] A landmark study by Rowe and Day[88] critically evaluated decades of studies for the metastatic potential of SCCs.

Factors of the patient that relate to a higher risk of metastasis include scar cancers, previous sites of irradiation, immunosuppression, location of the cancer, and recurrent tumors.[31,702] Scar carcinomas have a metastatic rate as high as 38% to 49%[494,514] and are discussed earlier in this chapter. Previous irradiation is associated with high metastatic risk both for those who received the treatment for acne and for those who have a squamous cell recurrence after previous radiotherapy. Patients with immunosuppression not only have a higher risk for development of squamous cell cancers but also are at higher risk for these cancers to metastasize.[90,703-706] Large tumors in immunosuppressed patients are at especially high risk for metastasis.[702]

Primary tumors arising in the oral commissure, lip, or ear are associated with a higher risk for metastasis. The lip is well known to have an increased risk for development of metastatic SCCs.[88,707,708] The oral commissure has the highest risk.[709] Other high-risk locations are the ears,[698,710] temple, dorsum of hands,[707]

scrotum,[711] penis,[712,713] and anus.[714] Cancers arising at these sites need evaluation of draining lymph nodes as part of the examination. In certain high-risk areas, such as the penis or lip, sentinel node evaluation may be necessary.[654,715]

Tumor factors for metastatic risk are size, depth, ulceration, and certain locations. Tumor size has been studied extensively, although depth of penetration, as for melanoma, may be a greater predictor of risk.[74] SCCs with a diameter of more than 2 cm have a metastatic rate of 30%.[88] Lip SCCs that metastasize are large and average 3.7 cm in diameter.[88] Another potential high-risk finding for metastasis is tumor ulceration.[716]

Microstaging of SCCs, as in melanomas, shows valuable prognostic information.[592] Depth of dermal penetration (Clark levels) is also a significant risk factor for metastasis of SCCs.[717,718] Invasion to Clark level IV or V has a high risk for metastasis.[74,466,718,719] Penetration of SCCs can also be measured in millimeters similar to the Breslow measurements in melanoma.[716] Those SCCs less that 4 mm in depth have a metastatic rate of 7% versus 46% for those that penetrated deeper than 4 mm.[720] In fact, only lesions greater than 4 mm recurred, and mortality resulted only from lesions deeper than 10 mm.[720] Another study evaluating tumors of the lip found that those deeper than 6 mm had a metastasis rate of 77%.[708] One study noted that all lesions causing mortality from lip cancers penetrated more than 10 mm.[708] SCCs with narrow penetration (<2 mm) have almost no risk of metastasis.[592] Other studies using the Breslow information have shown the Clark levels to be more predictive.[717]

HISTOLOGY

Histologic factors also make the risk for recurrence of certain SCCs high. The large review by Rowe et al[88] showed that the metastatic rate of poorly differentiated SCCs was 33% versus 9% for well-differentiated SCCs. Multivariate analysis has confirmed that poorly differentiated SCCs have increased local-regional recurrence.[721] Specific high-risk histologic findings include anaplastic, adenoid, spindle cell, and desmoplastic subtype squamous cells.[88,722,723] Desmoplastic SCCs of the skin are very high risk; they are six times more likely to metastasize (23% risk versus 4% overall risk) and have a much higher rate of local recurrence.[724]

LYMPH NODE EVALUATION AND THERAPEUTIC IMPLICATIONS

Patients with high-risk lesions at a minimum must undergo clinical evaluation of draining lymph nodes during the physical examination. Elective prophylactic lymph node dissections are rarely indicated for the treatment of basal or squamous cell skin cancers. Certain high-risk areas such as the lip, large size, or recurrence may warrant this approach.[725] A better method is sentinel node evaluation.[654,726,727] However, therapeutic lymph node dissection is indicated for node-positive lesions.[728] Sentinel lymph node analysis is a useful adjunct to treatment of SCCs of the lip larger than 2 cm.[654]

Lymph node metastases may arise during the period after treatment of the original cancer. In lip cancers, 5% to 13% of patients who initially presented as node negative subsequently develop adenopathy; this risk rises to 30% in locally recurrent lip cancer.[697]

TREATMENT

Surgery or radiotherapy is the recommended treatment of metastatic SCC. When squamous cell regional metastases are found at the initial evaluation, aggressive treatment is necessary. Multiple lesions are usually treated by nodal dissection followed by postoperative radiotherapy.[468,729,730] The parotid is a frequent location for metastatic SCCs, and parotidectomies are frequently needed in treatment of large tumors in the parotid and ear areas.[729,731] Evaluation by careful palpation or magnetic resonance imaging is necessary.

Conclusion

The mean survival rate for metastatic BCC after initial diagnosis is only 8 months.[681] Patients with operable SCC metastases have a mean survival of 53.8 months compared with the mean survival of 12.2 months for inoperable disease.[465] Cumulative 5-year survival in another series was 61% after surgery for metastases.[732]

DISCLAIMER

Tables 116-10 and 116-13 to 116-20 and Figures 116-10 and 116-11 adapted with permission from The NCCN 1.2004 Basal and Squamous Cell Skin Cancer Guidelines, *The Complete Library of NCCN Clinical Practice Guidelines in Oncology* [CD-ROM]. Jenkintown, Pennsylvania: © National Comprehensive Cancer Network, March 2005. To view the most recent and complete version of the guidelines, go online to www.nccn.org.

These Guidelines are a work in progress that will be refined as often as new significant data become available.

The NCCN Guidelines are a statement of consensus of its authors regarding their views of currently accepted approaches to treatment. Any clinician seeking to apply or consult any NCCN guideline is expected to use independent medical judgment in the context of individual circumstances to determine any patient's care or treatment. The National Comprehensive Cancer Network makes no warranties of any kind whatsoever regarding their content, use or application and disclaims any responsibility for their application or use in any way.

REFERENCES

1. Jenson AB, Geyer S, Sundberg JP, Ghim S: Human papillomavirus and skin cancer. J Invest Dermatol 2001;6:203-206.
2. Harwood CA, McGregor JM, Proby CM, Breuer J: Human papillomavirus and the development of non-melanoma skin cancer. J Clin Pathol 1999;52:249-253.
3. Fitzpatrick TB: The validity and practicality of sun-reactive skin types I through VI. Arch Dermatol 1988;124:869-871.
4. Fitzpatrick TB: The skin cancer cascade: from ozone depletion to melanoma—some definitions and some new interpretation, 1996. J Dermatol 1996;23:816-820.
5. Schwartz RA: Premalignant keratinocytic neoplasms. J Am Acad Dermatol 1996;35(pt 1):223-242.
6. Hutchinson J: Arsenic cancer. Br Med J 1887;2:1280.
7. Tromovitch TA, Stegman SJ: Microscopically controlled excision of skin tumors. Arch Dermatol 1974;110:231-232.
8. Stegman SJ, Tromovitch TA: Fresh tissue chemosurgery for tumors of the nose. Eye Ear Nose Throat Mon 1976;55:26-30, 32.
9. Leffell DJ, Brash DE: Sunlight and skin cancer. Sci Am 1996;275:52-53, 56-59.
10. Vitasa BC, Taylor HR, Strickland PT, et al: Association of non-melanoma skin cancer and actinic keratosis with cumulative solar ultraviolet exposure in Maryland watermen. Cancer 1990;65:2811-2817.
11. Forbes PD: Photocarcinogenesis: an overview. J Invest Dermatol 1981;77:139-143.
12. Cockerell CJ: Histopathology of incipient intraepidermal squamous cell carcinoma ("actinic keratosis"). J Am Acad Dermatol 2000;42(pt 2):11-17.
13. Marks R: Epidemiology of non-melanoma skin cancer and solar keratoses in Australia: a tale of self-immolation in Elysian fields. Australas J Dermatol 1997;38(suppl 1):S26-S29.
14. Dodson JM, DeSpain J, Hewett JE, Clark DP: Malignant potential of actinic keratoses and the controversy over treatment. A patient-oriented perspective. Arch Dermatol 1991;127:1029-1031.
15. Montgomery H, Dorffel J: Verruca senilis und keratoma senile. Arch Dermatol Syph (Berlin) 1939;29:387-408.
16. Green A, Beardmore G, Hart V, et al: Skin cancer in a Queensland population. J Am Acad Dermatol 1988;19:1045-1052.
17. Callen JP: Squamous cell carcinoma of the skin. Prim Care 1978;5:299-311.
18. Ponten F, Lundeberg J: Principles of tumor biology and pathogenesis of BCCs and SCCs. In Bolognia JL, Jorizzo JL, Rapini RP, eds: Dermatology. London, Mosby, 2003:1663-1676.
19. Harris CC: Molecular epidemiology of basal cell carcinoma. J Natl Cancer Inst 1996;88:315-317.
20. Drake LA, Ceilley RI, Cornelison RL, et al: Guidelines of care for actinic keratoses. Committee on Guidelines of Care. J Am Acad Dermatol 1995;32:95-98.
21. Moy RL: Clinical presentation of actinic keratoses and squamous cell carcinoma. J Am Acad Dermatol 2000;42(pt 2):8-10.
22. Silverstone H, Gordon D: Regional studies in skin cancer. 2. Wet tropical and subtropical coasts of Queensland. Med J Aust 1966;2:733-740.
23. Abel EA, Cox AJ, Farber EM: Epidermal dystrophy and actinic keratoses in psoriasis patients following oral psoralen photochemotherapy (PUVA). Follow-up study. J Am Acad Dermatol 1982;7:333-340.

24. Jerant AF, Johnson JT, Sheridan CD, Caffrey TJ: Early detection and treatment of skin cancer. Am Fam Physician 2000;62:357-368, 375-376, 381-382.

25. Sober AJ, Burstein JM: Precursors to skin cancer. Cancer 1995;75(suppl):645-650.

26. Marks VJ: Actinic keratosis. A premalignant skin lesion. Otolaryngol Clin North Am 1993;26:23-35.

27. Gloster HM Jr, Brodland DG: The epidemiology of skin cancer. Dermatol Surg 1996;22:217-226.

28. Rady P, Scinicariello F, Wagner RF Jr, Tyring SK: p53 mutations in basal cell carcinomas. Cancer Res 1992;52:3804-3806.

29. Ziegler A, Leffell DJ, Kunala S, et al: Mutation hotspots due to sunlight in the p53 gene of nonmelanoma skin cancers. Proc Natl Acad Sci USA 1993;90:4216-4220.

30. van der Riet P, Karp D, Farmer E, et al: Progression of basal cell carcinoma through loss of chromosome 9q and inactivation of a single p53 allele. Cancer Res 1994;54:25-27.

31. Skidmore RA Jr, Flowers FP: Nonmelanoma skin cancer. Med Clin North Am 1998;82:1309-1323, vi.

32. Grodstein F, Speizer FE, Hunter DJ: A prospective study of incident squamous cell carcinoma of the skin in the nurses' health study. J Natl Cancer Inst 1995;87:1061-1066.

33. Reizner GT, Chuang TY, Elpern DJ, et al: Basal cell carcinoma in Kauai, Hawaii: the highest documented incidence in the United States. J Am Acad Dermatol 1993;29(pt 1):184-189.

34. Miller SJ, Moresi M: Actinic keratosis, basal cell carcinoma and squamous cell carcinoma. In Bolognia JL, Jorizzo JL, Rapini RP, eds: Dermatology. London, Mosby, 2003:1677-1696.

35. Stern RS: The mysteries of geographic variability in nonmelanoma skin cancer incidence. Arch Dermatol 1999;135:843-844.

36. Altman A, Rosen T, Tschen JA, et al: Basal cell epithelioma in black patients. J Am Acad Dermatol 1987;17(pt 1):741-745.

37. Halder RM, Bang KM: Skin cancer in blacks in the United States. Dermatol Clin 1988;6:397-405.

38. Scotto J, Fears TR, Fraumeni JF: Incidence of Non-Melanoma Skin Cancer in the United States. Bethesda, Md, U.S. Dept. of Health and Human Services, National Institutes of Health, 1983. NIH publication no. 83-2433.

39. Halder RM, Bridgeman-Shah S: Skin cancer in African Americans. Cancer 1995;75(suppl):667-673.

40. Munyao TM, Othieno Abinya NA: Cutaneous basal cell carcinoma in Kenya. East Afr Med J 1999;76:97-100.

41. Johnson TM, Rowe DE, Nelson BR, Swanson NA: Squamous cell carcinoma of the skin (excluding lip and oral mucosa). J Am Acad Dermatol 1992;26(pt 2):467-484.

42. Chorun L, Norris JE, Gupta M: Basal cell carcinoma in blacks: a report of 15 cases. Ann Plast Surg 1994;33:90-95.

43. Suchniak JM, Baer S, Goldberg LH: High rate of malignant transformation in hyperkeratotic actinic keratoses. J Am Acad Dermatol 1997;37(pt 1):392-394.

44. English DR, Armstrong BK, Kricker A, et al: Demographic characteristics, pigmentary and cutaneous risk factors for squamous cell carcinoma of the skin: a case-control study. Int J Cancer 1998;76:628-634.

45. Green A, Battistutta D: Incidence and determinants of skin cancer in a high-risk Australian population. Int J Cancer 1990;46:356-361.

46. Davis MM, Hanke CW, Zollinger TW, et al: Skin cancer in patients with chronic radiation dermatitis. J Am Acad Dermatol 1989;20:608-616.

47. Marks R, Jolley D, Dorevitch AP, Selwood TS: The incidence of non-melanocytic skin cancers in an Australian population: results of a five-year prospective study. Med J Aust 1989; 150:475-478.

48. Stenbeck KD, Balanda KP, Williams MJ, et al: Patterns of treated non-melanoma skin cancer in Queensland—the region with the highest incidence rates in the world. Med J Aust 1990;153:511-515.

49. Hogan DJ, To T, Gran L, et al: Risk factors for basal cell carcinoma. Int J Dermatol 1989;28:591-594.

50. Chuang TY, Popescu A, Su WP, Chute CG: Basal cell carcinoma. A population-based incidence study in Rochester, Minnesota. J Am Acad Dermatol 1990;22:413-417.

51. Chuang TY, Reizner GT, Elpern DJ, et al: Nonmelanoma skin cancer in Japanese ethnic Hawaiians in Kauai, Hawaii: an incidence report. J Am Acad Dermatol 1995;33:422-426.

52. Cox NH: Basal cell carcinoma in young adults. Br J Dermatol 1992;127:26-29.

53. Dahl E, Aberg M, Rausing A, Rausing EL: Basal cell carcinoma. An epidemiologic study in a defined population. Cancer 1992;70:104-108.

54. Hogan DJ, Lane PR: Re: A prospective study of incident squamous cell carcinoma of the skin in the Nurses' Health Study. J Natl Cancer Inst 1996;88:56.

55. Harvey I, Frankel S, Marks R, et al: Non-melanoma skin cancer and solar keratoses. I. Methods and descriptive results of the South Wales Skin Cancer Study. Br J Cancer 1996;74:1302-1307.

56. Diepgen TL, Mahler V: The epidemiology of skin cancer. Br J Dermatol 2002;146(suppl 61):1-6.

57. Espana A, Redondo P, Fernandez AL, et al: Skin cancer in heart transplant recipients. J Am Acad Dermatol 1995;32:458-465.

58. Foote JA, Harris RB, Giuliano AR, et al: Predictors for cutaneous basal—and squamous—cell carcinoma among actinically damaged adults. Int J Cancer 2001;95:7-11.

59. Green A, Battistutta D, Hart V, et al: Skin cancer in a subtropical Australian population: incidence and lack of association with occupation. The Nambour Study Group. Am J Epidemiol 1996;144:1034-1040.

60. Karagas MR, Stukel TA, Greenberg ER, et al: Risk of subsequent basal cell carcinoma and squamous cell carcinoma of the skin among patients with prior skin cancer. Skin Cancer Prevention Study Group. JAMA 1992;267:3305-3310.

61. Harris RB, Griffith K, Moon TE: Trends in the incidence of nonmelanoma skin cancers in southeastern Arizona, 1985-1996. J Am Acad Dermatol 2001;45:528-536.

62. Reizner GT, Chuang TY, Elpern DJ, et al: Bowen's disease (squamous cell carcinoma in situ) in Kauai, Hawaii. A population based incidence report. J Am Acad Dermatol 1994;31:596-600.

63. Berg D, Otley CC: Skin cancer in organ transplant recipients: epidemiology, pathogenesis, and management. J Am Acad Dermatol 2002;47:1-17, quiz 18-20.

64. Ron E, Preston DL, Kishikawa M, et al: Skin tumor risk among atomic-bomb survivors in Japan. Cancer Causes Control 1998;9:393-401.

65. Sadamori N, Mine M, Honda T: Incidence of skin cancer among Nagasaki atomic bomb survivors. J Radiat Res (Tokyo) 1991;32(suppl 2):217-225.

66. Urbach F: Incidence of nonmelanoma skin cancer. Dermatol Clin 1991;9:751-755.

67. Miller DL, Weinstock MA: Nonmelanoma skin cancer in the United States: incidence. J Am Acad Dermatol 1994;30(pt 1):774-778.

68. Preston DS, Stern RS: Nonmelanoma cancers of the skin. N Engl J Med 1992;327:1649-1662.

69. Czarnecki D, Collins N, Meehan C, et al: Squamous cell carcinoma in southern and northern Australia. Int J Dermatol 1992;31:492-493.

70. Katz AD, Urbach F, Lilienfeld AM: The frequency and risk of metastases in squamous cell carcinoma of the skin. Cancer 1957;10:1162-1166.

71. Harvey RA, Chaglassian T, Knapper W, Goulian D: Squamous cell carcinoma of the skin in adolescence. Report of a case. JAMA 1977;238:513.

72. Aubry F, MacGibbon B: Risk factors of squamous cell carcinoma of the skin. A case-control study in the Montreal region. Cancer 1985;55:907-911.

73. Miller RW: Delayed effects of external radiation exposure: a brief history. Radiat Res 1995;144:160-169.

74. Kwa RE, Campana K, Moy RL: Biology of cutaneous squamous cell carcinoma. J Am Acad Dermatol 1992;26:1-26.

75. Stern RS, Lunder EJ: Risk of squamous cell carcinoma and methoxsalen (psoralen) and UV-A radiation (PUVA). A meta-analysis. Arch Dermatol 1998;134:1582-1585.

76. Katz KA, Marcil I, Stern RS: Incidence and risk factors associated with a second squamous cell carcinoma or basal cell carcinoma in psoralen + ultraviolet A light–treated psoriasis patients. J Invest Dermatol 2002;118:1038-1043.

77. Marks R, Staples M, Giles GG: Trends in non-melanocytic skin cancer treated in Australia: the second national survey. Int J Cancer 1993;53:585-590.

78. Chuang TY, Popescu NA, Su WP, Chute CG: Squamous cell carcinoma. A population-based incidence study in Rochester, Minn. Arch Dermatol 1990;126:185-188.

79. Weinstock MA: Nonmelanoma skin cancer mortality in the United States, 1969 through 1988. Arch Dermatol 1993;129:1286-1290.

80. Osterlind A, Hjalgrim H, Kulinsky B, Frentz G: Skin cancer as a cause of death in Denmark. Br J Dermatol 1991;125:580-582.

81. Berg D, Otley CC: Skin cancer in organ transplant recipients: epidemiology, pathogenesis, and management. J Am Acad Dermatol 2002;47:1-17.

82. Otley CC, Pittelkow MR: Skin cancer in liver transplant recipients. Liver Transpl 2000;6:253-262.

83. Fortina AB, Caforio AL, Piaserico S, et al: Skin cancer in heart transplant recipients: frequency and risk factor analysis. J Heart Lung Transplant 2000;19:249-255.

84. Ramsay HM, Fryer AA, Reece S, et al: Clinical risk factors associated with nonmelanoma skin cancer in renal transplant recipients. Am J Kidney Dis 2000;36:167-176.

85. Wang CY, Brodland DG, Su WP: Skin cancers associated with acquired immunodeficiency syndrome. Mayo Clin Proc 1995;70:766-772.

86. de Villiers EM, Lavergne D, McLaren K, Benton EC: Prevailing papillomavirus types in non-melanoma carcinomas of the skin in renal allograft recipients. Int J Cancer 1997;73:356-361.

87. Euvrard S, Kanitakis J, Pouteil-Noble C, et al: Comparative epidemiologic study of premalignant and malignant epithelial cutaneous lesions developing after kidney and heart transplantation. J Am Acad Dermatol 1995;33(pt 1):222-229.

88. Rowe DE, Carroll RJ, Day CL Jr: Prognostic factors for local recurrence, metastasis, and survival rates in squamous cell carcinoma of the skin, ear, and lip. Implications for treatment modality selection. J Am Acad Dermatol 1992;26:976-990.

89. Penn I: Tumors after renal and cardiac transplantation. Hematol Oncol Clin North Am 1993;7:431-445.

90. Euvrard S, Kanitakis J, Pouteil-Noble C, et al: Aggressive squamous cell carcinomas in organ transplant recipients. Transplant Proc 1995;27:1767-1768.

91. Gandara Rey J, Garcia Garcia A, Blanco Carrion A, et al: Cellular immune alterations in fifty-two patients with oral lichen planus. Med Oral 2001;6:246-262.

92. Gooptu C, Marks N, Thomas J, James MP: Squamous cell carcinoma associated with lupus vulgaris. Clin Exp Dermatol 1998;23:99-102.

93. Miyagawa S, Minowa R, Yamashina Y, et al: Development of squamous cell carcinoma in chronic discoid lupus erythematosus: a report of two patients with anti-Ro/SSA antibodies. Lupus 1996;5:630-632.

94. Sherman RN, Lee CW, Flynn KJ: Cutaneous squamous cell carcinoma in black patients with chronic discoid lupus erythematosus. Int J Dermatol 1993;32:677-679.

95. Powell JJ, Wojnarowska F: Lichen sclerosus. Lancet 1999;353:1777-1783.

96. Gawkrodger DJ, Stephenson TJ, Thomas SE: Squamous cell carcinoma complicating lichen planus: a clinico-pathological study of three cases. Dermatology 1994;188:36-39.

97. Weber F, Bauer JW, Sepp N, et al: Squamous cell carcinoma in junctional and dystrophic epidermolysis bullosa. Acta Derm Venereol 2001;81:189-192.

98. Bosch RJ, Gallardo MA, Ruiz del Portal G, et al: Squamous cell carcinoma secondary to recessive dystrophic epidermolysis bullosa: report of eight tumours in four patients. J Eur Acad Dermatol Venereol 1999;13:198-204.

99. Bastin KT, Steeves RA, Richards MJ: Radiation therapy for squamous cell carcinoma in dystrophic epidermolysis bullosa: case reports and literature review. Am J Clin Oncol 1997;20:55-58.

100. Powell J, Robson A, Cranston D, et al: High incidence of lichen sclerosus in patients with squamous cell carcinoma of the penis. Br J Dermatol 2001;145:85-89.

101. Kinlen LJ: Incidence of cancer in rheumatoid arthritis and other disorders after immunosuppressive treatment. Am J Med 1985;78:44-49.

102. Alam M, Ratner D: Cutaneous squamous-cell carcinoma. N Engl J Med 2001;344:975-983.

103. Hannuksela-Svahn A, Pukkala E, Karvonen J: Basal cell skin carcinoma and other nonmelanoma skin cancers in Finland from 1956 through 1995. Arch Dermatol 1999;135:781-786.

104. Bang KM, Halder RM, White JE, et al: Skin cancer in black Americans: a review of 126 cases. J Natl Med Assoc 1987;79:51-58.

105. Weinstock MA: Death from skin cancer among the elderly: epidemiological patterns. Arch Dermatol 1997;133:1207-1209.

106. Fewkes J: Do dark-skinned people get skin cancer? Skin Cancer Found J 1999;33-34.

107. Hoy WE: Nonmelanoma skin carcinoma in Albuquerque, New Mexico: experience of a major health care provider. Cancer 1996;77:2489-2495.

108. Gorlin RJ: Nevoid basal cell carcinoma syndrome. Dermatol Clin 1995;13:113-125.

109. Shanley S, Ratcliffe J, Hockey A, et al: Nevoid basal cell carcinoma syndrome: review of 118 affected individuals. Am J Med Genet 1994;50:282-290.

110. Evans DG, Farndon PA, Burnell LD, et al: The incidence of Gorlin syndrome in 173 consecutive cases of medulloblastoma. Br J Cancer 1991;64:959-961.

111. Kimonis VE, Goldstein AM, Pastakia B, et al: Clinical manifestations in 105 persons with nevoid basal cell carcinoma syndrome. Am J Med Genet 1997;69:299-308.

112. McKenna DB, Murphy GM: Skin cancer chemoprophylaxis in renal transplant recipients: 5 years of experience using low-dose acitretin. Br J Dermatol 1999;140:656-660.

113. Grossman L: Epidemiology of ultraviolet-DNA repair capacity and human cancer. Environ Health Perspect 1997;105(suppl 4):927-930.

114. Rahbari H, Mehregan AH: Basal cell epithelioma (carcinoma) in children and teenagers. Cancer 1982;49:350-353.

115. Epstein E Jr: Genetic determinants of basal cell carcinoma risk. Med Pediatr Oncol 2001;36:555-558.

116. Gorlin RJ: Nevoid basal cell carcinoma (Gorlin) syndrome: unanswered issues. J Lab Clin Med 1999;134:551-552.

117. Bazex A, Dupre A, Christol B: Genodermatose complexe de type indeterminé associant une hypotrichose, un etat atrophodermique generalise et des degenerescences cutanees multiples (epitheliomes basocellulaires). Bull Soc Fr Dermatol Syphiligr 1964;71:206-209.

118. Hauck RM, Manders EK: Familial syndromes with skin tumor markers. Ann Plast Surg 1994;33:102-111.

119. Buxtorf K, Hubscher E, Panizzon R: Bazex syndrome. Dermatology 2001;202:350-352.

120. Bolognia JL: Bazex syndrome: acrokeratosis paraneoplastica. Semin Dermatol 1995;14:84-89.

121. Michaelsson G, Olsson E, Westermark P: The Rombo syndrome: a familial disorder with vermiculate atrophoderma, milia, hypotrichosis, trichoepitheliomas, basal cell carcinomas and peripheral vasodilation with cyanosis. Acta Derm Venereol 1981;61:497-503.

122. Johnson SC, Bennett RG: Occurrence of basal cell carcinoma among multiple trichoepitheliomas. J Am Acad Dermatol 1993;28(pt 2):322-326.

123. Ashinoff R, Jacobson M, Belsito DV: Rombo syndrome: a second case report and review. J Am Acad Dermatol 1993;28:1011-1014.

124. van Steensel MA, Jaspers NG, Steijlen PM: A case of Rombo syndrome. Br J Dermatol 2001;144:1215-1218.

125. Alessi E, Sala F: Nevus sebaceus. A clinicopathologic study of its evolution. Am J Dermatopathol 1986;8:27-31.

126. Alessi E, Wong SN, Advani HH, Ackerman AB: Nevus sebaceus is associated with unusual neoplasms. An atlas. Am J Dermatopathol 1988;10:116-127.

127. Morioka S: The natural history of nevus sebaceus. J Cutan Pathol 1985;12:200-213.

128. Person JR, Bentkover S, Longcope C: Androgen receptors are increased in nevus sebaceus. J Am Acad Dermatol 1986;15:120-122.

129. Dunkin CS, Abouzeid M, Sarangapani K: Malignant transformation in congenital sebaceous naevi in childhood. J R Coll Surg Edinb 2001;46:303-306.

130. Smith KJ, Barrett TL, Skelton HG: Tumors arising in nevus sebaceus. J Am Acad Dermatol 2001;45:791-792, discussion 794.

131. Cribier B, Scrivener Y, Grosshans E: Tumors arising in nevus sebaceus: a study of 596 cases. J Am Acad Dermatol 2000;42(pt 1):263-268.

132. Massa LR, Stone MS: An unusual hematopoietic proliferation seen in a nevus sebaceous. J Am Acad Dermatol 2000;42(pt 2):881-882.

133. Bonvalet D, Barrandon Y, Foix C, Civatte J: Benign adnexal tumors of late occurrence in verrucoid-sebaceous nevus (Jadassohn). Apropos of 7 cases [in French]. Ann Dermatol Venereol 1983;110:337-342.

134. Li DF, Iwasaki H, Kikuchi M, et al: Dermatofibroma: superficial fibrous proliferation with reactive histiocytes. A multiple immunostaining analysis. Cancer 1994;74:66-73.

135. McKenna KE, Somerville JE, Walsh MY, et al: Basal cell carcinoma occurring in association with dermatofibroma. Dermatology 1993;187:54-57.

136. Rahbari H, Mehregan AH: Adnexal displacement and regression in association with histiocytoma (dermatofibroma). J Cutan Pathol 1985;12:94-102.

137. Han KH, Huh CH, Cho KH: Proliferation and differentiation of the keratinocytes in hyperplastic epidermis overlying dermatofibroma: immunohistochemical characterization. Am J Dermatopathol 2001;23:90-98.

138. Willis D, Rapini RP, Chernosky ME: Linear basal cell nevus. Cutis 1990;46:493-494.

139. Aloi FG, Tomasini CF, Isaia G, Grazia Bernengo M: Unilateral linear basal cell nevus associated with diffuse osteoma cutis, unilateral anodontia, and abnormal bone mineralization. J Am Acad Dermatol 1989;20(pt 2):973-978.

140. Curry SS, Gaither DH, King LE Jr: Squamous cell carcinoma arising in dissecting perifolliculitis of the scalp. A case report and review of secondary squamous cell carcinomas. J Am Acad Dermatol 1981;4:673-678.

141. Kraemer KH, Lee MM, Scotto J: Xeroderma pigmentosum. Cutaneous, ocular, and neurologic abnormalities in 830 published cases. Arch Dermatol 1987;123:241-250.

142. Cleaver JE, Bootsma D: Xeroderma pigmentosum: biochemical and genetic characteristics. Annu Rev Genet 1975;9:19-38.

143. Kraemer KH, Lee MM, Andrews AD, Lambert WC: The role of sunlight and DNA repair in melanoma and nonmelanoma skin cancer. The xeroderma pigmentosum paradigm. Arch Dermatol 1994;130:1018-1021.

144. van Steeg H, Kraemer KH: Xeroderma pigmentosum and the role of UV-induced DNA damage in skin cancer. Mol Med Today 1999;5:86-94.

145. Goyal JL, Rao VA, Srinivasan R, Agrawal K: Oculocutaneous manifestations in xeroderma pigmentosa. Br J Ophthalmol 1994;78:295-297.

146. King RA, Summers CG: Albinism. Dermatol Clin 1988;6:217-228.

147. Oetting WS, King RA: Molecular basis of oculocutaneous albinism. J Invest Dermatol 1994;103(suppl):131S-136S.

148. Lookingbill DP, Lookingbill GL, Leppard B: Actinic damage and skin cancer in albinos in northern Tanzania: findings in 164 patients enrolled in an outreach skin care program. J Am Acad Dermatol 1995;32:653-658.

149. Perry PK, Silverberg NB: Cutaneous malignancy in albinism. Cutis 2001;67:427-430.

150. Okoro AN: Albinism in Nigeria. A clinical and social study. Br J Dermatol 1975;92:485-492.

151. Luande J, Henschke CI, Mohammed N: The Tanzanian human albino skin. Natural history. Cancer 1985;55:1823-1828.

152. Lutzner MA: Epidermodysplasia verruciformis. An autosomal recessive disease characterized by viral warts and skin cancer. A model for viral oncogenesis. Bull Cancer 1978;65:169-182.

153. Lutzner MA: Papillomaviruses and skin cancer in Africa. IARC Sci Publ 1984;3:607-623.

154. Majewski S, Jablonska S: Do epidermodysplasia verruciformis human papillomaviruses contribute to malignant and benign epidermal proliferations? Arch Dermatol 2002;138:649-654.

155. Surentheran T, Harwood CA, Spink PJ, et al: Detection and typing of human papillomaviruses in mucosal and cutaneous biopsies from immunosuppressed and immunocompetent patients and patients with epidermodysplasia verruciformis: a unified diagnostic approach. J Clin Pathol 1998;51:606-610.

156. Cooper KD, Androphy EJ, Lowy D, Katz SI: Antigen presentation and T-cell activation in epidermodysplasia verruciformis. J Invest Dermatol 1990;94:769-776.

157. Majewski S, Malejczyk J, Jablonska S, et al: Natural cell-mediated cytotoxicity against various target cells in patients with epidermodysplasia verruciformis. J Am Acad Dermatol 1990;22:423-427.

158. Lutzner MA, Blanchet-Bardon C, Orth G: Clinical observations, virologic studies, and treatment trials in patients with epidermodysplasia verruciformis, a disease induced by specific human papillomaviruses. J Invest Dermatol 1984;83(suppl):18s-25s.

159. Kaspar T, Wagner RF Jr, Jablonska S, et al: Prognosis and treatment of advanced squamous cell carcinoma secondary to epidermodysplasia verruciformis: a worldwide analysis of 11 patients. J Dermatol Surg Oncol 1991;17:237-240.

160. Horn HM, Tidman MJ: The clinical spectrum of dystrophic epidermolysis bullosa. Br J Dermatol 2002;146:267-274.

161. Eady RA: Epidermolysis bullosa: scientific advances and therapeutic challenges. J Dermatol 2001;28:638-640.

162. Ciccarelli AO, Rothaus KO, Carter DM, Lin AN: Plastic and reconstructive surgery in epidermolysis bullosa: clinical experience with 110 procedures in 25 patients. Ann Plast Surg 1995;35:254-261.

163. McGrath JA, Schofield OM, Mayou BJ, et al: Epidermolysis bullosa complicated by squamous cell carcinoma: report of 10 cases. J Cutan Pathol 1992;19:116-123.

164. Choi GS, Lee ES, Kim SC, Lee S: Epidermolysis bullosa acquisita localized to the face. J Dermatol 1998;25:19-22.

165. Briggaman RA, Wheeler CE Jr: Epidermolysis bullosa dystrophica-recessive: a possible role of anchoring fibrils in the pathogenesis. J Invest Dermatol 1975;65:203-211.

166. McGrath JA, Schofield OM, Ishida-Yamamoto A, et al: Cultured keratinocyte allografts and wound healing in severe recessive dystrophic epidermolysis bullosa. J Am Acad Dermatol 1993;29:407-419.

167. Unemori EN, Mauch C, Hoeffler W, et al: Constitutive activation of the collagenase promoter in recessive dystrophic epidermolysis bullosa fibroblasts: role of endogenously activated AP-1. Exp Cell Res 1994;211:212-218.

168. Karelina TV, Hruza GJ, Goldberg GI, Eisen AZ: Localization of 92-kDa type IV collagenase in human skin tumors: comparison with normal human fetal and adult skin. J Invest Dermatol 1993;100:159-165.

169. Ferguson-Smith J: A case of multiple primary squamous-celled carcinomata of the skin in a young man with spontaneous healing. Br J Dermatol 1934;46:267-272.

170. Ferguson-Smith MA, Wallace DC, James ZH, Renwick JH: Multiple self-healing squamous epithelioma. Birth Defects Orig Artic Ser 1971;7:157-163.

171. Rajka G: Multiple keratoacanthoma (self-healing squamous epithelioma according to Ferguson-Smith). Acta Derm Venereol 1971;51:232-233.

172. Krunic AL, Garrod DR, Hunter JA, Clark RE: Desmoglein in multiple self-healing squamous epithelioma of Ferguson-Smith—comparison of staining patterns with actinic keratoacanthoma and squamous cell carcinoma of the skin. Arch Dermatol Res 1998;290:319-324.

173. Fosko SW: Predisposing genetic syndromes and clinical settings. In Miller SJ, Maloney ME, eds: Cutaneous Oncology: Pathophysiology, Diagnosis, and Management. Malden, Mass, Blackwell Science, 1998:457-467.

174. Goudie DR, Yuille MA, Leversha MA, et al: Multiple self-healing squamous epitheliomata (ESS1) mapped to chromosome 9q22-q31 in families with common ancestry. Nat Genet 1993;3:165-169.

175. Thomson MS: A hitherto undescribed familial disease. Br J Dermatol 1923;35:455-462.

176. Vennos EM, James WD: Rothmund-Thomson syndrome. Dermatol Clin 1995;13:143-150.

177. Wang LL, Levy ML, Lewis RA, et al: Clinical manifestations in a cohort of 41 Rothmund-Thomson syndrome patients. Am J Med Genet 2001;102:11-17.

178. Anbari KK, Ierardi-Curto LA, Silber JS, et al: Two primary osteosarcomas in a patient with Rothmund-Thomson syndrome. Clin Orthop 2000;378:213-223.

179. el-Khoury JM, Haddad SN, Atallah NG: Osteosarcomatosis with Rothmund-Thomson syndrome. Br J Radiol 1997;70:215-218.

180. Mohaghegh P, Hickson ID: DNA helicase deficiencies associated with cancer predisposition and premature ageing disorders. Hum Mol Genet 2001;10:741-746.

181. Vasseur F, Delaporte E, Zabot MT, et al: Excision repair defect in Rothmund Thomson syndrome. Acta Derm Venereol 1999;79:150-152.

182. Shinya A, Nishigori C, Moriwaki S, et al: A case of Rothmund-Thomson syndrome with reduced DNA repair capacity. Arch Dermatol 1993;129:332-336.

183. Grant SG, Wenger SL, Latimer JJ, et al: Analysis of genomic instability using multiple assays in a patient with Rothmund-Thomson syndrome. Clin Genet 2000;58:209-215.

184. Cleaver JE: DNA damage and repair in light-sensitive human skin disease. J Invest Dermatol 1970;54:181-95.

185. Fosko SW: Predisposing genetic syndromes and clinical settings. In Miller SJ, Maloney ME, eds: Cutaneous Oncology: Pathophysiology, Diagnosis, and Management. Malden, Mass, Blackwell Science, 1998:457-467.

186. Drachtman RA, Alter BP: Dyskeratosis congenita. Dermatol Clin 1995;13:33-39.

187. Dokal I: Dyskeratosis congenita: recent advances and future directions. J Pediatr Hematol Oncol 1999;21:344-350.

188. Ogden GR, Connor E, Chisholm DM: Dyskeratosis congenita: report of a case and review of the literature. Oral Surg Oral Med Oral Pathol 1988;65:586-591.

189. Caceres-Rios H, Tamayo-Sanchez L, Duran-Mckinster C, et al: Keratitis, ichthyosis, and deafness (KID syndrome): review of the literature and proposal of a new terminology. Pediatr Dermatol 1996;13:105-113.

190. van Steensel MA, van Geel M, Nahuys M, et al: A novel connexin 26 mutation in a patient diagnosed with keratitis-ichthyosis-deafness syndrome. J Invest Dermatol 2002;118:724-727.

191. Hazen PG, Walker AE, Stewart JJ, et al: Keratitis, ichthyosis, and deafness (KID) syndrome: management with chronic oral ketoconazole therapy. Int J Dermatol 1992;31:58-59.

192. Hazen PG, Carney P, Lynch WS: Keratitis, ichthyosis, and deafness syndrome with development of multiple cutaneous neoplasms. Int J Dermatol 1989;28:190-191.

193. Brosh RM Jr, Bohr VA: Roles of the Werner syndrome protein in pathways required for maintenance of genome stability. Exp Gerontol 2002;37:491-506.

194. Duvic M, Lemak NA: Werner's syndrome. Dermatol Clin 1995;13:163-168.

195. Shen J, Loeb LA: Unwinding the molecular basis of the Werner syndrome. Mech Ageing Dev 2001;122:921-944.

196. Tsuchiya H, Tomita K, Ohno M, et al: Werner's syndrome combined with quintuplicate malignant tumors: a case report and review of literature data. Jpn J Clin Oncol 1991;21:135-142.

197. Khraishi M, Howard B, Little H: A patient with Werner's syndrome and osteosarcoma presenting as scleroderma. J Rheumatol 1992;19:810-813.

198. Goto M: Werner's syndrome: from clinics to genetics. Clin Exp Rheumatol 2000;18:760-766.

199. Goto M, Miller RW, Ishikawa Y, Sugano H: Excess of rare cancers in Werner syndrome (adult progeria). Cancer Epidemiol Biomarkers Prev 1996;5:239-246.

200. Yu CE, Oshima J, Fu YH, et al: Positional cloning of the Werner's syndrome gene. Science 1996;272:258-262.

201. Bohr VA, Brosh RM Jr, von Kobbe C, et al: Pathways defective in the human premature aging disease Werner syndrome. Biogerontology 2002;3:89-94.

202. Lilic D: New perspectives on the immunology of chronic mucocutaneous candidiasis. Curr Opin Infect Dis 2002;15:143-147.

203. Kirkpatrick CH: Chronic mucocutaneous candidiasis. Pediatr Infect Dis J 2001;20:197-206.

204. McGurk M, Holmes M: Chronic muco-cutaneous candidiasis and oral neoplasia. J Laryngol Otol 1988;102:643-645.

205. Butturini A, Gale RP, Verlander PC, et al: Hematologic abnormalities in Fanconi anemia: an International Fanconi Anemia Registry study. Blood 1994;84:1650-1655.

206. Alter BP: Aplastic anemia, pediatric aspects. Oncologist 1996;1:361-366.

207. Grompe M, D'Andrea A: Fanconi anemia and DNA repair. Hum Mol Genet 2001;10:2253-2259.

208. Tekin M, Bodurtha JN, Riccardi VM: Cafe au lait spots: the pediatrician's perspective. Pediatr Rev 2001;22:82-90.

209. Oksuzoglu B, Yalcin S: Squamous cell carcinoma of the tongue in a patient with Fanconi's anemia: a case report and review of the literature. Ann Hematol 2002;81:294-298.

210. Somers GR, Tabrizi SN, Tiedemann K, et al: Squamous cell carcinoma of the tongue in a child with Fanconi anemia: a case report and review of the literature. Pediatr Pathol Lab Med 1995;15:597-607.

211. Lustig JP, Lugassy G, Neder A, Sigler E: Head and neck carcinoma in Fanconi's anaemia—report of a case and review of the literature. Eur J Cancer B Oral Oncol 1995;31B:68-72.

212. Cramer SF, Mandel MA, Hauler R, et al: Squamous cell carcinoma arising in a linear epidermal nevus. Arch Dermatol 1981;117:222-224.

213. Levin A, Amazon K, Rywlin AM: A squamous cell carcinoma that developed in an epidermal nevus. Report of a case and a review of the literature. Am J Dermatopathol 1984;6:51-55.
214. Schamroth JM, Zlotogorski A, Gilead L: Porokeratosis of Mibelli. Overview and review of the literature. Acta Derm Venereol 1997;77:207-213.
215. Lozinski AZ, Fisher BK, Walter JB, Fitzpatrick PJ: Metastatic squamous cell carcinoma in linear porokeratosis of Mibelli. J Am Acad Dermatol 1987;16(pt 2):448-451.
216. James WD, Rodman OG: Squamous cell carcinoma arising in porokeratosis of Mibelli. Int J Dermatol 1986;25:389-391.
217. Sarkany I: Porokeratosis mibelli with basal cell epithelioma. Proc R Soc Med 1973;66:435-436.
218. Chernosky ME, Freeman RG: Disseminated superficial actinic porokeratosis (DSAP). Arch Dermatol 1967;96:611-624.
219. Leache A, Soto de Delas J, Vazquez Doval J, et al: Squamous cell carcinoma arising from a lesion of disseminated superficial actinic porokeratosis. Clin Exp Dermatol 1991;16:460-462.
220. Cort DF, Abdel-Aziz AH: Epithelioma arising in porokeratosis of Mibelli. Br J Plast Surg 1972;25:318-28.
221. Reed RJ, Leone P: Porokeratosis—a mutant clonal keratosis of the epidermis. I. Histogenesis. Arch Dermatol 1970;101:340-347.
222. Jacob A: Observations respecting an ulcer of peculiar character which attacks the eyelids and other parts of the face. Dublin Hoop Rep 1827;4:231.
223. Lang PG, Maize JC: Basal cell carcinoma. In Friedman RJ, ed: Cancer of the Skin. Philadelphia, WB Saunders, 1991:35-73.
224. Maloney ME, Jones DB, Sexton FM: Pigmented basal cell carcinoma: investigation of 70 cases. J Am Acad Dermatol 1992;27:74-78.
225. Stern JB, Haupt HM, Smith RR: Fibroepithelioma of Pinkus. Eccrine duct spread of basal cell carcinoma. Am J Dermatopathol 1994;16:585-587.
226. Nguyen AV, Whitaker DC, Frodel J: Differentiation of basal cell carcinoma. Otolaryngol Clin North Am 1993;26:37-56.
227. Goldberg DP: Assessment and surgical treatment of basal cell skin cancer. Clin Plast Surg 1997;24:673-686.
228. Fitzpatrick JE, Whalen EA: Basal cell carcinoma or not? Histological variants and mimics of the most common cutaneous malignancy. Semin Cutan Med Surg 1999;18:15-24.
229. Lowe L, Rapini RP: Newer variants and simulants of basal cell carcinoma. J Dermatol Surg Oncol 1991;17:641-648.
230. Mohs FE, Snow SN, Kivett WT, et al: Anatomic rubber stamps of the face and body to document procedures in dermatologic surgery: one picture is worth a thousand words. J Dermatol Surg Oncol 1990;16:280-291.
231. Miller E: The metabolism and pharmacology of 5-fluorouracil. J Surg Oncol 1971;3:309-315.
232. Wolberg WH: The effect of 5-fluorouracil on DNA-thymine synthesis in human tumors. Cancer Res 1969;29:2137-2144.
233. Klein E, Stoll HL Jr, Milgrom H, et al: Tumors of the skin. XII. Topical 5-fluorouracil for epidermal neoplasms. J Surg Oncol 1971;3:331-349.
234. Stoll HL, Klein E, Case RW: Tumors of the skin. VII. Effects of varying the concentration of locally administered 5-fluorouracil on basal cell carcinoma. J Invest Dermatol 1967;47:219-224.
235. Sherertz EF, McTiernan RG: Topical tretinoin enhances percutaneous absorption of 5-fluorouracil in vitro. J Am Acad Dermatol 1987;17:692-694.
236. Strange PR, Lang PG Jr: Long-term management of basal cell nevus syndrome with topical tretinoin and 5-fluorouracil. J Am Acad Dermatol 1992;27(pt 2):842-845.
237. Brenner S, Wolf R, Dascalu DI: Topical tretinoin treatment in basal cell carcinoma. J Dermatol Surg Oncol 1993;19:264-266.
238. Jansen GT, Dillaha CJ, Honeycutt WM: Bowenoid conditions of the skin: treatment with topical 5-fluorouracil. South Med J 1967;60:185-188.
239. Raaf JH, Krown SE, Pinsky CM, et al: Treatment of Bowen's disease with topical dinitrochlorobenzene and 5-fluorouracil. Cancer 1976;37:1633-1642.
240. Breza T, Taylor R, Eaglstein WH: Noninflammatory destruction of actinic keratoses by fluorouracil. Arch Dermatol 1976;112:1256-1258.
241. Litwin MS, Ryan RF, Reed RJ, Krementz ET: Topical chemotherapy of advanced cutaneous malignancy with 5-fluorouracil creme. J Surg Oncol 1971;3:351-365.
242. Litwin MS, Ryan RF, Ichinose H, et al: Proceedings: use of 5-fluorouracil in the topical therapy of skin cancer: a review of 157 patients. Proc Natl Cancer Conf 1972;7:549-561.
243. Pearlman DL: Weekly pulse dosing: effective and comfortable topical 5-fluorouracil treatment of multiple facial actinic keratoses. J Am Acad Dermatol 1991;25:665-667.
244. Epstein E: Does intermittent "pulse" topical 5-fluorouracil therapy allow destruction of actinic keratoses without significant inflammation? J Am Acad Dermatol 1998;38:77-80.
245. Yamaguchi K, Arai Y, Kanda Y, Akagi K: Germline mutation of dihydropyrimidine dehydrogenese gene among a Japanese population in relation to toxicity to 5-fluorouracil. Jpn J Cancer Res 2001;92:337-342.
246. Bollag W, Holdener EE: Retinoids in cancer prevention and therapy. Ann Oncol 1992;3:513-526.
247. Lotan RM: Squamous differentiation and retinoids. Cancer Treat Res 1995;74:43-72.
248. Sun SY, Lotan R: Retinoids and their receptors in cancer development and chemoprevention. Crit Rev Oncol Hematol 2002;11:41-55.
249. Lotan R, Clifford JL: Nuclear receptors for retinoids: mediators of retinoid effects on normal and malignant cells. Biomed Pharmacother 1991;45:145-156.
250. Lotan R: Squamous cell differentiation markers in normal, premalignant, and malignant epithelium: effects of retinoids. J Cell Biochem Suppl 1993;17F:167-174.
251. Lotan R: Retinoids as modulators of tumor cells invasion and metastasis. Semin Cancer Biol 1991;2:197-208.
252. Zouboulis CC: Retinoids—which dermatological indications will benefit in the near future? Skin Pharmacol Appl Skin Physiol 2001;14:303-315.
253. Saade M, Debahy NE, Houjeily S: Clinical remission of xeroderma pigmentosum-associated squamous cell carcinoma with isotretinoin and chemotherapy: case report. J Chemother 1999;11:313-317.
254. Anolik JH, Di Giovanna JJ, Gaspari AA: Effect of isotretinoin therapy on natural killer cell activity in patients with xeroderma pigmentosum. Br J Dermatol 1998;138:236-241.
255. Kraemer KH: Lessons learned from xeroderma pigmentosum. Photochem Photobiol 1996;63:420-422.
256. Saitou M, Sugai S, Tanaka T, et al: Inhibition of skin development by targeted expression of a dominant-negative retinoic acid receptor. Nature 1995;374:159-162.
257. Peck GL, DiGiovanna JJ, Sarnoff DS, et al: Treatment and prevention of basal cell carcinoma with oral isotretinoin. J Am Acad Dermatol 1988;19(pt 2):176-185.
258. Moshell AN: Prevention of skin cancer in xeroderma pigmentosum with oral isotretinoin. Cutis 1989;43:485-490.
259. DiGiovanna JJ: Retinoid chemoprevention in the high-risk patient. J Am Acad Dermatol 1998;39(pt 3):S82-85.
260. Lippman SM, Kavanagh JJ, Paredes-Espinoza M, et al: 13-cis-Retinoic acid and interferon alpha-2a: effective combination therapy for advanced squamous cell carcinoma of the skin. J Natl Cancer Inst 1992;84:235-241.
261. Jacobs DG, Deutsch NL, Brewer M: Suicide, depression, and isotretinoin: is there a causal link? J Am Acad Dermatol 2001;45:S168-S175.
262. Byrne A, Hnatko G: Depression associated with isotretinoin therapy. Can J Psychiatry 1995;40:567.

263. Citrome L: Safety of Accutane with possible depression. Postgrad Med 1998;104:38.

264. DiGiovanna JJ: Posttransplantation skin cancer: scope of the problem, management, and role for systemic retinoid chemoprevention. Transplant Proc 1998;30:2771-2775, discussion 2776-2778.

265. Horn MA, Gordon KB: Chemoprevention of skin cancer. Cancer Treat Res 2001;106:255-282.

266. Stratton SP: Prevention of non-melanoma skin cancer. Curr Oncol Rep 2001;3:295-300.

267. Peck GL, Gross EG, Butkus D, DiGiovanna JJ: Chemoprevention of basal cell carcinoma with isotretinoin. J Am Acad Dermatol 1982;6(pt 2 suppl):815-823.

268. Watson AB: Preventative effect of etretinate therapy on multiple actinic keratoses. Cancer Detect Prev 1986;9:161-165.

269. Odom R: Managing actinic keratoses with retinoids. J Am Acad Dermatol 1998;39(pt 3):S74-S78.

270. Kelly JW, Sabto J, Gurr FW, Bruce F: Retinoids to prevent skin cancer in organ transplant recipients. Lancet 1991;338:1407.

271. Robinson TA, Kligman AM: Treatment of solar keratoses of the extremities with retinoic acid and 5-fluorouracil. Br J Dermatol 1975;92:703-706.

272. Bhawan J, Gonzalez-Serva A, Nehal K, et al: Effects of tretinoin on photodamaged skin. A histologic study. Arch Dermatol 1991;127:666-672.

273. Fields KA: Skin breakthroughs in the year 2000. Int J Fertil Womens Med 2000;45:175-181.

274. Buechner S, Wernli M, Bachmann F, et al: Intralesional interferon in basal cell carcinoma: how does it work? Recent Results Cancer Res 2002;160:246-250.

275. Tangrea JA, Edwards BK, Taylor PR, et al: Long-term therapy with low-dose isotretinoin for prevention of basal cell carcinoma: a multicenter clinical trial. Isotretinoin-Basal Cell Carcinoma Study Group. J Natl Cancer Inst 1992;84:328-332.

276. Lippman SM, Kalvakolanu DV, Lotan R: Retinoids and interferons in non-melanoma skin cancer. J Investig Dermatol Symp Proc 1996;1:219-222.

277. Dogan B, Harmanyeri Y, Baloglu H, Oztek I: Intralesional alfa-2a interferon therapy for basal cell carcinoma. Cancer Lett 1995;91:215-219.

278. LeGrice P, Baird E, Hodge L: Treatment of basal cell carcinoma with intralesional interferon alpha-2a. N Z Med J 1995;108:206-207.

279. Edwards L, Berman B, Rapini RP, et al: Treatment of cutaneous squamous cell carcinomas by intralesional interferon alfa-2b therapy. Arch Dermatol 1992;128:1486-1489.

280. Wickramasinghe L, Hindson TC, Wacks H: Treatment of neoplastic skin lesions with intralesional interferon. J Am Acad Dermatol 1989;20:71-74.

281. Kowalzick L, Rogozinski T, Wimheuer R, et al: Intralesional recombinant interferon beta-1a in the treatment of basal cell carcinoma: results of an open-label multicentre study. Eur J Dermatol 2002;12:558-561.

282. Shin DM, Glisson BS, Khuri FR, et al: Phase II and biologic study of interferon alfa, retinoic acid, and cisplatin in advanced squamous skin cancer. J Clin Oncol 2002;20:364-370.

283. Schroeder TL, Sengelmann RD: Squamous cell carcinoma in situ of the penis successfully treated with imiquimod 5% cream. J Am Acad Dermatol 2002;46:545-548.

284. Petrow W, Gerdsen R, Uerlich M, et al: Successful topical immunotherapy of bowenoid papulosis with imiquimod. Br J Dermatol 2001;145:1022-1023.

285. Smith KJ, Germain M, Skelton H: Squamous cell carcinoma in situ (Bowen's disease) in renal transplant patients treated with 5% imiquimod and 5% 5-fluorouracil therapy. Dermatol Surg 2001;27:561-564.

286. Hengge UR, Stark R: Topical imiquimod to treat intraepidermal carcinoma. Arch Dermatol 2001;137:709-711.

287. Drehs MM, Cook-Bolden F, Tanzi EL, Weinberg JM: Successful treatment of multiple superficial basal cell carcinomas with topical imiquimod: case report and review of the literature. Dermatol Surg 2002;28:427-429.

288. Stanley MA: Imiquimod and the imidazoquinolones: mechanism of action and therapeutic potential. Clin Exp Dermatol 2002;27:571-577.

289. Syed TA: A review of the applications of imiquimod: a novel immune response modifier. Expert Opin Pharmacother 2001;2:877-882.

290. Beutner KR, Geisse JK, Helman D, et al: Therapeutic response of basal cell carcinoma to the immune response modifier imiquimod 5% cream. J Am Acad Dermatol 1999;41:1002-1007.

291. Hannuksela-Svahn A, Nordal E, Christensen OB: Treatment of multiple basal cell carcinomas in the scalp with imiquimod 5% cream. Acta Derm Venereol 2000;80:381-382.

292. Kagy MK, Amonette R: The use of imiquimod 5% cream for the treatment of superficial basal cell carcinomas in a basal cell nevus syndrome patient. Dermatol Surg 2000;26:577-578, discussion 578-579.

293. Marks R, Gebauer K, Shumack S, et al: Imiquimod 5% cream in the treatment of superficial basal cell carcinoma: results of a multicenter 6-week dose-response trial. J Am Acad Dermatol 2001;44:807-813.

294. Mackenzie-Wood A, Kossard S, de Launey J, et al: Imiquimod 5% cream in the treatment of Bowen's disease. J Am Acad Dermatol 2001;44:462-470.

295. Pehoushek J, Smith KJ: Imiquimod and 5% fluorouracil therapy for anal and perianal squamous cell carcinoma in situ in an HIV-1-positive man. Arch Dermatol 2001;137:14-16.

296. Braun DP, Taylor SG 4th, Harris JE: Modulation of immunity in cancer patients by prostaglandin antagonists. Prog Clin Biol Res 1989;288:439-448.

297. Earnest DL, Hixson LJ, Alberts DS: Piroxicam and other cyclooxygenase inhibitors: potential for cancer chemoprevention. J Cell Biochem Suppl 1992;16I:156-166.

298. Kelloff GJ, Boone CW, Steele VE, et al: Mechanistic considerations in chemopreventive drug development. J Cell Biochem Suppl 1994;20:1-24.

299. Rivers JK, Arlette J, Shear N, et al: Topical treatment of actinic keratoses with 3.0% diclofenac in 2.5% hyaluronan gel. Br J Dermatol 2002;146:94-100.

300. Wolf JE Jr, Taylor JR, Tschen E, Kang S: Topical 3.0% diclofenac in 2.5% hyaluronan gel in the treatment of actinic keratoses. Int J Dermatol 2001;40:709-713.

301. Mason R, Dalton J: Novel topical therapy of solar keratosis. In Moschella SL, ed: Dermatology Update. New York, Elsevier, 2001:1-7.

302. Sibata CH, Colussi VC, Oleinick NL, Kinsella TJ: Photodynamic therapy in oncology. Expert Opin Pharmacother 2001;2:917-927.

303. Leshin B, White WL: Malignant neoplasms of keratinocytes. In Arndt KA, LeBoit PE, Robinson JK, Wintroub BU: Cutaneous Medicine and Surgery: An Integrated Program in Dermatology. Philadelphia, WB Saunders, 1996:1378-1391.

304. Jesionek A, Von Tappeiner H: Zur Behandlung der Hautcarcinome mit fluorescierenden Stoffen. Arch Klin Med 1905;82:223.

305. Hopper C: Photodynamic therapy: a clinical reality in the treatment of cancer. Lancet Oncol 2000;1:212-219.

306. Jeffes EW III, Tang EH: Actinic keratosis. Current treatment options. Am J Clin Dermatol 2000;1:167-179.

307. Jeffes EW, McCullough JL, Weinstein GD, et al: Photodynamic therapy of actinic keratoses with topical aminolevulinic acid hydrochloride and fluorescent blue light. J Am Acad Dermatol 2001;45:96-104.

308. Karrer S, Szeimies RM, Hohenleutner U, Landthaler M: Role of lasers and photodynamic therapy in the treatment of cutaneous malignancy. Am J Clin Dermatol 2001;2:229-237.

309. Grapengiesser S, Ericson M, Gudmundsson F, et al: Pain caused by photodynamic therapy of skin cancer. Clin Exp Dermatol 2002;27:493-497.

310. Kubler AC, Haase T, Staff C, et al: Photodynamic therapy of primary nonmelanomatous skin tumours of the head and neck. Lasers Surg Med 1999;25:60-68.

311. Fink-Puches R, Soyer HP, Hofer A, et al: Long-term follow-up and histological changes of superficial nonmelanoma skin cancers treated with topical delta-aminolevulinic acid photodynamic therapy. Arch Dermatol 1998;134:821-826.

312. Soler AM, Warloe T, Berner A, Giercksky KE: A follow-up study of recurrence and cosmesis in completely responding superficial and nodular basal cell carcinomas treated with methyl 5-aminolaevulinate-based photodynamic therapy alone and with prior curettage. Br J Dermatol 2001;145:467-471.

313. Haller JC, Cairnduff F, Slack G, et al: Routine double treatments of superficial basal cell carcinomas using aminolaevulinic acid-based photodynamic therapy. Br J Dermatol 2000;143:1270-1275.

314. Cappugi P, Campolmi P, Mavilia L, et al: Topical 5-aminolevulinic acid and photodynamic therapy in dermatology: a minireview. J Chemother 2001;13:494-502.

315. Wong TW, Sheu HM, Lee JY, Fletcher RJ: Photodynamic therapy for Bowen's disease (squamous cell carcinoma in situ) of the digit. Dermatol Surg 2001;27:452-456.

316. Thissen MR, Schroeter CA, Neumann HA: Photodynamic therapy with delta-aminolaevulinic acid for nodular basal cell carcinomas using a prior debulking technique. Br J Dermatol 2000;142:338-339.

317. Rifkin R, Reed B, Hetzel F, Chen K: Photodynamic therapy using SnET2 for basal cell nevus syndrome: a case report. Clin Ther 1997;19:639-641.

318. Walter AW, Pivnick EK, Bale AE, Kun LE: Complications of the nevoid basal cell carcinoma syndrome: a case report. J Pediatr Hematol Oncol 1997;19:258-262.

319. Pariser DM, Lowe NJ, Stewart DM, et al: Photodynamic therapy with topical methyl aminolevulinate for actinic keratosis: results of a prospective randomized multicenter trial. J Am Acad Dermatol 2003;48:227-232.

320. Grabski WJ, Salasche SJ, Mulvaney MJ: Razor-blade surgery. J Dermatol Surg Oncol 1990;16:1121-1126.

321. Brooks NA: Curettage and shave excision. A tissue-saving technic for primary cutaneous carcinoma worthy of inclusion in graduate training programs. J Am Acad Dermatol 1984;10(pt 1):279-284.

322. Diwan R, Skouge JW: Basal cell carcinoma. Curr Probl Dermatol 1990;2:70-91.

323. Nouri K, Spencer JM, Taylor JR, et al: Does wound healing contribute to the eradication of basal cell carcinoma following curettage and electrodesiccation? Dermatol Surg 1999;25:183-187, discussion 187-188.

324. Chiller K, Passaro D, McCalmont T, Vin-Christian K: Efficacy of curettage before excision in clearing surgical margins of nonmelanoma skin cancer. Arch Dermatol 2000;136:1327-1332.

325. Sheridan AT, Dawber RP: Curettage, electrosurgery and skin cancer. Australas J Dermatol 2000;41:19-30.

326. Alexiades-Armenakas M, Ramsay D, Kopf AW: The appropriateness of curettage and electrodesiccation for the treatment of basal cell carcinomas. Arch Dermatol 2000;136:800.

327. Nordin P, Larko O, Stenquist B: Five-year results of curettage-cryosurgery of selected large primary basal cell carcinomas on the nose: an alternative treatment in a geographical area underserved by Mohs' surgery. Br J Dermatol 1997;136:180-183.

328. Silverman MK, Kopf AW, Grin CM, et al: Recurrence rates of treated basal cell carcinomas. Part 2. Curettage-electrodesiccation. J Dermatol Surg Oncol 1991;17:720-726.

329. Ratner D, Skouge JW: Surgical management of local disease. In Miller SJ, Maloney ME, eds: Cutaneous Oncology: Pathophysiology, Diagnosis, and Management. Malden, Mass, Blackwell Science, 1998:664-671.

330. Graham GF: Cryosurgery in the management of cutaneous malignancies. Clin Dermatol 2001;19:321-327.

331. Zouboulis CC: Cryosurgery in dermatology. Eur J Dermatol 1998;8:466-474.

332. Kuflik EG: Cryosurgery updated. J Am Acad Dermatol 1994;31:925-944, quiz 944-946.

333. Mazur P: Cryobiology: the freezing of biological systems. Science 1970;168:939-949.

334. Wilkes TD, Fraunfelder FT: Principles of cryosurgery. Ophthalmic Surg 1979;10:21-30.

335. Limmer BL, Clark D: Nonsurgical management of primary skin malignancies. Otolaryngol Clin North Am 1993;26:167-183.

336. Breitbart EW, Schaeg G: Electron microscopic investigations of the cryolesion. Clin Dermatol 1990;8:30-38.

337. Yamada S, Tsubouchi S: Rapid cell death and cell population recovery in mouse skin epidermis after freezing. Cryobiology 1976;13:317-327.

338. Mazur P: Freezing of living cells: mechanisms and implications. Am J Physiol 1984;247(pt 1):C125-C142.

339. Torre D: Cryosurgical instrumentation and depth dose monitoring. Clin Dermatol 1990;8:48-60.

340. Gage AA, Meenaghan MA, Natiella JR, Greene GW Jr: Sensitivity of pigmented mucosa and skin to freezing injury. Cryobiology 1979;16:348-361.

341. Gage AA: What temperature is lethal for cells? J Dermatol Surg Oncol 1979;5:459-460, 464.

342. Torre D: Understanding the relationship between lateral spread of freeze and depth of freeze. J Dermatol Surg Oncol 1979;5:51-53.

343. Torre D: Cryosurgical treatment of epitheliomas using the cone-spray technique. J Dermatol Surg Oncol 1977;3:432-436.

344. Zouboulis CC, Zouridaki E, Rosenberger A, Dalkowski A: Current developments and uses of cryosurgery in the treatment of keloids and hypertrophic scars. Wound Repair Regen 2002;10:98-102.

345. Ahmed I, Berth-Jones J, Charles-Holmes S, et al: Comparison of cryotherapy with curettage in the treatment of Bowen's disease: a prospective study. Br J Dermatol 2000;143:759-766.

346. Wood JR, Anderson RL: Complications of cryosurgery. Arch Ophthalmol 1981;99:460-463.

347. Zacarian SA: Cryosurgery of cutaneous carcinomas. An 18-year study of 3,022 patients with 4,228 carcinomas. J Am Acad Dermatol 1983;9:947-956.

348. Martinez JC, Otley CC: The management of melanoma and nonmelanoma skin cancer: a review for the primary care physician. Mayo Clin Proc 2001;76:1253-1265.

349. Kuflik EG, Gage AA: The five-year cure rate achieved by cryosurgery for skin cancer. J Am Acad Dermatol 1991;24(pt 1):1002-1004.

350. Graham GF, Clark LC: Statistical analysis in cryosurgery of skin cancer. Clin Dermatol 1990;8:101-107.

351. Holt PJ: Cryotherapy for skin cancer: results over a 5-year period using liquid nitrogen spray cryosurgery. Br J Dermatol 1988;119:231-240.

352. Hauben DJ, Zirkin H, Mahler D, Sacks M: The biologic behavior of basal cell carcinoma: analysis of recurrence in excised basal cell carcinoma. Part II. Plast Reconstr Surg 1982;69:110-116.

353. Liu FF, Maki E, Warde P, et al: A management approach to incompletely excised basal cell carcinomas of skin. Int J Radiat Oncol Biol Phys 1991;20:423-428.

354. Gooding CA, White G, Yatsuhashi M: Significance of marginal extension in excised basal-cell carcinoma. N Engl J Med 1965;273:923-924.
355. Pascal RR, Hobby LW, Lattes R, Crikelair GF: Prognosis of "incompletely excised" versus "completely excised" basal cell carcinoma. Plast Reconstr Surg 1968;41:328-332.
356. Rakofsky SI: The adequacy of the surgical excision of basal cell carcinoma. Ann Ophthalmol 1973;5:596-600.
357. Shanoff LB, Spira M, Hardy SB: Basal cell carcinoma: a statistical approach to rational management. Plast Reconstr Surg 1967;39:619-624.
358. Taylor GA, Barisoni D: Ten years' experience in the surgical treatment of basal-cell carcinoma. A study of factors associated with recurrence. Br J Surg 1973;60:522-525.
359. Rowe DE, Carroll RJ, Day CL Jr: Long-term recurrence rates in previously untreated (primary) basal cell carcinoma: implications for patient follow-up. J Dermatol Surg Oncol 1989;15:315-328.
360. Dellon AL, Potvin C, Chretien PB, Rogentine CN: The immunobiology of skin cancer. Plast Reconstr Surg 1975;55:341-354.
361. Richmond JD, Davie RM: The significance of incomplete excision in patients with basal cell carcinoma. Br J Plast Surg 1987;40:63-67.
362. Menn H, Robins P, Kopf AW, Bart RS: The recurrent basal cell epithelioma. A study of 100 cases of recurrent, re-treated basal cell epitheliomas. Arch Dermatol 1971;103:628-631.
363. Rowe DE, Carroll RJ, Day CL Jr: Mohs surgery is the treatment of choice for recurrent (previously treated) basal cell carcinoma. J Dermatol Surg Oncol 1989;15:424-431.
364. McIntosh GS, Osborne DR, Li AK, Hobbs KE: Basal cell carcinoma—a review of treatment results with special reference to cryotherapy. Postgrad Med J 1983;59:698-701.
365. Marchac D, Papadopoulos O, Duport G: Curative and aesthetic results of surgical treatment of 138 basal-cell carcinomas. J Dermatol Surg Oncol 1982;8:379-387.
366. Silverman MK, Kopf AW, Bart RS, et al: Recurrence rates of treated basal cell carcinomas. Part 3. Surgical excision. J Dermatol Surg Oncol 1992;18:471-476.
367. Dubin N, Kopf AW: Multivariate risk score for recurrence of cutaneous basal cell carcinoma. Arch Dermatol 1983;119:373-377.
368. Mehta H: Surgical management of carcinoma of eyelids and periorbital skin. Br J Ophthalmol 1979;63:578-585.
369. Bart RS, Schrager D, Kopf AW, et al: Scalpel excision of basal cell carcinomas. Arch Dermatol 1978;114:739-742.
370. Rigel DS, Robins P, Friedman RJ: Predicting recurrence of basal-cell carcinomas treated by microscopically controlled excision: a recurrence index score. J Dermatol Surg Oncol 1981;7:807-810.
371. Torres A, Seeburger J, Robison D, Glogau R: The reliability of a second biopsy for determining residual tumor. J Am Acad Dermatol 1992;27:70-73.
372. Thissen MR, Neumann MH, Schouten LJ: A systematic review of treatment modalities for primary basal cell carcinomas. Arch Dermatol 1999;135:1177-1183.
373. Boeta-Angeles L, Bennett RG: Features associated with recurrence. In Miller SJ, Maloney ME, eds: Cutaneous Oncology: Pathophysiology, Diagnosis, and Management. Malden, Mass, Blackwell Science, 1998:xxiii, 998.
374. Wolf DJ, Zitelli JA: Surgical margins for basal cell carcinoma. Arch Dermatol 1987;123:340-344.
375. Albright SD III: Treatment of skin cancer using multiple modalities. J Am Acad Dermatol 1982;7:143-171.
376. Macomber WB, Wang MK, Sullivan JG: Cutaneous epithelioma: a study of 853 lesions. Plast Reconstr Surg 1959;24:545-562.
377. Griffith BH, McKinney P: An appraisal of the treatment of basal cell carcinoma of the skin. Plast Reconstr Surg 1973;51:565-571.
378. Bisson MA, Dunkin CS, Suvarna SK, Griffiths RW: Do plastic surgeons resect basal cell carcinomas too widely? A prospective study comparing surgical and histological margins. Br J Plast Surg 2002;55:293-297.
379. Miller SJ: The National Comprehensive Cancer Network (NCCN) guidelines of care for nonmelanoma skin cancers. Dermatol Surg 2000;26:289-292.
380. Brodland DG, Zitelli JA: Surgical margins for excision of primary cutaneous squamous cell carcinoma. J Am Acad Dermatol 1992;27(pt 1):241-248.
381. Johnson TM, Tromovitch TA, Swanson NA: Combined curettage and excision: a treatment method for primary basal cell carcinoma. J Am Acad Dermatol 1991;24:613-617.
382. Dellon AL, DeSilva S, Connolly M, Ross A: Prediction of recurrence in incompletely excised basal cell carcinoma. Plast Reconstr Surg 1985;75:860-871.
383. Dellon AL: Histologic study of recurrent basal cell carcinoma. Plast Reconstr Surg 1985;75:853-859.
384. De Silva SP, Dellon AL: Recurrence rate of positive margin basal cell carcinoma: results of a five-year prospective study. J Surg Oncol 1985;28:72-74.
385. Darmstadt GL, Steinman HK: Mohs' micrographic surgery of the head and neck. West J Med 1990;152:153-158.
386. Drake LA, Dinehart SM, Goltz RW, et al: Guidelines of care for Mohs micrographic surgery. American Academy of Dermatology. J Am Acad Dermatol 1995;33(pt 1):271-278.
387. Swanson NA: Mohs surgery. Technique, indications, applications, and the future. Arch Dermatol 1983;119:761-773.
388. Nelson BR, Railan D, Cohen S: Mohs' micrographic surgery for nonmelanoma skin cancers. Clin Plast Surg 1997;24:705-718.
389. Sussman LA, Liggins DF: Incompletely excised basal cell carcinoma: a management dilemma? Aust N Z J Surg 1996;66:276-278.
390. Koplin L, Zarem HA: Recurrent basal cell carcinoma. A review concerning the incidence, behavior, and management of recurrent basal cell carcinoma, with emphasis on the incompletely excised lesion. Plast Reconstr Surg 1980;65:656-664.
391. Saldanha G, Fletcher A, Slater DN: Basal cell carcinoma: a dermatopathological and molecular biological update. Br J Dermatol 2003;148:195-202.
392. Kumar P, Orton CI, McWilliam LJ, Watson S: Incidence of incomplete excision in surgically treated basal cell carcinoma: a retrospective clinical audit. Br J Plast Surg 2000;53:563-566.
393. Ghauri RR, Gunter AA, Weber RA: Frozen section analysis in the management of skin cancers. Ann Plast Surg 1999;43:156-160.
394. Sexton M, Jones DB, Maloney ME: Histologic pattern analysis of basal cell carcinoma. Study of a series of 1039 consecutive neoplasms. J Am Acad Dermatol 1990;23(pt 1):1118-1126.
395. Griffiths RW: Audit of histologically incompletely excised basal cell carcinomas: recommendations for management by re-excision. Br J Plast Surg 1999;52:24-28.
396. Lewis P: Frederic Mohs, 92, inventor of cancer surgery technique. New York Times 2002:7.
397. de Rosa G, Vetrani A, Zeppa P, et al: Comparative morphometric analysis of aggressive and ordinary basal cell carcinoma of the skin. Cancer 1990;65:544-549.
398. Abide JM, Nahai F, Bennett RG: The meaning of surgical margins. Plast Reconstr Surg 1984;73:492-497.
399. Robins P: Mohs micrographic surgery. In McCarthy JG, ed: Plastic Surgery. Philadelphia, WB Saunders, 1990:3652-3662.
400. Clark D: Cutaneous micrographic surgery. Otolaryngol Clin North Am 1993;26:185-202.
401. Zachary CB, Rest EB, Furlong SM, et al: Rapid cytokeratin stains enhance the sensitivity of Mohs micrographic surgery for squamous cell carcinoma. J Dermatol Surg Oncol 1994;20:530-535.

402. Siegle RJ, MacMillan J, Pollack SV: Infiltrative basal cell carcinoma: a nonsclerosing subtype. J Dermatol Surg Oncol 1986;12:830-836.

403. Dixon AY, Lee SH, McGregor DH: Histologic evolution of basal cell carcinoma recurrence. Am J Dermatopathol 1991;13:241-247.

404. Freeman RG: Histopathologic considerations in the management of skin cancer. J Dermatol Surg 1976;2:215-221.

405. Lang PG Jr, Maize JC: Histologic evolution of recurrent basal cell carcinoma and treatment implications. J Am Acad Dermatol 1986;14(pt 1):186-196.

406. Binstock JH, Stegman SJ, Tromovitch TA: Large, aggressive basal-cell carcinomas of the scalp. J Dermatol Surg Oncol 1981;7:565-569.

407. Gormley DE, Hirsch P: Aggressive basal cell carcinoma of the scalp. Arch Dermatol 1978;114:782-783.

408. Eliezri YD, Cohen PR: Cancer recurrence following Mohs micrographic surgery: a mechanism of tumor persistence. Plast Reconstr Surg 1992;90.121-125.

409. Hunt MJ, Halliday GM, Weedon D, et al: Regression in basal cell carcinoma: an immunohistochemical analysis. Br J Dermatol 1994;130:1-8.

410. Mohs FE, Mikhail GR: Mohs Micrographic Surgery. Philadelphia, WB Saunders, 1991.

411. Mohs FE: Chemosurgery for the microscopically controlled excision of cutaneous cancer. Head Neck Surg 1978;1:150-166.

412. Rapini RP: Potential pitfalls and abuses of Mohs surgery. In Gross GA, Steinman HK, Rapini RP, eds: Mohs Surgery: Fundamentals and Techniques. St. Louis, Mosby, 1999:221-229.

413. Steinman HK: Mohs surgical techniques. In Gross GA, Steinman HK, Rapini RP, eds: Mohs Surgery: Fundamentals and Techniques. St. Louis, Mosby, 1999:49-72.

414. Stegman SJ: Personal communication to W.F. Kivett, 1985.

415. Bennett RG: The meaning and significance of tissue margins. Adv Dermatol 1989;4:343-355, discussion 356-357.

416. Kivett WF: Training in pathology for plastic surgical residents. Plast Reconstr Surg 1991;87:994-995.

417. Parker RG, Withers HR: Principles of radiation oncology. In Haskell CM, ed: Cancer Treatment. Philadelphia, WB Saunders, 1995:23-31.

418. Morrison WH, Garden AS, Ang KK: Radiation therapy for nonmelanoma skin carcinomas. Clin Plast Surg 1997;24:719-729,

419. Shiu MH, Chu F, Fortner JG: Treatment of regionally advanced epidermoid carcinoma of the extremity and trunk. Surg Gynecol Obstet 1980;150:558-562.

420. Everall JD, Dowd PM: Influence of environmental factors excluding ultraviolet radiation on the incidence of skin cancer. Bull Cancer 1978;65:241-247.

421. Casson PR, Robins P: Malignant tumors of the skin. In McCarthy JG, ed: Plastic Surgery. Philadelphia, WB Saunders, 1990:3614-3662.

422. Shore RE, Albert RE, Reed M, et al: Skin cancer incidence among children irradiated for ringworm of the scalp. Radiat Res 1984;100:192-204.

423. Shore RE: Radiation-induced skin cancer in humans. Med Pediatr Oncol 2001;36:549-554.

424. van Vloten WA, Hermans J, van Daal WA: Radiation-induced skin cancer and radiodermatitis of the head and neck. Cancer 1987;59:411-414.

425. Van Daal WA, et al: Radiation-induced head and neck tumours: is the skin as sensitive as the thyroid gland? Eur J Cancer Clin Oncol 1983;19:1081-1086.

426. Conway H, Hugo NE: Radiation dermatitis and malignancy. Plast Reconstr Surg 1966;38:255-268.

427. Mark RJ, Poen J, Tran LM, et al: Postirradiation sarcomas. A single-institution study and review of the literature. Cancer 1994;73:2653-2662.

428. Avril MF, Auperin A, Margulis A, et al: Basal cell carcinoma of the face: surgery or radiotherapy? Results of a randomized study. Br J Cancer 1997;76:100-106.

429. Finizio L, Vidali C, Calacione R, et al: What is the current role of radiation therapy in the treatment of skin carcinomas? Tumori 2002;88:48-52.

430. Silverman MK, Kopf AW, Gladstein AH, et al: Recurrence rates of treated basal cell carcinomas. Part 4. X-ray therapy. J Dermatol Surg Oncol 1992;18:549-554.

431. Reymann F, Kopp H: Treatment of basal cell carcinoma of the skin with ultrasoft X-rays. Dermatologica 1978;156:40-47.

432. Westgate SJ: Radiation therapy for skin tumors. Otolaryngol Clin North Am 1993;26:295-309.

433. Akhtar S, Oza KK, Wright J: Merkel cell carcinoma: report of 10 cases and review of the literature. J Am Acad Dermatol 2000;43(pt 1):755-767.

434. Chuang TY, Brashear R: Risk factors of non-melanoma skin cancer in United States veterans patients: a pilot study and review of literature. J Eur Acad Dermatol Venereol 1999;12:126-132.

435. Karagas MR, McDonald JA, Greenberg ER, et al: Risk of basal cell and squamous cell skin cancers after ionizing radiation therapy. For The Skin Cancer Prevention Study Group. J Natl Cancer Inst 1996;88:1848-1853.

436. Pastore G, Antonelli R, Fine W, et al: Late effects of treatment of cancer in infancy. Med Pediatr Oncol 1982;10:369-375.

437. Gladstein AH: Efficacy, simplicity, and safety of X-ray therapy of basal-cell carcinomas on periocular skin. J Dermatol Surg Oncol 1978;4:586-593.

438. Smith SP, Grande DJ: Basal cell carcinoma recurring after radiotherapy: a unique, difficult treatment subclass of recurrent basal cell carcinoma. J Dermatol Surg Oncol 1991;17:26-30.

439. Cobbett J: Recurrence of rodent ulcers after radiotherapy. Br J Surg 1965;52:947-949.

440. Hayes H: Basal cell carcinoma: the East Grinstead experience. Plast Reconstr Surg 1962;30:273-280.

441. Rank B, Wakefield A: Surgery of basal cell carcinoma. Br J Surg 1958;45:531-547.

442. Churchill-Davidson I, Johnson E: Rodent ulcers: an analysis of 711 lesions treated by radiotherapy. Br Med J 1954;1:1465-1468.

443. Hansen P, Jensen M: Late results following radiotherapy of skin cancer. Acta Radiol Ther Phys Biol 1968;7:307-319.

444. Chen YJ, Kuo JV, Ramsinghani NS, Al-Ghazi MS: Intensity-modulated radiotherapy for previously irradiated, recurrent head-and-neck cancer. Med Dosim 2002;27:171-176.

445. Caccialanza M, Piccinno R, Grammatica A: Radiotherapy of recurrent basal and squamous cell skin carcinomas: a study of 249 re-treated carcinomas in 229 patients. Eur J Dermatol 2001;11:25-28.

446. Fischbach AJ, Sause WT, Plenk HP: Radiation therapy for skin cancer. West J Med 1980;133:379-382.

447. Lovett RD, Perez CA, Shapiro SJ, Garcia DM: External irradiation of epithelial skin cancer. Int J Radiat Oncol Biol Phys 1990;19:235-242.

448. Petrovich Z, Parker RG, Luxton G, et al: Carcinoma of the lip and selected sites of head and neck skin. A clinical study of 896 patients. Radiother Oncol 1987;8:11-17.

449. Locke J, Karimpour S, Young G, et al: Radiotherapy for epithelial skin cancer. Int J Radiat Oncol Biol Phys 2001;51:748-755.

450. Knox JM, Freeman RG, Duncan WC, Heaton CL: Treatment of skin cancer. South Med J 1967;60:241-246.

451. Parker RG: Selective use of radiation therapy for neoplasms of the skin. Clin Plast Surg 1980;7:337-348.

452. Chahbazian CM, Brown GS: Radiation therapy for carcinoma of the skin of the face and neck. Special considerations. JAMA 1980;244:1135-1137.

453. Bart RS, Kopf AW, Gladstein AH: Treatment of morphea-type basal cell carcinomas with radiation therapy. Arch Dermatol 1977;113:783-786.

454. Fitzpatrick PJ, Thompson GA, Easterbrook WM, et al: Basal and squamous cell carcinoma of the eyelids and their treatment by radiotherapy. Int J Radiat Oncol Biol Phys 1984;10:449-454.

455. Mendenhall WM, Parsons JT, Mendenhall NP, et al: Carcinoma of the skin of the head and neck with perineural invasion. Head Neck 1989;11:301-308.

456. Goepfert H, Dichtel WJ, Medina JE, et al: Perineural invasion in squamous cell skin carcinoma of the head and neck. Am J Surg 1984;148:542-547.

457. Veness MJ, Biankin S: Perineural spread leading to orbital invasion from skin cancer. Australas Radiol 2000;44:296-302.

458. McCord MW, Mendenhall WM, Parsons JT, et al: Skin cancer of the head and neck with incidental microscopic perineural invasion. Int J Radiat Oncol Biol Phys 1999;43:591-595.

459. McCord MW, Mendenhall WM, Parsons JT, et al: Skin cancer of the head and neck with clinical perineural invasion. Int J Radiat Oncol Biol Phys 2000;47:89-93.

460. Csaky KG, Custer P: Perineural invasion of the orbit by squamous cell carcinoma. Ophthalmic Surg 1990;21:218-220.

461. Petrovich Z, Kuisk H, Langholz B, et al: Treatment of carcinoma of the skin with bone and/or cartilage involvement. Am J Clin Oncol 1988;11:110-113.

462. Petrovich, Z, Kuisk H, Langholz B, et al: Treatment results and patterns of failure in 646 patients with carcinoma of the eyelids, pinna, and nose. Am J Surg 1987;154:447-450.

463. Yamamoto T, Kurosaka M, Soejima T, Fujii M: Contrast-enhanced three-dimensional helical CT for soft tissue tumors in the extremities. Skeletal Radiol 2001;30:384-387.

464. Thomas WO, Harper LL, Wong SG, et al: Surgical management of giant nonmelanoma skin neoplasia. South Med J 1998;91:190-195.

465. Joseph MG, Zulueta WP, Kennedy PJ: Squamous cell carcinoma of the skin of the trunk and limbs: the incidence of metastases and their outcome. Aust N Z J Surg 1992;62:697-701.

466. Haydon RC III: Cutaneous squamous carcinoma and related lesions. Otolaryngol Clin North Am 1993;26:57-71.

467. Johnson JT, Barnes EL, Myers EN, et al: The extracapsular spread of tumors in cervical node metastasis. Arch Otolaryngol 1981;107:725-729.

468. Olsen KD, Caruso M, Foote RL, et al: Primary head and neck cancer. Histopathologic predictors of recurrence after neck dissection in patients with lymph node involvement. Arch Otolaryngol Head Neck Surg 1994;120:1370-1374.

469. Rothman GB, Eiselle DW: Surgery and radiation therapy for advanced disease. In Miller SJ, Maloney ME, eds: Cutaneous Oncology: Pathophysiology, Diagnosis, and Management. Malden, Mass, Blackwell Science, 1998:553-557.

470. Wilder RB, Kittelson JM, Shimm DS: Basal cell carcinoma treated with radiation therapy. Cancer 1991;68:2134-2137.

471. Medina JE, Byers RM: Supraomohyoid neck dissection: rationale, indications, and surgical technique. Head Neck 1989;11:111-122.

472. Loeffler JS, Larson DA, Clark JR, et al: Treatment of perineural metastasis from squamous carcinoma of the skin with aggressive combination chemotherapy and irradiation. J Surg Oncol 1985;29:181-183.

473. Weiss MH, Harrison LB, Isaacs RS: Use of decision analysis in planning a management strategy for the stage N0 neck. Arch Otolaryngol Head Neck Surg 1994;120:699-702.

474. Taylor BW Jr, Brant TA, Mendenhall NP, et al: Carcinoma of the skin metastatic to parotid area lymph nodes. Head Neck 1991;13:427-433.

475. Jecker P, Hartwein J: Metastasis to the parotid gland: is a radical surgical approach justified? Am J Otolaryngol 1996;17:102-105.

476. Guix B, Finestres F, Tello J, et al: Treatment of skin carcinomas of the face by high-dose-rate brachytherapy and custom-made surface molds. Int J Radiat Oncol Biol Phys 2000;47:95-102.

477. Allan E, Stanton A, Pye D, et al: Fractionated high dose rate brachytherapy moulds—a precise treatment for carcinoma of the pinna. Radiother Oncol 1998;48:277-281.

478. Frankel DH, Hanusa BH, Zitelli JA: New primary nonmelanoma skin cancer in patients with a history of squamous cell carcinoma of the skin. Implications and recommendations for follow-up. J Am Acad Dermatol 1992;26(pt 1):720-726.

479. Hong WK, Lippman SM, Itri LM, et al: Prevention of second primary tumors with isotretinoin in squamous-cell carcinoma of the head and neck. N Engl J Med 1990;323:795-801.

480. Marghoob A, Kopf AW, Bart RS, et al: Risk of another basal cell carcinoma developing after treatment of a basal cell carcinoma. J Am Acad Dermatol 1993;28:22-28.

481. Evans RD, Kopf AW, Lew RA, et al: Risk factors for the development of malignant melanoma—I: review of case-control studies. J Dermatol Surg Oncol 1988;14:393-408.

482. Epstein E: Value of follow-up after treatment of basal cell carcinoma. Arch Dermatol 1973;108:798-800.

483. Silverman MK, Kopf AW, Grin CM, et al: Recurrence rates of treated basal cell carcinomas. Part 1. Overview. J Dermatol Surg Oncol 1991;17:713-718.

484. Dzubow LM, Rigel DS, Robins P: Risk factors for local recurrence of primary cutaneous squamous cell carcinomas. Treatment by microscopically controlled excision. Arch Dermatol 1982;118:900-902.

485. Treves N, Pack GT: The development of cancer in burn scars. Surg Gynecol Obstet 1930;51:749-782.

486. Marjolin JN: Ulcère. In Adelon NP, ed: Dictionnaire de médecine. Paris, Bechet, 1828:31-50.

487. De Costa JC: Carcinomatous changes in an area of chronic, ulceration, or Marjolin's ulcer. Ann Surg 1903;37:496-502.

488. Steffen C: Marjolin's ulcer. Report of two cases and evidence that Marjolin did not describe cancer arising in scars of burns. Am J Dermatopathol 1984;6:187-193.

489. Nancarrow JD: Cicatrial cancer in the South-West of England: a regional plastic surgery unit's experience over a 20-year period. Br J Surg 1983;70:205-208.

490. Fleming MD, Hunt JL, Purdue GF, Sandstad J: Marjolin's ulcer: a review and reevaluation of a difficult problem. J Burn Care Rehabil 1990;11:460-469.

491. Koga Y, Sawada Y: Basal cell carcinoma developing on a burn scar. Burns 1997;23:75-77.

492. Stromberg BV, Klingman R, Schluter WW: Basal cell burn carcinoma. Ann Plast Surg 1990;24:186-188.

493. Novick M, Gard DA, Hardy SB, Spira M: Burn scar carcinoma: a review and analysis of 46 cases. J Trauma 1977;17:809-817.

494. Stromberg BV, Keiter JE, Wray RC, Weeks PM: Scar carcinoma: prognosis and treatment. South Med J 1977;70:821-822.

495. Barr LH, Menard JW: Marjolin's ulcer. The LSU experience. Cancer 1983;52:173-175.

496. Dumurgier C, Pujol G, Chevalley J, et al: Pressure sore carcinoma: a late but fulminant complication of pressure sores in spinal cord injury patients: case reports. Paraplegia 1991;29:390-395.

497. Kaplan RP: Cancer complicating chronic ulcerative and scarifying mucocutaneous disorders. Adv Dermatol 1987;2:19-46.

498. Noodleman FR, Pollack SV: Trauma as a possible etiologic factor in basal cell carcinoma. J Dermatol Surg Oncol 1986;12:841-846.

499. Bostwick J III, Pendergrast WJ Jr, Vasconez LO: Marjolin's ulcer: an immunologically privileged tumor? Plast Reconstr Surg 1976;57:66-69.

500. Castillo J, Goldsmith HS: Burn scar carcinoma. CA Cancer J Clin 1968;18:140-142.

501. Hill LL, Ouhtit A, Loughlin SM, et al: Fas ligand: a sensor for DNA damage critical in skin cancer etiology. Science 1999; 285:898-900.

502. Baliarsing AS: Will Fas gene help to diagnose burn scar squamous cell carcinoma? Plast Reconstr Surg 2001;108:575.

503. Abbas JS, Beecham JE: Burn wound carcinoma: case report and review of the literature. Burns Incl Therm Inj 1988;14:222-224.

504. Sirsat MV, Shrikhande SS: Histopathologic study of the effects of solar radiation on the skin and its relationship to carcinoma. Indian J Cancer 1967;4:185-193.

505. Bartle EJ, Sun JH, Wang XW, Schneider BK: Cancers arising from burn scars. A literature review and report of twenty-one cases. J Burn Care Rehabil 1990;11:46-49.

506. Mosborg DA, Crane RT, Tami TA, Parker GS: Burn scar carcinoma of the head and neck. Arch Otolaryngol Head Neck Surg 1988;114:1038-1040.

507. Turegun M, Nisanci M, Guler M: Burn scar carcinoma with longer lag period arising in previously grafted area. Burns 1997;23:196 197.

508. Chowdri NA, Darzi MA: Postburn scar carcinomas in Kashmiris. Burns 1996;22:477-482.

509. Edwards MJ, Hirsch RM, Broadwater JR, et al: Squamous cell carcinoma arising in previously burned or irradiated skin. Arch Surg 1989;124:115-117.

510. Hahn SB, Kim DJ, Jeon CH: Clinical study of Marjolin's ulcer. Yonsei Med J 1990;31:234-241.

511. Arons MS, Lynch JB, Rodin AE, Lewis SR: Scar tissue carcinoma. II. Special reference to burn scar carcinoma. Surg Forum 1965;16:488-489.

512. Arons MS, Rodin AE, Lynch JB, et al: Scar tissue carcinoma. II. An experimental study with special reference to burn scar carcinoma. Ann Surg 1966;163:445-460.

513. Smith J, Mello LF, Nogueira Neto NC, et al: Malignancy in chronic ulcers and scars of the leg (Marjolin's ulcer): a study of 21 patients. Skeletal Radiol 2001;30:331-337.

514. Lifeso RM, Rooney RJ, el-Shaker M: Post-traumatic squamous-cell carcinoma. J Bone Joint Surg Am 1990;72:12-18.

515. Ames FC, Hickey RC: Squamous cell carcinoma of the skin of the extremities. Int Adv Surg Oncol 1980;3:179-199.

516. Kasse AA, Betel E, Dem A, et al: Cancers in the scars of thermal burns (apropos of 67 cases) [in French]. Dakar Med 1999;44:206-210.

517. Lifeso RM, Bull CA: Squamous cell carcinoma of the extremities. Cancer 1985;55:2862-2867.

518. Rahimizadeh A, Shelton R, Weinberg H, Sadick N: The development of a Marjolin's cancer in a human immunodeficiency virus-positive hemophilic man and review of the literature. Dermatol Surg 1997;23:560-563.

519. Schwartz RA: Keratoacanthoma. J Am Acad Dermatol 1994;30:1-19.

520. Straka BF, Grant-Kels JM: Keratoacanthoma. In Baker D, ed: Cancer of the Skin. Philadelphia, WB Saunders, 1991:390-407.

521. Popkin GL: Tumors of the skin: a dermatologist's viewpoint. In McCarthy JG, ed: Plastic Surgery. Philadelphia, WB Saunders, 1990:3560-3613.

522. Hamm JC, DeFranzo AJ, Argenta LC, White W: Keratoacanthoma necessitating metacarpal amputation. J Hand Surg Am 1990;15:980-986.

523. Hsi ED, Svoboda-Newman SM, Stern RA, et al: Detection of human papillomavirus DNA in keratoacanthomas by polymerase chain reaction. Am J Dermatopathol 1997;19:10-15.

524. Lu S, Syrjanen SL, Havu VK, Syrjanen S: Known HPV types have no association with keratoacanthomas. Arch Dermatol Res 1996;288:129-132.

525. Janecka IP, Wolff M, Crikelair GF, Cosman B: Aggressive histological features of keratoacanthoma. J Cutan Pathol 1977;4:342-348.

526. Kwittken J: A histologic chronology of the clinical course of the keratocarcinoma (so-called keratoacanthoma). Mt Sinai J Med 1975;42:127-135.

527. Goldenhersh MA, Olsen TG: Invasive squamous cell carcinoma initially diagnosed as a giant keratoacanthoma. J Am Acad Dermatol 1984;10(pt 2):372-378.

528. Beham A, Regauer S, Soyer HP, Beham-Schmid C: Keratoacanthoma: a clinically distinct variant of well differentiated squamous cell carcinoma. Adv Anat Pathol 1998;5:269-280.

529. Waring AJ, Takata M, Rehman I, Rees JL: Loss of heterozygosity analysis of keratoacanthoma reveals multiple differences from cutaneous squamous cell carcinoma. Br J Cancer 1996;73:649-653.

530. Chuang TY, Reizner GT, Elpern DJ, et al: Keratoacanthoma in Kauai, Hawaii. The first documented incidence in a defined population. Arch Dermatol 1993;129:317-319.

531. Sullivan JJ: Keratoacanthoma: the Australian experience. Australas J Dermatol 1997;38(suppl 1):S36-S39.

532. Letzel S, Drexler H: Occupationally related tumors in tar refinery workers. J Am Acad Dermatol 1998;39(pt 1):712-720.

533. Cramer SF: Subungual keratoacanthoma. A benign bone-eroding neoplasm of the distal phalanx. Am J Clin Pathol 1981;75:425-429.

534. Cribier B, Asch P, Grosshans E: Differentiating squamous cell carcinoma from keratoacanthoma using histopathological criteria. Is it possible? A study of 296 cases. Dermatology 1999;199:208-212.

535. Godbolt AM, Sullivan JJ, Weedon D: Keratoacanthoma with perineural invasion: a report of 40 cases. Australas J Dermatol 2001;42:168-171.

536. Moriyama M, Watanabe T, Sakamoto N, et al: A case of giant keratoacanthoma of the auricle. Auris Nasus Larynx 2000;27:185-188.

537. de Visscher JG, van der Wal JE, Starink TM, et al: Giant keratoacanthoma of the lower lip. Report of a case of spontaneous regression. Oral Surg Oral Med Oral Pathol Oral Radiol Endod 1996;81:193-196.

538. Saito M, Sasaki Y, Yamazaki N, Shimizu H: Self-involution of giant keratoacanthoma on the tip of the nose. Plast Reconstr Surg 2003;111:1561-1562.

539. Pagani WA, Lorenzi G, Lorusso D: Surgical treatment for aggressive giant keratoacanthoma of the face. J Dermatol Surg Oncol 1986;12:282-284.

540. Hale DS, Dockery GL: Giant keratoacanthoma of the plantar foot: a report of two cases. J Foot Ankle Surg 1993;32:75-84.

541. Goldschmidt H, Sherwin WK: Radiation therapy of giant aggressive keratoacanthomas. Arch Dermatol 1993;129:1162-1165.

542. Edelman BA, Jacobs JB, Rotterdam H, Auerbach R: Giant keratoacanthoma: an atypical presentation. Otolaryngol Head Neck Surg 1990;103:472-475.

543. Schaller M, Korting HC, Wolff H, et al: Multiple keratoacanthomas, giant keratoacanthoma and keratoacanthoma centrifugum marginatum: development in a single patient and treatment with oral isotretinoin. Acta Derm Venereol 1996; 76:40-42.

544. Spieth K, Gille J, Kaufmann R: Intralesional methotrexate as effective treatment in solitary giant keratoacanthoma of the lower lip. Dermatology 2000;200:317-319.

545. Grob JJ, Suzini F, Richard MA, et al: Large keratoacanthomas treated with intralesional interferon alfa-2a. J Am Acad Dermatol 1993;29(pt 1):237-241.

546. Baran R, Goettmann S: Distal digital keratoacanthoma: a report of 12 cases and a review of the literature. Br J Dermatol 1998;139:512-515.

547. Oliwiecki S, Peachey RD, Bradfield JW, et al: Subungual keratoacanthoma—a report of four cases and review of the literature. Clin Exp Dermatol 1994;19:230-235.

548. Cohen PR: Metastatic tumors to the nail unit: subungual metastases. Dermatol Surg 2001;27:280-293.

549. Patel MR, Desai S: Subungual keratoacanthoma in the hand. J Hand Surg Am 1989;14:139-142.

550. Muir EG, Bell AJ, Barlow KA: Multiple primary carcinomata of the colon, duodenum, and larynx associated with keratoacanthomata of the face. Br J Surg 1967;54:191-195.

551. Torre D: Multiple sebaceous tumors. Arch Dermatol 1968;98:549-551.

552. Lynch HT, Leibowitz R, Smyrk T, et al: Colorectal cancer and the Muir-Torre syndrome in a Gypsy family: a review. Am J Gastroenterol 1999;94:575-580.

553. Machin P, et al: Microsatellite instability and immunostaining for MSH-2 and MLH-1 in cutaneous and internal tumors from patients with the Muir-Torre syndrome. J Cutan Pathol 2002;29:415-420.

554. Spielvogel RL, DeVillez RL, Roberts LC: Oral isotretinoin therapy for familial Muir-Torre syndrome. J Am Acad Dermatol 1985;12:475-480.

555. Consigli JE, Gonzalez ME, Morsino R, et al: Generalized eruptive keratoacanthoma (Grzybowski variant). Br J Dermatol 2000;142:800-803.

556. Gjersvik P, Egass E, Clausen OP: Grzybowski's generalized eruptive keratocanthomas: a case report. Eur J Dermatol 2000; 10:135-1358.

557. Grine RC, Hendrix JD, Greer KE: Generalized eruptive keratoacanthoma of Grzybowski: response to cyclophosphamide. J Am Acad Dermatol 1997;36(pt 1):786-787.

558. Street ML, White JW Jr, Gibson LE: Multiple keratoacanthomas treated with oral retinoids. J Am Acad Dermatol 1990;23(pt 1):862-866.

559. Benoldi D, Alinovi A: Multiple persistent keratoacanthomas: treatment with oral etretinate. J Am Acad Dermatol 1984;10: 1035-1038.

560. Sanchez Yus E, Simon P, Requena L, et al: Solitary keratoacanthoma: a self-healing proliferation that frequently becomes malignant. Am J Dermatopathol 2000;22:305-310.

561. Hodak E, Jones RE, Ackerman AB: Solitary keratoacanthoma is a squamous-cell carcinoma: three examples with metastases. Am J Dermatopathol 1993;15:332-342, discussion 343-352.

562. Piscioli F, Boi S, Zumiani G, Cristofolini M: A gigantic, metastasizing keratoacanthoma. Report of a case and discussion on classification. Am J Dermatopathol 1984;6:123-129.

563. Gray RJ, Meland NB: Topical 5-fluorouracil as primary therapy for keratoacanthoma. Ann Plast Surg 2000;44:82-85.

564. Goette DK: Treatment of keratoacanthoma with topical fluorouracil. Arch Dermatol 1983;119:951-953.

565. Peris K, Micantonio T, Fargnoli MC: Successful treatment of keratoacanthoma and actinic keratoses with imiquimod 5% cream. Eur J Dermatol 2003;13:413-414, author reply 415.

566. Dendorfer M, Oppel T, Wollenberg A, Prinz JC: Topical treatment with imiquimod may induce regression of facial keratoacanthoma. Eur J Dermatol 2003;13:80-82.

567. Morse LG, Kendrick C, Hooper D, et al: Treatment of squamous cell carcinoma with intralesional 5-fluorouracil. Dermatol Surg 2003;29:1150-1153, discussion 1153.

568. de Visscher JG, van der Wal KG, Blanken R, Willemse F: Treatment of giant keratoacanthoma of the skin of the lower lip with intralesional methotrexate: a case report. J Oral Maxillofac Surg 2002;60:93-95.

569. de la Torre C, Losada A, Cruces MJ: Keratoacanthoma centrifugum marginatum: treatment with intralesional bleomycin. J Am Acad Dermatol 1997;37:1010-1011.

570. Hurst LN, Gan BS: Intralesional methotrexate in keratoacanthoma of the nose. Br J Plast Surg 1995;48:243-246.

571. Singal A, Mohanty S, Bhattacharya SN, et al: Unusual multiple keratoacanthoma in a child successfully treated with 5-fluorouracil. J Dermatol 1997;24:546-548.

572. Melton JL, Nelson BR, Stough DB, et al: Treatment of keratoacanthomas with intralesional methotrexate. J Am Acad Dermatol 1991;25(pt 1):1017-1023.

573. Parker CM, Hanke CW: Large keratoacanthomas in difficult locations treated with intralesional 5-fluorouracil. J Am Acad Dermatol 1986;14(pt 1):770-777.

574. Sayama S, Tagami H: Treatment of keratoacanthoma with intralesional bleomycin. Br J Dermatol 1983;109:449-452.

575. Grekin RC, Salmon PJ: Surgical management of local disease. In Miller SJ, Maloney ME, eds: Cutaneous Oncology: Pathophysiology, Diagnosis, and Management. Malden, Mass, Blackwell Science, 1998:506-517.

576. Santos-Dias A: CO₂ laser surgery in hemophilia treatment. J Clin Laser Med Surg 1992;10:297-301.

577. Elgart GW: Seborrheic keratoses, solar lentigines, and lichenoid keratoses. Dermatoscopic features and correlation to histology and clinical signs. Dermatol Clin 2001;19:347-357.

578. Maloney ME: Arsenic in dermatology. Dermatol Surg 1996;22:301-304.

579. Guo HR, Yu HS, Hu H, Monson RR: Arsenic in drinking water and skin cancers: cell-type specificity (Taiwan, ROC). Cancer Causes Control 2001;12:909-916.

580. Shannon RL, Strayer DS: Arsenic-induced skin toxicity. Hum Toxicol 1989;8:99-104.

581. Faber M, Hagedorn M: A light and electron microscopic study of bowenoid papulosis. Acta Derm Venereol 1981;61:397-403.

582. Gross G, Hagedorn M, Ikenberg H, et al: Bowenoid papulosis. Presence of human papillomavirus (HPV) structural antigens and of HPV 16-related DNA sequences. Arch Dermatol 1985;121:858-863.

583. Guillet GY, Braun L, Masse R, et al: Bowenoid papulosis. Demonstration of human papillomavirus (HPV) with anti-HPV immune serum. Arch Dermatol 1984;120:514-516.

584. Jaeger AB, Gramkow A, Hjalgrim H, et al: Bowen disease and risk of subsequent malignant neoplasms: a population-based cohort study of 1147 patients. Arch Dermatol 1999;135:790-793.

585. Horn TD, Moresi MM: Histology. In Miller SJ, Maloney ME, eds: Cutaneous Oncology: Pathophysiology, Diagnosis, and Management. Malden, Mass, Blackwell Science, 1998:481-493.

586. Smith KJ, Tuur S, Corvette D, et al: Cytokeratin 7 staining in mammary and extramammary Paget's disease. Mod Pathol 1997;10:1069-1074.

587. Vanstapel MJ, Gatter KC, De Wolf-Peeters C, et al: Immunohistochemical study of mammary and extra-mammary Paget's disease. Histopathology 1984;8:1013-1023.

588. Ragi G, Turner MS, Klein LE, Stoll HL Jr: Pigmented Bowen's disease and review of 420 Bowen's disease lesions. J Dermatol Surg Oncol 1988;14:765-769.

589. Nadji M, Morales AR, Girtanner RE, et al: Paget's disease of the skin. A unifying concept of histogenesis. Cancer 1982;50: 2203-2206.

590. Kariniemi AL, Forsman L, Wahlstrom T, et al: Expression of differentiation antigens in mammary and extramammary Paget's disease. Br J Dermatol 1984;110:203-210.

591. Gatter KC, Pulford KA, Vanstapel MJ, et al: An immunohistological study of benign and malignant skin tumours: epithelial aspects. Histopathology 1984;8:209-227.

592. Breuninger H, Black B, Rassner G: Microstaging of squamous cell carcinomas. Am J Clin Pathol 1990;94:624-627.

593. Cullen SI: Topical fluorouracil therapy for precancers and cancers of the skin. J Am Geriatr Soc 1979;27:529-535.

594. Sturm HM: Bowen's disease and 5-fluorouracil. J Am Acad Dermatol 1979;1:513-522.

595. Bargman H, Hochman J: Topical treatment of Bowen's disease with 5-fluorouracil. J Cutan Med Surg 2003;7:101-105.

596. Danielsen AG, Sand C, Weismann K: Treatment of Bowen's disease of the penis with imiquimod 5% cream. Clin Exp Dermatol 2003;28(suppl 1):7-9.

597. Chen K, Shumack S: Treatment of Bowen's disease using a cycle regimen of imiquimod 5% cream. Clin Exp Dermatol 2003;28(suppl 1):10-12.

598. Wu JK, Siller G, Whitehead K: Treatment of Bowen's disease and basal cell carcinoma of the nose with imiquimod 5% cream. Australas J Dermatol 2003;44:123-125.

599. Redondo P, Lloret P: Topical imiquimod for Bowenoid papulosis in an HIV-positive woman. Acta Derm Venereol 2002;82:212-213.

600. Cook-Bolden F, Weinberg JM: Topical imiquimod 5% cream in the treatment of Bowen's disease of the penis. J Am Acad Dermatol 2002;46:146-147.

601. Allison RR, Mang TS, Wilson BD: Photodynamic therapy for the treatment of nonmelanomatous cutaneous malignancies. Semin Cutan Med Surg 1998;17:153-163.

602. Lee CT, Tham SN, Tan T: Initial experience with CO_2 laser in treating dermatological conditions. Ann Acad Med Singapore 1987;16:713-715.

603. Gerber GS: Carcinoma in situ of the penis. J Urol 1994;151:829-833.

604. Gordon KB, Robinson J: Carbon dioxide laser vaporization for Bowen's disease of the finger. Arch Dermatol 1994;130:1250-1252.

605. Gordon KB, Garden JM, Robinson JK: Bowen's disease of the distal digit. Outcome of treatment with carbon dioxide laser vaporization. Dermatol Surg 1996;22:723-728.

606. Tantikun N: Treatment of Bowen's disease of the digit with carbon dioxide laser. J Am Acad Dermatol 2000;43:1080-1083.

607. Hunter GA, Donald GF, Burry JN: Bowen's disease: a clinical and histological re-evaluation. Australas J Dermatol 1967;9:132-135.

608. Breuninger H, Schaumburg-Lever G: Control of excisional margins by conventional histopathological techniques in the treatment of skin tumours. An alternative to Mohs' technique. J Pathol 1988;154:167-171.

609. Lim JK, Stewart MM, Pennington DG: Microscopically controlled excision of skin cancer. Med J Aust 1992;156:486-488.

610. Marchesa P, Fazio VW, Oliart S, et al: Perianal Bowen's disease: a clinicopathologic study of 47 patients. Dis Colon Rectum 1997;40:1286-1293.

611. Moritz DL, Lynch WS: Extensive Bowen's disease of the penile shaft treated with fresh tissue Mohs micrographic surgery in two separate operations. J Dermatol Surg Oncol 1991;17:374-378.

612. Ongenae K, Van De Kerckhove M, Naeyaert JM: Bowen's disease of the nail. Dermatology 2002;204:348-350.

613. Cleary RK, Schaldenbrand JD, Fowler JJ, et al: Treatment options for perianal Bowen's disease: survey of American Society of Colon and Rectal Surgeons Members. Am Surg 2000;66:686-688.

614. Brown SR, Skinner P, Tidy J, et al: Outcome after surgical resection for high-grade anal intraepithelial neoplasia (Bowen's disease). Br J Surg 1999;86:1063-1066.

615. Panizzon RG: Radiotherapy of skin tumors. Recent Results Cancer Res 2002;160:234-239.

616. Gordon KB, Roenigk HH, Gendleman M: Treatment of multiple lesions of Bowen disease with isotretinoin and interferon alfa. Efficacy of combination chemotherapy. Arch Dermatol 1997;133:691-693.

617. Ramrakha-Jones VS, Herd RM: Treating Bowen's disease: a cost minimization study. Br J Dermatol 2003;148:1167-1172.

618. Toker C: Trabecular carcinoma of the skin. Arch Dermatol 1972;105:107-110.

619. Argenyi ZB: Neural and neuroendocrine neoplasms (other than neurofibromatosis). In Bolognia JL, Jorizzo JL, Rapini RP, eds: Dermatology. London, Mosby, 2003:1843-1861.

620. Haag ML, Glass LF, Fenske NA: Merkel cell carcinoma. Diagnosis and treatment. Dermatol Surg 1995;21:669-683.

621. Sibley RK, Dahl D: Primary neuroendocrine (Merkel cell?) carcinoma of the skin. II. An immunocytochemical study of 21 cases. Am J Surg Pathol 1985;9:109-116.

622. Sibley RK, Dehner LP, Rosai J: Primary neuroendocrine (Merkel cell?) carcinoma of the skin. I. A clinicopathologic and ultrastructural study of 43 cases. Am J Surg Pathol 1985;9:95-108.

623. Gould VE, Moll R, Moll I, et al: Neuroendocrine (Merkel) cells of the skin: hyperplasias, dysplasias, and neoplasms. Lab Invest 1985;52:334-353.

624. Hoefler H, Kerl H, Rauch HJ, Denk H: New immunocytochemical observations with diagnostic significance in cutaneous neuroendocrine carcinoma. Am J Dermatopathol 1984;6:525-530.

625. Gollard R, Weber R, Kosty MP, et al: Merkel cell carcinoma: review of 22 cases with surgical, pathologic, and therapeutic considerations. Cancer 2000;88:1842-1851.

626. Medina-Franco H, Urist MM, Fiveash J, et al: Multimodality treatment of Merkel cell carcinoma: case series and literature review of 1024 cases. Ann Surg Oncol 2001;8:204-208.

627. Boyle F, Pendlebury S, Bell D: Further insights into the natural history and management of primary cutaneous neuroendocrine (Merkel cell) carcinoma. Int J Radiat Oncol Biol Phys 1995;31:315-323.

628. An KP, Ratner D: Merkel cell carcinoma in the setting of HIV infection. J Am Acad Dermatol 2001;45:309-312.

629. Smith PD, Patterson JW: Merkel cell carcinoma (neuroendocrine carcinoma of the skin). Am J Clin Pathol 2001;115(suppl):S68-S78.

630. Gruber S, Wilson L: Merkel cell carcinoma In Miller SJ, Maloney ME, eds: Cutaneous Oncology: Pathophysiology, Diagnosis, and Management. Malden, Mass, Blackwell Science, 1998:710-721.

631. Plunkett TA, Subrumanian R, Leslie MD, Harper PG: Management of Merkel cell carcinoma. Expert Rev Anticancer Ther 2001;1:441-445.

632. Ott MJ, Tanabe KK, Gadd MA, et al: Multimodality management of Merkel cell carcinoma. Arch Surg 1999;134:388-392, discussion 392-393.

633. Coit DG: Merkel cell carcinoma. Ann Surg Oncol 2001;8(suppl):99S-102S.

634. Poulsen M, Harvey J: Is there a diminishing role for surgery for Merkel cell carcinoma of the skin? A review of current management. ANZ J Surg 2002;72:142-146.

635. O'Connor WJ, Roenigk RK, Brodland DG: Merkel cell carcinoma. Comparison of Mohs micrographic surgery and wide excision in eighty-six patients. Dermatol Surg 1997;23:929-933.

636. Connelly TJ, Cribier B, Brown TJ, Yanguas I: Complete spontaneous regression of Merkel cell carcinoma: a review of the 10 reported cases. Dermatol Surg 2000;26:853-856.

637. Bischof M, van Kampen M, Huber P, Wannenmacher M: Merkel cell carcinoma: the role of radiation therapy in general management. Strahlenther Onkol 1999;175:611-615.

638. Zeitouni NC, Cheney RT, Delacure MD: Lymphoscintigraphy, sentinel lymph node biopsy, and Mohs micrographic surgery in the treatment of Merkel cell carcinoma. Dermatol Surg 2000;26:12-18.

639. Ames SE, Krag DN, Brady MS: Radiolocalization of the sentinel lymph node in Merkel cell carcinoma: a clinical analysis of seven cases. J Surg Oncol 1998;67:251-254.

640. Koops HS, Doting MH, de Vries J, et al: Sentinel node biopsy as a surgical staging method for solid cancers. Radiother Oncol 1999;51:1-7.

641. Mehrany K, Otley CC, Weenig RH, et al: A meta-analysis of the prognostic significance of sentinel lymph node status in Merkel cell carcinoma. Dermatol Surg 2002;28:113-117.

642. Petrasch S: Management of hematologic systemic diseases and rare tumor entities with manifestations in the oromaxillofacial area [in German]. Mund Kiefer Gesichtschir 1998;2:172-180.

643. Yiengpruksawan A, Coit DG, Thaler HT, et al: Merkel cell carcinoma. Prognosis and management. Arch Surg 1991;126:1514-1519.

644. Wynne CJ, Kearsley JH: Merkel cell tumor. A chemosensitive skin cancer. Cancer 1988;62:28-31.

645. Allen PJ, Zhang ZF, Coit DG: Surgical management of Merkel cell carcinoma. Ann Surg 1999;229:97-105.

646. Skelton HG, Smith KJ, Hitchcock CL, et al: Merkel cell carcinoma: analysis of clinical, histologic, and immunohistologic features of 132 cases with relation to survival. J Am Acad Dermatol 1997;37(pt 1):734-739.

647. Crown J, Lipzstein R, Cohen S, et al: Chemotherapy of metastatic Merkel cell cancer. Cancer Invest 1991;9:129-132.

648. Lawenda BD, Thiringer JK, Foss RD, Johnstone PA: Merkel cell carcinoma arising in the head and neck: optimizing therapy. Am J Clin Oncol 2001;24:35-42.

649. Queirolo P, Gipponi M, Peressini A, et al: Merkel cell carcinoma of the skin. Treatment of primary, recurrent, and metastatic disease: review of clinical cases. Anticancer Res 1997;17:673-677.

650. Baker SR: Risk factors in multiple carcinomas of the lip. Otolaryngol Head Neck Surg 1980;88:248-251.

651. Scully C, Porter S: Orofacial disease: update for the dental clinical team: 3. White lesions. Dent Update 1999;26:123-129.

652. Casiglia J, Woo SB: A comprehensive review of oral cancer. Gen Dent 2001;49:72-82.

653. Sciubba JJ: Oral cancer. The importance of early diagnosis and treatment. Am J Clin Dermatol 2001;2:239-251.

654. Altinyollar H, Berberoglu U, Celen O: Lymphatic mapping and sentinel lymph node biopsy in squamous cell carcinoma of the lower lip. Eur J Surg Oncol 2002;28:72-74.

655. Zitsch RP III, Park CW, Renner GJ, Rea JL: Outcome analysis for lip carcinoma. Otolaryngol Head Neck Surg 1995;113:589-596.

656. Kopelson PL, Nguyen QH, Moy RL: Verruca vulgaris and radiation exposure are associated with squamous cell carcinoma of the finger. J Dermatol Surg Oncol 1994;20:38-41.

657. McKee PH, Wilkinson JD, Black MM, Whimster IW: Carcinoma (epithelioma) cuniculatum: a clinico-pathological study of nineteen cases and review of the literature. Histopathology 1981;5:425-436.

658. Kao GF, Graham JH, Helwig EB: Carcinoma cuniculatum (verrucous carcinoma of the skin): a clinicopathologic study of 46 cases with ultrastructural observations. Cancer 1982;49:2395-2403.

659. Demian SD, Bushkin FL, Echevarria RA: Perineural invasion and anaplastic transformation of verrucous carcinoma. Cancer 1973;32:395-401.

660. Yoshimura Y, Mishima K, Obara S, et al: Treatment modalities for oral verrucous carcinomas and their outcomes: contribution of radiotherapy and chemotherapy. Int J Clin Oncol 2001;6:192-200.

661. Foroudi F, Turner S: Verrucous scrotal carcinoma: a radioresponsive tumor. J Urol 1999;162:1694-1695.

662. Ferlito A, Rinaldo A, Mannara GM: Is primary radiotherapy an appropriate option for the treatment of verrucous carcinoma of the head and neck? J Laryngol Otol 1998;112:132-139.

663. Jyothirmayi R, Sankaranarayanan R, Varghese C, et al: Radiotherapy in the treatment of verrucous carcinoma of the oral cavity. Oral Oncol 1997;33:124-128.

664. Tharp ME 2nd, Shidnia H: Radiotherapy in the treatment of verrucous carcinoma of the head and neck. Laryngoscope 1995;105(pt 1):391-396.

665. Reinecke L, Thornley AL: Case report: radiotherapy—an effective treatment for vaginal verrucous carcinoma. Br J Radiol 1993;66:375-378.

666. Swanson NA, Taylor WB: Plantar verrucous carcinoma. Literature review and treatment by the Mohs' chemosurgery technique. Arch Dermatol 1980;116:794-797.

667. Kraus FT, Perezmesa C: Verrucous carcinoma. Clinical and pathologic study of 105 cases involving oral cavity, larynx and genitalia. Cancer 1966;19:26-38.

668. Schwartz RA: Verrucous carcinoma of the skin and mucosa. J Am Acad Dermatol 1995;32:1-21, quiz 22-24.

669. Cuesta KH, Palazzo JP, Mittal KR: Detection of human papillomavirus in verrucous carcinoma from HIV-seropositive patients. J Cutan Pathol 1998;25:165-170.

670. Creasman C, Haas PA, Fox TA Jr, Balazs M: Malignant transformation of anorectal giant condyloma acuminatum (Buschke-Loewenstein tumor). Dis Colon Rectum 1989;32:481-487.

671. Trombetta LJ, Place RJ: Giant condyloma acuminatum of the anorectum: trends in epidemiology and management: report of a case and review of the literature. Dis Colon Rectum 2001;44:1878-1886.

672. Greif C, Bauer A, Wigger-Alberti W, Elsner P: Giant condylomata acuminata (Buschke-Lowenstein tumor) [in German]. Dtsch Med Wochenschr 1999;124:962-964.

673. Grussendorf-Conen EI: Anogenital premalignant and malignant tumors (including Buschke-Lowenstein tumors). Clin Dermatol 1997;15:377-388.

674. Rhea WG Jr, Bourgeois BM, Sewell DR: Condyloma acuminata: a fatal disease? Am Surg 1998;64:1082-1087.

675. Panje WR, Ceilley RI: The influence of embryology of the midface on the spread of epithelial malignancies. Laryngoscope 1979;89:1914-1920.

676. Dufresne RG Jr, Curlin MU: Actinic cheilitis. A treatment review. Dermatol Surg 1997;23:15-21.

677. Shumack SP, Commens CA: Disseminated superficial actinic porokeratosis: a clinical study. J Am Acad Dermatol 1989;20:1015-1022.

678. Frigy AF, Cooper PH: Benign lichenoid keratosis. Am J Clin Pathol 1985;83:439-443.

679. Lattes R, Kessler RW: Metastasizing basal cell epithelioma of the skin. Cancer 1951;4:866-878.

680. Sacco M, Mohit-Tabatabai M: Metastatic basal cell carcinoma. Contemp Surg 1994;44:339-342.

681. von Domarus H, Stevens PJ: Metastatic basal cell carcinoma. Report of five cases and review of 170 cases in the literature. J Am Acad Dermatol 1984;10:1043-1060.

682. Snow SN, Sahl W, Lo JS, et al: Metastatic basal cell carcinoma. Report of five cases. Cancer 1994;73:328-335.

683. Feakins RM, Lowe DG: Basal cell carcinoma of the vulva: a clinicopathologic study of 45 cases. Int J Gynecol Pathol 1997;16:319-324.

684. Mizushima J, Ohara K: Basal cell carcinoma of the vulva with lymph node and skin metastasis—report of a case and review of 20 Japanese cases. J Dermatol 1995;22:36-42.

685. Winkelmann SE, Llorens AS: Metastatic basal cell carcinoma of the vulva. Gynecol Oncol 1990;38:138-140.

686. Staley TE, Nieh PT, Ciesielski TE, Cieplinski W: Metastatic basal cell carcinoma of the scrotum. J Urol 1983;130:792-794.

687. Shertz WT, Balogh K: Metastasizing basal cell carcinoma of the nipple. Arch Pathol Lab Med 1986;110:761-762.

688. White WB, Schneiderman H, Sayre JT: Basal cell carcinoma of the anus: clinical and pathological distinction from cloacogenic carcinoma. J Clin Gastroenterol 1984;6:441-446.

689. Murphy KJ: Metastatic basal cell carcinoma with squamous appearances in the naevoid basal cell carcinoma syndrome. Br J Plast Surg 1975;28:331-334.

690. Lichtenstein HL, Lee JC: Amyloidosis associated with metastazing basal cell carcinoma. Cancer 1980;46:2693-2696.

691. Beck HI, Andersen JA, Birkler NE, Ottosen PD: Giant basal cell carcinoma with metastasis and secondary amyloidosis: report of case. Acta Derm Venereol 1983;63:564-567.

692. Berardi RS, Korba J, Melton J, Chen H: Pulmonary metastasis in nevoid basal cell carcinoma syndrome. Int Surg 1991;76:64-66.

693. Winkler PA, Guyuron B: Multiple metastases from basal cell naevus syndrome. Br J Plast Surg 1987;40:528-531.

694. Nangia R, Sait SN, Block AW, Zhang PJ: Trisomy 6 in basal cell carcinomas: Trisomy 6 in basal cell carcinomas correlates with metastatic potential: a dual color fluorescence in situ hybridization study on paraffin sections. Cancer 2001;91:1927-1932.

695. Patel MS, Thigpen JT, Vance RB, et al: Basal cell carcinoma with lung metastasis diagnosed by fine-needle aspiration biopsy. South Med J 1999;92:321-324.

696. Ames FC, Hickey RC: Metastasis from squamous cell skin cancer of the extremities. South Med J 1982;75:920-923, 932.

697. Zitsch RP III: Carcinoma of the lip. Otolaryngol Clin North Am 1993;26:265-277.

698. Bernstein SC, Lim KK, Brodland DG, Heidelberg KA: The many faces of squamous cell carcinoma. Dermatol Surg 1996;22:243-254.

699. Jackson A: Prevention, early detection and team management of skin cancer in primary care: contribution to the health of the nation objectives. Br J Gen Pract 1995;45:97-101.

700. Baker NJ, Webb AA, Macpherson D: Surgical management of cutaneous squamous cell carcinoma of the head and neck. Br J Oral Maxillofac Surg 2001;39:87-90.

701. Lund HZ: How often does squamous cell carcinoma of the skin metastasize? Arch Dermatol 1965;92:635-637.

702. Nguyen P, Vin-Christian K, Ming ME, Berger T: Aggressive squamous cell carcinomas in persons infected with the human immunodeficiency virus. Arch Dermatol 2002;138:758-763.

703. Jensen P, Hansen S, Moller B, et al: Skin cancer in kidney and heart transplant recipients and different long-term immunosuppressive therapy regimens. J Am Acad Dermatol 1999;40(pt 1):177-186.

704. Gupta AK, Cardella CJ, Haberman HF: Cutaneous malignant neoplasms in patients with renal transplants. Arch Dermatol 1986;122:1288-1293.

705. Hoxtell EO, Mandel JS, Murray SS, et al: Incidence of skin carcinoma after renal transplantation. Arch Dermatol 1977;113:436-438.

706. Dinehart SM, Chu DZ, Maners AW, Pollack SV: Immunosuppression in patients with metastatic squamous cell carcinoma from the skin. J Dermatol Surg Oncol 1990;16:271-274.

707. Dinehart SM, Pollack SV: Metastases from squamous cell carcinoma of the skin and lip. An analysis of twenty-seven cases. J Am Acad Dermatol 1989;21(pt 1):241-248.

708. Frierson HF Jr, Cooper PH: Prognostic factors in squamous cell carcinoma of the lower lip. Hum Pathol 1986;17:346-354.

709. Teichgraeber JF, Larson DL: Some oncologic considerations in the treatment of lip cancer. Otolaryngol Head Neck Surg 1988;98:589-592.

710. Estrem SA, Renner GJ: Special problems associated with cutaneous carcinoma of the ear. Otolaryngol Clin North Am 1993;26:231-245.

711. Andrews PE, Farrow GM, Oesterling JE: Squamous cell carcinoma of the scrotum: long-term followup of 14 patients. J Urol 1991;146:1299-1304.

712. Derakhshani P, Neubauer S, Braun M, et al: Results and 10-year follow-up in patients with squamous cell carcinoma of the penis. Urol Int 1999;62:238-244.

713. Adeyoju AB, Thornhill J, Corr J, et al: Prognostic factors in squamous cell carcinoma of the penis and implications for management. Br J Urol 1997;80:937-939.

714. Pintor MP, Northover JM, Nicholls RJ: Squamous cell carcinoma of the anus at one hospital from 1948 to 1984. Br J Surg 1989;76:806-810.

715. Horenblas S: Lymphadenectomy for squamous cell carcinoma of the penis. Part 1: diagnosis of lymph node metastasis. BJU Int 2001;88:467-472.

716. Petter G, Haustein UF: Squamous cell carcinoma of the skin—histopathological features and their significance for the clinical outcome. J Eur Acad Dermatol Venereol 1998;11:37-44.

717. Cherpelis BS, Marcusen C, Lang PG: Prognostic factors for metastasis in squamous cell carcinoma of the skin. Dermatol Surg 2002;28:268-273.

718. Immerman SC, Scanlon EF, Christ M, Knox KL: Recurrent squamous cell carcinoma of the skin. Cancer 1983;51:1537-1540.

719. Asarch RG: A review of the lymphatic drainage of the head and neck: use in evaluation of potential metastases. J Dermatol Surg Oncol 1982;8:869-872.

720. Friedman HI, Cooper PH, Wanebo HJ: Prognostic and therapeutic use of microstaging of cutaneous squamous cell carcinoma of the trunk and extremities. Cancer 1985;56:1099-1105.

721. Eroglu A, Berberoglu U, Berreroglu S: Risk factors related to locoregional recurrence in squamous cell carcinoma of the skin. J Surg Oncol 1996;61:124-130.

722. Weidner N, Foucar E: Adenosquamous carcinoma of the skin. An aggressive mucin- and gland-forming squamous carcinoma. Arch Dermatol 1985;121:775-779.

723. Ikegawa S, Saida T, Takizawa Y, et al: Vimentin-positive squamous cell carcinoma arising in a burn scar. A highly malignant neoplasm composed of acantholytic round keratinocytes. Arch Dermatol 1989;125:1672-1676.

724. Breuninger H, Schaumburg-Lever G, Holzschuh J, Horny HP: Desmoplastic squamous cell carcinoma of skin and vermilion surface: a highly malignant subtype of skin cancer. Cancer 1997;79:915-919.

725. Zitsch RP III, Lee BW, Smith RB: Cervical lymph node metastases and squamous cell carcinoma of the lip. Head Neck 1999;21:447-453.

726. Retsas S: Sentinel-lymph-node biopsy. N Engl J Med 1999;340:318-319.

727. Reschly MJ, Messina JL, Zaulyanov LL, et al: Utility of sentinel lymphadenectomy in the management of patients with high-risk cutaneous squamous cell carcinoma. Dermatol Surg 2003;29:135-140.

728. Heller KS, Shah JP: Carcinoma of the lip. Am J Surg 1979;138:600-603.

729. Chu A, Osguthorpe JD: Nonmelanoma cutaneous malignancy with regional metastasis. Otolaryngol Head Neck Surg 2003;128:663-673.

730. Martinez JC, Otley CC, Stasko T, et al: Defining the clinical course of metastatic skin cancer in organ transplant recipients: a multicenter collaborative study. Arch Dermatol 2003;139:301-306.

731. Teymoortash A, Dunne AA, Werner JA: Parotideal lymph node metastasis in squamous cell carcinoma of the skin. Eur J Dermatol 2002;12:376-380.

732. Khurana VG, Mentis DH, O'Brien CJ, et al: Parotid and neck metastases from cutaneous squamous cell carcinoma of the head and neck. Am J Surg 1995;170:446-450.

733. Fleming ID, Amonette R, Monaghan T, Fleming MD: Principles of management of basal and squamous cell carcinoma of the skin. Cancer 1995;75(suppl):699-704.

734. Salasche S: Features associated with recurrence. In Miller SJ, Maloney ME, eds: Cutaneous Oncology: Pathophysiology, Diagnosis, and Management. Malden, Mass, Blackwell Science, 1998:494-99.

735. Robins P, Nix M: Analysis of persistent disease on the ear following Mohs surgery. Head Neck Surg 1984;6:998-1006.

736. Bailin PL, Levine HL, Wood BG, Tucker HM: Cutaneous carcinoma of the auricular and periauricular region. Arch Otolaryngol 1980;106:692-696.

737. Levine H: Cutaneous carcinoma of the head and neck: management of massive and previously uncontrolled lesions. Laryngoscope 1983;93:87-105.

738. Ashby MA, Smith J, Ainslie J, McEwan L: Treatment of nonmelanoma skin cancer at a large Australian center. Cancer 1989;63:1863-1871.

739. Freeman RG, Duncan C: Recurrent skin cancer. Arch Dermatol 1973;107:395-399.
740. Breuninger H, Dietz K: Prediction of subclinical tumor infiltration in basal cell carcinoma. J Dermatol Surg Oncol 1991;17:574-578.
741. Burg G, Hirsch RD, Konz B, Braun-Falco O: Histographic surgery: accuracy of visual assessment of the margins of basal-cell epithelioma. J Dermatol Surg 1975;1:21-24.
742. Niparko JK, Swanson NA, Baker SR, et al: Local control of auricular, periauricular, and external canal cutaneous malignancies with Mohs surgery. Laryngoscope 1990;100(pt 1):1047-1051.
743. Sweet RD: The treatment of basal cell carcinoma by curettage. Br J Dermatol 1963;75:137-148.
744. Kopf AW, Bart RS, Schrager D, et al: Curettage-electrodesiccation treatment of basal cell carcinomas. Arch Dermatol 1977;113:439-443.
745. Suhge d'Aubermont PC, Bennett RG: Failure of curettage and electrodesiccation for removal of basal cell carcinoma. Arch Dermatol 1984;120:1456-1460.
746. Egloff DV, Bosse JP, Papillon J, Perras C: Immediate flap reconstruction after excision of basal cell carcinoma of the face. Ann Plast Surg 1979;3:28-34.
747. Lauritzen RE, Johnson RE, Spratt JS Jr: Pattern of recurrence in basal cell carcinoma. Surgery 1965;57:813-816.
748. Steinkogler FJ, Scholda CD: The necessity of long-term follow up after surgery for basal cell carcinomas of the eyelid. Ophthalmic Surg 1993;24:755-758.
749. Rank BK, Wakefield AR: Surgery of basal-cell carcinoma. Br J Surg 1958;45:531-547.
750. Graham PG, McGavran MH: Basal-cell carcinomas and sebaceous glands. Cancer 1964;17:803-806.
751. Lobo DV, Chu P, Grekin RC, Berger TG: Nonmelanoma skin cancers and infection with the human immunodeficiency virus. Arch Dermatol 1992;128:623-627.
752. Horton CE, Crawford HH, Love HG, Loeffler RA: The malignant potential of burn scar. Plast Reconstr Surg 1958;22:348-353.
753. Lawrence EA: Carcinoma arising in the scars of thermal burns. Surg Gynecol Obstet 1952;94:579-588.
754. Epstein E: Malignant sun-induced squamous-cell carcinoma of the skin. J Dermatol Surg Oncol 1983;9:505-506.
755. Cappello JC, Donick II: Squamous cell carcinoma as a complication of chronic osteomyelitis. J Foot Surg 1981;20:136-141.
756. Mohs FE, Lathrop TG: Modes of spread of cancer of skin. AMA Arch Derm Syphilol 1952;66:427-439.
757. Hirsch P: Recurrence rates of treated basal cell carcinomas. J Dermatol Surg Oncol 1993;19:175-176.
758. Del Regato JA, Vuksanovic M: Radiotherapy of carcinomas of the skin overlying the cartilages of the nose and ear. Radiology 1962;79:203-208.
759. Kuflik EG: Cryosurgery for tumors of the ear. J Dermatol Surg Oncol 1985;11:1165-1168.
760. Niazi ZB, Lamberty BG: Perineural infiltration in basal cell carcinomas. Br J Plast Surg 1993;46:156-157.
761. Barrett TL, Greenway HT Jr, Massullo V, Carlson C: Treatment of basal cell carcinoma and squamous cell carcinoma with perineural invasion. Adv Dermatol 1993;8:277-304, discussion 305.
762. Cottel WI: Perineural invasion by squamous-cell carcinoma. J Dermatol Surg Oncol 1982;8:589-600.
763. Mohs FE, Zitelli JA: Microscopically controlled surgery in the treatment of carcinoma of the scalp. Arch Dermatol 1981;117:764-769.
764. Mohs FE, Snow SN: Microscopically controlled surgical treatment for squamous cell carcinoma of the lower lip. Surg Gynecol Obstet 1985;160:37-41.
765. Mohs FE: Micrographic surgery for the microscopically controlled excision of eyelid cancers. Arch Ophthalmol 1986;104:901-909.
766. Broders AC: Squamous epithelioma of the lip. JAMA 1920;74:656-664.
767. Broders AC: Squamous epithelioma of the lip. Ann Surg 1921;73:141-160.
768. Thackray AC: Histological classification of rodent ulcers and its bearing on their prognosis. Br J Cancer 1951;5:213-224.
769. Emmett AJ: Surgical analysis and biological behaviour of 2277 basal cell carcinomas. Aust N Z J Surg 1990;60:855-863.
770. Steinman HK: Indications for Mohs surgery. In Gross GA, Steinman HK, Rapini RP, eds: Mohs Surgery: Fundamentals and Techniques. St. Louis, Mosby, 1999:9-14.
771. Zitelli JA, Mohs FE, Larson P, Snow S: Mohs micrographic surgery for melanoma. Dermatol Clin 1989;7:833-843.
772. Zitelli JA, Brown C, Hanusa BH: Mohs micrographic surgery for the treatment of primary cutaneous melanoma. J Am Acad Dermatol 1997;37(pt 1):236-245.
773. Mohs FE, Jones DL, Koranda FC: Microscopically controlled surgery for carcinomas in patients with nevoid basal cell carcinoma syndrome. Arch Dermatol 1980;116:777-779.
774. Brown MD, Zachary CB, Grekin RC, Swanson NA: Genital tumors: their management by micrographic surgery. J Am Acad Dermatol 1988;18(pt 1):115-122.
775. Hobbs ER, Wheeland RG, Bailin PL, et al: Treatment of dermatofibrosarcoma protuberans with Mohs micrographic surgery. Ann Surg 1988;207:102-107.
776. Larson PO: Keratoacanthomas treated with Mohs' micrographic surgery (chemosurgery). A review of forty-three cases. J Am Acad Dermatol 1987;16(pt 1):1040-1044.
777. Brown MD, Swanson NA: Treatment of malignant fibrous histiocytoma and atypical fibrous xanthomas with micrographic surgery. J Dermatol Surg Oncol 1989;15:1287-1292.
778. Pitcher ME, Fish S, Thomas JM: Management of soft tissue sarcoma. Br J Surg 1994;81:1136-1139.
779. Burns MK, Chen SP, Goldberg LH: Microcystic adnexal carcinoma. Ten cases treated by Mohs micrographic surgery. J Dermatol Surg Oncol 1994;20:429-434.
780. Dzubow LM: Sebaceous carcinoma of the eyelid: treatment with Mohs surgery. J Dermatol Surg Oncol 1985;11:40-44.
781. Yount AB, Bylund D, Pratt SG, Greenway HT: Mohs micrographic excision of sebaceous carcinoma of the eyelids. J Dermatol Surg Oncol 1994;20:523-529.
782. Coldiron BM, Goldsmith BA, Robinson JK: Surgical treatment of extramammary Paget's disease. A report of six cases and a reexamination of Mohs micrographic surgery compared with conventional surgical excision. Cancer 1991;67:933-938.
783. Mohs FE, Blanchard L: Microscopically controlled surgery for extramammary Paget's disease. Arch Dermatol 1979;115:706-708.
784. Chesser RS, Bertler DE, Fitzpatrick JE, Mellette JR: Primary cutaneous adenoid cystic carcinoma treated with Mohs micrographic surgery toluidine blue technique. J Dermatol Surg Oncol 1992;18:175-176.
785. Boyer JD, Zitelli JA, Brodland DG, D'Angelo G: Local control of primary Merkel cell carcinoma: review of 45 cases treated with Mohs micrographic surgery with and without adjuvant radiation. J Am Acad Dermatol 2002;47:885-892.
786. O'Connor WJ, Brodland DG: Merkel cell carcinoma. Dermatol Surg 1996;22:262-267.
787. Dhawan SS, Nanda VS, Grekin S, Rabinovitz HS: Apocrine adenocarcinoma: case report and review of the literature. J Dermatol Surg Oncol 1990;16:468-470.
788. Davidson TM: Otolaryngology perspective of Mohs surgery. In Gross GA, Steinman HK, Rapini RP, eds: Mohs Surgery: Fundamentals and Techniques. St. Louis, Mosby, 1999:245-260.
789. Chute CG, Chuang TY, Bergstralh EJ, Su WP: The subsequent risk of internal cancer with Bowen's disease. A population-based study. JAMA 1991;266:816-819.

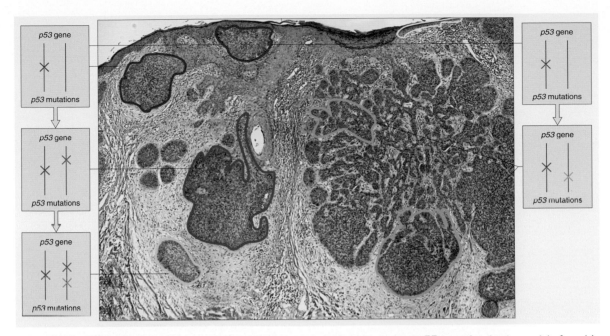

COLOR PLATE 116-1. Subclones within a basal cell carcinoma. A common *p53* mutation (red cross) is found in different parts of the tumor. Despite indistinguishable morphologic features, different parts of individual basal cell carcinomas have acquired additional mutations in the *p53* gene (blue, yellow, and green crosses). Boxes illustrate the two *p53* alleles. Note normal *p53* status (outlined in yellow) in overlying epidermal keratinocytes. (From Miller SJ, Moresi M: Actinic keratosis, basal cell carcinoma and squamous cell carcinoma. In Bolognia JL, Jorizzo JL, Rapini RP, eds: Dermatology. London, Mosby, 2003:1677-1696.)

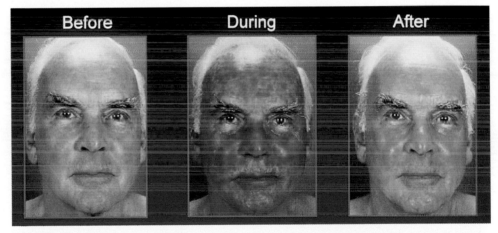

COLOR PLATE 116-2. Unretouched photographs of a patient with actinic keratosis. In the far left photograph, multiple, diffuse actinic keratoses can be seen on the patient's skin. After 7 to 10 days of 5-fluorouracil (Efudex) treatment (center photograph), abnormal cells are shed, the skin reddens, and then the skin crusts and peels. In some patients, inflammation may be a sign of allergic reaction. Finally, after therapy (photograph at far right), the diseased skin is replaced by healthy, normal-appearing skin. (Reprinted with permission of ICN Pharmaceuticals, Inc.)

Management of Regional Metastatic Disease of the Head and Neck: Diagnosis and Treatment

STEPHAN ARIYAN, MD, MBA

SPREAD OF CANCER

CLINICAL EVALUATION
   Diagnostic Work-up
   Biopsy
   Diagnostic Imaging Tests

RADICAL NECK DISSECTION
   Classic Radical Neck Dissection
   Functional Radical Neck Dissection

There have been significant advances in the treatment modalities for cancers of the head and neck. More extensive resections are now possible because of the advances in reconstruction with musculocutaneous flaps and bone flaps and the reliable microsurgical transplantation of tissues in one stage. These techniques allow more vascular tissue to be transported to sites of previous irradiation, permitting intraoperative application of additional radiation therapy by means of radioactive seeds at the time of resection of advanced cancers in patients with a poor prognosis for cure. These more advanced resections required developments in the rehabilitation of these patients.

The development of these various therapeutic modalities (surgery, therapeutic radiation, and chemotherapy), concomitant with that of the treatment of head and neck cancer, mandates a close communication among the various specialists managing these patients with cancer. Many medical centers have already developed multidisciplinary tumor boards to evaluate these patients and to recommend appropriate treatment plans. It is the author's belief that these tumor boards should not recommend any one "decision" on management because cancer is different in each patient, and the possible combinations of primary site, TNM variables, and ancillary medical problems lead to innumerable possibilities of staging.

Most of the studies of head and neck cancers have been retrospective because no single institution can generate significant numbers of comparable patients in a short enough time to make valid comparisons between different modalities for any given tumor site and stage. Tumor boards should therefore evaluate each patient for the individual problem and make recommendations according to previous experiences within the various specialty disciplines. This group should be advisory, providing a consensus of opinion and permitting minority opinions as well. The ultimate decision should still rest with the physician who has the primary responsibility for the individual care of that specific patient.

Finally, there are a large number of patients with cancers too advanced for any hope of cure. On occasion, aggressive treatments (such as with intraoperative adjuvant radiation therapy[1]) have permitted long-term disease-free survival, opening up new avenues in treating patients for cure. In certain circumstances, some of these patients have no hope for cure but may be candidates for resections, adjuvant radiotherapy, or chemotherapy, if only for local control to be achieved. Physicians have a responsibility to provide patients with comfort from their disability and their pain and to give them the opportunity to die with dignity in the company of their families and loved ones. Even though such treatments will not lead to increased survival, they may allow the patients to return to their homes and to spend the rest of their time in their chosen environment rather than in a hospital or nursing home.

SPREAD OF CANCER

Cancer of the head and neck area generally grows locally, with direct invasion first. As the tumor grows, the cancer cells may spread along the lymphatic channels to reach the regional draining lymph nodes in the neck. This lymphatic spread to different chains of lymph nodes varies according to the anatomic site of the primary tumor (Fig. 117-1). An understanding of this course of events is important because the decisions for treatment of these cancers are predicated on the prognosis of the individual case, which may be predicted by the staging classification. This classification is determined in turn by the extent of the primary lesion and the presence or absence of clinically palpable nodes in the neck.

CERVICAL LYMPH NODES. Tumor cells may travel along lymphatic channels to reach the regional nodes, where they may begin to replace the lymph nodes. Those nodes become enlarged because of reactive response to the cancer cells, reactive response to the bacteria in the oral cavity that invade the tumor ulcer to cause a local infection, or tumor replacement of the lymph node parenchyma. In general, lymph nodes need to enlarge to at least 1 cm in diameter before they can become clinically detectable. A 1-cm node completely replaced by cancer harbors 10^9 tumor cells. Cancer volume should be thought of in terms of logs rather than in absolute numbers because the treatment of

cancer by radiation therapy or chemotherapy kills tumor cells in "logs of kill" rather than in arithmetical kill.

The clinical examination finding of a "fixed" lymph node (i.e., one that cannot be moved around by the examining fingers) is believed to represent the continued growth of the tumor within the lymph node, which has broken through the capsule and grown into and become attached to the adjacent structures. However, this fixation may in fact result from inflammation of the lymph node as a response either to the tumor cells by the host's immune defense mechanism or to the infection from bacterial invasion of the ulcer in the primary tumor. Although preoperative irradiation has been shown to convert a fixed lymph node to a "freely movable" one, this change has also been seen in a number of patients treated with systemic antibiotics (or topical antibiotics by mouthwashes) without any radiation therapy.

UNKNOWN PRIMARY. A clinically positive lymph node may sometimes be diagnosed in the neck, but the site of the primary tumor cannot be identified. The examinations of these patients may or may not have been entirely adequate, and a complete and thorough examination with direct and indirect endoscopies and random biopsies will reveal the primary tumor in 60% to 70% of the initial cases. Of the remaining 40% of tumors, one third are also eventually found clinically or at autopsy,[2,3] whereas 25% remain undiagnosed. The most common sites are the nasopharynx, base of the tongue, tonsils, and piriform sinus. These unknown primary tumors are believed to be the result of a very small primary lesion that metastasized early or spontaneous regression of a primary tumor by the host's immune defense mechanism. Regardless of the true etiology, the consensus is to treat these patients with a definitive surgical resection of the cervical lymph nodes or with radiation therapy to the neck because such treatment leads to a 25% to 30% cure rate at 5 years.

NEGATIVE LYMPH NODES. Clinically positive (palpable) nodes removed by a neck dissection are shown to harbor no tumor cells in 20% to 25% of the cases. These "false-positive" nodes may result from the absence of tumor cells, with the lymph nodes enlarged by "reactive inflammation," or malignant cells may be too scarce to be detected by microscopic examination. Pathologists scanning cut sections of a lymph node are viewing millions of lymphocytes within the node, looking for abnormal (malignant) cells in the microscopic field. They will be able to detect 1 abnormal cell among 10 normal cells, perhaps even 1 abnormal cell in 100; but they will not be able to detect 1 abnormal cell among 1000 normal cells. Because any gram of tissue in the body (a 1-cm lymph node) contains 10^9 cells, 1 abnormal cell in 1000 would yield 10^6 (1

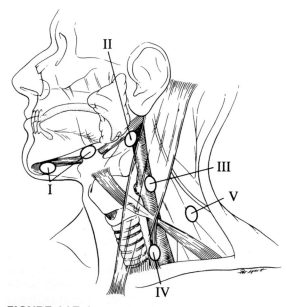

FIGURE 117-1. Classification of nodal metastases to the various zones: I, submandibular; II, jugulodigastric; III, midjugular; IV, supraclavicular; V, posterior cervical. (From Ariyan S, Chicarilli ZN: Cancer of the upper aerodigestive system. In McCarthy JG, ed: Plastic Surgery. Philadelphia, WB Saunders, 1990:3412.)

million) tumor cells in a lymph node that would be read as "negative," unless these cells were all clustered together.[4]

Therefore, the only definitive statement that can be made about a histologic examination of a lymph node is a report of a positive finding of tumor. A negative report can give only relative assurance that the node is free of tumor. It is for this reason that some patients with histologically free margins may still have recurrence of tumor at the primary site. This would also explain the 7.5% recurrence rate of tumor in the neck within 2 years after elective neck dissection in histologically negative necks reported from the Mayo Clinic by DeSanto et al.[5] These authors stated that "even pathologic staging is not completely accurate" and speculated that "there would have to be undetected disease within the neck for recurrences." This must be kept in mind when postoperative radiation therapy is considered as an adjuvant to surgery in patients with a statistically high chance of recurrence in spite of a histologically favorable report.

HEMATOGENOUS SPREAD. Metastatic lymph nodes do not *cause* distant organ spread but are rather *indicators* of the aggressiveness of the cancer and the potential for distant metastases. Although tumor cells may be spread into the blood stream as a result of biopsies or manipulation of the cancer during the surgical removal, studies have shown no correlation between positive blood samples or wound washings and subsequent recurrences or distant metastases.[6,7] It is more likely that the primary tumor is constantly shedding malignant cells in the blood stream at intervals throughout its growth for some time before the diagnosis of malignancy is even made. If these cells that are shed are aggressive enough to survive, they will eventually grow and become evident as metastatic disease in the future. If they survive but remain dormant with no new growth, they would most likely never be detected, and such patients would be considered cured.

The most frequent sites of distant organ spread are the lungs, bones, and liver. Although distant metastases are detected clinically in 5% to 25% of the patients with oropharyngeal cancers,[8] autopsy studies have demonstrated that 10% to 50% of such patients have distant organ metastases,[9-11] virtually to every organ in the body. Thus, the initial work-up should include liver function tests and radiographs of the lungs and any painful bone sites to determine the proper staging of these tumors before the treatment modality is chosen for each patient.

CLINICAL EVALUATION

In general, the patient with a cancer of the oropharyngeal area is a middle-aged man in his fifth or sixth

decade. The patient usually has a long history of smoking cigarettes and chronic alcoholism. Although proof of causal relationships does not exist between smoking, alcohol intake, and head and neck cancers, a number of reports do illustrate an association of those habits with these cancers. There are also some inconsistencies, with the incidence rate of head and neck cancer remaining steady in spite of increasing consumption of alcohol, especially wines, in the United States and the United Kingdom during the past 2 decades. This merely shows the complex interrelationships of these habits and oral hygiene with the end result of oropharyngeal diseases.

Although a patient may occasionally be an otherwise healthy, gainfully employed individual with temperate habits, the most frequently seen patients with head and neck cancers have poor oral hygiene and generally take poor care of their health. They often exhibit poor nutrition and have high blood pressure, diabetes, chronic lung disease, and sometimes cirrhosis of the liver. These coexisting conditions often complicate not only the decision to perform extensive operations to resect these cancers but also the postoperative course of the patients who have agreed to undergo surgical treatment.

The social network of these patients is also significant for their eventual care. These patients have often so neglected their health and well-being that the cancers are sometimes too far advanced to attempt a treatment for cure. The operations may be debilitating or disabling, and some patients might not have anyone to care for them or aid them after their definitive treatment. An overall view of the management of these individuals is essential, rather than the treatment of the cancer per se.

Diagnostic Work-up

The work-up of the patient with head and neck cancer includes a thorough examination with proper biopsies to determine the extent of the disease and to classify and stage the cancer properly. The occurrence of malignant-appearing benign lesions, such as necrotizing sialometaplasia,[12] and the benign appearance of early malignant neoplasms both serve to preclude accurate clinical assessment of oral and pharyngeal lesions. Regardless of the clinical experience and expertise of the treating physician, diagnostic errors are unavoidable, and only a systematic work-up will ensure the proper evaluations. Hence, in all cases, biopsy is the essential definitive diagnostic maneuver.

Biopsy

The significant majority of the patients have a proven malignant neoplasm by a biopsy of the site of the primary tumor. In these patients, all clinically suspicious lymph nodes in the neck (as determined before the biopsy) are considered to be clinical spread of the tumor to the regional draining lymph nodes.

Biopsy of the tumor may be either incisional or excisional. Incisional biopsy (i.e., removal of a representative portion of the lesion as well as a small segment of adjacent normal tissue) is the most satisfactory technique for intraoral lesions. Incisional biopsy results in minimal disturbance of tissue planes and appropriately leaves the residual lesion in situ, thereby allowing either accurate re-examination for radiotherapy planning or definitive radical excision. Excisional biopsy should be reserved for solitary lesions that are small (<1 cm), easily accessible, and superficial. In all excisional biopsies, strict attention must be paid to both the perimeter and the deep margins with respect to microscopic adequacy of the excision.

FINE-NEEDLE ASPIRATION. Open biopsy of a suspicious neck node or of any mass in the head and neck region should absolutely be deferred until an exhaustive diagnostic work-up has been completed in an effort to find the unknown primary lesion. Because a primary cancer can be discovered in all but 10% to 15% of patients who are initially seen with such masses, adherence to this policy avoids treatment delays, inappropriate incisions, and local recurrences as a result of seeding.

Whereas open biopsies are to be condemned, the technique of thin- or fine-needle aspiration biopsy has been firmly established in the diagnostic work-up of the patient with head and neck cancer. Fine-needle aspiration biopsy defines the disorder (tumor versus inflammation) and identifies the cell type or tissue of origin, thereby obviating cost-ineffective and often unsuccessful investigations.

On the other hand, sometimes a patient has a mass in the neck for which the primary site cannot be readily identified. This situation necessitates a thorough work-up. In these patients, an open neck biopsy must be deferred until an exhaustive examination is made to determine the source of the neck mass. Martin and Ellis[13] introduced the concept of a tissue core biopsy with a large-bore needle, but this technique had the shortcoming of occasional needle track recurrences. A fine-needle aspiration biopsy with a 22-gauge needle,[14] however, has been found to be a reliable technique for diagnosis, with a low risk of tumor spread in the neck. Fine-needle aspiration biopsy is a simple technique that can be performed readily in the office and can provide the pathologist with glass slide smears for cytologic examination and samples for a paraffin block.[15] In reports of large numbers of cases, the accuracy and reproducibility have been found to be 90% to 95%.[15,16]

SENTINEL NODE BIOPSIES. This technique of localization of the lymph nodes draining specific areas of skin has been employed successfully for the detection of metastatic nodes in melanoma (see Chapter 114). The success is based on the rich lymphatics in the dermis of skin that readily transport the radiocolloid material to the draining lymph nodes. Because head and neck cancers are epithelial malignant neoplasms in origin, this method of radiolocalization was evaluated in several studies.[17,18] These researchers found that the injected technetium sulfur colloid in the mucosa surrounding the oral carcinomas was readily taken up by the regional nodes. However, they noted that after the tumors had been resected, the changes in the anatomy render the uptake of the colloid unreliable for any meaningful localization.[17]

Diagnostic Imaging Tests

Head and neck cancers are epithelial surface tumors. Therefore, useful radiographic studies are limited to evaluations of the surface mucosa, most commonly by use of contrast material such as in barium swallow examination of the hypopharynx or the esophagus. On occasion, a xeroradiogram can provide a view of the mucosal lining that is far superior to routine soft tissue radiographs of the neck.

COMPUTED TOMOGRAPHY AND RELATED STUDIES. Computed tomographic (CT) scanning is also helpful in the evaluation of cervical lymph node metastases, and criteria have been developed that provide for differentiation of normal or "reactive" nodes from those involved with metastatic tumor.[19,20] The criteria for lymph nodes positive for harboring tumor include discrete masses measuring 15 mm or more in diameter; ill-defined or irregular borders to nodal masses; and groups of three or more nodes, each in the range of 6 to 15 mm in diameter.

NUCLEAR MAGNETIC RESONANCE IMAGING. Magnetic resonance (MR) imaging appears to be superior to CT scanning in several respects. Techniques for MR imaging allow a better definition of soft tissue and the extent of tumor invasion into the various tissue planes. As such, MR imaging is superior to CT scanning for soft tissue delineation. The use of MR imaging of the posterior fossa was first reported by Young et al[21] to illustrate these advantages. In a subsequent study, Randell et al[22] compared MR imaging with CT scanning in a series of 26 patients with tumors in the posterior fossa. MR imaging was shown overall to be more sensitive than CT scanning for mass effects, demonstrating some tumors that were not visualized at all by CT scanning; on the other hand, CT scanning was better for demonstrating calcification or bone invasion by tumor. MR imaging is also excellent for evaluating the neck for large metastatic nodes and determining the extent of tumor invasion of adjacent muscles, vessels, and nerves.

RADICAL NECK DISSECTION

The intent of an operation for cancer of the neck is to remove all of the tissue that potentially harbors the cancer cells. Crile[23] advocated a radical neck dissection to remove these tumors in the cervical lymphatics to achieve better cure rates. The three incisions commonly used to elevate the neck skin are the McFee incision, the double opposing flaps, and a posterior neck incision (Fig. 117-2). The McFee incision has a better blood supply by virtue of being a bipedicled flap, but it is more tedious to elevate properly with its underlying platysma muscle while preserving the superficial cervical fascia. The double opposing flaps are easier to dissect and provide excellent exposure of the neck contents, but the triangular flaps may become ischemic and result in partial necrosis, particularly if the neck has been previously irradiated. Overall, the posterior neck incision (Fig. 117-2B; also see Fig. 117-3E and F) appears to be the most advantageous.[24] The incision is made from the mastoid area down to the shoulder, running approximately 2 cm behind the anterior border of the trapezius muscle before extending medially below the clavicle. If the incision is placed in front of the border of the muscle, the contraction phase of the healing wound can result in a linear web from the mastoid to the shoulder. On the other hand, the

incision placed overlying the muscle allows the scar to heal by adherence to the underlying trapezius without the contracture or webbing in the neck.

Classic Radical Neck Dissection

Once the skin flaps are elevated, the lymphatic contents are incised along the anterior border of the trapezius muscle, and the dissection is carried anteriorly and superiorly (Fig. 117-3). The inferior belly of the omohyoid is transected, and the muscle is retracted with the specimen. As the deep cervical fascia overlying the brachial plexus is reached, the cervical contents can be peeled and swept forward by means of an operative sponge. The spinal accessory nerve is transected as it enters the trapezius muscle.

The two heads of the sternocleidomastoid muscle are then transected from the sternum and clavicle, and the specimen is further dissected anteriorly to the internal jugular vein. The vagus nerve is identified and preserved before the jugular vein is doubly clamped, transected, and ligated with sutures. Dissection along this area of the jugular vein may reveal clear fluid, which is a result of disruptions of the thoracic duct. These lymphatic ducts usually need to be transected and ligated twice because they take a C-shaped loop

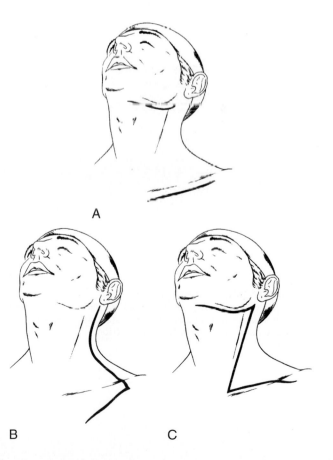

FIGURE 117-2. Neck incisions illustrating the McFee incision *(A),* the Ariyan incision *(B),* and the double opposing flaps *(C).* (From Ariyan S, Chicarilli ZN: Cancer of the upper aerodigestive system. In McCarthy JG, ed: Plastic Surgery. Philadelphia, WB Saunders, 1990:3412.)

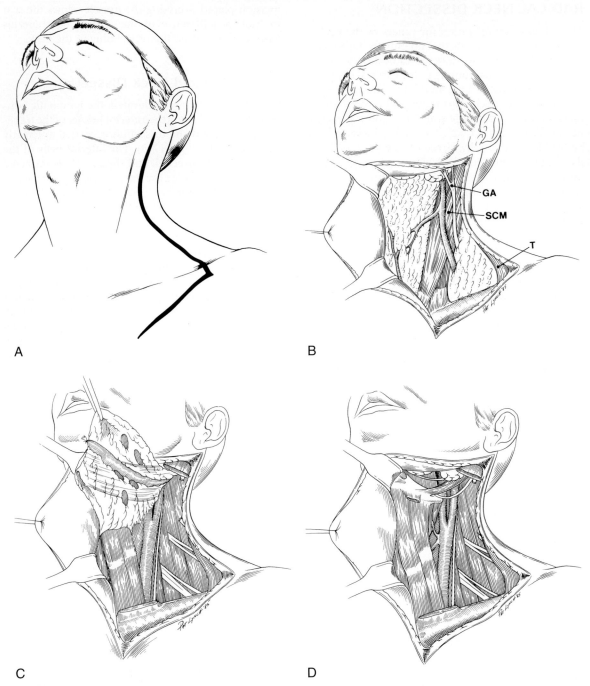

A

B

C

D

FIGURE 117-3. Illustrations of the neck dissections. The incision is made along 2 cm behind the anterior border of the trapezius muscle *(A)*, and the neck flap is elevated with the platysma muscle *(B)*. The classic radical neck dissection, when indicated, can remove the sternocleidomastoid muscle *(C)* together with the jugular vein and the spinal accessory nerve *(D)* as one block dissection.

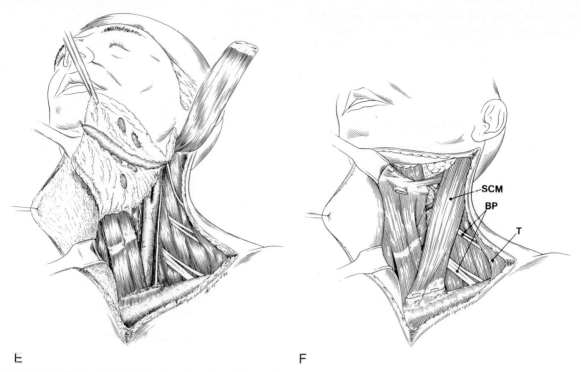

E

F

FIGURE 117 3, cont'd. The functional neck dissection elevates and preserves the sternocleidomastoid muscle *(E)* to remove the cervical nodal contents, after which the muscle is sutured back at its sternal and clavicular insertions *(F)*. BP, brachial plexus; GA, great auricular nerve; SCM, sternocleidomastoid muscle; T, trapezius. (From Ariyan S: Radical neck dissection. Surg Clin North Am 1986;66:133.)

cephalad and return on themselves to their junction with the jugular vein. Although the thoracic duct is often mentioned with regard to a left-sided neck dissection, a right lymphatic duct can also be identified in right-sided neck dissections if it is looked for carefully. Proper identification and ligations of these ducts should prevent postoperative problems with a lymphocele or a chylous fistula.

As the dissection proceeds cephalad, the branches of the jugular vein are ligated and transected, the cutaneous sensory nerves of the cervical plexus are transected, and the block dissection is continued to the submandibular area. At this point, the marginal mandibular branch of the facial nerve is identified and preserved as it crosses the facial vessels parallel to and about 2 cm below the margin of the mandible at the antegonial notch. This notch is the location of the facial vessels crossing the mandible, and the mandibular branch crosses these vessels just deep to the platysma muscle.

As the neck contents are further dissected, the omohyoid muscle is detached from the hyoid bone. As the dissection is continued over the carotid bifurcation, the carotid sinus is blocked by the gentle injection of 1% plain lidocaine (Xylocaine) by means of a 27- to 30-gauge needle into the loose adventitia over this bifurcating vessel. This blocks the carotid sinus reflex, which

can cause serious degrees of brachycardia due to the manipulation of the carotid artery during the dissection.

Continued dissection makes it possible to identify the hypoglossal nerve as it crosses the carotid artery while preserving it. The contents of the submandibular triangle are removed after the lingual nerve is identified and preserved. As this dissection continues along the angle of the mandible, the tail of the parotid gland is transected at the anterior border of the sternocleidomastoid muscle. The jugular vein at the base of the skull is doubly clamped, transected, ligated, and then suture ligated. After transection of the sternocleidomastoid muscle from its attachment at the mastoid, the block dissection of the cervical contents is completed.

The neck is then irrigated well with sterile water to lyse the blood and clots, helping to identify any sites of small bleeding vessels that should then be cauterized. Large suction catheters are then placed in the neck, not to drain the blood but to suction the neck flaps down to the wound bed to decrease the amount of bleeding. If the neck wound is bleeding actively at the time of the closure, the suction catheters cannot remove the blood effectively, and the clots will elevate the neck flap, which will lead to further bleeding and formation of a large hematoma. Also, it is imperative to wake the patient from the anesthesia slowly and gently because if the patient struggles against the endotracheal tube, the bucking and coughing will lead to the Valsalva maneuver, which will in turn increase the venous pressure and lead to bleeding under the neck flaps.

Functional Radical Neck Dissection

Although Crile[23] advocated the radical resection of all the neck contents for squamous cell carcinoma, he did not remove the spinal accessory nerve, and he included the sternocleidomastoid muscle merely to get better exposure of the anatomy to protect the branches of the facial nerve during the dissection. Few would argue against a classic radical neck dissection in a patient who has spread of the tumor through the capsule of the lymph nodes and adherence to the surrounding soft tissues; but little justification exists for the routine removal of all of the structures in the neck in every case.

Suarez[25] demonstrated that cervical lymph nodes lie within the space enveloped by the cervical fascia and are not found in vessel walls or in the muscles overlying them. Thus, there is little rationale for entering the carotid sheath to remove the jugular vein while sparing the carotid artery, vagus nerve, and sympathetic chain or for removing the spinal accessory nerve while preserving the hypoglossal and lingual nerves. Bocca and Pignataro[26] popularized the "functional" neck dissection when they reported several hundred cases of neck dissection in which they spared the jugular vein and preserved the sternocleidomastoid muscle by retracting the muscle and dissecting the lymphatic contents deep to it, without altering the disease-free rates.

ANATOMY. Experimentation with fresh and preserved cadaver dissections shows that the sternocleidomastoid muscle has three blood supplies.[27-29] Superiorly, the blood supply is from a branch of the occipital artery; in the midportion, the blood supply is from the superior thyroid; and from below, the supply is from the thyrocervical trunk (Fig. 117-4). The investing layer of the cervical fascia extends across the posterior cervical triangle, splits to envelop the sternocleidomastoid muscle by its two layers, and re-forms into one layer to extend across the anterior cervical triangle (Fig. 117-5). The lymph nodes are incorporated in the soft tissue between this layer of the fascia and the deep cervical fascia and are not found in the carotid sheath or the fascia of the sternocleidomastoid muscle. If the sternocleidomastoid muscle is dissected and elevated from the neck, the deeper half of the split cervical fascia would remain continuous with the cervical fascia covering the anterior and posterior cervical triangles, permitting the same composite dissection

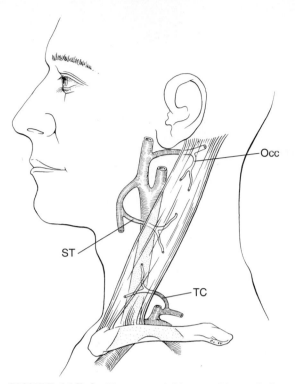

FIGURE 117-4. The sternocleidomastoid muscle has three blood supplies: superiorly from the occipital artery (Occ), in the middle from the superior thyroid (ST), and inferiorly from the thyrocervical trunk (TC). (From Ariyan S: Radical neck dissection. Surg Clin North Am 1986;66:133.)

of the lymphatics and lymph nodes that a classic radical lymphadenectomy in the neck does (Fig. 117-6).

TECHNIQUE.[24] Once the preferred incisions are made and the neck flaps are elevated together with the platysma muscle, incise the superficial layer of the split cervical fascia along the anterior and posterior borders of the entire length of the sternocleidomastoid muscle to elevate the muscle on its superior blood supply (see Fig. 117-3A, E, and F). Take care to preserve the blood supply from the occipital artery to the superior portion of the muscle.

Begin to remove the lymphatic contents from the posterior triangle, as already described for the classic radical neck dissection. During the dissection, identify the spinal accessory nerve as it enters the anterior border of the trapezius muscle. Split the contents of the posterior cervical triangle as the spinal accessory nerve is dissected free between the trapezius and the sternocleidomastoid muscles. The spinal accessory nerve is frequently found not to pass *through* the sternocleidomastoid muscle but rather to traverse along the *undersurface* of this muscle and give a motor branch to this muscle.

As the dissection proceeds anteriorly and superiorly, incise the carotid sheath along the entire length of the carotid artery and internal jugular vein and remove the sheath together with the block dissection of the cervical lymphatics. Dissect the upper portion of the neck and submandibular triangle with a technique similar to that of the classic neck dissection, with preservation of the marginal mandibular nerve, the hypoglossal nerve, and the lingual nerve. After completion of the block dissection, return the sternocleidomastoid muscle to its original position and suture the sternal and clavicular heads back to the sites of their origins. Close the neck flaps over large suction catheters placed in the operative wound.

CONCLUSIONS

It is important to consider that some of these patients have a cancer too advanced to cure with any

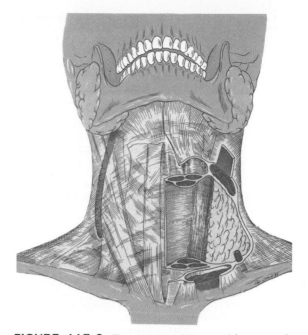

FIGURE 117-6. The sternocleidomastoid muscle is outside the lymph node-bearing tissue of the neck. (From Ariyan S: Radical neck dissection. Surg Clin North Am 1986;66:133.)

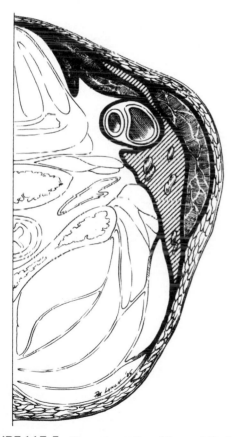

FIGURE 117-5. The cross section of the neck illustrates the posterior cervical fascia splitting to incorporate the sternocleidomastoid muscle within its split sheaths and then re-forming to proceed as the anterior cervical fascia. This fascia and the deep investing fascia envelop the lymph nodes in the neck. (From Ariyan S: Radical neck dissection. Surg Clin North Am 1986;66:133.)

probability. It is our responsibility as physicians not only to cure the patients when we are able but also to comfort patients and relieve them of pain when we cannot. Some patients with advanced, incurable cancers have the tumor growing through the skin of the face and neck; if not cared for, they will eventually require long-term hospitalization because of the pain or the odor from the secondarily infected necrotic tumor and die in a lonely ward. It is within our capability to operate on some of these patients, albeit for palliation alone, to comfort them and provide the dignity of spending whatever short time they have at home with their loved ones.

REFERENCES

1. Son YH, Ariyan S: Intraoperative adjuvant radiotherapy for advanced cancers of the head and neck: a preliminary report. Am J Surg 1985;150:480.
2. Barrie JR, Krappen WH, Strong EW: Cervical node metastases of unknown origin. Am J Surg 1970;120:466.
3. MacComb WS: Diagnosis and treatment of metastatic cervical cancerous nodes from unknown primary site. Am J Surg 1972;124:441.
4. Ariyan S, Krizek TJ, Mitchell MS: Identification of squamous cell carcinoma of the head and neck by tissue culture and immunologic testing. Plast Reconstr Surg 1977;59:386.
5. DeSanto LW, Holt JJ, Beahrs OH, et al: Neck dissection: is it worthwhile? Laryngoscope 1982;92:502.
6. Arons MS, Smith RR, Myers MH: Significance of cancer cells in operative wounds. Cancer 1961;14:1041.

7. Griffiths JD, McKinna JA, Rowbotham HD, et al: Carcinoma of the colon and rectum: circulating malignant cells and five-year survival. Cancer 1973;31:226.

8. Merino OR, Lindberg RD, Fletcher GH: An analysis of distant metastases from squamous cell carcinoma of the upper respiratory and digestive tracts. Cancer 1977;40:145.

9. Dennington ML, Carter DR, Meyers AD: Distant metastases in head and neck epidermoid carcinoma. Laryngoscope 1980;90:196.

10. Papac RJ: Distant metastases from head and neck cancer. Cancer 1984;53:342.

11. Probert JC, Thompson RW, Bagshaw MA: Patterns of spread of distant metastases in head and neck cancer. Cancer 1974;33:127.

12. Gahhos F, Enriquez RE, Bahn SL, Ariyan S: Necrotizing sialometaplasia: report of five cases. Plast Reconstr Surg 1983;71:650.

13. Martin HE, Ellis EB: Biopsy by needle puncture and aspiration. Ann Surg 1930;92:169.

14. Einhorn J, Franzen S: Thin needle biopsy in the diagnosis of thyroid disease. Acta Radiol 1962;58:321.

15. Goldberg NH, Cuono CB, Ariyan S, Enriquez RE: Improved reliability in tumor diagnosis by fine needle aspiration. Plast Reconstr Surg 1981;67:492.

16. Young JEM, Archibald SD, Shier KJ: Needle aspiration cytologic biopsy in head and neck masses. Am J Surg 1981;142:484.

17. Chiesa F, Mauri S, Grana C, et al: Is there a role for sentinel node biopsy in early N0 tongue tumors? Surgery 2000;128:16.

18. Alex JC, Sasaki CT, Krag DN, et al: Sentinel lymph node radiolocalization in head and neck squamous cell carcinoma. Laryngoscope 2000;110:198.

19. Mancuso AA, Harnsberger HR, Muraki AS, Stevens MH: Computed tomography of cervical and retropharyngeal lymph nodes: normal anatomy, variants of normal, and application in staging head and neck cancer. Part 1: normal anatomy. Radiology 1983;148:709.

20. Mancuso AA, Maceri D, Pice D, Hanafee WN: C17 of cervical lymph node cancer. Am J Roentgenol 1981;136-381.

21. Young JEM, Archibald SD, Shier KJ: Needle aspiration cytologic biopsy in head and neck masses. Am J Surg 1981;142:484.

22. Randell CP, Collins AG, Young IR, et al: Nuclear magnetic resonance imaging of posterior fossa tumors. Am J Neuroradiol 1983;4:1027.

23. Crile GW: Excision of cancer of the head and neck: with special reference to plan of dissection based on one hundred and thirty-two operations. JAMA 1906;47:1780.

24. Ariyan S: Functional neck dissection. Plast Reconstr Surg 1980;65:768.

25. Suarez D: El problema de las metastasis lingfaticas y alejados del cancer de laringe e hipofaringe. Rev Otorhinolaryngol 1963;23:83.

26. Bocca E, Pignataro D: A conservative technique in radical neck dissection. Ann Otol Rhinol Laryngol 1967;76:975.

27. Ariyan S: One-stage reconstruction for defects of the mouth using the sternomastoid myocutaneous flap. Plast Reconstr Surg 1979;63:618.

28. Ariyan S: One-stage repair of the cervical esophagostome with two myocutaneous flaps from the neck and shoulder. Plast Reconstr Surg 1979;63:426.

29. Ariyan S: Pectoralis major, sternomastoid, and other musculocutaneous flaps for head and neck reconstruction. Clin Plast Surg 1980;7:89.

Index

Note: **Boldface** roman numerals indicate volume. Page numbers followed by f refer to figures; page numbers followed by t refer to tables.

i

Tongue *(Continued)*
reconstruction of, III:924-925, 927-928, 929f, 941, 942f-944f. *See also* Oral cavity reconstruction.
rectus abdominis flap for, III:941, 942f-944f
skin graft for, III:927-928, 929f
trauma to, III:37
tumors of, V:166-167, 166f
Tongue flap, for lower lip reconstruction, V:383, 385, 385f
Tongue-lip adhesion procedure, in Robin sequence, IV:514-515, 516f
Tonic-clonic movements, ketamine-related, I:175
Tonsillar pillars, V:165, 165f
Tonsilloadenoidectomy, in craniofacial clefts, IV:422
Tonsils, V:165, 165f
Tooth (teeth). *See also* Orthodontics; Orthognathic surgery.
aesthetic analysis of, II:4t, 13, 13f-15f, 23-24, 25f
anatomy of, III:920, 921f
cephalometric analysis of, II:23-24, 25f
cracks in, with laser resurfacing, II:375-376
examination of
in craniosynostoses, IV:497
in temporomandibular joint dysfunction, III:542
preoperative, I:168
fracture of, in children, III:407, 409
fracture-related fixation of, III:118, 120 128, 155
acrylic splints in, III:127, 129f
anatomy for, III:118, 120-122, 120f-122f
arch bar method wiring in, III:123-126, 124f-127f
Eyelet method wiring in, III:122-123, 123f
Gilmer method wiring in, III:122, 122f
intermaxillary fixation screw in, III:128, 130f
monomaxillary vs. bimaxillary, III:128
orthodontic bands in, III:127, 128f
wiring techniques in, III:122 128, 122f-127f
implantation of
after mandibular reconstruction, III:985-986, 986f, 987f
osseointegrated, I:524, 524f
recombinant bone morphogenetic proteins with, I:662-663
injury to
in children, III:405-409, 406f-408f
with orthognathic surgery, II:684
malocclusion of
class I, II:649, 650f
class II, II:649, 650f
class III, II:649, 650f
in condylar process fracture, III:515
in mandibular fracture, III:185-186, 187f
in maxillary fracture, III:239, 240f, 252-253, 252f
in panfacial fracture, III:257, 257f

Tooth (teeth) *(Continued)*
in pediatric facial fracture, III:411-412
in zygoma fracture, III:213
transverse dimension of, II:649, 650f
vertical dimension of, II:649, 650f
with condylar process fracture, III:515
overbite of, II:13, 15f
overjet of, II:13, 15f
reimplantation of
in children, III:406f, 409
in mandibular fracture treatment, III:155
roots of, in mandibular fracture treatment, III:187
Torsoplasty, circumferential, VI:171-172, 172f, 173f
Torticollis, III:398, 1032-1033, 1033f, IV:98-99
Torus mandibularis, V:11
Torus palatinus, V:11
Total anterior tenoarthrolysis, in Dupuytren disease, VII:752
Total body surface area, in burn assessment, I:813-814, 814f, 815f
Tourniquet, for hand surgery, VII:115-118, 116f
Toxic epidermal necrolysis, I:793-799
ABCs in, I:797
classification of, I:793-794, 794t
clinical presentation of, I:795-796, 796f
corticosteroid therapy in, I:798
cyclosporine in, I:799
definition of, I:793-794
differential diagnosis of, I:796-797
drugs in, I:794-795, 798
epidemiology of, I:794-795
infection in, I:795-796, 799
intravenous immune globulin in, I:799
nutrition in, I:798 799
ocular care in, I:799
ocular sequelae of, I:796
oral hygiene in, I:798
pathogenesis of, I:795
plasmapheresis in, I:799
prognosis for, I:799
sequelae of, I:796
treatment of, I:797-799, 798f
wound care in, I:797-798, 798f
Toxic shock syndrome, VII:762
after laser resurfacing, II:372
TP53 gene, VII:988
Trace metal deficiency, wound healing and, I:221
Trachea
arterial supply of, Color Plate I:15-13, I:343-344, 343t
embryology of, III:1026-1027
endoscopic clip for, in fetal diaphragmatic hernia, I:1124
ligation of, in fetal diaphragmatic hernia, I:1123-1124
occlusion of, in fetal diaphragmatic hernia, I:1123-1124
stenosis of, in pediatric facial trauma, III:398
Tracheal intubation, I:176-177
in children, III:395, 397-398, 397f
Tracheoesophageal fistula, congenital, III:1026-1027

Tracheostomy
in burn treatment, I:829
in craniofacial microsomia, IV:523
in micrognathia, III:777
in obstructive sleep apnea, III:786, 791-794, 793f, 794f
in pediatric facial trauma, III:397
scar after, revision of, I:255, 257f, 258, 258f
Tragus deformity, after face lift, II:732-734, 733f, 734f
TRAM flap. *See* Transverse rectus abdominis myocutaneous (TRAM) flap.
Tramadol, in complex regional pain syndrome/reflex sympathetic dystrophy, VII:860
Transblepharoplasty, II:63-64
Transconjunctival blepharoplasty, II:122-124, 124f
Transcutaneous electrical nerve stimulation
in complex regional pain syndrome/reflex sympathetic dystrophy, VII:855
in hand therapy, VIII:572
Transcutaneous oxygen tension, in foot, VI:1414-1415
TransCyte
in burn treatment, I:824t, 825
in wound healing, I:1018
Transference, I:70 71
Transforming growth factor-β
exogenous, I:664-665
in bone repair, I:656t, 663-665
in fetal wound healing, I:218
in wound healing, I:212t, 215-216, 1018
osteogenic protein 1 with, I:663
Transforming growth factor-β3, in palatal fusion, IV:8
Transoral resection, in oral cavity cancer, V:177, 177f, 178f
Transplantation, I:269-285
antibody screening for, I:274
basal cell carcinoma and, V:396
crossmatching for, I:274
historical perspective on, I:269-270
immunologic screening for, I:273-274
immunologic tolerance in, I:278-279, 285
anergy and, I:279
clonal deletion and, I:278-279
suppression and, I:279
immunology of, I:270-279
B lymphocytes in, I:271-272
blood group antigens in, I:271
complement in, I:272
dendritic cells in, I:272
granulocytes in, I:271
immunoglobulins in, I:272
macrophages in, I:272
major histocompatibility complex in, I:270-271
minor histocompatibility antigens in, I:271
natural killer cells in, I:271
rejection cascade in, I:271-273
skin-specific antigens in, I:271
T lymphocytes in, I:272-273